Differential Diagnosis in Head and Neck Imaging

Differential Diagnosis in Head and Neck Imaging

A Systematic Approach to the Radiologic Evaluation of the Head and Neck Region and the Interpretation of Difficult Cases

Thomas J. Vogl, MD

Jörn Balzer, MD
Martin Mack, MD
Wolfgang Steger, MD

Department of Radiology
Johann Wolfgang Goethe-University
Frankfurt, Germany

With a foreword by Roland Felix

309 illustrations in
621 separate panels
178 tables

Thieme
Stuttgart · New York 1999

Library of Congress Cataloging-in-Publication Data
Radiologische Differentialdiagnostik in der Kopf-Hals-Region.
English.
Differential diagnosis in head and neck imaging : a systematic approach to the radiologic evaluation of the head and neck region and the interpretation of difficult cases / Thomas J. Vogl . . . [et al.] : with a foreword by Roland Felix.
p. cm.
ISBN 3-13-115411-X, — ISBN 0-86577-811-6. — ISBN 3-13-115411-X
1. Head—Imaging. 2. Neck—Imaging. 3. Head—Diseases—Diagnosis. 4. Neck—Diseases—Diagnosis. 5. Diagnosis, Differential. I. Vogl, Thomas J. II. Title.
[DNLM: 1. Head—pathology. 2. Neck—pathology. 3. Diagnosis, Differential. 4. Diagnostic Imaging—methods. WE 705R129 1998]
RC 936.R2913 1998
617.5'10754—dc21
DNLM/DLC 98-36571
for Library of Congress CIP

Translated by Terry C. Telger, Ft. Worth, Texas, USA.

This book is an authorized translation of the German edition published and copyrighted 1998 by Georg Thieme Verlag, Stuttgart, Germany.
Title of the German edition: Radiologische Differentialdiagnostik in der Kopf-Hals-Region.

Important Note: Medicine is an ever-changing science undergoing continual development. Research and clinical experience are continually expanding our knowledge, in particular our knowledge of proper treatment and drug therapy. Insofar as this book mentions any dosage or application, readers may rest assured that the authors, editors and publishers have made every effort to ensure that such references are in accordance with *the state of knowledge at the time of production of the book.*

Nevertheless this does not involve, imply, or express any guarantee or responsibility on the part of the publishers in respect of any dosage instructions and forms of application stated in the book. *Every user is requested to examine carefully* the manufacturers' leaflets accompanying each drug and to check, if necessary in consultation with a physician or specialist, whether the dosage schedules mentioned therein or the contraindications stated by the manufacturers differ from the statements made in the present book. Such examination is particularly important with drugs that are either rarely used or have been newly released on the market. Every dosage schedule or every form of application used is entirely at the user's own risk and responsibility. The authors and publishers request every user to report to the publishers any discrepancies or inaccuracies noticed.

Typesetting by Druckhaus Götz GmbH,
D-71636 Ludwigsburg
(CCS-Textline [Linotronic 630])

Printed in Germany by Grammlich, Pliezhausen

ISBN 3-13-115411-X (GTV)
ISBN 0-86577-811-6 (TNY)

Foreword

For more than a decade, my colleague Thomas J. Vogl has actively explored the issues and problems associated with diagnostic imaging of the head and neck region. Working closely with the coeditors of this book and with colleagues from various clinical disciplines, he has published numerous articles on various specific issues in diagnostic imaging as well as several monographs dealing with specific imaging procedures.

Today, however, the complex spectrum of clinical requirements makes it necessary to go beyond the implementation of imaging studies and tailor the diagnostic workup to the specific clinical problem. The traditional staged workup should be replaced by a rapid, cost-effective, well tolerated evaluation that will ensure maximum success. Today this can be accomplished only by providing the most skillful clinical and radiologic diagnosis and differential diagnosis.

Differential Diagnosis in Head and Neck Imaging does full justice to these goals and brings us a significant step closer to the optimization of head and neck imaging. I wish the book all the success it deserves.

Berlin, fall, 1998 Roland Felix

Preface

With its complex anatomy and diversity of landmarks, the head and neck region poses a special challenge to clinical and radiologic diagnosis. Sound therapeutic decision making requires the use of modern imaging procedures to define the precise location and extent of pathologic processes and delineate the involvement of adjacent structures. Other important information is derived from the vascularity of a lesion, its internal structure, its homogeneity, and the nature of its margins. All these criteria will suggest a radiologic differential diagnosis that forms the basis for an accurate interpretation of the findings.

This book offers a systematic approach to differential diagnosis based on the experience gained in more than 4000 comparative clinical and radiologic examinations. To use the book, first locate the chapter dealing with the anatomic region of interest. That chapter will outline the regional anatomy and types of pathology that may be encountered and will systematically guide the user through the process of making an accurate differential diagnosis.

The images presented in each chapter are intended to illustrate the differentiating criteria that are applied to various types of pathology. Besides demonstrating the key elements of an accurate differential diagnosis, the images also show how radiologic tissue characterization is not possible for all lesions, but that imaging can direct the biopsy procedures that may be needed to establish a diagnosis.

The idea for this book evolved from numerous continuing-education settings and is based specifically on a lecture at Humboldt University entitled "The challenge of radiologic differential diagnosis."

I would like to express thanks to Dr. Thomas Scherb and Dr. Clifford Bergman of Thieme Verlag for their critical input and committed support. I would also like to thank my clinical partners, including my friends and colleagues at the Ear, Noses, and Throat Clinic in Munich—especially Prof. Dr. G. Grevers and Prof. Dr. E. Kastenbauer who have vigorously supported my research and clinical work for many years. I acknowledge the help of Prof. Dr. V. Jahnke of the Rudolf Virchow Medical Center who made it possible for me to continue my work in Berlin. I would also like to express special thanks to Prof. Dr. D. J. Bier, Director of the Oral Surgery Clinic, and to our esteemed department chair, Prof. Dr. R. Felix who was kind enough to write the foreword for this book.

My coeditors and I hope that the readers will find our approach helpful and instructive. We also hope that the book will enable less experienced examiners to make an accurate diagnosis that is supported by sound differential diagnostic criteria.

Berlin, fall, 1998

Thomas J. Vogl
Jörn Balzer
Martin Mack
Wolfgang Steger

Contents

General Part

Special Part

General Part

1 Introduction

Concept and Approach

The goal of this book is to present a systematic approach to the radiologic differential diagnosis of head and neck disorders. This approach should enable the radiologist to make an accurate diagnosis from available radiographic, computed tomographic, and magnetic resonance findings while noting the range of possible differential diagnoses and distinguishing benign from malignant disease. The radiologist should further be able to differentiate a circumscribed lesion from the local manifestation of a systemic disease.

The general section of this book deals with specific clinical and radiologic criteria that are useful in evaluations of the head and neck region. It outlines diagnostically important groups of disorders such as anatomic variations and malformations, tumors, inflammatory lesions, traumatic lesions, and therapy-induced changes. It is shown how an awareness of the clinical problem is essential for accurate image interpretation.

General diagnostic techniques are subdivided into clinical examinations and imaging studies. The principal imaging modalities are *conventional radiography*, *computed tomography (CT)*, *magnetic resonance imaging (MRI)* and *magnetic resonance angiography (MRA)*, *digital subtraction angiography (DSA)*, and *ultrasound imaging* including *color duplex sonography*.

The clinical section of the book shows how the various diagnostic criteria, including the clinical presentation and radiologic findings, can be systematically applied to make a precise differential diagnosis for specific subregions of the head and neck.

Following the introduction of diagnostic radiography around the turn of the century, rapid advances were made in evaluations of the facial skeleton, skull base, and neck. Many of the standard radiographic positions introduced in the early part of this century (e.g., Schüller's projection in 1905, Stenvers' projection in 1917) are still in use today.

Angiography soon developed as an important adjunct for studying vascularized lesions. The advent of DSA in 1978 permitted an accurate portrayal of the morphologic and hemodynamic characteristics of blood vessels and vascularized tumors. Meanwhile, ultrasound imaging became established as a routine procedure that was particularly useful in evaluating diseases of the neck and facial soft tissues.

Perhaps the most significant advance in the diagnosis of head and neck lesions was the advent of sectional imaging modalities such as CT and MRI. These techniques were unique in that they furnished a complete view of anatomic and pathologic processes in the head and neck, unobscured by superimposed structures.

Diagnostic imaging must satisfy the clinical requirements for accurate diagnosis and treatment planning within an interdisciplinary context. Increasingly, refined microsurgical techniques and innovations in radiotherapy and chemotherapy are placing more rigorous demands on imaging evaluations of the head and neck region.

Based on an awareness of the specific clinical problem or presumptive clinical diagnosis, the radiologist must select the most informative, least invasive imaging study from the many options that are available. Every study has a two-fold objective: to accurately depict the location and extent of a lesion and to identify the nature of the lesion with adequate sensitivity and specificity based on an assessment of characteristic imaging features. In the sections that follow, we shall attempt to convey an effective diagnostic strategy for various pathologic processes occurring in specific subregions of the head and neck.

A comprehensive analysis of the topographic and imaging characteristics of a lesion and a knowledge of the differential diagnostic spectrum are the keys to making an accurate radiologic diagnosis.

Systematic Approach to the Analysis of Radiologic Findings in the Head and Neck Region

The primary goal of this book is to train the reader in image interpretation while laying the informational groundwork for a systematic analysis of diagnostic imaging procedures in the head and neck region.

A helpful mnemonic in image interpretation is the "5 D's" used to describe and evaluate circumscribed osseous lesions: *detect*, *describe*, *discuss*, *differential diagnosis*, and *diagnosis*.

"**Detect**" refers to the basic task of identifying a lesion or disease. This is best accomplished by a systematic analysis that starts by scrutinizing all essential structures for possible sites where a lesion may originate. Classic lesions of the head and neck region may arise from a variety of anatomic structures (Table 1.**1**).

"**Describe**" means localizing the lesion to bone, joints, soft tissues, neurovascular structures, etc. and documenting its precise relation to other involved or adjacent structures. This includes characterizing the disease as focal, regional, or generalized and detecting solitary or multiple sites of involvement.

"**Discuss**" refers to the initial interpretation of the radiologic findings.

"**Differential diagnosis**" is a significant step that involves identifying, listing, and considering the range of possible differential diagnoses.

"**Diagnosis**," the final step, means rendering a definitive judgment based on a consideration of all possible criteria and the overall constellation of findings.

Table 1.**1** Sites of origin for diseases of the head and neck region

Bone: ➤ Cortex (e.g., bony walls: maxilla) ➤ Cancellous bone (e.g., petrous apex)
Joints: ➤ Temporomandibular joint (synovium, cortical bone, soft tissues, cartilage)
Mucous membranes: ➤ Mucosa ➤ Submucosa
Blood vessels: ➤ Arteries ➤ Veins
Lymphatic system: ➤ Vessels ➤ Lymph nodes
Nervous system: ➤ Nerves and ganglia
Salivary glands: ➤ Parotid gland ➤ Submandibular gland ➤ Sublingual gland
Soft tissues: ➤ Connective tissue ➤ Fasciae ➤ Tendons

Clinical Examination Techniques

For the physician considering clinical issues of differential diagnosis, the history and physical examination are of fundamental importance. Standard examination methods such as inspection, palpation, indirect ENT examinations, and classic audiometric tests are essential in the detection of head and neck disorders.

Clinical examination techniques relating to clinical otology and the diagnosis of skull base disorders include inspection and palpation of the auricle and its surroundings, palpation of the regional lymph nodes, otoscopic examination, audiologic studies, and vestibular and eustachian-tube function testing. Some cases may also require smears and bacteriologic testing, and more extensive lesions of the skull base may warrant a comprehensive cranial nerve examination.

In the differential diagnosis of hearing disorders, inspection, palpation, and otoscopy are supplemented by tuning fork tests (Weber, Renne, and Gelle tests), pure-tone audiometry, spoken voice testing, and speech audiometry. Sensorineural hearing loss is evaluated by testing for recruitment and by performing the Fowler test. Other potentially useful studies are auditory fatigue testing and the measurement of acoustic impedance. In patients with balance disorders, the clinical examination includes specialized studies such as thermal testing, torsion chair testing, and evaluation of the oculomotor and somatic systems. This is particularly important in complex evaluations for disorders such as vertigo.

For diseases of the facial region, key emphasis is placed on otorhinolaryngologic examinations of the facial soft tissues, paranasal sinuses, oral cavity, maxilla, mandible, and parotid region.

The major tools for evaluating the nose, paranasal sinuses, and nasopharynx are endoscopy, rhinomanometry, rhinorheography, and sinuscopy (anteroscopy). Magnifying endoscopes can be used for evaluations of the mouth and pharynx.

The major salivary glands can be evaluated by determining the salivary flow rate (sialometry), which yields information on saliva production and the function of the affected gland. Salivary chemistry can furnish additional information on the biochemical composition of the saliva.

The larynx and hypopharynx can be evaluated by classic indirect examination with a laryngeal mirror (indirect laryngoscopy) as a prelude to instrumental laryngeal exploration, but indirect magnification laryngoscopy may be preferred owing to its magnified field of view. Direct microlaryngoscopy is also available for endolaryngeal measures and manipulations.

In patients with voice and speech disorders, extensive clinical testing procedures are needed to aid in the assessment of vocal function and phonation.

2 Diagnostic Imaging Techniques

Today, an optimum radiologic workup of head and neck disorders can be accomplished only through the discriminating use of the imaging modalities and techniques listed in Table 2.**1**.

With the advent of modern sectional imaging methods such as computed tomography (CT) and magnetic resonance imaging (MRI), there has been a radical change in the primary indications for conventional radiographic examinations and other imaging procedures. At present, conventional radiography still has some value in the initial workup of trauma cases and in the evaluation of inflammatory disorders of the head and neck region. Below we shall review the most important imaging techniques and their optimal technical parameters for head and neck applications. The requirements for specific subregions will be discussed in the chapters dealing with the assessment of those regions.

Table 2.**1** Imaging procedures in the head and neck region

Conventional radiography:
- Tomography, oral contrast cineradiography

CT:
- Spiral CT
- High-resolution CT
- CTA
- CT-guided biopsy

MRI:
- MRI
- MRA
- MR spectroscopy
- Interventional MRI

Sonography:
- Doppler sonography
- Color duplex sonography

DSA:
- Diagnostic DSA
- Interventional procedures

(Nuclear-medicine imaging procedures)

Conventional Radiography

The following technical parameters are recommended for conventional radiographic examinations of the skull and skull base: kilovoltage 70 to 85 kV, constant tube current 50 mAs, 200-speed film-screen combination, 0.6 mm focal spot size, and grid technique. The path of the central ray conforms to traditional standard requirements. The exposure time should be less than 100 ms. Conventional lateral views of the skull can be obtained at 65 to 80 kV and a lower tube current, with otherwise identical technical parameters. Skull radiographs in women should deliver a gonadal dose of less than 0.2 μSv and less than 4 mSv to the red bone marrow of the skull.

Axial View of the Skull Base

For this projection the head is hyperextended and the central ray is approximately perpendicular to the orbitomeatal plane. The axial view demonstrates the *anterior*, *middle*, and *posterior cranial fossae*. The *foramina lacerum*, *ovale*, and *spinosum* form a medial-to-lateral series of apertures in the middle fossa. The posterior fossa encompasses the *foramen magnum*. Between the middle and posterior fossae, the bony structures of the petrous pyramid and the mastoid air cells can be evaluated.

Posteroanterior (PA) Skull View

For this view the patient lies prone or sits upright in front of the stand with the forehead resting against the cassette. This standard projection demonstrates the *bony structures of the calvarium* and the cranial sutures. It also defines the bony contours of the *orbits*, the *frontal sinus*, and the *nasal cavity*. The *petrous ridge*, *petrous apex*, and *mastoid* are visible at a more caudal level. This projection provides a general survey view of the skull that is useful for detecting asymmetries and disproportions (e.g., in patients with congenital malformations).

Lateral Skull View

The lateral skull view is taken with the patient prone, the side to be examined close to the film, and the median plane of the skull parallel to the tabletop. This gives a laterally projected view of the bony structures and sutures of the calvarium and the structures of the skull base (*pituitary fossa*, *dorsum sellae*, and *frontal bone*). The *nasal bone* and *frontal sinus* are visible anteriorly. The lateral skull film also consistently demonstrates the *craniocervical junction* and the upper cervical vertebrae.

Schüller View

The Schüller view is obtained by angling the central ray 30° cranially with respect to the horizontal plane. This view is used to evaluate the *mastoid process* and *mastoid air cells*, the *external auditory canal*, the tympanic cavity, and the *condyle of the mandible*. Abnormalities are best appreciated by making a side-to-side comparison.

Stenvers View

The Stenvers view is a special oblique projection used to demonstrate the *petrous ridge*, *petrous apex*, and the *internal auditory canal* and its contents (semicircular canals, cochlea). The central ray is angled 45° posteriorly and 12° caudally. Typical abnormalities disclosed by this view include osteolytic lesions of the petrous ridge and apex, a right-left discrepancy of more than 2 mm between the bilateral Stenvers views, and expansion of the internal auditory canal to more than 8 mm.

Mayer View

The Mayer projection of the temporal bone, obtained by angling the tube 45° cephalad, is useful for evaluating the *mastoid* and the *mandibular condyle*. While this view has similar applications to those of the Schüller view, it is obtained only in exceptional cases.

Sectional Imaging Modalities

Computed Tomography (CT)

CT provides better delineation of the bony structures of the skull base and facial skeleton than conventional radiography. Its superior resolution and absence of superimposed structures offer significant advantages for the evaluation of neoplastic and traumatic lesions, with the result that CT has largely supplanted conventional motion-controlled tomography in the head and neck region. CT is also excellent for demonstrating sites of bone destruction and lymph node enlargement (malignant lymphomas, metastases). Another advantage of CT is its ability to characterize tissue structures by *densitometry*. Bony structures have attenuation values as high as 100 Hounsfield units (HU) (metal), while water has an attenuation of 0 HU, and air is assigned a value of -1000 HU. Thus, various soft tissues such as muscle, glands, connective tissue, and tumors have positive attenuation values while fatty tissue has negative attenuation values. By selecting a bone or soft-tissue "window," the examiner can highlight CT image details that are relevant to a particular inquiry.

Routine examinations should employ a slice thickness of 3 to 5 mm and should include a topogram (scout view) that may or may not display the programmed image planes. Studies evaluating for inner ear pathology (e.g., otosclerosis) should employ high-resolution thin-section CT scanning (HRCT) with a slice thickness of 1 mm. This technique can define the ossicular chain, the semicircular canals, the foramen ovale, and the tympanic membrane. CT evaluations for neoplastic lesions often require the intravenous injection of an iodinated contrast agent to heighten the contrast of the tumor with its surroundings and improve vascular delineation. The total volume of contrast agent depends on the imaging volume in the region under study and is usually between 100 and 180 mL.

Spiral (helical) CT scanning (Table 2.**2**) is particularly helpful in trauma patients, as it provides the same image quality as conventional CT while significantly shortening the imaging time. Spiral CT can scan an entire volume of interest without discontinuities in a single breath hold, concluding the examination for the patient and providing data sets that can be quantitatively and qualitatively analyzed. Postprocessing yields sectional images in any desired slice thickness, regardless of the table speed. The spiral CT scanner should have the capability for single or dual helical scanning. Current systems can generate 24 to110 images from a single helical CT scan exposure.

Intravenous contrast is of key importance in spiral CT studies. The contrast volume, injection rate, and delay time before initiating the scan should be individually determined.

A contrast volume of 150 mL, an injection rate of up to 2 mL per second, and a delay of about 20 seconds appear to be adequate for most examinations of the skull base. Owing to its advantages, spiral CT is increasingly used in evaluations of nontraumatic conditions, particularly inflammatory and neoplastic dis-

Table 2.**2** Definition of characteristic parameters of spiral CT

	Volume	**Injection rate**	**Delay**
Contrast agent	100–150 mL	2–5 mL/s	5–70 s
	Slice thickness	**Table feed**	**Reconstruction interval**
Spiral technique	1–5 mm	1–5 mm	1–2

orders. One shortcoming of spiral CT scanning in the head and neck is its high susceptibility to motion artifacts, which can be a significant problem in trauma patients. If certain of the images show poor quality, it may be necessary to rescan the zones obscured by artifacts.

The chapters dealing with specific subregions present scanning protocols that optimally coordinate scan parameters such as slice thickness, table feed, and reconstruction interval (pitch factor). Another mode of CT reconstruction is CT angiography (CTA), which is useful for visualizing the extracranial carotid system. This technique is currently limited by time-consuming reconstruction algorithms, however, and is best suited for studies of the carotid bifurcation.

The usefulness of CT is most seriously limited in the skull base region, where bone artifacts can hamper interpretation. This circumstance, plus the frequent inability of CT to provide acceptable soft tissue differentiation, will often necessitate the use of MRI for evaluations of malignant or inflammatory infiltration.

The radiation exposure associated with a cranial CT examination is approximately 5 mSv to the red bone marrow of the skull and 10 μSv to the female gonads (from scattered radiation).

The spiral CT examination can be tailored by varying the delay time as a function of the patient's cardiac output, the region under study, and the contrast injection rate. A reduced slice thickness is recommended for examinations of the larynx and hypopharynx to achieve maximum resolution of structural details.

In patients who cannot lie still, conventional CT scanning is advantageous owing to its reproducible quality and the ability to repeat the examination as needed.

Magnetic Resonance Imaging (MRI)

MRI is superior to CT in its differentiation of soft tissue structures, its arteriographic capabilities, and its ability to depict anatomic and pathologic structures in any desired spatial plane without repositioning the patient. Several components characterize the practical use of MRI: the *coil technology* that is used, the *sequence-specific parameters*, and the use of *contrast agents*. A head coil is used for imaging the skull base, and a routine imaging protocol in this region consists of T1- and T2-weighted spin-echo (SE) sequences, turbo spin-echo (TSE) sequences, as well as fast gradient-echo sequences (e.g., FLASH, FISP, GRASS) for the dynamic evaluation of contrast enhancement. A paramagnetic contrast agent such as gadolinium-DTPA (Gd-DTPA) (Magnevist, Schering) or Gd-DTPA-BMA (Omniscan, Nykomed), injected in an intravenous dose of 0.1 mL/kg w, is well tolerated in cases where there are no contraindications to contrast use.

T1-weighted sequences, with or without fat suppression, can precisely document the enhancement characteristics of normal and pathologic structures—an essential step in formulating an optimum differential diagnosis.

In patients with a presumptive diagnosis of a tumor mass, fast gradient-echo sequences should be performed immediately after contrast injection to document the enhancement characteristics of the lesion. In this dynamic MR study, a hypervascular mass will show an initially marked rise in signal intensity followed by a characteristic inversion of the time-intensity curve and then a stable plateau of marked enhancement. This effect is well documented by a contrast dose of 0.3 mol/kg body weight.

CISS sequences are a recent advance in MRI technology that can demonstrate the circulation of cerebrospinal fluid (CSF) and of endolymph within the semicircular canals and cochlea. Magnetic resonance angiography (MRA) is another noninvasive procedure that can specifically image venous flow in the head and neck region. The specific techniques are known as time-of-flight (TOF) and phase-contrast (PC) MRA. Special presaturation techniques can be used to provide a specific analysis of arterial or venous flow. Depending on the system used, heavily T2-weighted TSE or inversion-recovery sequences are available for imaging fluid-containing structures.

Both TOF and PC MRA offer advantages, depending on the type of equipment used. 3-D FISP sequences are particularly effective for arterial MRA in the region of the facial skeleton, cervical soft tissues, and skull base. The TONE TOF technique offers diagnostic advantages in intracerebral vascular studies. For arterial MRA studies, a venous presaturation pulse is applied at the level of the proximal skull base to suppress inflow signals from the sigmoid sinus, jugular bulb, and jugular vein. Venous MRA requires the application of a deep presaturation pulse, usually placed at the level of the aortic arch, to suppress arterial spins entering the image plane from the aortic region.

One of the most reliable protocols is the 2-D FLASH sequence, which can be optimally adapted to flow velocities in the venous circulation. This technique images venous flow exclusively, producing a high-intensity image of venous spins entering the image slice from the sigmoid sinus, jugular bulb, and jugular vein.

Image analysis in arterial and venous MRA can be done from individual documented images or from various views in a 3-D maximum intensity projection (MIP). The accurate interpretation of MRA requires a knowledge of potential pitfalls, including zones of increased signal intensity such as intralesional hemorrhage and protein-rich fluids and the artifacts that can occur at boundary surfaces. When these precautions are observed, clinical MRA is an important diagnostic tool for evaluating major vascular structures and their involvement by various primary or secondary disease processes.

Radionuclide Imaging

Nuclear medicine techniques are reserved for a few selected indications in the head and neck region such as the investigation of posttraumatic CSF rhinorrhea with ^{111}In-DTPA, which is administered by intrathecal injection and confirms CSF leakage by detection of the tracer in nasal secretions.

Radionuclide bone scanning with ^{99m}Tc can be used to screen for metastatic lesions. A positive scan shows sites of tracer uptake in the skull base region that require further evaluation by other imaging techniques.

Diagnostic Angiography and Interventional Treatment

A modern angiographic unit with DSA capability should be available whenever an invasive arterial procedure in the head and neck region is proposed. Usually the initial step after femoral puncture is to obtain a survey arteriogram of the internal and external carotid arteries. Following selective catheterization of the internal and external carotid branches, the vascular territories of interest are catheterized with thin-lumen catheters or propulsive systems, and small amounts of contrast material are injected. In interventional procedures, embolization can be performed using embolic materials such as particles, coils, balloons, or liquid agents, which have varying degrees of permanence. The main hazard in the facial region is the risk of occlusive material embolizing to vessels supplying the central nervous system (CNS), resulting in neurologic deficits.

In the region of the skull base, such procedures are used mainly for the evaluation and treatment of glomus tumors and other benign and malignant hypervascular tumors. Because these tumors are usually supplied by the external carotid artery, the selective visualization of that vessel is imperative. The frequent multifocal or bilateral occurrence of these tumors also requires a general assessment of the vertebral artery, internal carotid artery, maxillary artery, internal occipital artery, ascending pharyngeal artery, and posterior auricular artery.

Principles in the Interpretation of Normal Tissue Structures in Imaging Techniques

Interpretation of Normal Tissue Structures in MRI

This section deals with the typical MR signal characteristics of normal tissue structures in the head and neck region and bordering spaces based on signal intensities and morphologic features depicted on MR images. With its high soft-tissue differentiation and improved contrast resolution, MRI is the optimum imaging modality for most investigations. The following factors characterize the MR signal intensities of anatomic and pathologic structures:

- T1 and T2 relaxation times
- Proton density
- Spin flow
- Technical parameters (repetition time TR, echo delay time TE, flip angle α).

The MR sequences for basic image interpretation are T2-weighted SE sequences, proton-density images, and T1-weighted sequences. These should be supplemented by gradient-echo sequences and 3-D sequences to document the signal characteristics of essential structures. A knowledge of the signal characteristics that appear in the MR imaging protocols forms an important basis for the accurate differential diagnosis of head and neck lesions. Below we shall review the signal characteristics for various tissue groups and for most pathologic processes.

Muscle Tissue

Muscle tissue has low signal intensity on all SE and gradient-echo sequences. This creates a sharp contrast between muscle and surrounding hyperintense fat. Muscle is also well demarcated from cortical bone, connective tissue, capsular ligaments, and menisci, which appear as areas of signal void. The interpretation of muscle tissue on MR images should encompass the presence, size, conspicuity, and location of the muscles in question. When pathology is present, its PA and proximal-distal distribution should be precisely documented. Necrotic muscle is usually replaced by fat and connective tissue, which show a markedly increased signal intensity on T1- and T2-weighted SE sequences relative to healthy muscle. Muscular strains and ruptures show increased signal intensity on T2-weighted sequences (Table 2.**3**).

Table 2.**3** MR characteristics of muscle tissue

Low signal intensity in T1- and T2-weighted SE sequences

Identification:
- Location
- Volume
- Signal characteristics

Pathologic findings:
- Malformation
- Tumor mass
- Structural alteration
- Atrophy, hypertrophy
- Hemorrhage
- Fatty infiltration

Fatty Tissue

The subcutaneous space, the infratemporal fossa, and all significant anatomic compartments in the head and neck region contain fat that is characterized by high signal intensity in T1- and T2-weighted SE sequences. The intense fat signals clearly differentiate normal topographic structures from adjacent muscle, connective tissue, and vessels. Structural changes in muscle tissues may be associated with fatty involution, which acquires the same high signal intensity as fat. Varying concentrations of fat are found in the bone marrow of the mandibular ramus, portions of the temporal bone, the clivus, and the sphenoid bone (Table 2.**4**).

Cartilage

Articular Cartilage

MRI can noninvasively differentiate cartilaginous structures from adjacent soft tissues. Articular cartilage appears hyperintense to subcutaneous bone and menisci in SE sequences. In gradient-echo sequences (e.g., FLASH or FISP sequences), articular cartilage shows a high signal intensity that contrasts sharply with surrounding structures. MRI can define both the severity and extent of cartilage lesions such as erosion, thinning, fractures, and chondromalacia.

Table 2.**4** MR characteristics of fatty tissue

High signal intensity in T1- and T2-weighted SE sequences

Fibrocartilage

Normal fibrocartilage unaffected by degenerative or traumatic changes has low signal intensity in SE and gradient-echo sequences. This should distinguish these cartilaginous structures from the higher-intensity bilaminar zone of the temporomandibular joint. Foci of increased signal intensity within the articular disc provide early evidence of degenerative change. A tear appears as a linear hyperintensity causing contour disruption and communicating with the articular surface of the temporomandibular joint (Table 2.**5**).

Cortical and Cancellous Bone

Cortical and cancellous bone have markedly different sectional imaging appearances. For example, the essential structures of the temporomandibular joint such as the glenoid fossa and mandibular condyle feature a cortical layer devoid of MR signals and a medullary cavity of high signal intensity. *Cortical bone* shows a complete absence of signal in T1- and T2-weighted fast SE and gradient-echo sequences.

By contrast, the normal marrow of nonhematopoietic bone shows a uniformly high signal intensity in T2-weighted SE sequences. The bone marrow of adults consists of up to 70% lipids, more than 90% of which are triglycerides. The high proton content of these triglyceride molecules is responsible for the high signal intensity of the marrow. A significant decline in MR signal intensity must be interpreted as signifying a previous or current pathologic process. In the early stage of the pathologic process, the reduction of MR signal intensity correlates with a diminished proton concentration.

Table 2.**5** MR characteristics of cartilage

Articular cartilage:
- High signal intensity in T2-weighted SE sequences and gradient-echo sequences

Fibrocartilage:
- Low signal intensity in SE sequences
- Pathologic findings:
  —Malformation
  —Degeneration
  —Hemorrhage (associated with an increase in signal intensity)

The process may have an inflammatory, traumatic, or vascular cause. Pathologic changes are characterized by anoxia and edema, with loss of signal intensity usually commencing at the subarticular level and later becoming more pronounced due to calcification and trabecular fragmentation. *Cancellous bone structures* in the head and neck region contain varying proportions of hematopoietic marrow and yellow marrow. The signal registered in a particular MR sequence depends on the relative amount and structure of these components and on the scan parameters that are used.

Bone marrow displays moderate signal intensity on T1-weighted SE sequences. As the proportion of yellow marrow increases, the signal becomes more intense. Signal intensity decreases as water-containing cells become more numerous and displace the yellow marrow.

Cancellous bone changes are most clearly appreciated in proton-density SE sequences. These images heighten the contrast between the marrow and cortical bone and provide a better signal-to-noise ratio than T1-weighted images.

In T2-weighted SE sequences, structures like the mandibular condyle generally have a homogeneous imaging appearance. Signal intensity depends strongly on the amount of yellow marrow in the bone. A high content of yellow marrow correlates with high signal intensity caused by focal accumulations of fat within the normal cancellous bone.

In gradient-echo sequences with a prolonged repetition time, the normal cancellous bone cavity usually shows a low signal intensity, regardless of the flip angle. Signal intensity shows some dependence on the echo delay time (Table 2.**6**).

Table 2.**6** MR characteristics of bony structures

Cortical bone:
- Low signal intensity or signal void in T1- and T2-weighted SE and gradient-echo sequences

Cancellous bone:
- Hematopoietic marrow:
  - —Low signal intensity in T1- and T2-weighted images
  - —Pathologic changes in cancellous bone, focal or diffuse zones of decreased signal intensity
- Pathologic findings:
  - —Edema
  - —Tumor
  - —Hemorrhage

Special Part

3 Anterior Skull Base

The anterior skull base forms a bony boundary separating the nasopharynx from the frontal lobes of the brain. As such, it poses a special challenge to clinical and radiologic diagnosis. A number of primary osseous lesions can arise in this region, but more commonly the anterior skull base is infiltrated by lesions that have a nasopharyngeal or intracranial origin.

The *clinical examination* is based largely on inspection, palpation, biopsy, and function tests of the cranial nerves that supply this region. Because the anterior skull base is clinically inaccessible, lesions in this area are usually advanced when diagnosed and require accurate imaging evaluation to direct the further planning of treatment. An understanding of the complex anatomy of this region is essential for the optimum application of imaging procedures and the interpretation of differential diagnostic criteria.

Normal Anatomy

The *sphenoid bone* constitutes the bony foundation of the anterior skull base. This anatomically complex structure forms the floor of the middle skull base and parasellar cavernous sinus. It contains the sella turcica, which lodges the pituitary, and is pierced by numerous foramina that transmit neurovascular structures.

In shape, the sphenoid bone resembles a bird with outstretched wings. It consists of a *body*, paired *greater wings* and *lesser wings* that spread laterally from the body, and two *pterygoid processes* that extend downward from the junction of the body with the greater wings (Fig. 3.**1**). The body of the sphenoid is cubical and contains two air-filled cavities, the sphenoid sinuses.

The posterior border of the sphenoid bone is formed by the dorsum sellae and the laterally situated posterior clinoid processes, which give attachment to the tentorium.

The *sphenoid sinus* is located in the body of the bone and is generally subdivided into two air-filled cavities by a thin, vertical bony septum. These cavities are often asymmetric and may extend laterally into the lesser and greater sphenoid wings or inferolaterally to the pterygoid plate. The sphenoid sinus communicates anterosuperiorly with the nasal fossa via two apertures that open into the sphenoethmoid recess.

The *greater wing* of the sphenoid curves laterally and slightly upward from the body. The greater wings form part of the floor of the middle cranial fossa, supporting the anterolateral portions of the brain, and contain a number of neurovascular foramina. The wing is bounded inferiorly by the lateral part of the inferior orbital fissure and medially by the lateral part of the superior orbital fissure.

The *lesser wings* articulate with the posterior edge of the orbital roof of the frontal bone. The posteromedial portion of the wing forms a projection, the anterior clinoid process, which gives attachment to the anterior border of the tentorium. A fold of dura bridges the gap between the anterior and middle clinoid processes. This fold may calcify, forming a caroticoclinoid foramen. The optic canal, which transmits the optic nerve and ophthalmic artery, traverses the medial attachment of the lesser wing to the body of the sphenoid.

The triangular *orbital fissure* is bounded medially by the sphenoid body, superiorly by the lesser wing, and inferiorly by the orbital surface of the greater wing. This aperture gives passage to the oculomotor, trochlear, and abducent nerves, the orbital branches of the meningeal artery, sympathetic branches of the internal carotid plexus, branches of the lacrimal artery, and the ophthalmic vein.

The *pterygoid process* descends from the inferomedial part of the greater wing on each side. Each process consists of a medial and a lateral plate (Fig. 3.**1**) that are fused anteriorly. The pterygoid fossa forms a groove between the two surfaces and gives origin to the medial pterygoid muscle. The anterior surface of the pterygoid process forms the posterior wall of the pterygopalatine fossa.

The *lateral pterygoid plate* forms part of the medial wall of the infratemporal fossa and gives attachment to the lateral pterygoid muscle. The medial plate forms the lateral wall of the pterygoid fossa to which the medial pterygoid muscle is attached. The upper part of the anterior border of the plate forms the posterior boundary of the pterygomaxillary fissure. The pharyngobasilar fascia is attached to the posterior margin of the medial plate, and the superior pharyngeal constrictor muscle arises farther inferiorly. The lower end of the medial plate forms a hook-like process, the pterygoid hamulus, around which winds the tendon of the tensor veli palatini muscle.

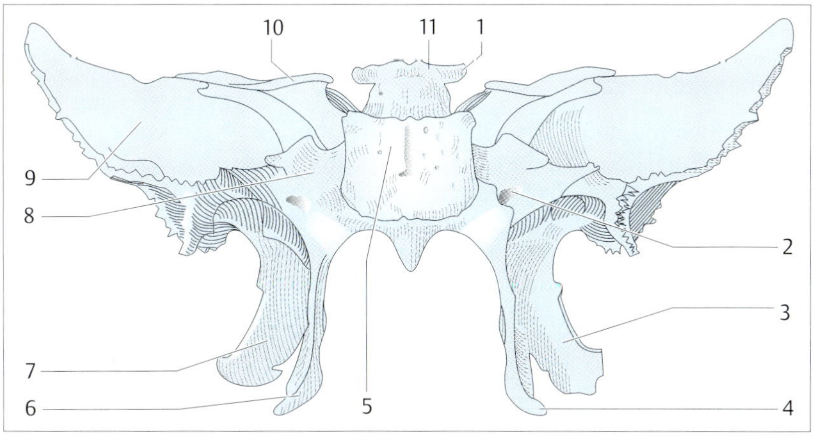

Fig. 3.**1** **Sphenoid bone, posterior aspect**

1 Posterior clinoid process
2 Pterygoid canal
3 Pterygoid fossa
4 Pterygoid hamulus
5 Body of sphenoid
6 Medial plate
7 Lateral plate
8 Carotid sulcus
9 Greater wing
10 Lesser wing
11 Dorsum sellae

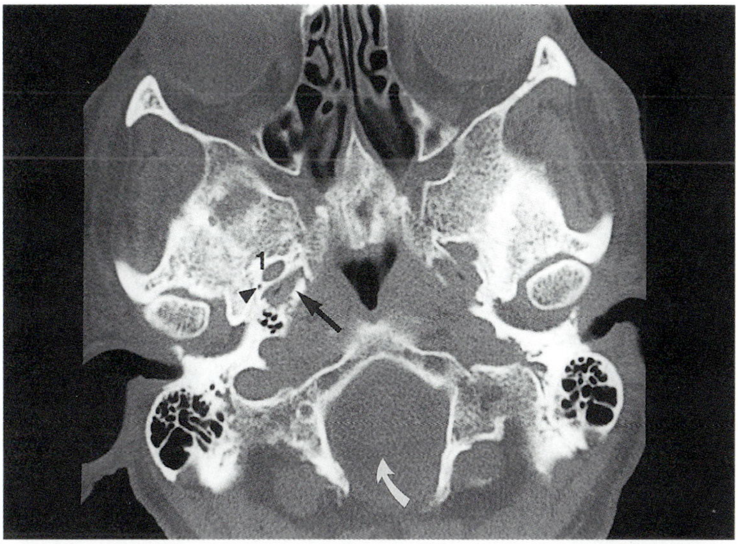

a

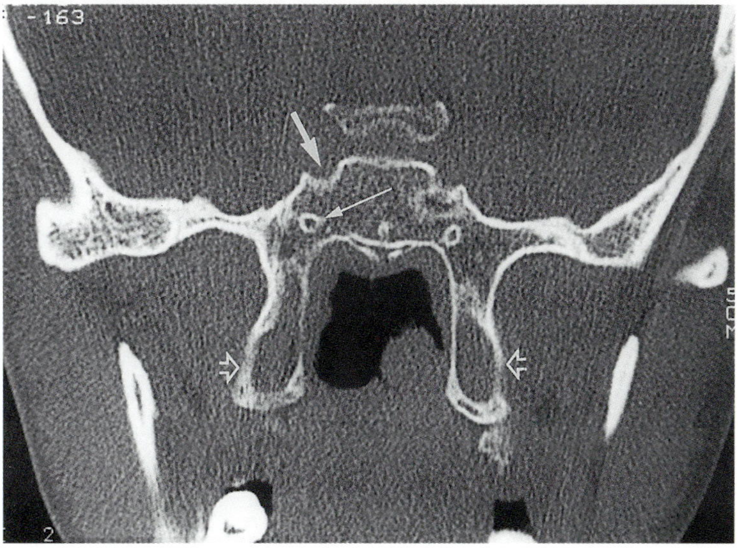

b

Figs. 3.**2** **a, b** **Normal topographic anatomy of the anterior skull base.** (**a**) Axial noncontrast CT scan (1 mm, bone window) demonstrates the normal apertures of the skull base: the foramen ovale (1), carotid canal (arrow), foramen spinosum (arrowhead), and foramen magnum (curved arrow). (**b**) Coronal noncontrast CT scan (1 mm, bone window) demonstrates the pterygoid canal (thin arrow) within the sphenoid, the carotid sulcus (thicker arrow), and the pterygoid process (open arrows).

Basal Foramina (Tables 3.1 and 3.2)

Foramen Rotundum

The foramen rotundum lies below and lateral to the superior orbital fissure at the base of the greater wing of the sphenoid bone. The foramen is bounded medially by the lateral wall of the sphenoid sinus, and the whole of the foramen may lie within the sinus in some individuals. The foramen rotundum runs laterally downward in a slightly oblique course. It unites the middle cranial fossa with the pterygopalatine fossa and transmits the maxillary nerve and emissary veins.

The maxillary nerve supplies sensory innervation to the midfacial skin. The artery of the foramen rotundum arises in the pterygopalatine fossa as the terminal branch of the internal maxillary artery and accompanies the maxillary nerve. This vessel establishes an important anastomosis between the cavernous branches of the internal carotid artery and the internal maxillary artery. The foramen rotundum is best appreciated on coronal CT scans.

Foramen Ovale

The foramen ovale, located in the medial part of the greater wing of the sphenoid bone, transmits the accessory meningeal artery and emissary veins (Fig. 3.**2a**). The intracranial opening of the foramen is posterolateral to the foramen rotundum, and its extracranial opening is at the base of the lateral pterygoid plate.

The foramen ovale is visible on axial and coronal CT scans, which can demonstrate both interindividual and intraindividual (side-to-side) variations in the normal diameter of the foramen. Lesions that spread through the foramen ovale are best visualized on coronal MR images.

The mandibular nerve contains both sensory and motor fibers. It supplies motor innervation to the masseter, temporal, and pterygoid muscles and sensory innervation to the skin over the temporal region, lower face, lips, mandible, temporomandibular joint, and part of the dura.

Table 3.**1** Neural foramina of the skull base and transmitted neurovascular structures

Foramen	Location	Transmitted nerves	Transmitted vessels
Cribriform plate	Anterior cranial fossa	Olfactory nerves Anterior ethmoid nerve	Anterior ethmoid artery Anterior ethmoid vein
Optic canal	Lesser wing of sphenoid bone	Optic nerve	Ophthalmic artery
Superior orbital fissure	Between lesser and greater sphenoid wings	Oculomotor nerve (III) Trochlear nerve (IV) Ophthalmic nerve (V_1) Abducent nerve (VI)	Superior ophthalmic vein
Foramen rotundum	Middle cranial fossa, inferior to superior orbital fissure	Maxillary nerve (V_2)	Artery of foramen rotundum Emissary vein
Foramen ovale	Middle cranial fossa, lateral to sella	Mandibular nerve (V_3)	Accessory meningeal branch of maxillary artery Emissary veins
Foramen spinosum	Posterolateral to foramen ovale	Meningeal branch of mandibular nerve	Middle meningeal artery Recurrent meningeal branch
Foramen lacerum	Base of pterygoid plate	Greater petrosal nerve Lesser petrosal nerve	Branches of ascending pharyngeal artery
Pterygoid (vidian) canal	In sphenoid bone inferomedial to foramen rotundum	Vidian nerve (nerve of pterygoid canal)	Vidian artery (artery of pterygoid canal)
Carotid canal	In petrous part of temporal bone	Sympathetic plexus	Internal carotid artery
Jugular foramen	Posterolateral to carotid canal	Pars nervosa: Glossopharyngeal nerve Jacobsen's nerve Pars vascularis: Vagus nerve Spinal accessory nerves Arnold's nerve	Pars nervosa: Inferior petrosal sinus Pars vascularis: Internal jugular vein

Table 3.2 Accessibility of neural foramina to various imaging procedures

Neural foramina	Technique and projection
Cribriform plate	CT, axial and coronal Tomography, AP and lateral
Optic canal	CT, axial and coronal MRI, axial and coronal Rhese projection of skull
Superior orbital fissure	CT, axial and coronal Tomography, AP and lateral
Foramen rotundum	CT, coronal Paranasal sinuses, OF Skull radiograph, PA
Pterygoid canal	CT, axial and coronal Tomography, AP
Foramen ovale	CT, axial and coronal MRI, coronal Axial skull radiograph
Foramen spinosum	CT, coronal
Foramen lacerum	CT, axial and coronal MRI, axial and coronal

The accessory meningeal artery may arise directly from the middle meningeal artery or from the internal maxillary artery just distal to the middle meningeal. It traverses the foramen ovale anterior to the mandibular nerve and supplies the pharynx and eustachian tube.

Foramen Spinosum

The foramen spinosum is a short canal in the posteromedial part of the greater sphenoid wing connecting the middle cranial fossa with the infratemporal fossa (Fig. 3.**2a**). The intracranial opening of the foramen lies posterolateral to the foramen ovale, and its extracranial opening is anterolateral to the eustachian tube. This foramen transmits the middle meningeal artery and vein and the meningeal branch of the mandibular nerve. It is best appreciated on coronal CT and MR images.

The middle meningeal artery arises from the proximal part of the internal maxillary artery and passes through the foramen to the skull base. In rare cases the middle meningeal artery springs directly from the ophthalmic artery, resulting in a small or absent foramen spinosum.

Foramen Lacerum

The extracranial part of this foramen is covered by cartilage (basal fibrocartilage). The foramen lacerum lies at the base of the medial pterygoid plate and is bounded anterolaterally by the greater sphenoid wing, posteriorly by the petrous apex, and medially by the body of the sphenoid and the basilar part of the occipital bone. The opening of the pterygoid canal lies farther back in the anterior part of the foramen lacerum.

The internal carotid artery does not pass through this foramen, as was once taught, but lies upon the cartilage covering its intracranial portion. An inconstant meningeal branch of the ascending pharyngeal artery and the greater and lesser petrosal nerves pierce the cartilage covering and are the only structures that traverse the foramen lacerum, which is visible on axial and coronal CT and MR images.

Pterygoid Canal

The pterygoid (vidian) canal (Figs. 3.**1** and 3.**2**), located at the base of the pterygoid process below and medial to the foramen rotundum in the body of the sphenoid, connects the pterygopalatine fossa with the foramen lacerum. In rare cases, the canal may traverse the floor of the sphenoid sinus. It transmits the vidian artery and the nerve of the pterygoid canal, a prolongation of the greater petrosal nerve past its union with the deep petrosal nerve. After leaving the canal, the nerve passes to the pterygopalatine ganglion and supplies autonomic innervation to the lacrimal gland and the mucosal surfaces of the nose, pharynx, and palate.

The vidian artery, a terminal branch of the internal maxillary artery, arises in the pterygopalatine fossa, passes around the sphenopalatine foramen, and accompanies the vidian nerve through the pterygoid canal. With its proximity to the foramen lacerum, the vidian artery provides an important collateral pathway for the internal carotid artery.

Sella Turcica

The bony portion of the sella turcica is formed by the sphenoid bone. It is bounded on each side by the cavernous sinusus and posteriorly by the dorsum sellae (Fig. 3.**1**) and clivus. The floor of the sella is formed by the roof of the sphenoid sinus. The sella derives its blood supply from the superior and inferior pituitary arteries, which arise from the internal carotid, and from a complex portal vascular system. The sella is drained by the cavernous sinuses. The pituitary is bordered by the optic chiasm rostrally and the sphenoid sinus inferiorly, and it is flanked by the cavernous sinuses. The internal carotid artery and abducent nerve pass through the cavernous sinus, whose lateral wall transmits the oculomotor, trochlear, ophthalmic, and maxillary nerves.

Cavernous Sinus

The cavernous sinuses are placed one on each side of the body of the sphenoid bone, extending from the apex of the orbital fissure anteriorly to the petrous apex posteriorly. Each sinus measures approximately 2 cm x 1 cm. The cavernous sinus is traversed by the internal carotid artery, which is surrounded by a plexus of connective tissue and sympathetic nerves. The abducent nerve runs inferolateral to the artery in its passage through the cavernous sinus, while the lateral wall of the sinus transmits (from above to below) the oculomotor, trochlear, ophthalmic, and maxillary nerves. Each of these nerves is ensheathed by connective tissue and is further isolated from the venous blood in the sinus by endothelium.

The sella above and the sphenoid sinus below are both medial to the cavernous sinus. The Meckel cavity, which contains the trigeminal ganglion, is adjacent to the posteroinferior part of the lateral sinus wall.

The tributaries of the cavernous sinus include the ophthalmic vein and the superficial, middle, and inferior cerebral veins. The cavernous sinus drains into the transverse sinus via the superior petrosal sinus, and into the internal jugular vein via the inferior petrosal sinus. It also drains into the pterygoid venous plexus by veins that traverse the sphenoidal foramen, into the emissary veins of the foramen ovale and foramen lacerum, and into the facial vein through the superficial ophthalmic vein. The two sinuses communicate with each other via the basilar plexus on the clivus and via the anterior and posterior intercavernous sinuses.

Blood is propelled through the cavernous sinus by the pulsations of the internal carotid artery, by gravitational effects, and by the position of the head.

Clivus

The clivus is the portion of the skull base situated between the foramen magnum and dorsum sellae. It is bounded anterolaterally by the petro-occipital fissure and more posteriorly by the synchondrosis between the basilar and exoccipital portions of the occipital bone. The anterior superior boundary of the clivus is formed by the body of the sphenoid and the sphenoid sinus while the inferior boundary is continuous with the anterior rim of the foramen magnum. The nasopharynx forms the extracranial boundary of the clivus.

The inferior petrosal sinus runs along the inferolateral border of the clivus. A venous plexus occurs on the intracranial surface of the clivus; this area relates closely to the pons and medulla oblongata.

Clinical Signs and Symptoms

The clinical symptoms associated with lesions of the anterior skull base depend on the origin of the lesion (nasopharyngeal or intracranial) and on the extent of cranial nerve involvement.

The most frequent clinical syndromes that characterize primary or secondary cranial nerve involvement in this region are listed in Table 3.**3**.

The main clinical symptoms produced by lesions of the anterior skull base are shown in Table 3.**4**. In many cases the symptoms are nonspecific and are based largely on morphologic changes. Supraorbital morphologic changes are the most conspicuous clinical signs and can have various causes:

- Tumors and malformations.
- Facial swelling.
- Skin disorders.
- Paralysis in the facial region.
- Motor paralysis.
- Functional disturbances and sensory paralysis.
- Pain in the skull base region.
- ENT diseases.
- Diseases of the teeth and jaws.
- Neuralgias.
- Intracranial disease.

Pathology of the anterior skull base may include tumors, malformations, morphologic changes, inflammatory lesions, degenerative processes, vascular lesions, trauma, and complications from therapeutic procedures.

The most common diseases, in order of increasing frequency, are:

- Malformations
- Tumors
- Inflammatory processes

The accurate assessment of a lesion of the anterior skull base starts with the history and clinical examination including rhinoscopy. Further evaluation consists of blood studies, a cerebrospinal fluid (CSF) examination if required, and diagnostic imaging. Imaging studies are essential, given the limitations of direct visual evaluation in this region, and are particularly useful for diagnosing therapy-induced changes and tumor recurrence.

Table 3.**3** Major clinical syndromes associated with lesions of the anterior skull base

Syndrome	Symptoms	Cranial nerve involvement
Olfactory nerve syndrome	Anosmia, visual deterioration	Olfactory nerve Optic nerve
Foster–Kennedy syndrome	Optic nerve atrophy, papilledema	Optic nerve Possible involvement of olfactory nerve
Orbital fissure syndrome	Ophthalmoplegia, ptosis, large pupil	Oculomotor nerve Trochlear nerve Ophthalmic nerve Abducent nerve
Orbital apex syndrome	Visual deterioration, ptosis, diplopia, exophthalmos, temporoparietal pain	Optic nerve Oculomotor nerve Trochlear nerve Trigeminal nerve Abducent nerve
Cavernous sinus syndrome (anterior syndrome)	Ophthalmoplegia, trigeminal hypesthesia, lack of pupillary response	Oculomotor nerve Possible involvement of abducent and ophthalmic nerves
Sphenoid wing syndrome	Temporal headache, exophthalmos, dysfunction of cranial nerves III, IV, V_1, and VI	Oculomotor nerve Trochlear nerve Ophthalmic nerve Abducent nerve
Jacob syndrome	Ophthalmoplegia, ptosis, visual deterioration to blindness, trigeminal paresthesia	Optic nerve Oculomotor nerve Trochlear nerve Trigeminal nerve Abducent nerve
Raeder syndrome	Incomplete Horner syndrome, periorbital pain	Sympathetic innervation of internal carotid artery
Carotid-cavernous sinus syndrome	Retroorbital headache, pulsatile exophthalmos, congested fundic veins, nasal mucosa and conjunctiva	Fistula between internal carotid artery and cavernous sinus

Table 3.**4** Clinical symptoms associated with diseases of the anterior skull base and their possible causes

Symptom	Cause	Example
Swelling, hematoma	Trauma, inflammation	Frontobasal fracture, sinusitis
Facial dysmorphias and skin changes	Congenital anomaly, trauma, tumor	Encephalocele, frontobasal fracture, nasopharyngeal tumor
Facial paralysis	Inflammation, trauma, tumor	Sinusitis, frontobasal fracture, basal skull fracture, nasopharyngeal tumor
Facial pain, headache, dysesthesia	Inflammation, trauma, tumor	Sinusitis, pituitary tumor, nasopharyngeal tumor, internal carotid aneurysm
Rhinorrhea	Inflammation, trauma, tumor	Sinusitis, frontobasal fracture, nasopharyngeal tumor
Epistaxis	Trauma, vascular pathology, tumor	Frontobasal fracture, carotid–cavernous fistula, aneurysm, nasopharyngeal tumor
Fetid nasal odor	Inflammation, tumor	Sinusitis, neoplasia
Conductive hearing loss	Inflammation, tumor	Sinusitis, nasopharyngeal and skull base tumors
Rhinophonia clausa	Inflammation, tumor	Sinusitis, nasopharyngeal tumor
Altered mental status, local brain symptoms, epileptic seizures	Inflammation, trauma, tumor	Seepage sinusitis, tumors of anterior skull base

Imaging Evaluation and Differential Diagnosis

The basic imaging study is *conventional radiography* using *occipitomental (OM) and occipitofrontal (OF) projections* and, in selected cases, *PA and lateral skull films*. Modern imaging is based on the use of unenhanced and contrast-enhanced *axial and coronal CT scans*. *MRI* has become the imaging modality of choice for visualizing the soft-tissue structures of the skull base. The limited indications for *conventional angiography* include, most notably, the diagnosis of vascularized tumors. *Radionuclide studies* such as CSF scintigraphy may be appropriate in selected cases.

Ultrasound

Ultrasound imaging has limited applications in this region and is used mainly to evaluate the paranasal sinuses. The posterior portion of the ethmoid sinus and the sphenoid sinus are inaccessible to ultrasound imaging, and the frontal sinus only to a limited degree. A common sonographic technique in this region is unidimensional *A-mode scanning* with a 3.5- to 5-MHz transducer.

This method can be used to evaluate mucosal swellings, secretions, cysts, mucoceles, pyoceles, and tumors of the paranasal sinuses, though it does not provide the morphologic detail or spatial information obtainable with conventional X-ray studies. Indications for ultrasonography in this region are acute and chronic diseases of the paranasal sinuses, monitoring of therapeutic response, and examinations in children and pregnant women.

Conventional Radiography

While the availability of CT and MRI have curtailed the role of X-ray films in evaluations of the skull base, trauma and inflammatory sinus disease are still considered *primary indications* for conventional radiography. Also, special views can furnish additional information in selected cases and are currently performed as adjuncts to sectional imaging procedures. Conventional tomography has *no* role in the present-day diagnosis of neoplastic processes, because they cannot accurately define the extent of tumor masses and entail a substantially higher radiation exposure than CT scans. This particularly applies to motion-controlled tomography, which has largely been supplanted by CT scanning in investigations of this region.

Table 3.**5** lists the principal radiographic techniques and their indications in the region of the anterior skull base.

Computed Tomography (CT)

CT examination of the anterior skull base usually employs a series of *axial* scans angled approximately 15° to 20° to the orbitomeatal line. This region can also be imaged on *semicoronal* slices with the head in maximal extension. In this technique the scan plane should intersect the orbitomeatal line at approximately a 70° angle, so that it is perpendicular to the clivus. If the patient cannot hyperextend the neck or if amalgam dental fillings cause serious image degradation, coronal sections can be reconstructed from *thin axial* CT slices.

The images should be documented using a *soft-tissue window* and, in selected cases, *bone window technique*. If osseous lesions are sought, a *high-resolution bone algorithm* with a high window setting (approximately 4000 HU) should be used. A slice thickness of 1 to 5 mm is generally recommended, and axial scan coverage should extend from the foramen magnum to the suprasellar cisterns. Intravenous contrast should be used in patients undergoing evaluation for soft-tissue masses. The primary advantages of CT over conventional radiographs in this region are its ability to provide nonsuperimposed views of bony structures, to define and differentiate soft-tissue structures, and to provide secondary reconstructions of extra planes or even 3-D images of the region under study.

Magnetic Resonance Imaging (MRI)

A *head coil* is routinely used for MRI of the anterior skull base. A *Helmholtz surface coil* also can be used for selected inquiries and for studies requiring high spatial resolution.

The standard examination of this region starts with a *scout sequence in three planes* followed by T1- and T2-weighted axial images. Good results are achieved with the parameters TR = 3000 ms, TE = 22 – 90 ms (double echo) for the T2-weighted sequence, and TR/TE = 700/15 ms for the T1-weighted sequence. The recommended slice thickness is 3 – 5 mm. After administration of the contrast agent gadolinium-DTPA (Gd-DTPA) in a standard dose of 0.1 mmol/kg, the T1-weighted sequence is repeated using the same parameters as in the noncontrast study. Additional T1-weighted sequences can be obtained in the coronal and even the sagittal plane, depending on the nature of the inquiry and the findings.

The inquiry and noncontrast findings may warrant *"special sequences"* that yield additional diagnostic information. These may include *noncontrast arterial and venous magnetic resonance angiography (MRA)*, a dynamic sequence to document enhancement patterns, and a fat suppression sequence before and after contrast administration.

Table 3.5 Conventional radiographic techniques and their indications in evaluations of the skull base

Technique	Indication
PA and lateral skull views	Evaluation of the cranial bones and the bony boundaries of the paranasal sinuses, orbits, and anterior skull base (e.g., for suspected fractures or tumors)
Lateral view of facial skeleton	Evaluation of AP tumor extent
OM view of paranasal sinuses (Walter view)	Evaluation of maxillary and sphenoid sinus
OF view of paranasal sinuses (Caldwell view)	Evaluation of frontal sinus and ethmoid cells
Axial Welin view	Evaluation of petrous apex, labyrinth, clivus and middle skull base (including sella and sphenoid sinus)
Lateral spot view of sella	Evaluation of shape, size and structure of sella
Rhese view	More accurate evaluation of posterior orbital region, optic nerve canal and adjacent structures
Lateral and AP tomograms	Evaluation of: ➤ circumscribed defects and thinning of bone ➤ bone inclusions (cysts, unerupted teeth) ➤ displacement of paranasal sinus walls ➤ wall deposits of bony or calcific density

Arterial and venous MRA can delineate major blood vessels in this region, define the location of tumors and vessels, reveal vascular displacement or compression by tumor, and demonstrate vascular pathology (e.g., fistulae, aneurysms). Tumor-feeding vessels also can be visualized in rare cases.

A dynamic enhancement study is useful for assessing the vascularity of a lesion as a means of narrowing the differential diagnosis. The *gadolinium-(Gd)-enhanced fat suppression sequence* is extremely useful for defining the extent of tumor infiltration into adjacent soft-tissue structures.

The axial images should cover the region from the suprasellar cisterns to the nasopharynx, and the coronal images should extend from the anterior frontal sinus to the rim of the foramen magnum.

Value of Different MR Sequences

The improved soft-tissue contrast and multiplanar imaging capability of MRI account for its superiority in evaluations of this region:

T1-Weighted Sequences

This type of sequence permits the assessment of tumor location, morphology, internal structure, and displacement of adjacent structures. Even minute structural changes in the hypointense CSF and ventricular system can be appreciated in T1-weighted sequences.

T2-Weighted Sequences

These sequences are useful for the characterization of pathologic tissue structures and inflammatory lesions, most notably the differentiation of solid and cystic tumor components and the detection of regressive changes associated with extra-axial tumors. With a heavily T2-weighted sequence, tumor can be distinguished from surrounding edema in approximately 75% of cases based on signal disparities. This sequence is also very useful in the evaluation of recurrent or residual tumor following treatment.

Gadolinium-Enhanced T1-Weighted Sequences

In most cases, injection of the paramagnetic contrast agent Gd-DTPA significantly improves the differentiation of tumor from surrounding structures on MR images. This contrast agent can penetrate a compromised blood-brain barrier and shorten the T1 relaxation time of tumor masses. Thus, axial and extra-axial lesions of the skull base can be accurately detected and classified by means of Gd-enhanced T1-weighted sequences.

Radionuclide Imaging

Bone scans and other radionuclide studies play an important role in evaluations for local or generalized involvement of bony structures in this region by primary and secondary lesions. Also, advanced techniques such as immunoscintigraphy can provide information on tumor histology or can be used in CSF scintigraphy, for example, to identify sites of CSF leakage.

Radionuclide Bone Scans

In patients with osteogenic systemic diseases and tumors, affected bone areas usually show intense tracer uptake 2 to 6 hours after the intravenous injection of ^{99m}Tc-MDP. While these accumulations are not pathognomonic for a specific disease, they are much more sensitive than radiodiagnostic procedures, especially in the detection of osteomyelitis. Radionuclide bone scans are indicated in patients who are clinically symptomatic but still have negative X-ray films. They are also useful in the follow-up of osteomyelitis and of treated malignancies with osseous involvement. In cases of tumor recurrence, the bone scan can document a (nonspecific) recurrence of increased tracer uptake at the same or different site at an early stage.

Radionuclide uptake is particularly marked at sites of bone destruction caused by malignant tumors, bone metastases, systemic malignant diseases (lymphoma, eosinophilic granuloma), benign bone tumors (osteoma, osteochondroma), Paget disease, fibrous bone dysplasia, and inflammatory processes (osteomyelitis, sinusitis with reactive bone involvement). These sites may continue to show a modest elevation of tracer uptake for many years.

Immunoscintigraphy

Highly differentiated tumors such as neuroblastoma can be detected by the use of radiolabeled metabolites or antimetabolites such as the guanethidine derivative metaiodobenzylguanidine (MIBG). These techniques provide a highly specific approach to tumor detection.

CSF Scintigraphy

This study is used in the diagnosis of primary (traumatic) or secondary (iatrogenic) CSF leakage. Following intrathecal administration of the radiotracer, separate readings are taken on each side, and the pattern of tracer uptake is documented. If a CSF leak is present, an increase in activity will be measured over the affected side. The leak is confirmed by measuring the activity of the extravasated CSF.

Imaging Findings

This section deals with the principal disorders of the anterior skull base—their morphologic characteristics, imaging features, and aspects of differential diagnosis. The spectrum of anterior skull base lesions ranges from congenital malformations, anatomic variations, and neoplastic processes to trauma-induced and posttherapeutic changes.

Congenital Variations and Malformations (Figs. 3.**3**, 3.**4a**, and Table 3.**6**)

The region of the facial skeleton, which includes the upper extension of the skull base, is one of the most important and distinctive features of the individual personality. Abnormalities in this region tend to be conspicuous. Possible morphologic changes must be accurately documented and described on the basis of clinical data and radiologic findings.

The most common malformations involving the skull base are *median and lateral clefts* and *frontal bone dysplasias*. Other types of malformation are *craniomandibulofacial dysostoses*, *craniosynostoses*, and *otomandibular* and *otopalatinodigital anomalies*. The goal of imaging in these cases is to provide a morphologic description of the anomaly, identify the bony structures involved, and determine the relation of the anomaly to neurovascular structures.

Craniosynostosis

Craniosynostosis (craniostenosis) denotes premature fusion of the cranial sutures, which normally occurs at approximately 30 years of age. It is approximately four times more prevalent in males than females. Craniosynostosis is subdivided into *primary* and *secondary* forms. The secondary forms are often an accompanying feature of a primary hematologic, metabolic, or osseous disease, and rare cases may have an iatrogenic cause (e.g., following shunt implantation for hydrocephalus). Various types of deformity may occur, depending on the sutures involved, including brachycephalus (frontal and lambdoid sutures) and plagiocephalus (unilateral frontal suture and lambdoid suture). Clinical evaluation and treatment planning are guided by biplane skull radiographs and particularly by high-resolution CT with 3-D surface reconstruction of the calvarium. MRI is used only in the evaluation of associated soft-tissue changes or anomalies.

Arachnoid Cyst (Fig. 3.**3**)

An arachnoid cyst is a *developmental anomaly of the subarachnoid space*. These lesions may undergo progressive expansion during antenatal development and chiefly involve the middle cranial fossa. The pathogenesis of the lesion is poorly understood, but a variety of theories have been proposed.

Arachnoid cysts show a density and signal intensity similar to intraventricular fluid on CT scans and MR images. Bony changes in the skull base are best demonstrated by cranial CT, which may show thinning of the temporal bone, elevation of the lesser sphenoid wing, and anterior displacement of the greater sphenoid wing.

MRI can accurately define the location and extent of the arachnoid cyst owing to its multiplanar capability.

Cephalocele (Fig. 3.**4**)

Cephalocele has a reported incidence of approximately 1–4 per 100,000 live births and accounts for 10% to 20% of all craniospinal anomalies. Approximately 75% of the lesions are occipital, 13% to 15 % are frontoethmoidal, 10% are sphenoidal, and 10% to 12% are parietal. An association with other malformation syndromes (e.g., spina bifida, Arnold–Chiari syndrome, etc.) is noted in approximately 60% of cases.

Cephaloceles can occur virtually anywhere in the neurocranium but are most common in the midline, the occipital region, the anterior skull base, and the vertex (Fig. 3.**4 a**). A cephalocele may protrude through the sphenoid bone due to persistence of the craniopharyngeal canal, which is assumed to be the remnant of a vascular supply channel through the sphenoid bone during antenatal development. A cephalocele in this region can also result from maldevelopment of the multiple, complex ossification centers of the anterior skull base. In these cases the dura is usually adherent to the periosteum at the external opening of the defect, and the bone dehiscence may occur at a suture, at the junction of several bones, or at the junction of several ossification centers in the same bone (e.g., the sphenoid bone). The outer covering of the cephalocele varies with the origin and location of the lesion.

The most common form of cephalocele is the sphenopharyngeal type, which may present clinically as a pharyngeal mass causing airway obstruction and may create a portal for CSF rhinorrhea and meningitis. Before the advent of CT, the radiologic diagnosis of cephalocele was based on the plain-film identification of a bony defect in the skull base combined with a soft-tissue mass. The cranial defect had to be quite large before it could be detected by this method.

CT scanning of the anterior skull base can clearly depict the bony margins of the defect and the soft-tissue component of the cephalocele while the lesion is still small. It may also show a faint sclerotic zone surrounding the bony defect. Small amounts of intrathecal contrast material can help differentiate a simple meningocele (herniation of meninges) from an encephalocele (herniation of meninges and brain substance) by outlining the cortical sulci of the encephalocele. While intrathecal contrast is seldom used today in the diagnosis of cephaloceles, it is the method of choice for investigating a suspected CSF fistula.

MRI has become the method of choice for identifying the contents of the sac and particularly for revealing herniated intracranial structures. In this way MRI can obviate the need for more invasive diagnostic procedures (Figs. 3.**4 b, c**). Cerebral angiography, performed as an adjunctive study, can furnish more detailed information on the vascular components of the cephalocele.

Osteopathies

The skull base is a frequent site of involvement by generalized osteopathies, notably *fibrous dysplasia*, *osteopetrosis*, and *Paget disease*.

The local radiologic features of bone dysplasias and sclerosis may resemble those of primary osteoplastic tumors. The differential diagnosis of these

Table 3.**6** Malformations of the anterior skull base

Findings	CT morphology	MRI morphology
Craniosynostosis	Bony lesion, possible bone expansion	Difficult to differentiate
Arachnoid cyst (Fig. 3.**3 a**)	Isodense to CSF, possible bone destruction	Cyst-equivalent signal intensity
Meningocele	Predominantly hypodense center (isodense to CSF); bony lesion	Soft-tissue mass; central cyst-equivalent signal intensity
Encephalocele (Fig. 3.**4 c**)	Predominantly isodense center (isodense to brain parenchyma); bony lesion	Soft-tissue mass; central signal predominantly isointense to brain

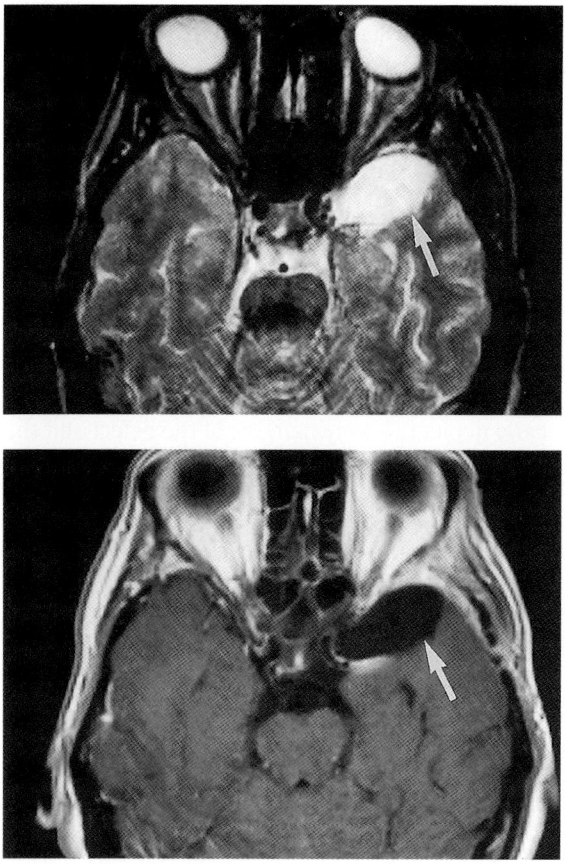

a

b

Figs. 3.**3 a, b** **Arachnoid cyst of the left temporal lobe.**
(**a**) Axial noncontrast T2-weighted MR image (SE, TR/TE = 3000/90 ms) demonstrates a hyperintense lesion (arrow) in the left temporal lobe. The lesion relates closely to the anterior skull base.
(**b**) Axial noncontrast T1-weighted MR image (SE, TR/TE = 700/15 ms) on the same plane shows the lesion (arrow) as a low-intensity mass that is isointense to CSF.

cases is advanced by supplementing skull films with other skeletal views, high-resolution CT (HRCT), and radionuclide bone scans. CT-guided biopsy may be warranted to establish a definitive diagnosis. MRI plays only a minor role in the evaluation of osteopathies due to the difficulty of distinguishing between osseous and air-containing structures in the anterior skull base.

On skull radiographs and CT, generalized osteopathies appear as areas of increased cranial bone density with associated expansion and deformity.

Osteopetrosis (Albers–Schönberg Disease)

Widening of the cortical bone, with consequent bone thickening, is the hallmark of this rare hereditary bone dysplasia. Osteopetrosis is marked histologically by varying persistence of calcified cartilage rests surrounded by exuberant osteoid masses. With cranial involvement, there is a predominant thickening of the skull base. The sphenoid, frontal, and ethmoid sinuses may be small, or even obliterated, due to thickening of the surrounding bone. The narrowing of nerve passages through the skull base (optic canal, foramen rotundum, foramen ovale) frequently leads to cranial-nerve encroachment and middle-ear involvement.

Foraminal narrowing is poorly demonstrated on plain skull films. Adequate evaluation requires axial and coronal CT scans. Besides smallness of the sphenoid, ethmoid, and frontal sinuses due to widening, sclerosis, and increased density of the cortical bone, CT may show thickening and increased density of the sphenoid wing and pterygoid processes along with sclerosis and obliteration of the mastoid air cells.

Idiopathic Sclerosing Hyperostosis

This osteopathy resembles osteopetrosis but involves an increase in bone mass that is confined to one bone. The maxilla is the site of predilection in cases of cranial involvement; the sphenoid bone is less commonly affected.

The disease presents radiologically as a circumscribed area of increased bone thickness and density. Solitary or multiple osteomas should be considered in the differential diagnosis.

Fibrous Dysplasia (Fig. 3.**5**)

Fibrous dysplasia is characterized histologically by *fibrosis of the bone marrow* (fibrous replacement of the medullary cavity) with associated local expansion of the bone. A common site of occurrence at the anterior skull base is the *frontotemporal-orbital region*, which may be involved in a setting of *monostotic* or *polyostotic* disease. The peak incidence is in school-age children, with approximately a 3 : 1 predominance of females over males.

Conventional X-ray films show widening and thickening of the affected site with scattered lucent areas. The overall mottled pattern of new bone formation is considered pathognomonic for fibrous dysplasia after Paget disease has been excluded.

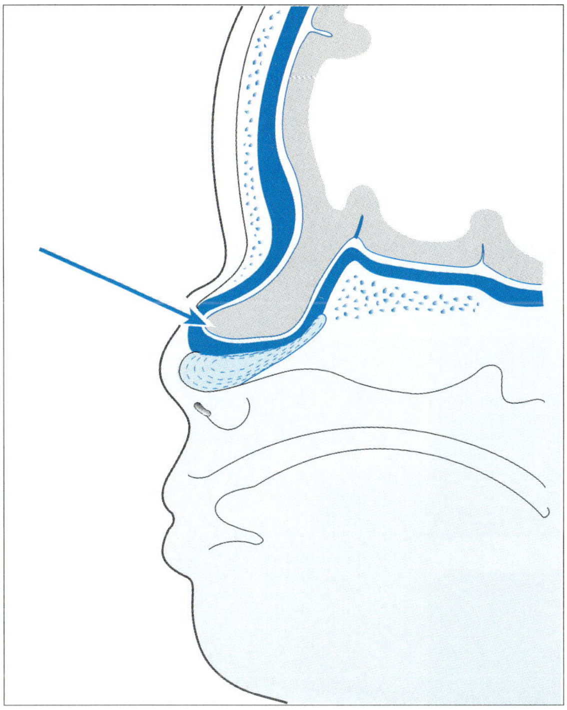

a

Figs. 3.**4 a–c** **Cephalocele and encephalocele:**
(**a**) Development of a cephalocele of the anterior skull base (arrow).
(**b, c**) **Encephalocele of the anterior skull base:**
(**b**) Axial noncontrast T2-weighted MR image (SE, TR/TE = 3000/90 ms) demonstrates a lesion of the anterior skull base. The scan clearly shows the herniation of brain substance, surrounded by CSF (arrows), into the nasal cavity.
(**c**) Noncontrast T1-weighted MR image (SE, TR/TE = 700/15 ms) in the coronal plane defines the extent of this encephalocele (arrow) with frontal brain tissue herniating into the nasal cavity.

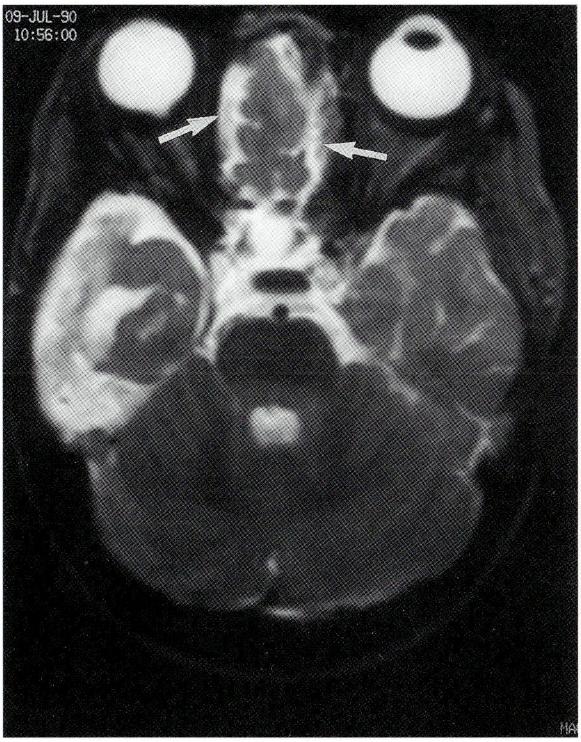

b

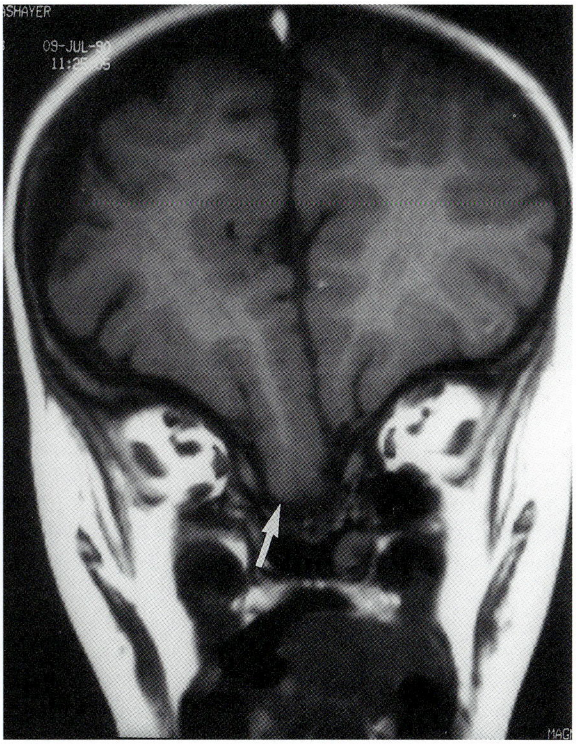

c

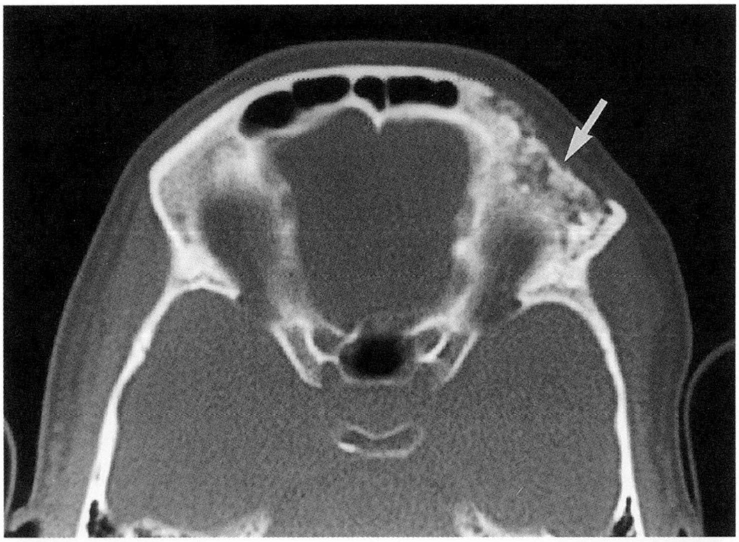

a

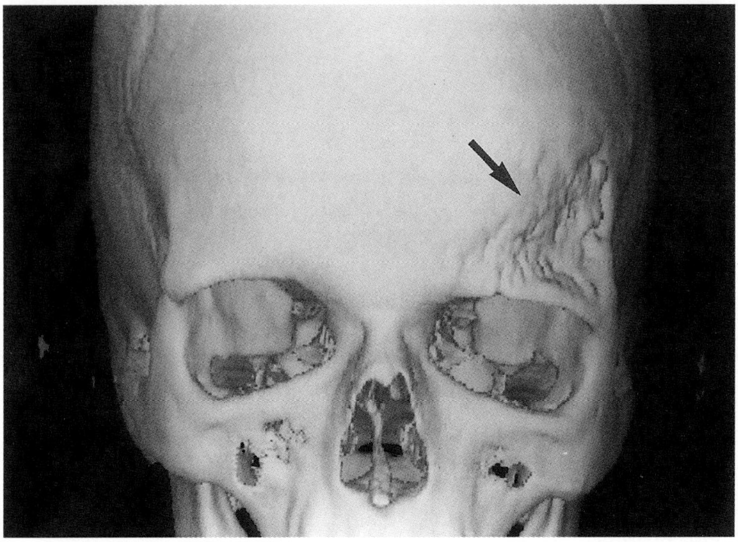

b

Figs. 3.**5** **a, b** **Fibrous dysplasia.**
(**a**) Axial noncontrast CT scan (1 mm, bone window) demonstrates a bony lesion of the left orbital roof causing local expansion and destruction of the bone (arrow).
(**b**) Axial noncontrast CT scan (1 mm, 3-D reconstruction) shows the precise location and extent of the fibrous dysplasia (arrow) in the region of the orbital roof.

CT scans in fibrous dysplasia show thickening and increased sclerosis of the affected bone with a ground-glass appearance. Cystic regions may be identified in the early stage of the disease (Fig. 3.**5**).

MRI shows bony expansion of the skull base and can occasionally differentiate cystic from sclerotic areas. The lesions of fibrous dysplasia have a low signal intensity on T1-weighted sequences, a low to high signal intensity on T2-weighted sequences, and show moderate to no enhancement after contrast administration.

Paget Disease

This generalized osteopathy is characterized histologically by processes of *bone destruction and excessive new bone formation* with *fibrosis of the medullary cavity*. Most patients are over 40 years of age, with males predominating. The process starts with a circumscribed and very aggressive destructive phase that causes deformation and expansion of the affected bone (osteitis deformans). The site of predilection in the skull is the calvaria, followed by the skull base, sella, and paranasal sinuses. As in Albers–Schönberg osteopetrosis, the narrowing of neural foramina can irritate or damage the transmitted cranial nerves. Involvement of the sella and skull base can lead to narrowing of the sphenoid and ethmoid sinuses. If the sphenoid or ethmoid sinus becomes obliterated, the differential diagnosis should include Albers–Schönberg osteopetrosis. The deformities of the anterior skull base and facial skeleton may create a leonine appearance (leontiasis ossea) in advanced cases.

Skull radiographs and CT scans show a mottled pattern of densities and patchy lucencies in the expanded calvaria. Early cases show pathognomonic areas of decalcification involving the frontal, parietal, and occipital bones.

MRI in Paget disease shows a juxtaposition of low-signal areas and signal voids on T1- and T2-weighted sequences as a manifestation of cortical thickening. There is a general expansion of the affected bone, and granulation tissue within the medullary space may appear as areas of low signal intensity on T1-weighted sequences and high signal intensity on T2-weighted sequences.

Histiocytosis X

Three forms of histiocytosis X are recognized:

- Letterer–Siwe syndrome (acute, fulminating, disseminated form)
- Hand–Schüller–Christian syndrome (chronic disseminated form)
- Eosinophilic granuloma (benign form).

The two latter forms account for approximately 14% to 40% and 60% to 80% of all cases, respectively, and commonly involve the skull base and orbits. The differential diagnosis of these syndromes should include metastasis, fibrous dysplasia, and Paget disease.

Hand–Schüller–Christian Syndrome

This disease appears between 5 and 10 years of age and affects both sexes equally. An association with exophthalmos, diabetes insipidus, and lytic skull lesions is found in 10% of cases. The orbits and sella turcica are the most common sites of involvement in the region of the anterior skull base.

On conventional radiographs and CT scans, the lesions appear as osteolytic areas that may have indistinct margins. CT and MRI may document an associated soft-tissue mass in rare cases.

On MRI, the destructive lesions appear isointense on T1-weighted images and show a high, heterogeneous signal intensity on T2-weighted images. The lesions show nonhomogeneous enhancement on post-contrast images. With involvement of the orbital margins, a contrast-enhanced sequence with fat suppression can accurately define the extent of intraorbital infiltration.

Eosinophilic Granuloma

Approximately 75% of patients are under age 20, with a 3 : 2 ratio of females to males. The most frequent site of involvement (approximately 50%) is the skull, predominantly the parietal bone and temporal bone. Involvement of the anterior skull base is rare, occurring in approximately 3% of cases.

Conventional radiographs show round to oval, punched-out defects that do not have sclerotic margins. Eosinophilic granuloma is more commonly associated with a soft-tissue mass than Hand–Schüller–Christian disease, and the mass is often palpable. A sclerotic border may appear around the lesion during the healing phase.

CT is decidedly superior to conventional radiographs for visualizing the destructive bone lesions. MRI depicts the soft-tissue component better than CT, the lesion appearing isointense on T1-weighted images and showing high, nonhomogeneous signal intensity on T2-weighted images. Contrast administration produces nonhomogeneous enhancement with central areas of low signal intensity (Fig. 3.**6**).

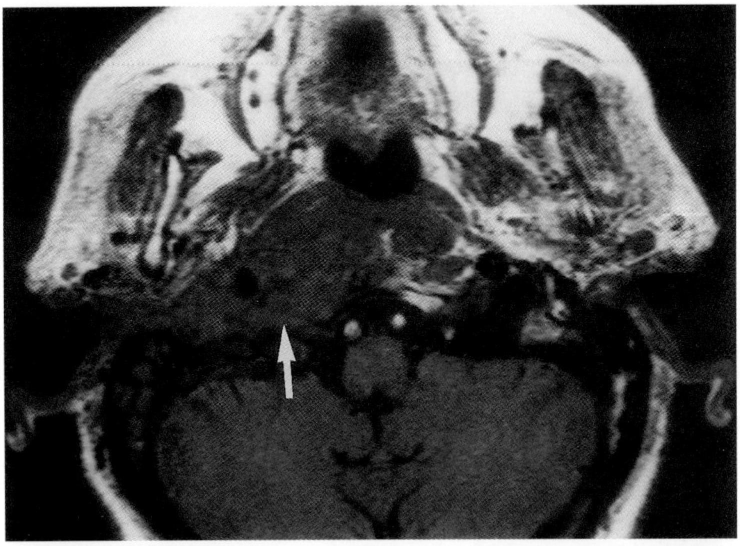

a

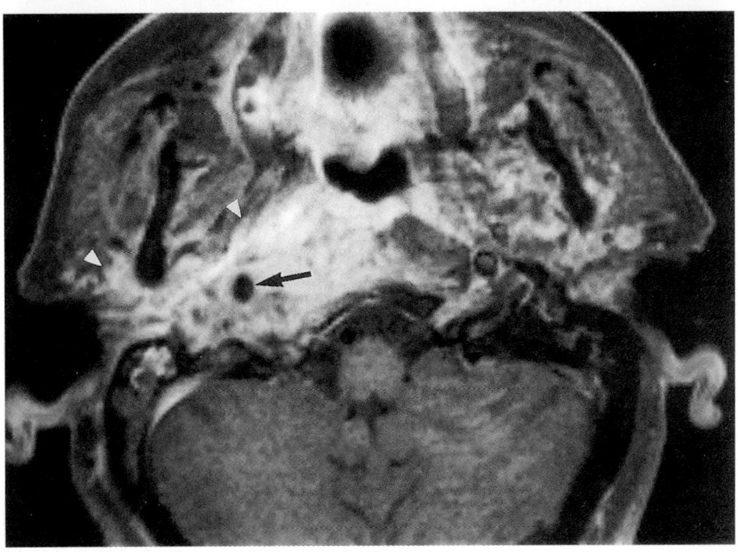

b

Figs. 3.**6 a, b** **Histiocytosis X of the anterior skull base and nasopharynx.**
(**a**) Axial noncontrast T1-weighted MR image (SE, TR/TE = 700/15 ms) shows a uniformly isointense mass in the parapharyngeal space extending to the anterior skull base.
(**b**) Axial gadolinium (Gd)-enhanced fat-saturated MR image (SE, TR/TE = 700/15 ms) shows predominantly homogeneous enhancement of the mass, which has encased the internal carotid artery (arrow) and has diffusely infiltrated surrounding structures (arrowheads).

Tumors (Tables 3.**7** and 3.**8**)

Meningioma (Fig. 3.**19 a**)

Meningioma of the anterior skull base is generally considered the third most common tumor of this region, accounting for approximately 17% of all intracranial mass lesions. The peak incidence is approximately 45 years of age, with a 2 : 1 to 4 : 1 ratio of females to males. Meningioma is a well-circumscribed, extra-axial tumor that most commonly occurs at the convexities, the sphenoid-bone area, the olfactory groove, the posterior cranial fossa, and along cranial nerves. Topographic (site-of-lesion) criteria form the basis for the correct diagnosis of meningiomas. Unlike other tumors of the anterior skull base, meningiomas always establish broad contact with adjacent bony structures. In many patients this is the main criterion that distinguishes meningiomas from other tumors of the anterior skull base such as esthesioneuroblastoma.

Meningioma appears isointense to brain on T1-weighted MR sequences, thus small tumors arising from arachnoid cell nests may not be appreciated on unenhanced images. Intravenous injection of the paramagnetic contrast agent Gd-DTPA always produces intense, homogeneous tumor enhancement due to shortening of the T1 relaxation time. HRCT scanning may be necessary in rare cases to establish the diagnosis, often showing circumscribed exostosis at the origin of the meningioma (Figs. 3.**7 a, b**). While large and medium-sized exostoses of the anterior skull base are visible on MR images, very small foci usually escape detection. The characteristics listed in Table 3.**7** are useful in the CT and MR diagnosis of meningioma.

Table 3.7 Characteristics of meningiomas on CT and MR images

Relation to surrounding structures	➤ Sessile lesion ➤ Extra-axial location ➤ Invasion of venous sinus system ➤ Rare: extension toward petrous apex
Conventional radiographs	➤ Hyperostosis ➤ Calcifications ➤ Blistering in paranasal sinuses
Noncontrast CT	➤ Isodense to hyperdense to brain parenchyma (approx. 95%) ➤ Circular or radial calcification pattern; differential diagnosis: osteoma ➤ Permeation of bone (intraosseous meningioma); differential diagnosis: fibrous dysplasia ➤ Hyperostosis ➤ Minimal perifocal edema; differential diagnosis: intra–axial lesion
Post-contrast CT	➤ Isodense, uniform enhancement
Noncontrast MRI	➤ T2-weighted images: isodense to hyperintense to white matter ➤ T1-weighted images: isodense to hypointense to white matter, heterogeneous appearance ➤ Homogeneous or heterogeneous appearance
Post-contrast MRI	➤ Intense, homogeneous contrast enhancement with an enhancement factor of approx. 148% ➤ "Dural tail": curved extension of enhancement along dural margin of meningioma, seen in approx. 60% of cases ➤ Enhancement dynamics: rapid enhancement during first 3 min

Table 3.8 Soft-tissue tumors of the anterior skull base

Findings	**CT morphology**	**MRI morphology**
Meningioma (Fig. 3.**19 a**)	Isodense to hypodense on plain scans, homogeneous enhancement on contrast scans	Isointense on plain images, homogeneous enhancement on contrast images
Metastases (Figs. 3.**14 a–f**)	Bone destruction, nonhomogeneous enhancement	Isodense to hyperintense on T2-weighted images, marked enhancement
Craniopharyngioma	Calcifications, cyst formation, variable enhancement pattern	Cyst-equivalent signal intensity, peripheral enhancement
Chordoma	Bone destruction, calcifications, bone fragments	Hyperintense on T2-weighted images, marked enhancement
Esthesioneuroblastoma (Fig. 3.**12**)	Bone destruction, rarely calcifications; intense enhancement	Nonhomogeneous signal intensity on T1- and T2-weighted images, intense enhancement
Chondroma	Predominantly soft-tissue mass, calcifications, ossification, moderate enhancement	Moderate signal intensity on T1-weighted images, high signal intensity on T2-weighted images; possible heterogeneous enhancement
Chondrosarcoma (Fig. 3.**13 a**)	Slightly hyperdense on plain scans, flocculent calcifications, moderate enhancement	High signal intensity on T2-weighted images, moderate enhancement

It seems almost paradoxical that MRI has become the imaging modality of first choice for the diagnosis of meningiomas, despite the fact that lesions may go undetected on noncontrast images. But use of the paramagnetic contrast agent Gd-DTPA and fast imaging sequences in multiplanar sections have significantly improved preoperative planning in the management of these tumors (Figs. 3.**7 b** and 3.**9 c**).

Differentiation is required from dural metastases and lymphomas due to their similar imaging characteristics.

Craniopharyngioma

Craniopharyngioma is a benign tumor that is most prevalent between 10 and 25 years of age. It reportedly accounts for 1.2% of all brain tumors and shows a slight predilection for males. Craniopharyngioma (Erdheim tumors, Rathke pouch tumor) arises from rests of the craniopharyngeal duct and may develop within the sella, on the pituitary stalk, or in the infundibular region. The tumor may be predominantly cystic or predominantly solid and usually has internal calcifications. The peak incidence is between age 10 and 15, although late manifestations can occur. Histologically, craniopharyngioma is a *slow-growing benign tumor* that has a good prognosis with adequate treatment. Depending on its size, the tumor may cause hypothalamic-pituitary dysfunction (growth hormone deficiency, diabetes insipidus), visual field defects, or obstructive hydrocephalus due to occlusion of the foramen of Monro.

Even noncontrast CT scans will show prominent intratumoral calcification. After the administration of contrast material, there is variable enhancement of the solid tumor components depending on the gross composition of the tumor.

Since most craniopharyngiomas are quite large when diagnosed, the tumor can often be identified on noncontrast T1-weighted MR images. Additionally, the tumor is conspicuous by the low signal intensity of its fluid-filled cystic components relative to the brain parenchyma. T2-weighted images depict the fluid-filled cysts even more clearly as well-defined areas of high signal intensity. Despite the conspicuity of these tumors on unenhanced MR images, the use of contrast material offers several advantages. First, contrast administration produces intense enhancement of the cyst walls, which may be poorly visualized on noncontrast images. Second, contrast enhancement makes it possible to differentiate the solid tumor component, which usually lies within the sella. The solid intrasellar tumor component appears isointense to the pons on noncontrast T1-weighted images, making it indistinguishable from normal pituitary tissue. When contrast is used, however, the intensely enhancing pituitary tissue is easily distinguished from the more weakly enhancing solid tumor component. This also explains the value of MRI in postoperative evaluations for residual or recurrent tumor. Because these tumors have a high rate of recurrence, the contrasting enhancement characteristics of normal pituitary tissue and craniopharyngiomas facilitate the detection of recurrent tumor on MR images.

In summary, MRI has a very high sensitivity in the preoperative and postoperative evaluation of craniopharyngiomas. The multiplanar capability of MRI also permits more accurate presurgical planning of the tumor excision (Table 3.**9**).

Table 3.**9** Signal characteristics of craniopharyngiomas relative to brain parenchyma in various MR imaging sequences

	T1-weighted unenhanced	T1-weighted, contrast-enhanced	T2-weighted
Cyst contents	↓	↓/↑	↑
Cyst wall	→	↑	→
Solid tumor component	↓	↑	↑

↓ = hypointense, → = isointense, ↑ = hyperintense

Chordoma

Chordomas arise from remnants of the embryonic notochord, with approximately 35% occurring in the skull-base region. There is approximately a 2 : 1 male preponderance with a peak incidence around 50 years of age. Sites of predilection in the skull base are the clivus and its immediate surroundings and the spheno-occipital synchondrosis. Although chordomas are slow-growing and rarely metastasize, their prognosis is poor because of their invasive growth and their invariable tendency to recur despite radical extirpation. Chordomas tend to spread downward into the nasopharynx and toward the clivus and occasionally may extend into the nasal cavity. These tumors typically cause *significant bone destruction* and contain *calcifications* and *bone fragments*. They show an expansile type of growth outside of bone.

Conventional radiographs may show apical erosion of the clivus or dens or anterior erosion of the atlas arch.

Axial noncontrast CT scanning is the technique of choice for documenting bone destruction and tumor calcifications and demonstrating intratumoral bone fragments. Following the injection of contrast material, the soft-tissue components generally show moderate enhancement. The degree of soft-tissue infiltration is difficult to evaluate, however, particularly in the nasopharyngeal region and parapharyngeal space.

On MRI, chordomas appear isointense or hypointense to muscle on T1-weighted images and hyperintense on T2-weighted images. After the administration of Gd-DTPA, marked contrast enhancement is observed. MRI is more accurate than CT in defining the extent of nasopharyngeal and other soft-tissue infiltration.

The differential diagnosis of this mass should include meningioma, metastasis to the skull base, plasmacytoma, nasopharyngeal carcinoma, chondrosarcoma, and giant cell tumor.

Esthesioneuroblastoma (Fig. 3.**12** and 7.**27**)

Esthesioneuroblastoma is a rare, highly malignant variant of neuroblastoma that arises from the neuroectoderm of the olfactory nerve ("olfactory neuroblastoma"). It is most common around 40 years of age (30 to 50 years) and affects both sexes equally.

Two characteristics of this tumor are its tendency to *penetrate the cribriform plate and infiltrate the sphenoid and maxillary sinuses* and its *high vascularity*. Growth is usually confined to the anterior skull base, anterior cranial fossa, and paranasal sinuses. With involvement of the anterior skull base, a brain abscess may develop. Distant metastases are found in approximately 20% of patients.

The most conspicuous change on plain radiographs is the osseous destruction of the anterior skull base and adjacent involved bone. A tumor obstructing the ethmoid cells may cause frontal sinus opacity with or without an air–fluid level.

Contrast-enhanced CT scans show marked tumor enhancement with associated destruction of the involved osseous boundaries of the anterior skull base. Intratumoral calcifications are occasionally seen.

On MRI, esthesioneuroblastoma is characterized by a heterogeneous internal structure, prolonged T1 and T2 relaxation times, and marked contrast enhancement (by a factor of approximately 2.3). This can make the tumor difficult to distinguish from normal mucosal tissue. A useful diagnostic feature is the immediate relation of the tumor to the olfactory filaments and cribriform plate. While MRI is not useful for assessing the extent of bone destruction, it is more accurate than CT in defining the extent of the tumor.

Differentiation from olfactory meningioma (Figs. 3.**8**, 3.**10**, 3.**11**) is aided by topography, i.e., by noting the exact location of the tumor and the structures to which it is related.

Chondroma

Chondroma is a slow-growing, histologically benign tumor that arises from the dura of the skull base at synchondroses and near the foramen lacerum. Like chondromas elsewhere in the body, this tumor is characterized by *expansile growth* and an *elastic consistency* with *regressive changes* such as mucus formation, cyst formation, calcification, and ossification. The tumor can destroy bone despite the calcification, but dural penetration and intracranial extension are rare. The peak incidence is between 10 and 30 years of age, with a slight female preponderance. Conventional radiographs and CT demonstrate the tumor as a circumscribed, lobulated, predominantly extraskeletal mass. Sites of ossification or ring-shaped calcifications are seen in 33% to 70% of cases. The adjacent bone shows deformation and reactive sclerosis.

On MRI, chondromas show moderate signal intensity on T1-weighted images and high signal intensity on T2-weighted images. Contrast administration causes marked homogeneous to nonhomogeneous enhancement, depending on the amount of calcification within the lesion.

Chondrosarcoma (Fig. 3.**13**)

Chondrosarcoma, the *malignant form of chondroma*, may arise directly from cartilage or enchondral bone or from tissue devoid of cartilaginous elements. Approximately 7% of all malignant and benign chondromas occur in the head and neck region. The development of this tumor is determined during embryonic life, since the bone of the anterior skull base has a cartilaginous origin.

This tumor is most prevalent around the age of 45 and is twice as common in males as females. It is characterized by its extension, its local infiltration of surrounding structures, and its high rate of recurrence following extirpation. Metastases from chondrosarcoma are rare, but when they occur they are much more aggressive than the primary tumor.

The extent of bone destruction and small calcifications are best appreciated on CT scans. Gadolinium-enhanced MRI is superior to CT in defining the precise extent of the tumor, the soft-tissue component, and the extent of infiltration.

Noncontrast CT scans usually show a slightly hyperdense mass with clumps of calcification and associated foci of nonspecific bone destruction. The mass enhances only slightly after the administration of contrast material. Gadolinium-enhanced MR images show a somewhat greater degree of contrast enhancement. In T2-weighted sequences, the mass shows a high signal intensity that may be isointense to CSF and is characteristic of this lesion. The tumor appears isointense to hypointense on T1-weighted images.

The differential diagnosis of chondrosarcoma includes chondroma, meningioma, plasmacytoma, chordoma, metastases from other tumors, and carcinoma spreading from adjacent regions.

Metastases

Overall, bony metastases are rare in the anterior skull base but are more common than primary malignant osseous lesions of this region. Carcinoma of the prostate, lung, and breast are the most common sources of metastatic seeding to the anterior skull base. CT is the imaging modality of choice for accurately depicting sites of bone destruction and differentiating lytic and osteoplastic tumor components. CT can precisely document the extent of osseous involvement (Figs.

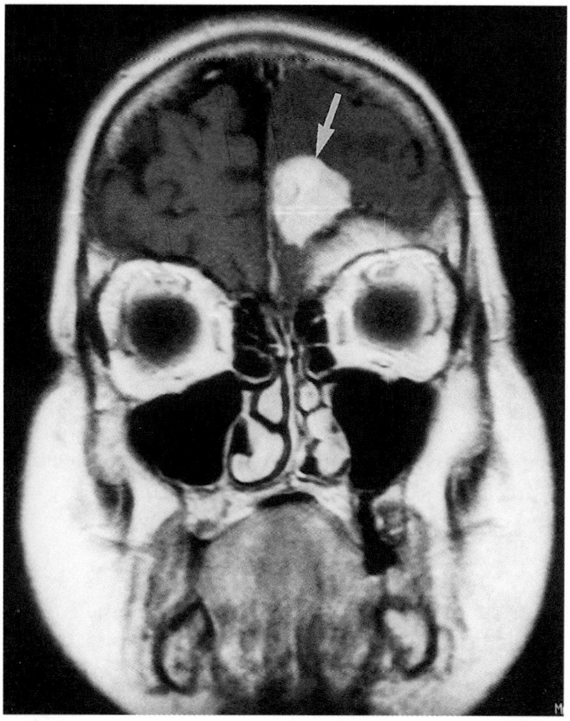

a

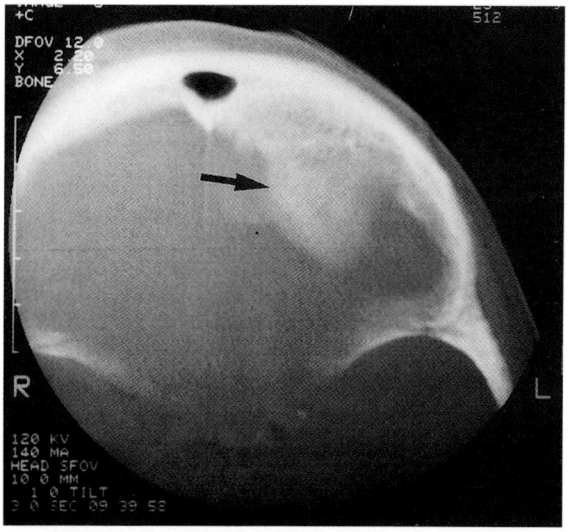

b

Figs. 3.**7 a, b** **Meningioma of the anterior calvaria.**
(**a**) Coronal noncontrast CT scan (1 mm, bone window) demonstrates a region of hyperostosis (arrow) involving the anterior calvaria on the left side.
(**b**) Coronal Gd-enhanced MR image (SE, TR/TE = 700/15 ms) on the same plane shows a homogeneously enhancing lesion in this area (arrow).

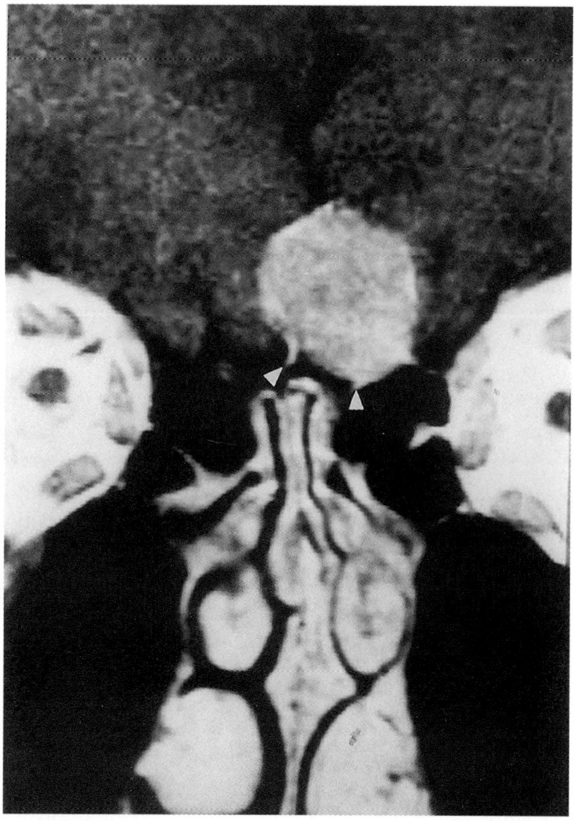

Fig. 3.**8** **Olfactory nerve meningioma.** Gd-enhanced MR image in the coronal plane (SE, TR/TE = 700/15 ms) shows the tumor as a smoothly marginated mass with two small basal extensions (arrowheads) following the olfactory nerve filaments.

Figs. 3.**9 a – e** **Meningioma of the right temporal region.** ▷
(**a**) Axial noncontrast MR image (SE, TR/TE = 700/15 ms) shows a barely perceptible mass in the area of the right sphenoid bone (arrow) with no evidence of bone destruction.
(**b**) Axial Gd-enhanced MR image (SE, TR/TE = 700/15 ms) shows marked, homogeneous enhancement of the meningioma, which is clearly demarcated from surrounding structures and causes marked impression on the orbit (arrow).
(**c**) Axial noncontrast CT scan (1 mm, bone window) documents the sphenoid bone destruction on the right side (arrow) by the meningioma.
(**d**) Coronal Gd-enhanced MR image (SE, TR/TE = 700/15 ms) shows intradural extension (arrowhead) and clearly demonstrates the impression on the orbit (arrow).
(**e**) Selective digital subtraction angiography (DSA) of the right external carotid artery (AP projection) demonstrates blood flow to the sphenoid meningioma from branches of the external carotid artery (arrow).

Fig. 3.**10** **Olfactory nerve meningioma.** Axial Gd-enhanced T1-weighted MR image (SE, TR/TE = 700/15 ms) shows a sharply circumscribed, uniformly enhancing mass (arrow) in the area of the interhemispheric fissure superior to the cribriform plate.

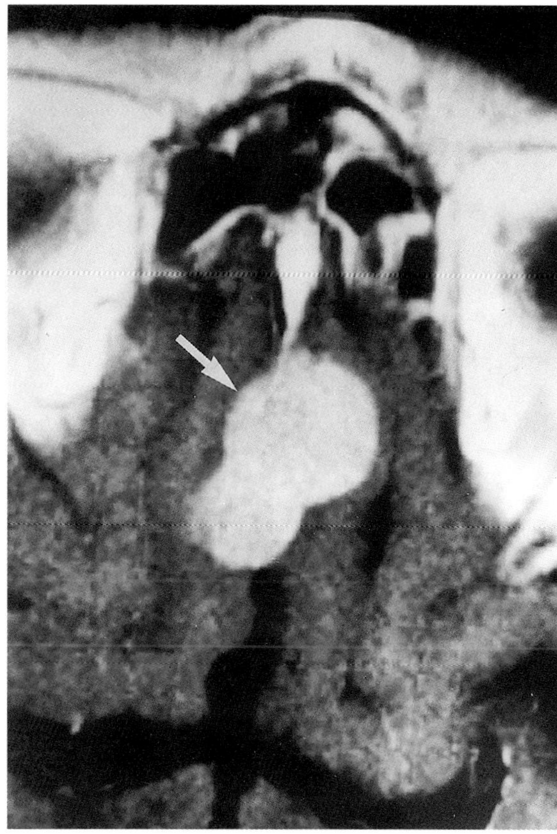

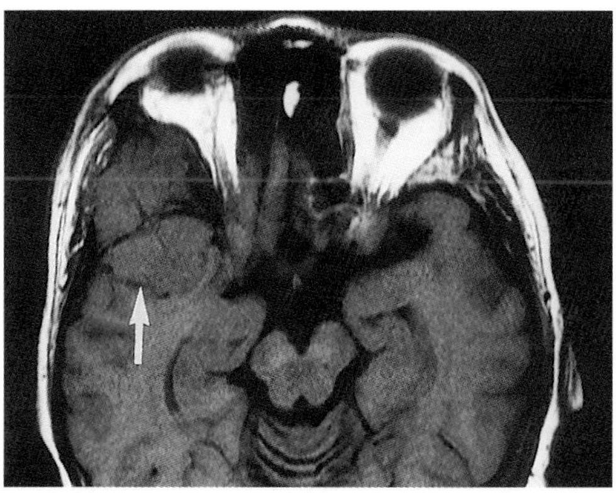

a

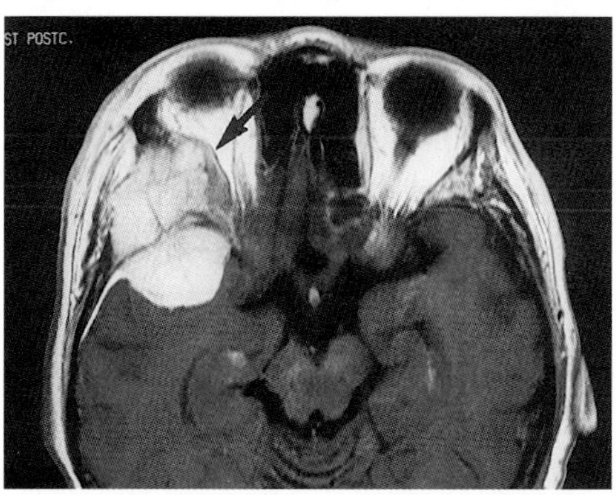

b

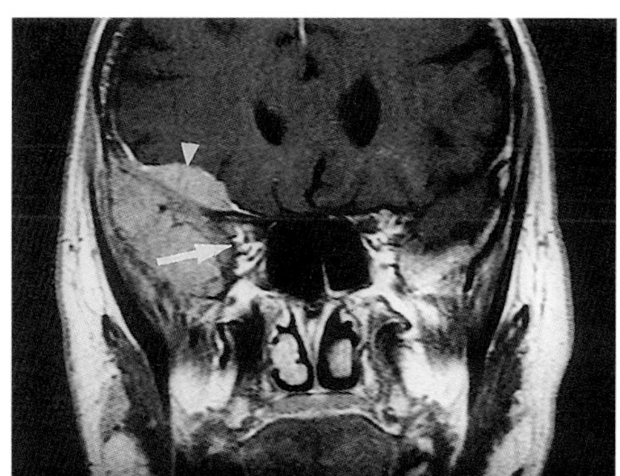

d

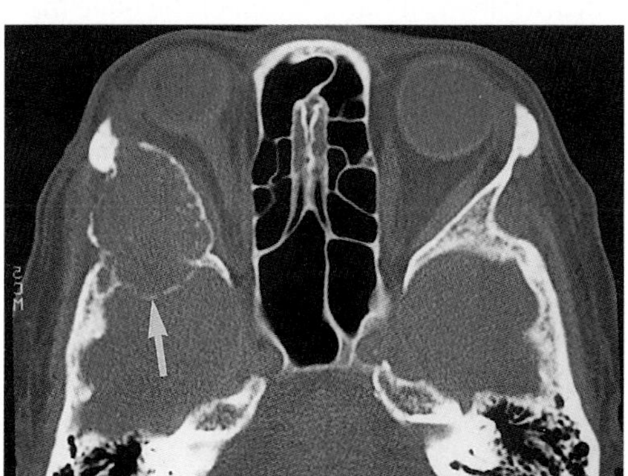

c

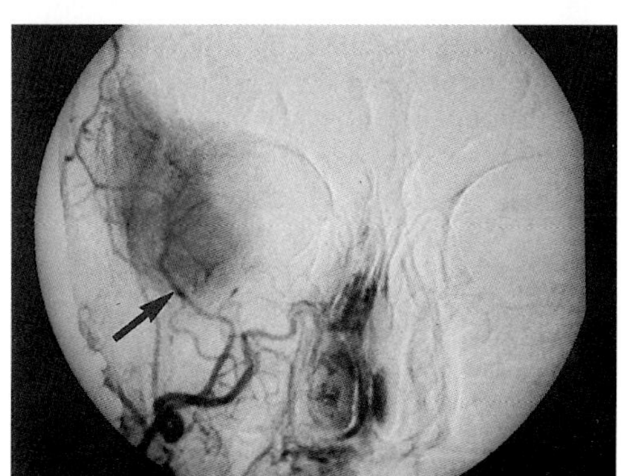

e

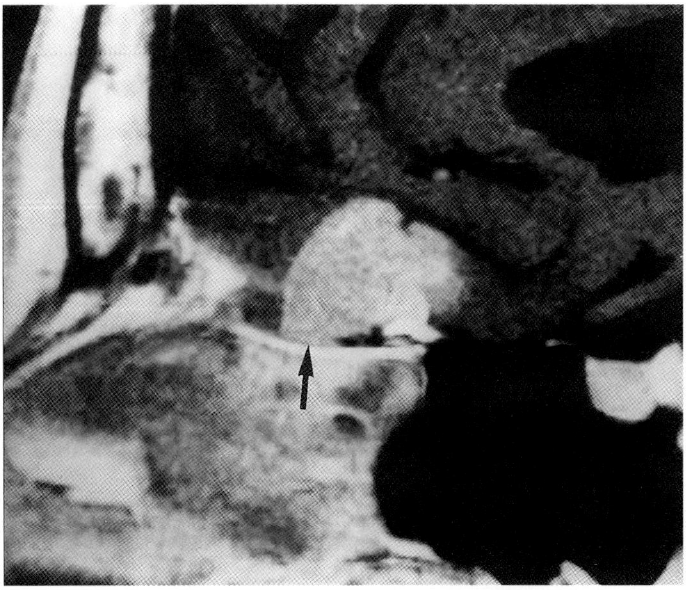

Fig. 3.**11** **Olfactory nerve meningioma.** Gd-enhanced MR image in the sagittal plane (SE, TR/TE = 700/15 ms) shows the mass in broad contact with the cribriform plate and in close relation to the olfactory nerve. The lesion does not transgress the cribriform plate.

3.**14a, b**). Contrast-enhanced scans can differentiate soft-tissue components and their infiltration into surrounding structures (Figs. 3.**14c–e**). On MRI, metastases of the skull base appear as ill-defined, isointense to slightly hyperintense lesions on T2-weighted images, and they appear isointense on T1-weighted images. Following the administration of Gd-DTPA, the metastases may show moderate to intense contrast enhancement (Figs. 3.**14f–h**). The infiltration of adjacent soft tissues is better appreciated on MRI than CT owing to the higher soft-tissue contrast of MRI. It can be difficult to distinguish between primary osseous lesions and metastases.

Primary Osseous Tumors

Osteoma

Osteoma is a *benign lesion* that most often arises in the paranasal sinuses. Its peak incidence is between 40 and 50 years of age, and it is twice as common in males as females.

On plain skull films as well as CT scans, osteoma appears as a smoothly marginated round lesion of extremely high density. It may also appear as an expansile mass with scalloped borders.

Because of its high density, osteoma appears on MR images as an area of extremely low signal intensity when surrounded by hyperintense structures (bone marrow, fat). Meningioma should be considered in the differential diagnosis of this lesion.

Osteoid Osteoma

Osteoid osteoma is a *benign osseous lesion* that, by definition, is 1.5 cm or less in diameter. Ninety percent of all lesions occur between 5 and 25 years of age, and males predominate by approximately a 2:1 ratio. Osteoid osteoma presents with characteristic pain symptoms that vary with the activity level and time of day. Some 95% to 98% of cases are marked by weeks or even years of unremitting local pain that worsens at night and with rest. Aspirin usually relieves the pain within 20 to 30 minutes.

In approximately 75% of cases, conventional radiographs and CT demonstrate a small, circumscribed, round or oval lucent nidus surrounded by a dense sclerotic zone. The remaining bone appears depleted of mineral salts, giving the impression of regional osteoporosis. The nidus enhances after the administration of contrast material.

On MRI, the nidus appears isointense to muscle on T1-weighted images and moderately hyperintense on T2-weighted images. In approximately 63% of cases, MRI also shows inflammation of the bone marrow surrounding the nidus, and approximately 47 % of cases show an inflammatory soft-tissue response with edema.

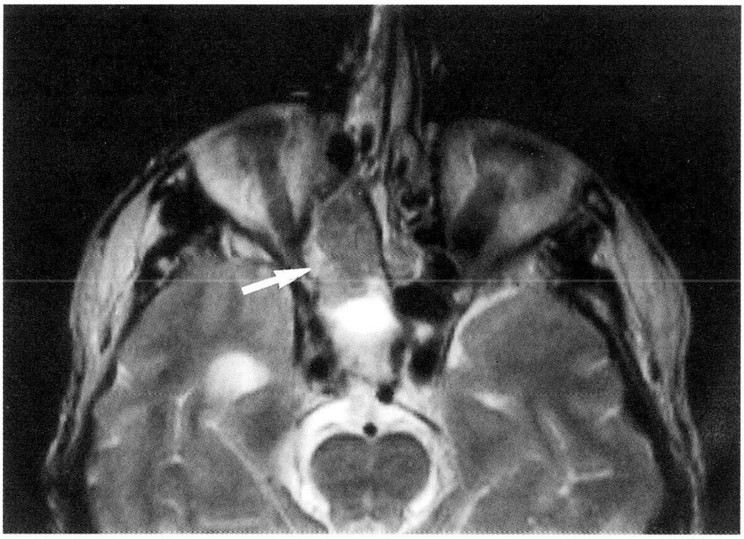

a

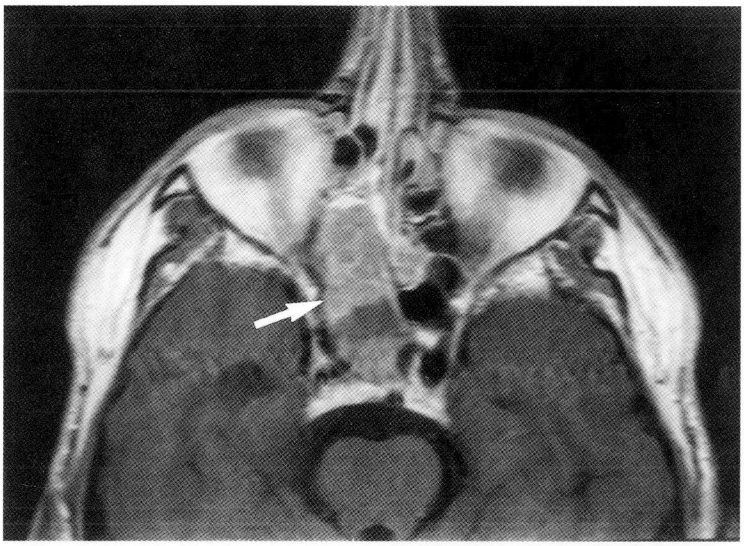

b

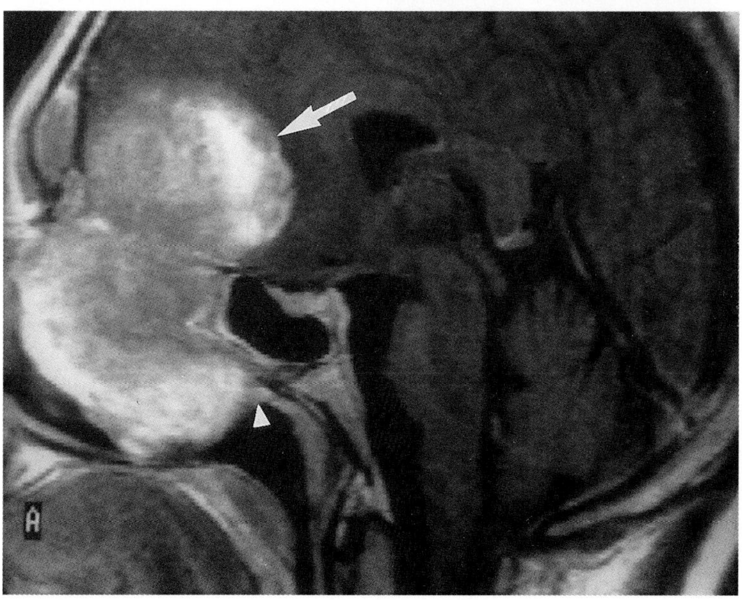

c

Figs. 3.**12 a – c** **Esthesioneuroblastoma.**
(**a**) Axial noncontrast T2-weighted MR image (SE, TR/TE = 3000/90 ms) shows a smoothly marginated, nonhomogeneous anterior skull-base mass extending into the paranasal sinuses (arrow).
(**b**) Axial Gd-enhanced T1-weighted MR image (SE, TR/TE = 700/15 ms) shows heterogeneous enhancement of the esthesioneuroblastoma (arrow).
(**c**) Gd-enhanced image (SE, TR/TE = 700/15 ms) on the sagittal plane defines the overall extent of the tumor (arrow) and shows possible infiltration of the paranasal sinus mucosae (arrow head).

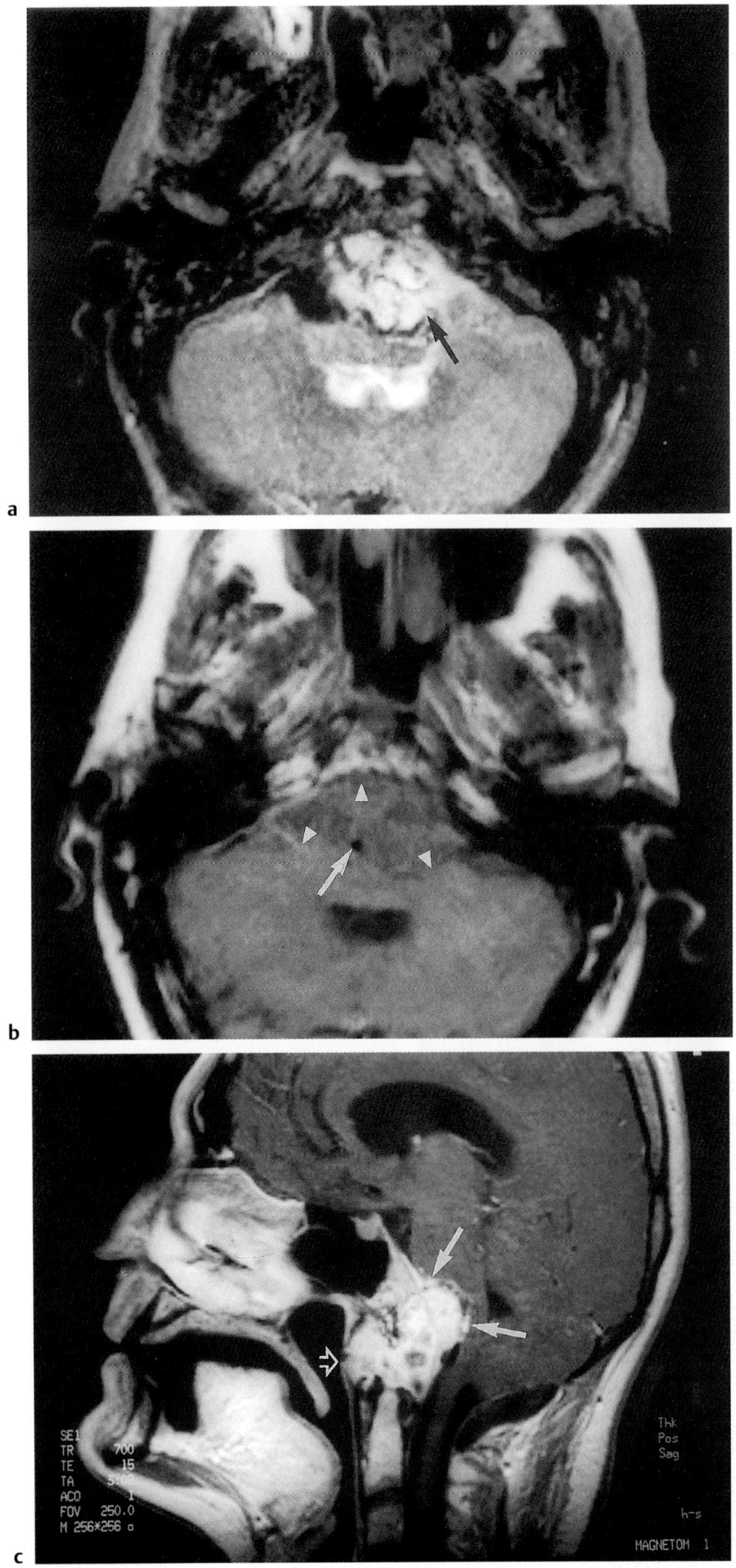

Figs. 3.**13 a – c** **Chondrosarcoma of the clivus.**
(**a**) Axial noncontrast T2-weighted MR image (SE, TR/TE = 3000/90 ms) shows a large, nonhomogeneous, predominantly hyperintense mass (arrow) in the clivus region with extension to the prepontine cistern.
(**b**) Axial noncontrast T1-weighted MR image (SE, TR/TE = 700/15 ms) shows a large, predominantly isointense mass (arrowheads) in the clivus region extending to the prepontine cistern and displacing the basilar artery (arrow).
(**c**) Sagittal Gd-enhanced MR image (SE, TR/TE = 700/15 ms) more accurately defines the extent of the tumor. Note the indentation of the brainstem (arrows) and the extension of tumor toward the nasopharynx (open arrow).

Inflammatory Lesions

Inflammatory lesions of the anterior skull base are usually secondary to a primary process of the paranasal sinuses, most commonly the frontal and ethmoid sinuses. Primary disease of the sphenoid sinus is comparatively rare. *Mucoceles* and *pyoceles* (Figs. 3.**15 a, b**) may develop as a complication of chronic sinusitis, trauma, neoplasia, or surgery. Other inflammatory lesions are *frontobasal abscess* and *osteomyelitis of the anterior skull base* , both of which are due predominantly to chronic inflammatory, traumatic, or iatrogenic processes.

Conventional radiographs may show a geographic, moth-eaten, or permeative pattern of bone destruction. Depending on the stage of the inflammation (acute or chronic), sclerotic zones may surround the sites of bone destruction, or sclerosis may be the predominant process in chronic cases. The films should also be evaluated for paranasal sinus opacification, with or without air–fluid levels, and for demonstrable soft-tissue swellings.

Three-phase radionuclide bone scans and leukocyte scintigraphy are appropriate when there is clinical suspicion of osteomyelitis. These studies are more sensitive and more specific than conventional radiographs.

The CT findings of osteomyelitis are similar to those in conventional radiographs: osseous defects with or without a sclerotic zone. CT is superior to conventional radiography in demonstrating the involvement of adjacent soft tissues and the underlying focus. Contrast-enhanced CT can accurately define the soft-tissue component of the inflammatory process and demonstrate any abscess formation.

On MRI, the inflammatory lesions have a high signal intensity on T2-weighted sequences and appear isointense to hypointense on T1-weighted sequences. Post-gadolinium images usually demonstrate a smoothly marginated mass with an enhancing rim; some lesions show homogeneous enhancement. Seepage sinusitis with secondary involvement of the meninges or brain parenchyma and the extraosseous spread of infection from an osteomyelitic focus are characterized by diffuse, usually localized contrast enhancement of the affected structures. Perifocal edema causes the affected structures to display a high signal intensity even on unenhanced T2-weighted images.

A neoplasm should always be excluded as part of the differential diagnosis.

Traumatic Lesions

Fractures of the *posterior wall of the frontal sinus, ethmoid roof, sphenoid sinus roof, orbit, cribriform plate,* and *lesser sphenoid wing* are classified clinically as *frontobasal fractures.*

Dural tears are considered an open brain injury because they establish a direct communication between the intracranial cavity and adjacent paranasal sinuses. Lateral fracture lines through the orbital roof represent a closed type of brain injury. The fracture lines in most frontobasal fractures have a sagittal orientation, although transverse fracture lines that breach the orbit may occur. Fractures involving the frontal or frontotemporal areas of the calvaria are also common.

The conventional radiographic workup includes biplane (PA and lateral) skull radiographs, the Rhese view, and OF and OM projections of the paranasal sinuses. Further imaging evaluation consists of axial and coronal CT scans using bone and soft-tissue algorithms. Besides accurately defining the course of the fracture line, this study can also confirm or exclude intracranial complications. In particular, CT scans should be evaluated for evidence of a communication between the cranial cavity and adjacent paranasal sinuses (open brain injury), fractures of the orbital roof (closed brain injury), subdural and epidural hematomas or bone fragments, intracranial hemorrhage, malignant brain edema, and pneumocephalus. Intravenous contrast is necessary for the diagnosis of a brain abscess or carotid-cavernous fistula.

As a rule, coronal CT scans are superior to conventional radiographs in the diagnosis of frontobasal skull fractures (Fig. 3.**16**). CT is better for demonstrating displaced intraorbital fragments and small intracranial air inclusions, and axial scans can reliably detect complications of greater and lesser sphenoid wing fractures such as optic sheath hematoma, subperiosteal hematoma, and avulsions of the optic nerve.

The prime radiographic signs of a frontobasal fracture are contour disruption, visible bone fragments, and dehiscence. The most useful indirect signs of a fracture are an air–fluid level in the paranasal sinus (hematosinus); soft-tissue changes in the paranasal sinuses and nasal cavity due to hematoma, edema, or CSF leakage; and intracranial or intraorbital air inclusions.

Besides its role in acute diagnosis, CT is also the method of choice for evaluating traumatic lesions and

Figs. 3.**14a–h** **Metastases:**

(**a**) Metastasis from breast carcinoma to the anterior skull base. Axial noncontrast CT scan (2 mm, bone window) shows marked bone destruction involving much of the anterior skull base including the orbital roof and paranasal sinuses (arrows).

(**b–e**) **Metastatic neuroblastoma of the anterior skull base:**

(**b**) Axial CT scan (1 mm, soft-tissue window) after intravenous contrast shows a large mass infiltrating both orbits (arrows) and the ethmoid sinus, with pronounced osteolysis (arrowheads) of the anterior skull base and right petrous bone.

(**c**) Axial post-contrast CT scan (soft-tissue window, 100 mL Ultravist 370) provides better delineation of the mass infiltrating both orbits (arrows).

(**d**) Sagittal reconstruction of the contrast-enhanced CT scan defines the extent of the neuroblastoma and clearly reveals its extracranial and intracranial components (arrows).

(**e**) On MIGB immunoscintigraphy (AP projection), the metastatic neuroblastoma appears as an area of markedly increased radiotracer uptake in the left sphenoid bone (arrow).

(f–h) Metastasis from bronchogenic carcinoma to the anterior skull base:

(**f**) Axial noncontrast T1-weighted MR image (SE, TR/TE = 700/15 ms) shows a large mass with indistinct margins (arrowheads) in the clivus region with possible infiltration of the cerebellopontine angle.

(**g**) Axial MR image (SE, TR/TE = 700/15 ms) after gadolinium injection more clearly defines the extent of the tumor and its infiltration toward the nasopharynx (arrow) and cerebellopontine angle (arrowheads). Small necrotic foci are visible at the center of the mass.

(**h**) Gd-enhanced MR image (SE, TR/TE = 700/15 ms) in the coronal plane clearly defines the craniocaudal extent of the tumor (arrows).

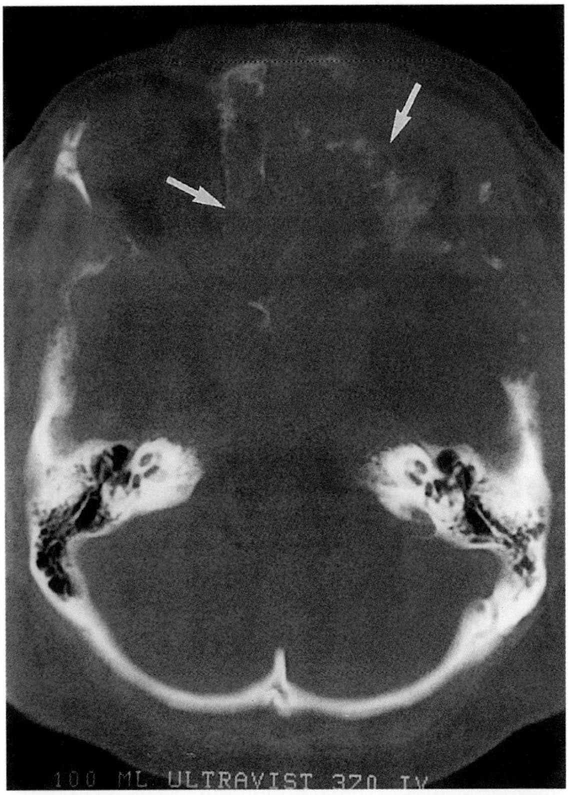

a

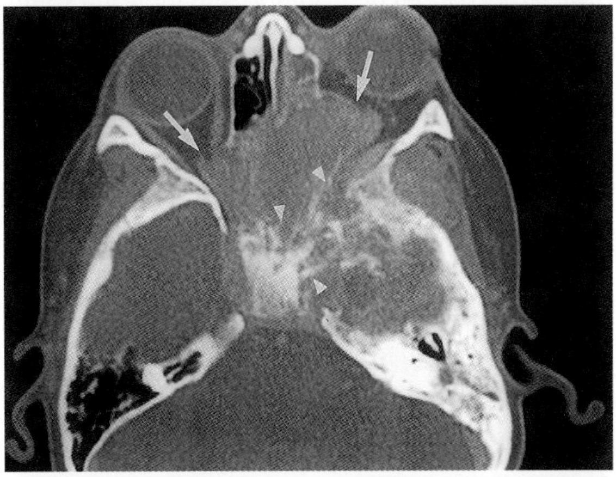

b

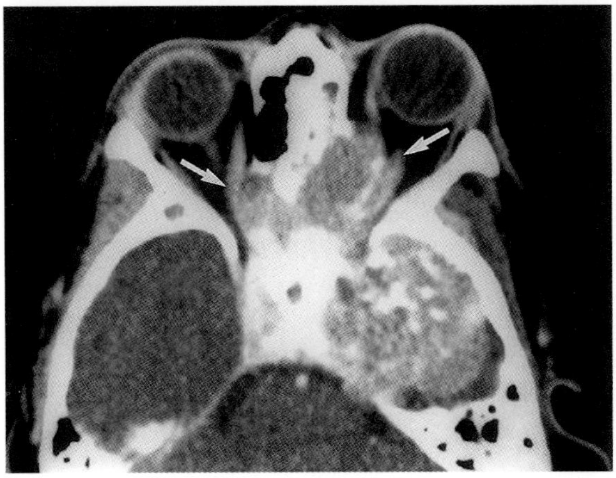

c

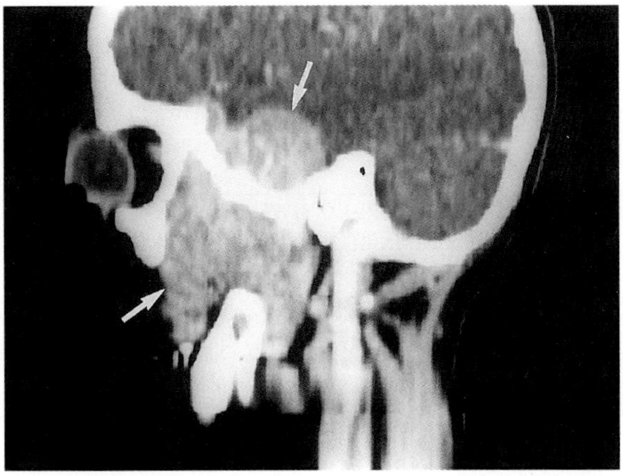

d

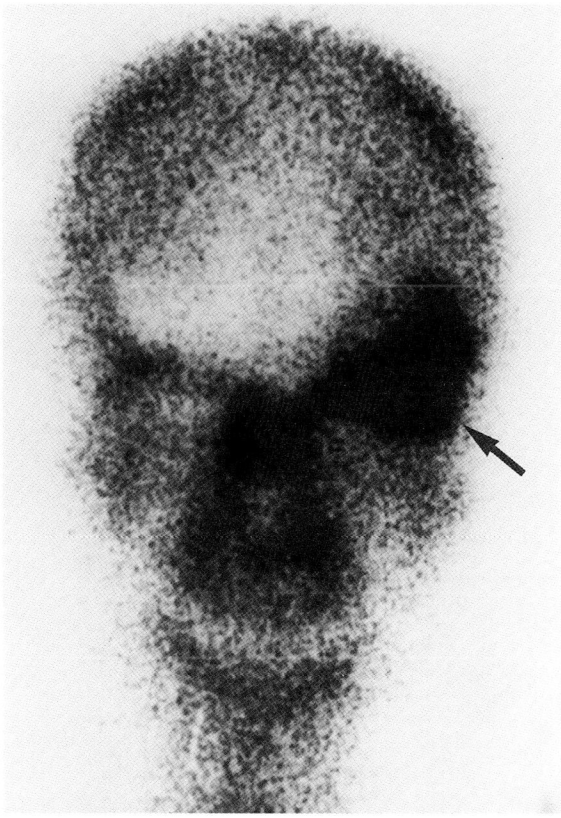

e

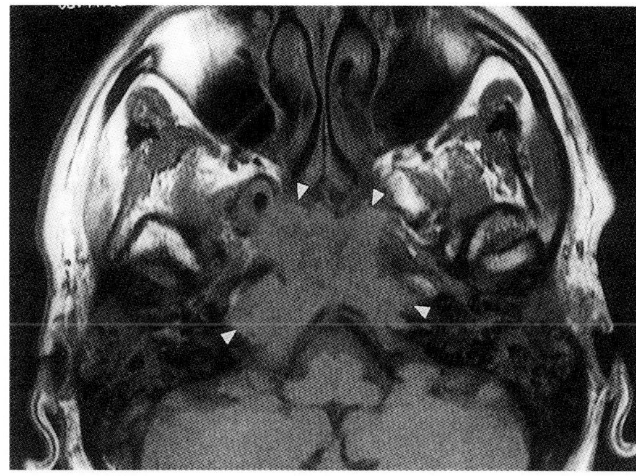

f

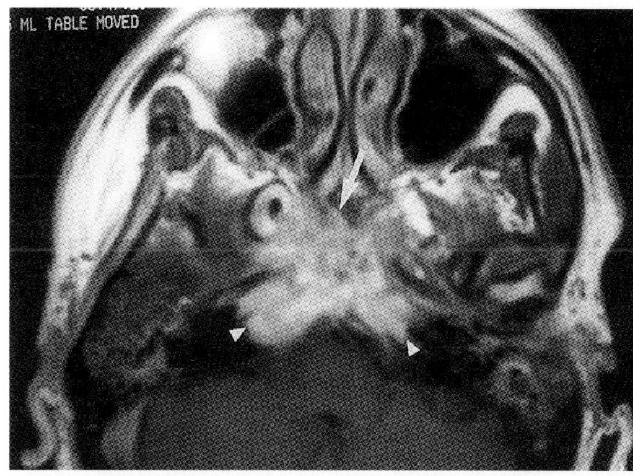

g

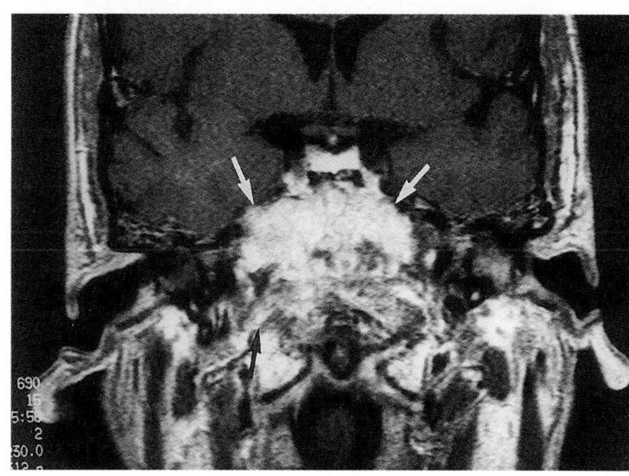

h

their complications. It can demonstrate fracture discontinuities causing functional compromise involving the orbit and other structures, frontal osteomyelitis, mucoceles, pyoceles, and ascending rhinogenic infections with intracranial complications (meningitis, encephalitis) secondary to CSF leakage. If a CSF fistula is suspected, CT should be performed after the intrathecal administration of contrast material to accurately define the site of the leak. Contrast-enhanced MRI is more sensitive than, and thus markedly superior to, postcontrast CT scans in the evaluation of meningitis and encephalitis. MRI is also more accurate in detecting and differentiating intracranial abscess. The only drawback of MRI relative to CT is the longer examination time, which may necessitate sedation or general anesthesia in some patients.

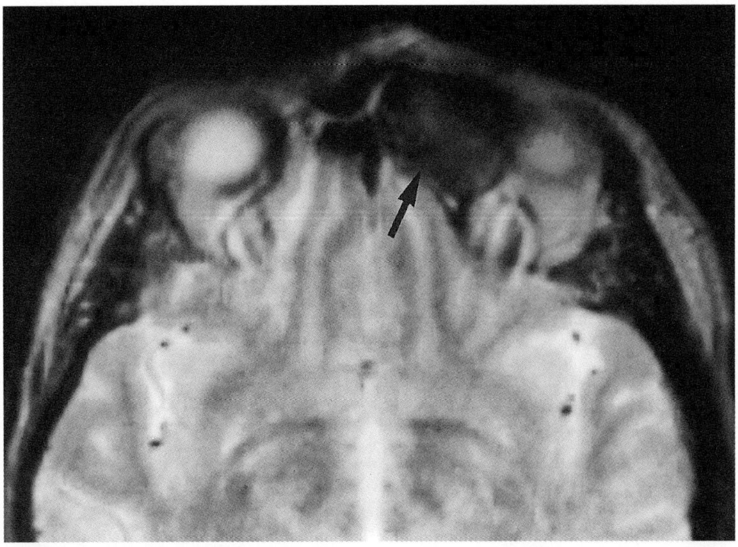
a

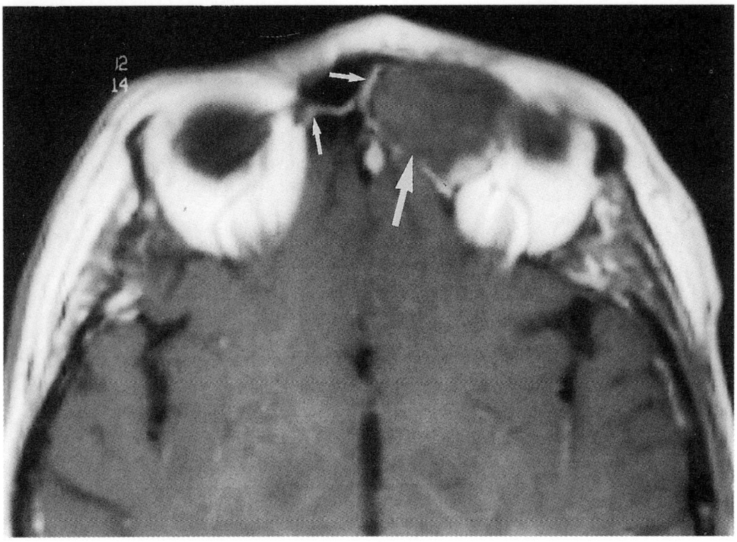

b

Figs. 3.**15 a, b** **Epidermoid cyst of the frontal sinus.**
(**a**) Axial noncontrast T2-weighted MR image (SE, TR/TE = 3000/90 ms). In this sequence the epidermoid cyst in the frontal sinus has a low signal intensity relative to brain (arrow). There is no evidence that the lesion has infiltrated adjacent structures.
(**b**) Axial Gd-enhanced MR image (SE, TR/TE = 700/15 ms). The lesion in the frontal sinus (large arrow) does not enhance after gadolinium injection, while the sinus mucosa shows normal enhancement (small arrows).

Iatrogenic Lesions

Primary lesions (malformations, tumors, trauma) must be differentiated from therapy-induced lesions that are secondary to a surgical procedure or to the radiotherapy or chemotherapy of recurrent or residual tumors.

MRI, with its variable weighting techniques, is markedly superior to radiographic studies in the follow-up of tumors with soft-tissue components. While the changes in signal intensity noted during early follow-up, particularly in T2-weighted sequences, are very nonspecific and are due mainly to posttherapeutic edema, an increase in T2-weighted signal intensity seen during intermediate to long-term follow-up, combined with contrast enhancement on the T1-weighted image, can be interpreted as signifying a residual or recurrent tumor.

The situation is different with primary osseous lesions that do not have a soft-tissue component. In these cases, radionuclide imaging combined with conventional radiography or CT is the preferred follow-up method for the detection of tumor recurrence.

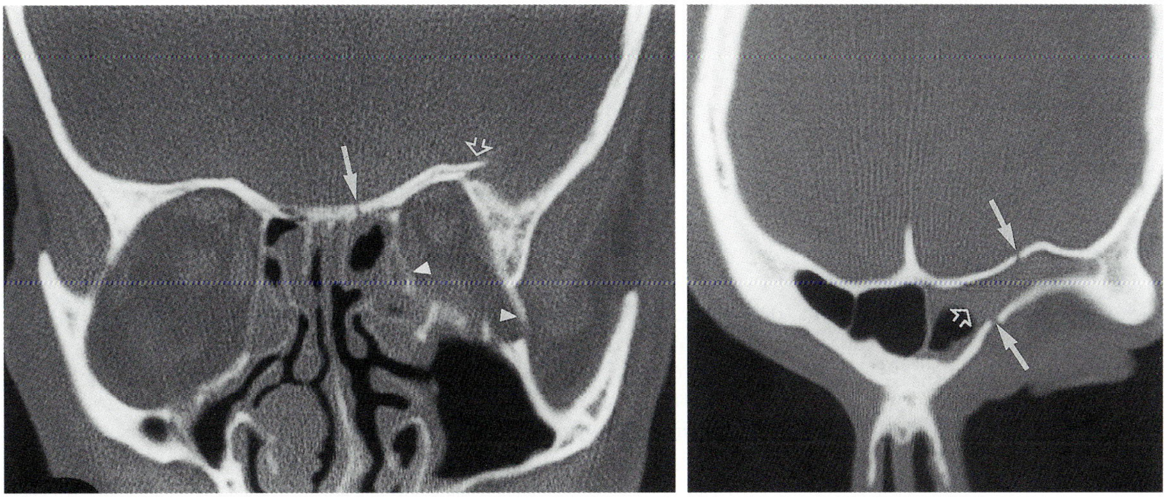

Figs. 3.**16** a, b **Frontobasal skull fracture.**
(**a**) Coronal noncontrast CT scan (2 mm, bone window) reveals a complex fracture of the anterior skull base involving the frontal part of the skull base (arrow), the left orbital roof (open arrow), and the lateral and medial orbital walls (arrowheads).
(**b**) Coronal noncontrast CT scan (2 mm, bone window) shows extension of the fracture line into the superior and inferior walls of the frontal sinus (arrows). The scan also shows bleeding into the frontal sinus (open arrow) as a secondary sign of the fracture.

Imaging Criteria and their Differential Diagnosis

This section deals with morphologic image criteria that are useful in the differential diagnosis of lesions of the anterior skull base. The appearance of a lesion in an imaging study forms the basis for formulating the differential diagnosis and establishing the final, definitive diagnosis.

Liquid Masses

Liquid masses and structures of the anterior skull base are a common imaging finding, particularly in the evaluation of diseases of the facial skeleton and paranasal sinuses. CT scanning in these patients must be able to differentiate an obstructed frontal or sphenoid sinus from an inflammatory or neoplastic complication.

Points of key interest in conventional X-ray films are asymmetries, density variations, and morphologic differences in adjacent bony structures. For example, thinning of the bony walls of a sinus may signify a mucocele requiring further investigation.

The criteria for interpreting CT findings include the density of a lesion, its margination, its relationship to surrounding structures, and the involvement of osseous structures. On contrast scans, it is important to describe the type of contrast enhancement (homogeneous, nonhomogeneous, no enhancement) and the pattern of the enhancement (peripheral or diffuse), giving special attention to meningeal enhancement associated with solid or inflammatory lesions.

On MRI, the identity of a liquid mass of the anterior skull base is determined by making a summary interpretation of T1- and T2-weighted sequence findings before and after contrast administration. Primary attention is given to the T2-weighted sequence, with its sensitivity to tissues that have a high water and protein content. The T1-weighted image with Gd enhancement is also useful for narrowing the differential diagnosis. Figure 3.**17** summarizes the main considerations in the differential diagnosis of liquid masses of the anterior skull base that are demonstrated by MRI. Cystic and liquid masses are best appreciated on T2-weighted sequences owing to their high signal intensity (Fig. 3.**18** and Table 3.**10**).

Air-Containing Masses

As with the paranasal sinuses (Chapter 7), it is important to differentiate variations such as pneumosinus dilatans and processes secondary to inflammatory, traumatic, or iatrogenic pathology when evaluating air-containing masses in the region of the anterior skull base. Given the limitations of MRI in differentiating air from bone, CT is the primary imaging modality for the evaluation of these lesions.

Most air-containing lesions of the anterior skull base are a result of trauma (e.g., frontobasal fractures) or prior surgery. These lesions require differentiation from variations such as pneumosinus dilatans. Inflammatory processes involving gas-forming microorganisms and tumor-associated structural defects with secondary air inclusions should also be considered in the differential diagnosis of air-containing masses (Table 3.**11**).

Tumor Masses

When a solid mass is detected in the anterior skull base by CT or MRI, one of the first questions to be addressed in differential diagnosis is the presence or absence of associated bone destruction. The clinical problem will direct the choice of imaging studies: MRI is the method of choice for neurologic investigations, while CT is the primary modality for investigating morphologic changes and other problems involving the upper facial skeleton. Besides visualizing the bone destruction caused by a solid mass, CT also aids in the detection of intratumoral calcifications and bone fragments. Tables 3.**12**–3.**15** list the criteria for identifying lesions that involve the anterior skull-base from above, intrinsically, or from below.

The accurate differential diagnosis of an anterior skull base lesion requires assessment of the following imaging findings:

- The topography of the lesion, i.e., its size, shape, and relation to surrounding structures.
- The morphology of the lesion (predominantly cystic, solid, calcified).
- Its enhancement characteristics (faint, moderate, marked or intense enhancement, also the pattern of enhancement).
- The margins of the lesion (sharp, indistinct, infiltrative).

An important factor in the differential diagnosis of a mass lesion, besides its margins, is its relation to surrounding structures (Fig. 3.**19**). By making this topographic assessment, the examiner can determine the site of origin of the lesion. Another useful guide is the accurate characterization of tumor morphology. MRI is better than CT for this purpose owing to its superior soft-tissue contrast. The interpretation of signal characteristics in different MR sequences and the analysis of enhancement dynamics are particularly helpful in establishing the identity of a solid mass on

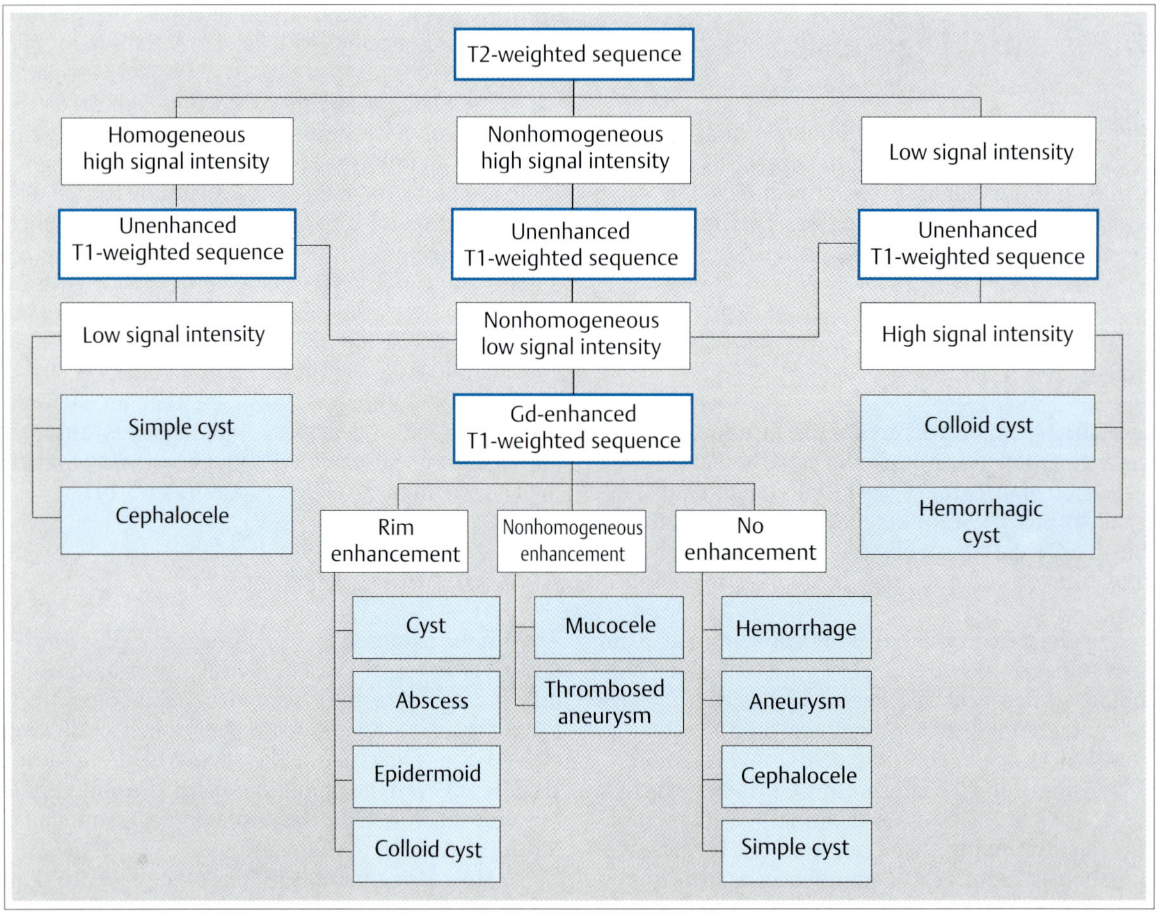

Fig. 3.**17** Differential diagnosis: MR imaging of liquid masses of the anterior skull base.

Table 3.**10** Liquid masses of the anterior skull base

Findings	Differential diagnostic criteria
Variation: ➤ Pneumosinus dilatans with fluid accumulation ➤ Cephalocele	Morphology, density, topography
Tumor: ➤ Cystic epidermoid ➤ Primary cyst ➤ Craniopharyngioma	Density characteristics, type and pattern of contrast enhancement
Inflammation: ➤ Mucocele ➤ Abscess	Location, morphology of bony boundaries, type of contrast enhancement, meningeal enhancement
Vascular: ➤ Aneurysm ➤ Hemorrhage	Signal or density characteristics, topography
Iatrogenic: ➤ CSF leak ➤ Seroma ➤ Surgical defect	Defects, morphology, signal or density characteristics

Table 3.**11** Air-containing masses of the anterior skull base

Findings	Differential diagnostic criteria
Variation: ➤ Pneumosinus dilatans	Morphology, density, topography
Tumor: ➤ Superinfected tumor	Defects, morphology, signal or density characteristics
Inflammation: ➤ Brain abscess ➤ Frontobasal abscess	Location, morphology of bony boundaries, type of contrast enhancement, meningeal enhancement
Trauma (Figs. 3.**16 a**, 3.**18 a–d**): ➤ Frontobasal fracture ➤ Calvarial fracture	Density characteristics, type and pattern of contrast enhancement
Iatrogenic: ➤ Surgical defect ➤ Prior surgery	Signal or density characteristics, topography, distribution pattern

Table 3.**12** Lesions involving the anterior skull base from above

Findings	Differential diagnostic criteria
Malformation:	
➤ Encephalocele (Fig. 3.**4 b**) ➤ Arachnoid cyst (Fig. 3.**3 a**)	Morphology, structure, density
Tumor:	
➤ Dermoid cyst	Density
➤ Meningioma	Location, enhancement
➤ Craniopharyngioma	Cystic internal structure
➤ Pituitary adenoma	Topography
➤ Neuroma	Enhancement
➤ Esthesioneuroblastoma (Fig. 3.**12**)	Topography, enhancement
➤ Brain tumor	Enhancement
Inflammation:	
➤ Mucocele	Location, density, enhancement
Trauma (Figs. 3.**16 a**, 3.**18 a**):	
➤ Hematoma	Density
Iatrogenic:	
➤ Hematoma	Density

MR images. MRI has an important role, moreover, in the evaluation of recurrent tumors and their differentiation from residual posttherapeutic changes.

Osseous Lesions

Osseous lesions of the anterior skull base are differentiated on the basis of circumscribed or generalized thinning of the calvaria, solitary or multiple sites of bone destruction, and generalized or geographic expansion of the affected bone.

When *generalized or geographic thinning* of the calvaria is noted in the anterior skull base, a normal variant must be differentiated from true pathology. Pathologic processes that may be associated with bone thinning include intracranial mass lesions (e.g., meningioma), circumscribed osteoporosis, and arachnoid cysts. *Solitary or multiple sites of bone destruction* require differentiation as normal (fissure, foramen, canal, pacchionian granulations), iatrogenic (craniotomy, craniectomy), or pathologic. An isolated site of bone destruction is most frequently caused by an eosinophilic granuloma or solitary metastasis. Geographic bone destruction may be caused by malignant tumors of the nasopharynx or paranasal sinuses that invade the anterior skull base by contiguous spread; usually these are nasopharyngeal and paranasal sinus carcinomas, neuroblastomas, or soft-

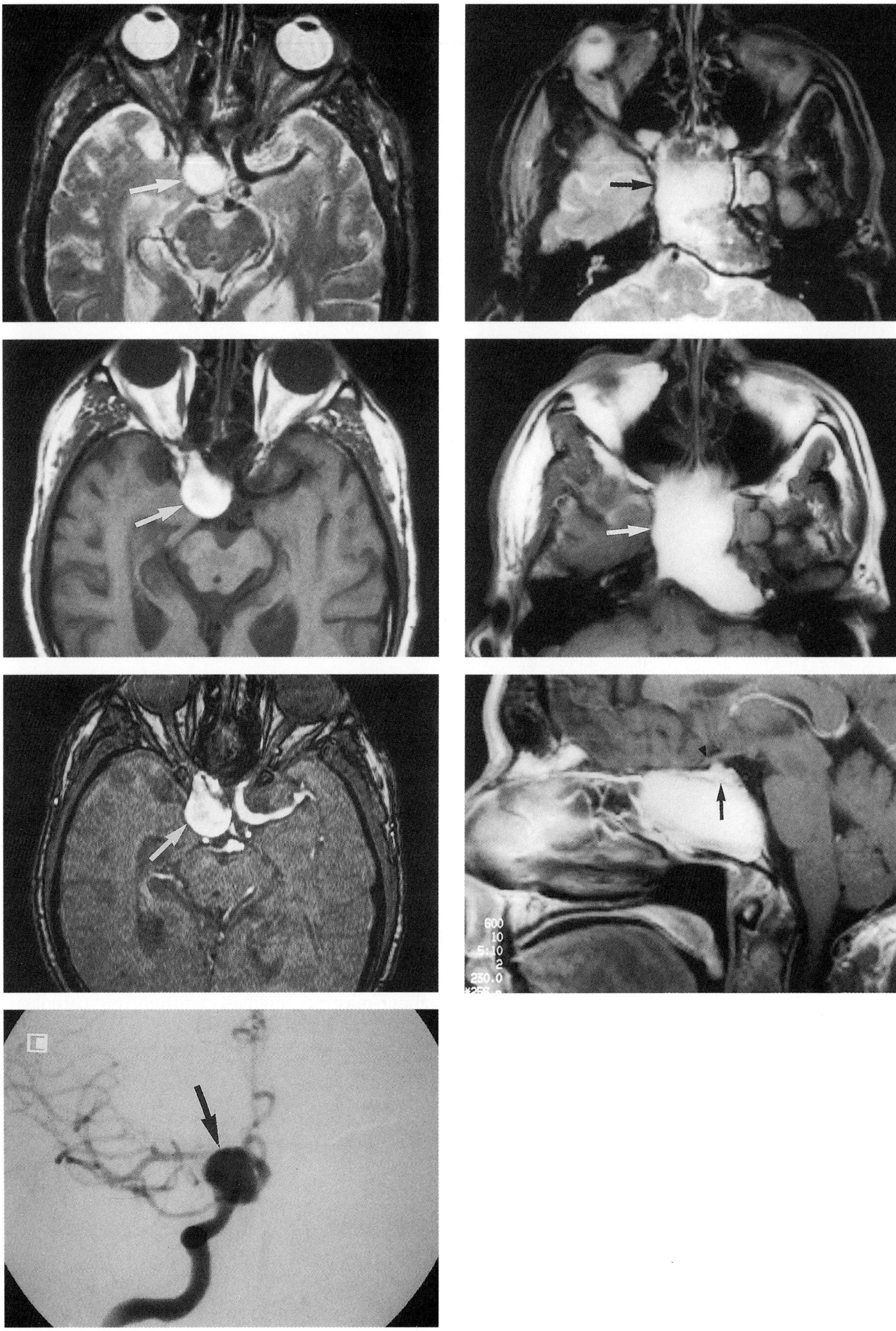

a e b f c g d

◁ Figs. 3.**18 a–g** **Liquid masses.**
(**a–d**) Aneurysm of the right internal carotid artery:
(**a**) Axial noncontrast T2-weighted MR image (SE, TR/TE = 3000/90 ms) demonstrates the aneurysm as a hyperintense mass (arrow). The lesion cannot be definitely localized to the internal carotid artery or middle cerebral artery on the right side.
(**b**) Axial noncontrast T1-weighted MR image (SE, TR/TE = 700/15 ms). The lesion also shows high signal intensity in this sequence (arrow), consistent with the slow blood flow in the aneurysm.
(**c**) Axial noncontrast arterial MR angiogram (TONE technique, TR/TE = 43/8 ms, flip angle $\alpha = 15°$). The lesion shows uniformly high signal intensity in the original MRA data set. Analysis of the individual image slices showed no signs of partial thrombosis in the aneurysm (arrow) and identified the origin of the lesion as the right internal carotid artery.
(**d**) Selective DSA of the right internal carotid artery (AP projection) corroborates MR findings, showing a right internal carotid artery aneurysm (arrow) with no evidence of thrombosis.
(**e–g**) **Cholesterol granuloma of the sphenoid sinus:**
(**e**) Axial noncontrast T2-weighted MR image (SE, TR/TE = 3000/90 ms) shows a cholesterol granuloma of the sphenoid sinus (arrow) as a hyperintense mass with a predominantly cystic signal intensity. The areas of low signal intensity are due to the varying protein content of the intracystic material.
(**f**) Axial noncontrast T1-weighted MR image (SE, TR/TE = 700/15 ms). T1 weighting displays the granuloma as a sharply circumscribed lesion of uniformly high signal intensity (arrow). Areas with different compositions are not differentiated in this sequence. The high signal intensity on the T1-weighted image is consistent with the high protein and cholesterol content of the cyst.
(**g**) Gd-enhanced sagittal MR image (SE, TR/TE = 700/15 ms) shows no significant enhancement of the sphenoid sinus lesion. The relation of the lesion to the optic chiasm (arrowhead) and pituitary (arrow) is more clearly appreciated on the sagittal plane.

tissue metastases. Osteoma and bone cysts are benign osseous lesions that may cause isolated bone destruction.

Less frequent causes are epidermoids, cephaloceles, arachnoid cysts, and meningiomas. Multiple sites of calvarial bone destruction are most likely caused by metastases. Other potential causes are osteoporosis, myeloma, hyperparathyroidism, and osteomyelitis (Table 3.**16**).

Table 3.**13** Intrinsic lesions of the anterior skull base

Findings	Differential diagnostic criteria
Tumor:	
➤ Metastasis (Figs. 3.**14 a–f**)	Bone destruction, bone morphology
➤ Fibrous dysplasia (Fig. 3.**5 b**)	Bone morphology, location, density, morphology
➤ Paget disease	Bone morphology
➤ Chondroma	Morphology, enhancement
➤ Osteoma	Bone destruction, soft-tissue infiltration
➤ Lymphoma	Location, density, morphology
➤ Histiocytosis X (Fig. 3.**6 a**)	Bone morphology, bone destruction
➤ Chondrosarcoma	Soft-tissue infiltration
➤ Osteopathy	
➤ Osteosarcoma	
Inflammation:	
➤ Osteomyelitis	Bone morphology
➤ Granuloma	Enhancement, bone destruction, soft-tissue infiltration
Trauma (Figs. 3.**16 a**, 3.**18 a**):	Density
➤ Hematoma	
Malformation:	
➤ Dysostosis	Location, morphology
Iatrogenic:	
➤ Residual lesions	Enhancement, morphology

Table 3.**14** Lesions involving the anterior skull base from below

Findings	Differential diagnostic criteria
Tumor:	
➤ Nasopharyngeal carcinoma	Density, morphology, location
➤ Polyposis	
➤ Papilloma	
➤ Angiofibroma (Fig. 6.**8 a**)	
➤ Sinus osteoma	
➤ Rhabdomyosarcoma (Fig. 6.**13 a**)	
Inflammation:	
➤ Mucocele	Location, density, morphology, enhancement
➤ Parapharyngeal abscess	
Iatrogenic:	
➤ Residual lesions	Density, enhancement
Malformation:	
➤ Rathke pouch tumor	Location, density
Trauma (Figs. 3.**16 a**, 3.**18 a**):	
➤ Frontobasal fracture with soft-tissue prolapse	Morphology

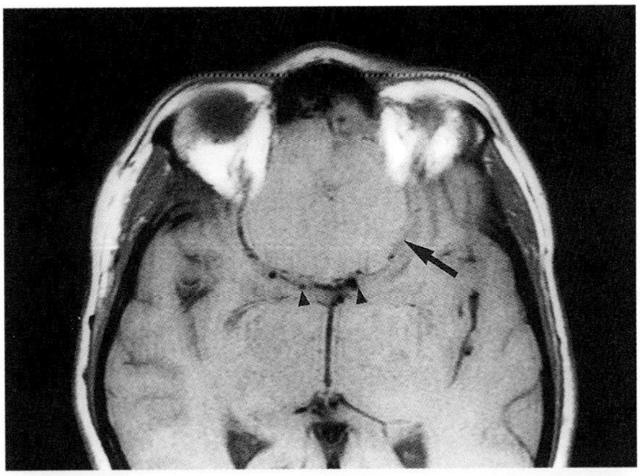

a

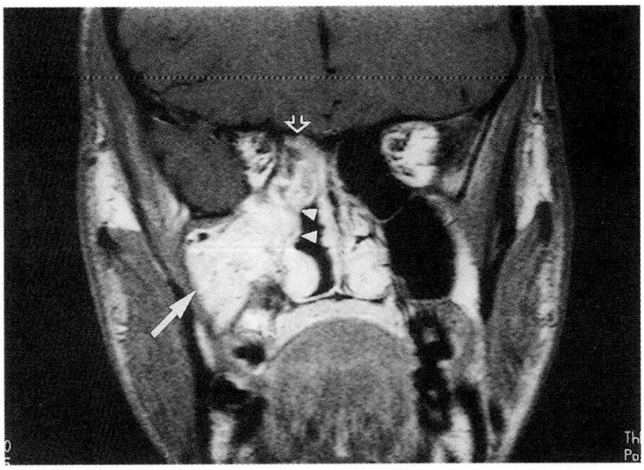

e

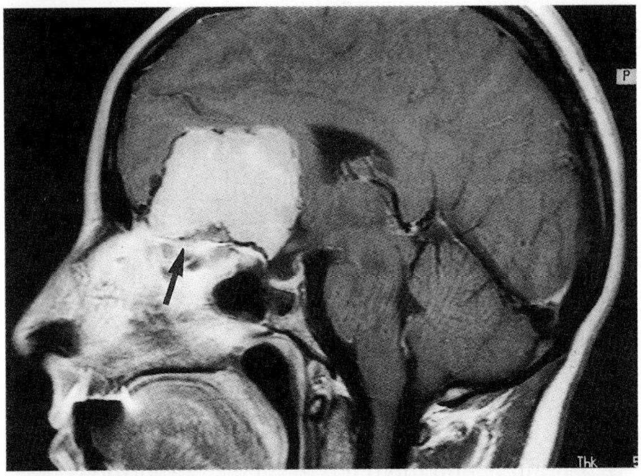

b

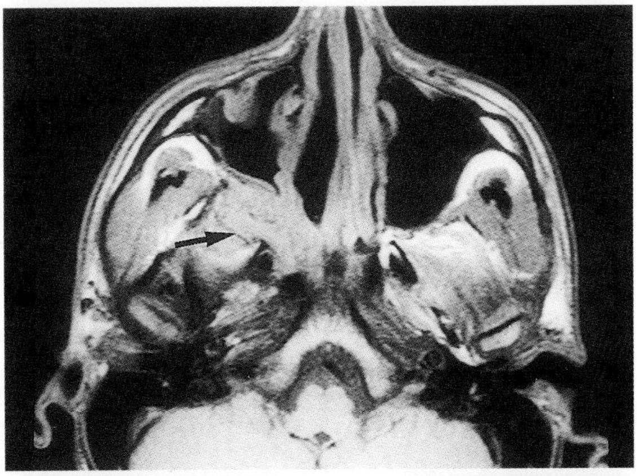

c

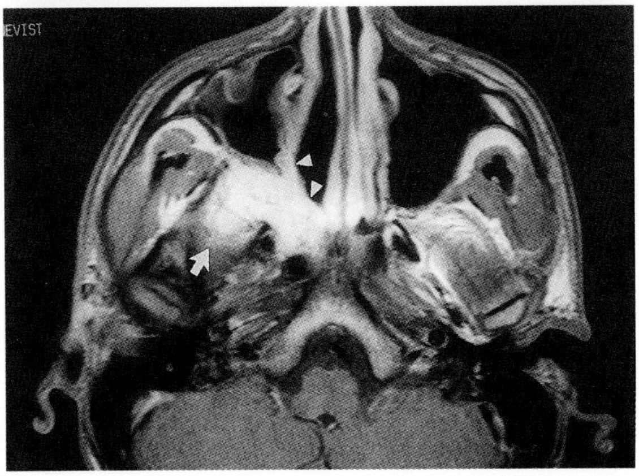

d

Figs. 3.**19a–e** **Tumor masses.**

(a, b) Olfactory nerve meningioma:

(**a**) Axial noncontrast T1-weighted MR image (SE, TR/TE = 700/15 ms) shows a uniformly isointense lesion (arrow) of the anterior skull base with a conspicuous mass effect displacing the anterior cerebral artery (arrowheads). There is no perifocal edema.

(**b**) Sagittal post-contrast T1-weighted MR image (SE, TR/TE = 700/15 ms). After gadolinium injection, the olfactory-nerve meningioma shows intense, homogeneous enhancement revealing the broad-based contact of the tumor with the olfactory filaments (arrow).

(c–e) Adenoid cystic carcinoma with infiltration of the skull base:

(**c**) Axial noncontrast T1-weighted MR image (SE, TR/TE = 700/15 ms) shows an extrinsic lesion invading the anterior skull base from below. The lesion appears as a circumscribed, isointense mass involving the right sphenoid (arrow). The infiltrative nature of this adenoid cystic carcinoma is difficult to appreciate in this image.

(**d**) Axial Gd-enhanced MR image (SE, TR/TE = 700/15 ms) shows an intensely and uniformly enhancing lesion with indistinct margins relative to the pterygoid muscle (arrow). Infiltration of the muscular layer of the nasal cavity is also apparent (arrowheads).

(**e**) Coronal Gd-enhanced MR image (SE, TR/TE = 700/15 ms) more accurately defines the craniocaudal extent of the tumor, which extends from the right parapharyngeal space (arrow) to the anterior skull base (open arrow). The tumor has infiltrated all of the right lateral nasal cavity (arrowheads).

Table 3.**15** MR signal characteristics of tumors of the anterior skull base

Tumor	T2-weighted image	T1-weighted image	Edema	Enhancement
Meningioma (Fig. 3.**19 a**)	↗	↙	+/–	↑↑
Carcinoma	↑	↓	++	↑ – ↑↑
Craniopharyngioma	↑↑	↑	+/–	↑
Chordoma	↑	↙	–	↑
Chondroma	↑↑	↓	+/–	↗
Chondrosarcoma	↑↑	↙	+	↑
Esthesioneuroblastoma (Fig. 3.**12 a**)	↗	↙	+/–	↑
Metastasis (Figs. 3.**14 a–f**)	↑	↓	+++	↑↑

↑ = High signal intensity/intense enhancement
↗ = Isointense to hyperintense/moderate enhancement
↙ = Hypointense to isointense
↓ = Low signal intensity/no enhancement
\+ = Moderate
++ = Marked
+++ = Intense
+/– = Minimal
– = None

Table 3.**16** Lesions causing bone destruction in the anterior skull base

Findings	Differential diagnostic criteria
Variation:	
➤ Arachnoid cyst (Fig. 3.**3 a**)	Signal characteristics, density,
➤ Cephalocele (Fig. 3.**4 b**)	topography, contents
Tumor:	
➤ Metastasis (Figs. 3.**4 a–f**)	Destruction, infiltration
➤ Secondary malignancy	Topography, destruction
➤ Osteoma	Density, signal characteristics
➤ Eosinophilic granuloma	Focality (unifocal)
➤ Plasmacytoma	Focality (multifocal)
➤ Epidermoid	Signal characteristics
Inflammation:	
➤ Osteomyelitis	Pattern, infiltration, destruction, sequestrum
Metabolism:	
➤ Hyperparathyroidism	Morphology

Expansion of the Bony Structures of the Skull Base

Bony expansion of the anterior skull base can be demonstrated by conventional biplane skull radiographs, axial and coronal CT scans, and in some cases by MRI using plain and Gd-enhanced T1- and T2-weighted sequences.

Meningioma and craniosynostosis are the most likely causes of bone expansion in the anterior skull base. Expansion can also result from lesions that involve the bone secondarily, such as nasopharyngeal carcinoma, or from rare benign tumors such as osteogenic, chondrogenic, and mesenchymal masses. It is essential to identify primary osteoplastic processes such as fibrous dysplasia, Paget disease, and osteomyelosclerosis (Table 3.**17**).

Structural Defects of the Bony Skull Base

Structural defects of the anterior skull base are usually detected by conventional radiography and CT, i.e., biplane skull films, paranasal sinuses views in the OM and OF projections, and axial and coronal CT scans using bone-window technique. When structural defects are noted, the following criteria should be listed, documented, and included in the examination report:

- ➤ Modeling characteristics to differentiate between traumatic, congenital, inflammatory, and neoplastic lesions.
- ➤ Margins (sharp, indistinct, variable structural heterogeneities).
- ➤ Density characteristics (homogeneous, lytic, soft-tissue components or calcifications, in rare cases fat inclusions).

Summary and Diagnostic Strategy

The clinical and radiologic evaluation of the anterior skull base requires sophisticated diagnostic equipment combined with detailed anatomic knowledge and clinical experience on the part of the examiner. With modern sectional imaging modalities (CT and MRI) supplanting conventional X-ray studies in evaluations of the anterior skull base, adequate diagnostic techniques are available but must be selectively applied in a manner that is appropriate for the individual patient.

The selection of the optimum primary imaging study depends on the nature of the clinical inquiry. It is common practice, however, to combine optimal CT scans with contrast-enhanced MR images. Arterial or

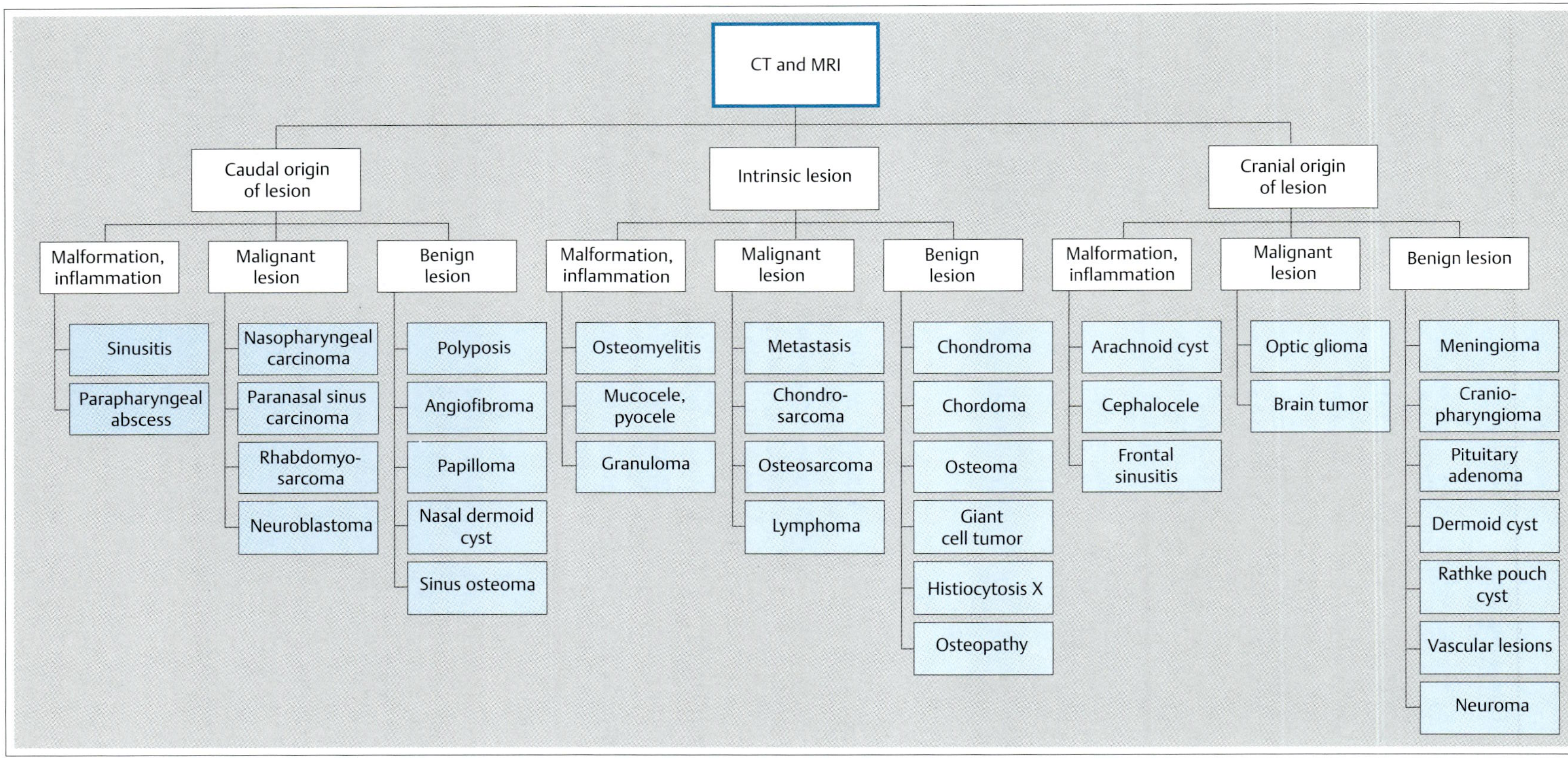

a

Figs. 3.**20 a, b** **Anterior skull base.**
(**a**) Differential diagnosis: lesions of the anterior skull base.
(**b**) Diagnostic strategy: MR imaging of the anterior skull base.

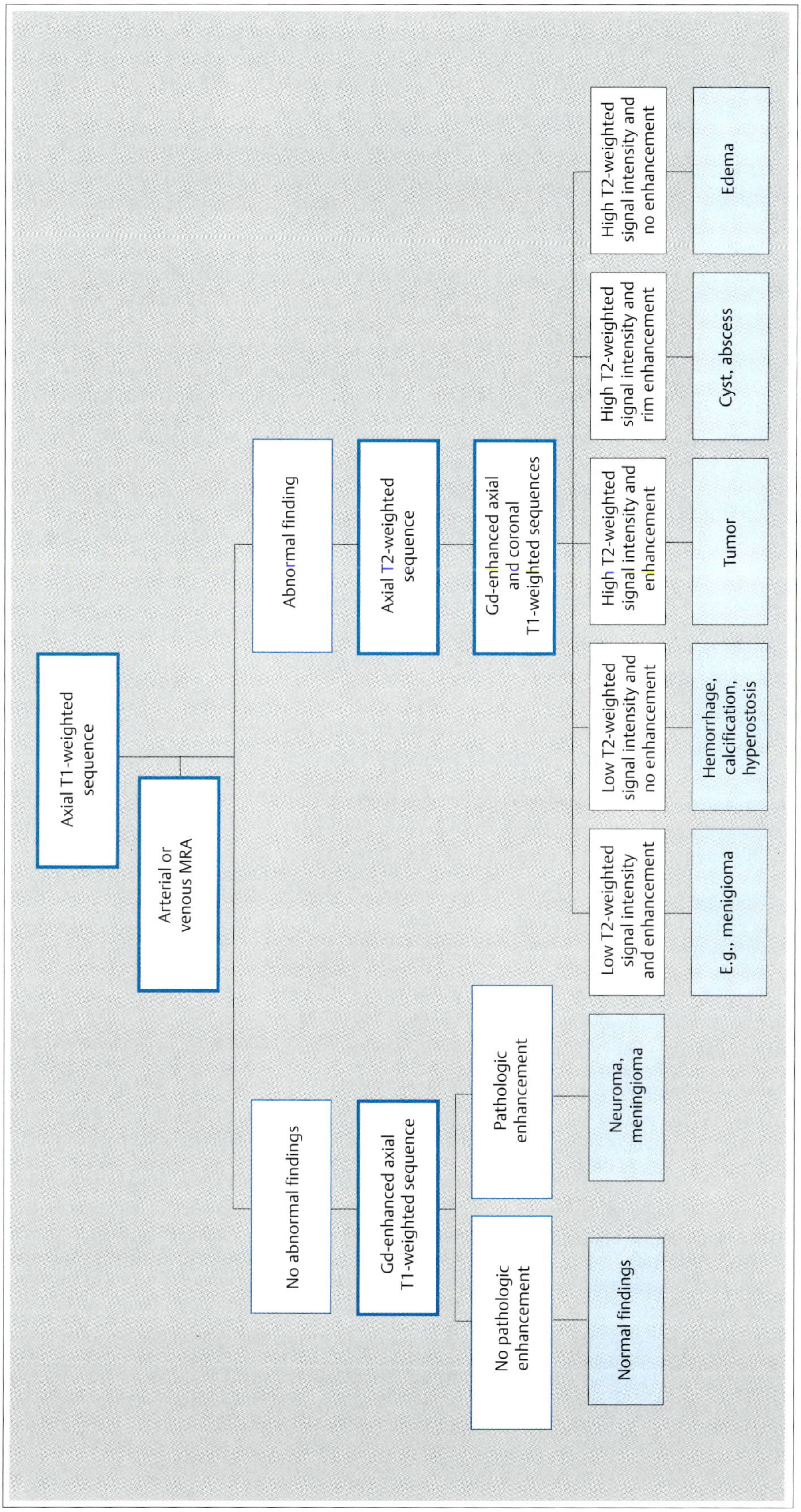
Axial T1-weighted sequence
Arterial or venous MRA
No abnormal findings
Abnormal finding
Gd-enhanced axial T1-weighted sequence
Axial T2-weighted sequence
Gd-enhanced axial and coronal T1-weighted sequences
No pathologic enhancement
Pathologic enhancement
Normal findings
Neuroma, meningioma
Low T2-weighted signal intensity and enhancement
Low T2-weighted signal intensity and no enhancement
High T2-weighted signal intensity and enhancement
High T2-weighted signal intensity and rim enhancement
High T2-weighted signal intensity and no enhancement
E.g., menigioma
Hemorrhage, calcification, hyperostosis
Tumor
Cyst, abscess
Edema

b

Table 3.**17** Lesions causing bone expansion in the anterior skull base

Findings	Differential diagnostic criteria
Variation:	
➤ Fibrous dysplasia (Fig. 3.**5 a**)	Morphology, age, sex, pattern
➤ Paget disease	
➤ Osteomyelosclerosis	
Tumor:	
➤ Osteoma	Contour, density, morphology
➤ Osteoid osteoma	
➤ Chondroma	Morphology
➤ Primary malignant tumors	Infiltration pattern
➤ Secondary malignant tumors	Topography, infiltration
Inflammation:	
➤ Chronic productive osteomyelitis	Pattern, peripheral reaction

venous MR angiography should be used adjunctively if there are vascular problems that also require investigation (Fig. 3.**20**).

References

1 Ahmadi, J., S. Destian, M. L. J. Apuzzo, H. D. Segall, C. S. Zee: Cystic fluid in craniopharyngeomas: MR Imaging and quantitative analysis. Radiology 182 (1992) 783-785
2 Castelijns, J. A., M. W. van den Brekel: Magnetic Resonance Imaging evaluation of extracranial head and neck tumors. Magn. Reson. Q. 9 (1993) 113-128
3 Chapman, S., R. Nakielny: Aids to Radiological Differential Diagnosis, 3rd ed. W. B. Saunders, London 1995
4 Dähnert, W.: Radiology Review Manual, 3rd ed. Williams & Wilkins, Baltimore 1996
5 Dillon, W. P.: Applications of Magnetic Resonance Imaging to the head and neck. Semin. US CT MR 7 (1986) 202-205
6 Dillon, W. P.: Magnetic Resonance Imaging of head and neck tumors. Cardiovasc Intervent Radiol. 8 (1986) 275-281
7 Freeman, M. P., R. M. Kessler, J. H. Allen, A. C. Price: Craniopharyngeoma: CT and MR Imaging in nine cases. J Comput Assist Tomogr. 11 (1987) 810-814
8 Frey, K. W., K. Mees, T. J. Vogl: Bildgebende Vefahren in der HNO-Heilkunde. Enke, Stuttgart 1989
9 Grodd, W., C. Claussen, K. Voigt: Intrakranielle Tumoren. In Reiser, M., W. Semmler: Magnetresonanztomographie. Springer, Berlin 1992
10 Han, J. S., R. G. Huss, J. E. Benson, B. Kaufmann, Y. S. Yoon et al.: MR Imaging of the skull base. J Comput Assist Tomogr. 8 (1984) 944-952
11 Harnsberger, H. R.: Handbook of Head and Neck Imaging, 2nd ed. Mosby Year Book, St. Louis 1995
12 Lufkin, R. B., W. N. Hanafee: MR reveals subtleties of head and neck pathology. Diagn Imag. 8 (1986) 98-104
13 Lufkin, R. B., W. N. Hanafee: MRI of the head and neck. Magn Reson Imaging 6 (1988) 69-88
14 Mafee, M. F., G. E. Valvassori et al.: High resolution and dynamic sequential computed tomography. Arch Otolaryngol. 109 (1983) 691-696
15 Mödder, U., M. Lenz: Schädelbasis, Felsenbein. In Reiser, M., W. Semmler: Magnetresonanztomographie. Springer, Berlin 1992
16 Mödder, U., M. Lenz: Klinische Radiologie: Gesichtsschädel, Felsenbein, Speicheldrüsen, Pharynx, Larynx, Halsweichteile. Diagnostik mit bildgebenden Verfahren. Springer, Berlin 1991
17 Naumann, H. H: Differentialdiagnostik in der Hals-Nasen-Ohren-Heilkunde. Thieme, Stuttgart 1990
18 Rosenfield, N. S., J. J. Abrahams: Brain MR in patients with Langerhans cell histiocytosis: finding and enhancement with Gd-DTPA. Pediatr Radiol. 20 (1990) 433-436
19 Rosseau, G., A. Mark, D. O. Davis: Gd-DTPA-enhancement Magnetic Resonance Imaging of the cavernous sinus. Acta neurochir., Suppl. 53 (1991) 113-116
20 Som, P. M., R. T. Bergeron: Head and Neck Imaging, 2nd ed. Mosby Year Book, St. Louis 1991 (pp. 467-496, 875-924)
21 Stark, D. D., W. G. Bradley jr.: Magnetic Resonance Imaging, Vol. I, 2nd ed Mosby Year Book, St. Louis 1992 (pp. 3-65, 253-334)
22 Valvassori, G. E., G. D. Potter, W. N. Hanafee, B. L. Carter, R. A. Buckingham: Radiology of the Ear, Nose and Throat. Thieme, Stuttgart 1982
23 Valvassori, G. E., R. A. Buckingham, B. L. Carter, W. N. Hanafee, M. F. Mafee: Head and Neck Imaging. Thieme, Stuttgart 1988
24 Vogl, T. J.: MRI of the Head and Neck. Springer, Berlin 1991
25 Vogl. T. J., S. Dresel: MR Imaging of the nasopharynx and the face: new developments. Curr Opin Radiol. 3 (1991) 61-66
26 Vogl, T. J., R. Felix: Head and neck tumors: MR-guided laser-induced thermotherapy (LITT). In Lufkin, R., R. Black: Interventional MRI. Med Publisher, Los Angeles 1994 (pp. 58-60)
27 Vogl, T. J., J. O. Balzer: Base of skull, nasopharynx, and parapharyngeal space. In Yousem, D. M.: Head and neck imaging. Neuroimaging Clin North Am. 6 (1996) 357-378
28 Vogl, T. J., S. Dresel, L. T. Bilaniuk, G. Grevers, K. Kang, J. Lissner: Tumors of the nasopharynx and adjacent areas: MR Imaging with Gd-DTPA AJNR 11 (1990): 187-194
29 Vogl, T. J., M. G. Mack, M. Juergens, C. Bergman, G. Grevers, T. F. Jacobsen, J. Lissner, R. Felix: Skull base tumors: Gadodiamide injection-enhanced MR imaging. Drop-out effect in the early enhancement pattern of paragangliomas versus different tumors. Radiology 188 (1993): 339-346
30 Vogl, T. J., M. Juergens, J. O. Balzer, M. G. Mack, C. Bergman, G. Grevers, J. Lissner, R. Felix: Glomus tumors of the skull base: combined MR angiography and spin-echo imaging. Radiology 192 (1994) 103-110

4 Middle Skull Base and Middle Ear

The clinical evaluation of the middle skull base is based on the assessment of differential diagnostic criteria in general clinical otology and on the investigation of hearing and balance disorders. The clinical symptoms of diseases of the middle skull base are diverse and depend on the location and infiltrative characteristics of the underlying pathology.

Normal Anatomy

It is convenient for imaging purposes to subdivide the middle skull base into the *middle ear*, *temporal bone*, *jugular fossa*, *internal auditory canal*, and *cerebellopontine angle*. With its ability to define bony details, computed tomography (CT) has become the primary imaging modality for evaluating diseases of the external and middle ear. Magnetic resonance imaging (MRI) has become the primary modality for imaging the inner ear, the internal auditory canal, and the cerebellopontine angle.

Below we shall review the anatomic and radiologic principles involved in the diagnosis of diseases involving the middle-ear cavity (tympanic cavity), external auditory canal, and mastoid. Both clinically and pathogenically, these regions comprise a structural system that is subject to primary involvement by various diseases. The clinical evaluation of this system includes general examination techniques such as inspection and palpation, instrumented procedures such as otoscopy, and a variety of tests for diseases of the auditory apparatus (sensorineural and conductive hearing loss) and vestibular apparatus. The standard imaging procedures of 15 years ago, plain radiography and conventional tomography, have now been completely replaced by high-resolution computed-tomography (HRCT).

The tympanic cavity is a well-defined anatomic compartment, but the presence of the tympanic membrane limits the clinical evaluation of various inflammatory and neoplastic diseases of the middle ear, necessitating the use of imaging procedures (Figs. 4.**1** – 4.**8**).

In this section we shall review the normal anatomic relationships that are important in the diagnosis and differential diagnosis of middle-ear pathology. The tympanic membrane separates the external ear canal (Figs. 4.**1** and 4.**4**) from the tympanic cavity proper, also called the mesotympanum. The points of attachment of the tympanic membrane can be clearly identified on axial and coronal CT scans. The membrane itself averages just 10 mm in its vertical diameter and 9 mm in its horizontal diameter. The manubrium and lateral process of the malleus are attached to the tympanic membrane (Fig. 4.**2**). As a rule, all portions of the tympanic membrane cannot be identified on CT scans, but generally this fact has little clinical importance.

The normal ossicular chain is composed of the malleus, incus, and stapes. The malleus consists of a head, neck, lateral short process, anterior process, and manubrium, the short process and manubrium being attached to the tympanic membrane. The head of the malleus articulates with the incus through a synovial joint. The incus consists of a body from which a short process and long process extend. These processes are very thin and cannot be consistently defined on one CT section. They are appreciated most clearly on coronal scans.

The stapes with its footplate and associated annular ligament is best seen on axial CT scans, which are also best for demonstrating the malleoincudal and incudostapedial joints (Fig. 4.**3**).

Ligaments define and maintain the anatomic relationships of the auditory ossicles. HRCT using a 1-mm slice thickness will resolve these structures in some patients. The superior, anterior, and lateral ligaments that suspend the malleus from the walls of the tympanic cavity are best appreciated on coronal CT scans.

The functional unit of the ossicular chain includes two muscles: the tensor tympani and the stapedius. The tensor tympani muscle is innervated by cranial nerve V, the stapedius muscle by cranial nerve VII (Fig. 4.**6**). The tensor tympani runs in its own bony canal parallel to the eustachian tube. Its tendon, which runs posterolaterally and inserts on the neck of the malleus, is consistently identifiable on axial and coronal CT scans. The stapedius muscle runs in a canal medial to the second genu of the facial nerve and is usually only visible on axial scans.

The tympanic cavity features a number of recesses and bony prominences. An important recess is the Prussak space, located above the tympanic membrane. This space communicates posteriorly with the epitympanum and is an important site of origin for acquired cholesteatoma (Fig. 4.**18**).

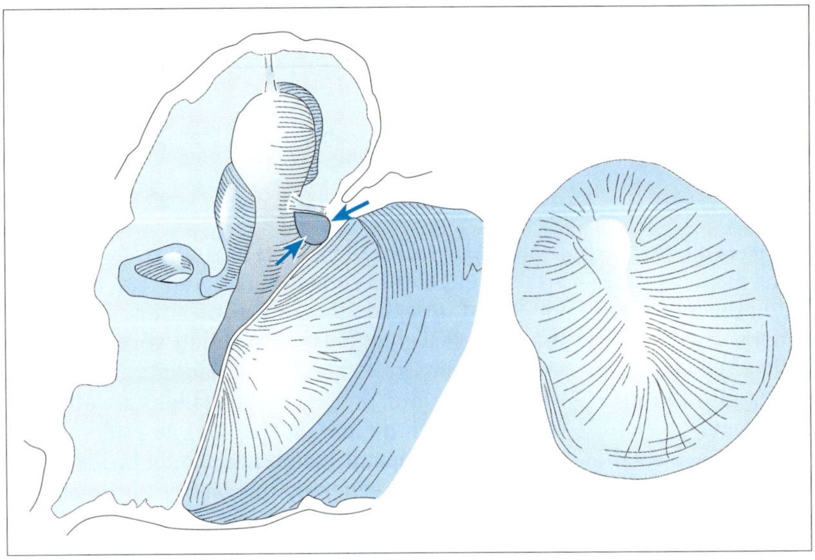

Fig. 4.**1** **Normal anatomy of the middle ear, showing the malleus, incus, stapes, and tympanic membrane.**

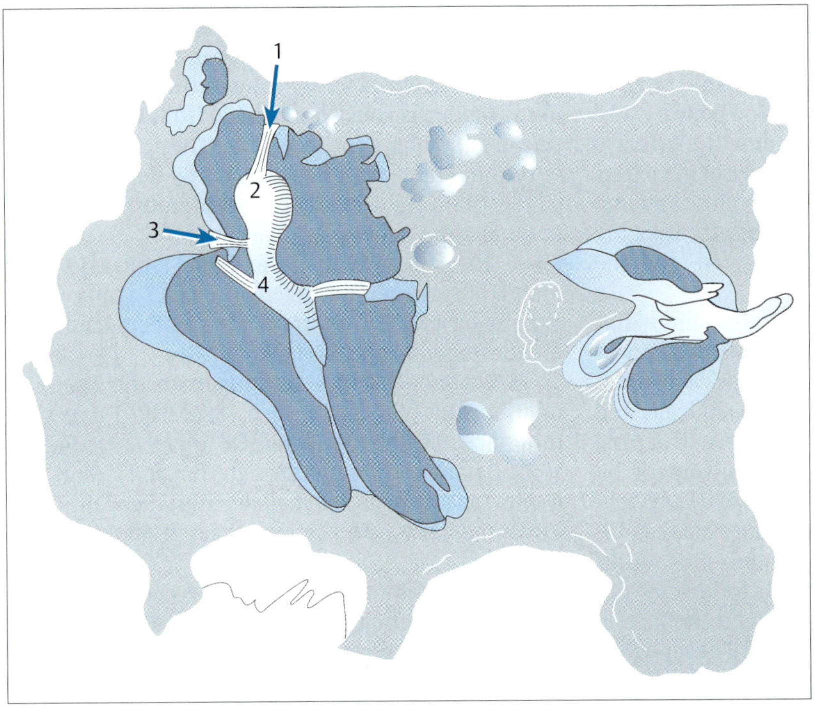

Fig. 4.**2** **Anatomic relationship of the malleus and its attachments.**

1 Superior ligament of the malleus
2 Head of the malleus
3 Lateral ligament of the malleus
4 Pars flaccida and process

Blood Supply and Innervation

A number of arteries supply the principal structures of the tympanic cavity (Fig. 4.**1**). The *inferior tympanic artery* is a branch of the ascending pharyngeal artery that passes through the Jacobson canal, accompanied by a homonymous nerve (Fig. 4.**7**) arising from cranial nerve IX, to supply the middle ear. The *anterior tympanic artery* runs posteriorly from the maxillary artery and enters the middle ear through the petrotympanic fissure, accompanied by the chorda tympani. The *stylomastoid artery* springs from occipital branches of the external carotid artery and runs through the stylomastoid foramen. The *superior tympanic artery* and *petrosal artery* are given off by the middle meningeal artery before it enters the cranial cavity through the foramen spinosum.

The mucosa of the middle ear derives its nerve supply principally from the tympanic plexus of cranial nerve IX (Fig. 4.**7**).

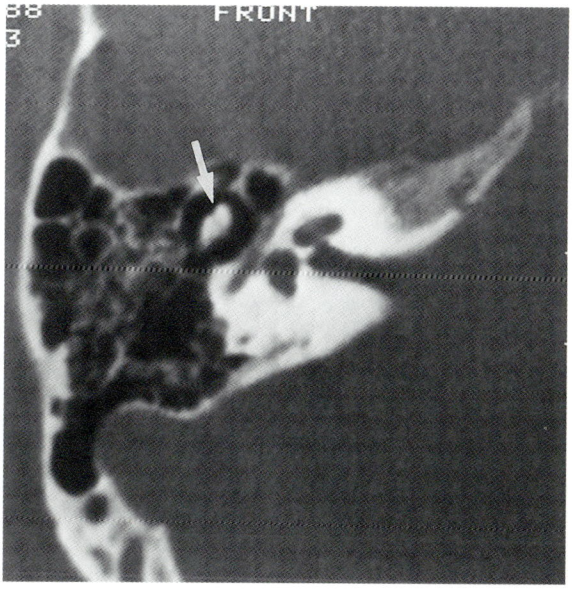

Fig. 4.**3** **Normal middle ear.** Axial CT scan documents the principal landmarks. Note the "ice-cream cone" configuration of the incus and malleus (arrow).

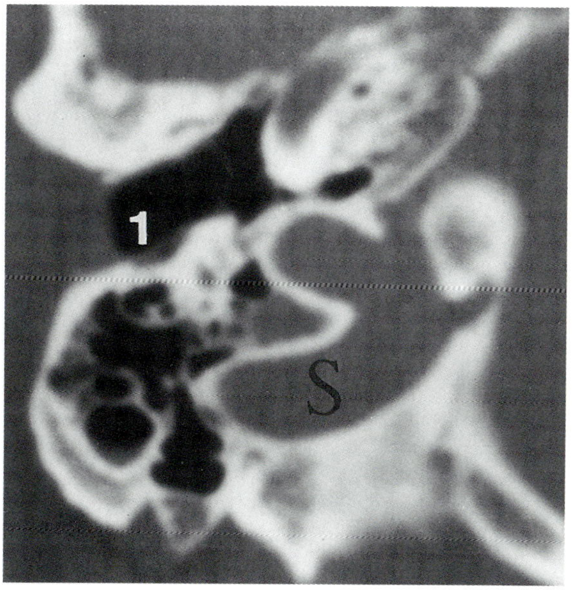

Fig. 4.**4** **Relationship of the sigmoid sinus to the middle ear cavity on the right side.**
1 External auditory canal
S Sigmoid sinus

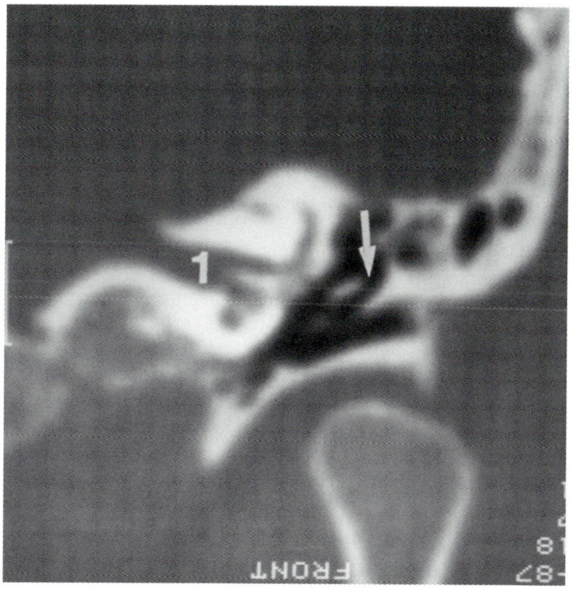

Fig. 4.**5** **Normal coronal section of the middle ear showing the internal auditory canal with Bill's bar and the ossicular chain** (arrows).
1 Internal auditory canal

Facial Nerve (Cranial Nerve VII)

The facial nerve (Fig. 4.**57**) arises from three nuclei in the brainstem. The *motor nucleus*, located in the lower pons, gives origin to the efferent branches that supply the facial muscles. These fibers also provide motor innervation to the posterior belly of the digastric muscle, the stapedius muscle, and the styloid muscle. The *superior salivary nucleus*, lying posterior to the motor nucleus, distributes branches to the lacrimal gland via the superficial petrosal nerve and to the sublingual gland via the chorda tympani. A third nucleus in the medulla gives rise to the *afferent gustatory fibers* (chorda tympani).

The facial nerve arises at the lower border of the pons in a recess between the olive and the superior cerebellar peduncle. It is subdivided into the following segments:

- Intracranial segment.
- Intracanalicular segment.
- Internal auditory canal (Fig. 4.**5**).
- Labyrinthine segment.
- Tympanic segment.
- Mastoid segment.
- Infraforaminal segment.

Within the internal auditory canal (Fig. 4.**5**), the facial nerve relates above to the superior boundary of the canal and below to the falciform crest that separates the facial nerve from cranial nerve VIII. Posteriorly, a vertical crest (Bill's bar, Fig. 4.**5**) separates the facial nerve from the superior vestibular nerve.

The course of the facial nerve can be traced indirectly on CT scans but is defined more clearly on multiplanar MR images, especially in the sagittal plane.

The degree of pneumatization of the temporal bone (Fig. 4.**11**, Table 4.**1**) is variable and depends on a number of factors:

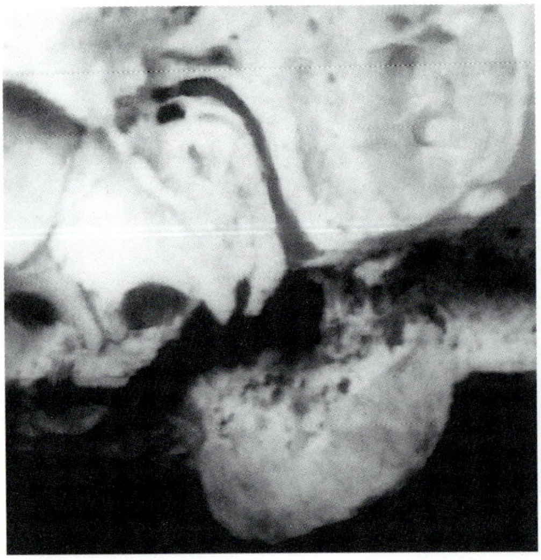

a

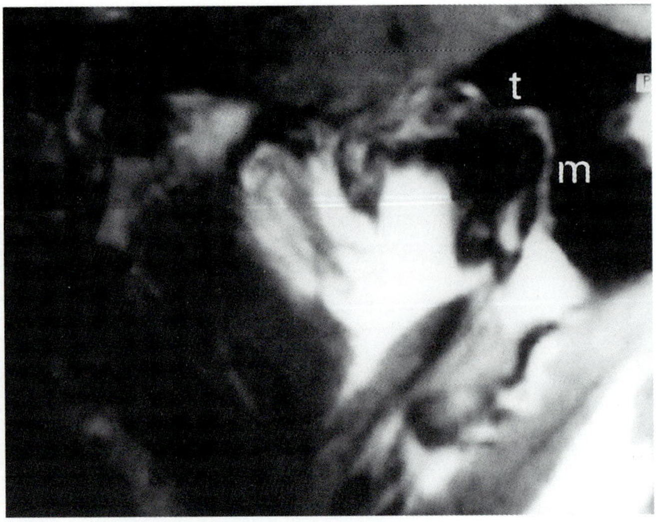

b

Figs. 4.**6 a, b** **Comparison of the tympanic and mastoid segments of the facial nerve:**
(**a**) in a specimen radiograph,
(**b**) in a sagittal T1-weighted MR image.
m Mastoid segment
t Tympanic segment

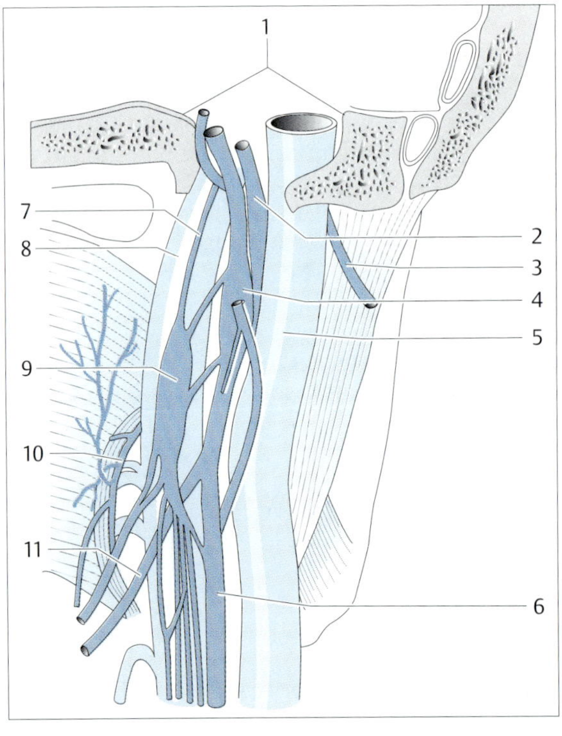

Fig. 4.**7** **Compartments of the jugular foramen.** The pars nervosa, located anteromedially, transmits the inferior petrosal sinus, glossopharyngeal nerve, and Jacob nerve. The pars vascularis, located posterolaterally, contains the jugular bulb, vagus nerve, Arnold nerve, and accessory nerve.
1 Jugular foramen
2 Inferior ganglion of glossopharyngeal nerve
3 Accessory nerve
4 Inferior ganglion of vagus nerve
5 Internal jugular vein
6 Vagus nerve
7 Internal carotid nerve
8 Internal carotid artery
9 Superior cervical ganglion of sympathetic trunk
10 Glossopharyngeal nerve
11 Superior laryngeal nerve

Table 4.1 Pneumatization of the temporal bone
Types: ➤ Completely pneumatized (Fig. 4.**5**) ➤ Partially pneumatized (Figs. 4.**12 a, b**) ➤ Sclerotic (nonpneumatized)
Regions: ➤ Middle ear: —Epitympanum —Mesotympanum —Hypotympanum —Protympanum ➤ Mastoid: —Antrum —Central portions (Fig. 4.**12**) —Peripheral portions (Fig. 4.**11**) ➤ Perilabyrinthine space: —Supralabyrinthine —Infralabyrinthine ➤ Petrous pyramid ➤ Accessory spaces

- Hereditary factors.
- Environment.
- Nutrition.
- Eustachian tube function.
- Frequency of bacterial infections.

The degree of pneumatization ranges from a normal air-cell system to partial or complete nonpneumatization (sclerosis) in which only the antrum and portions of the central mastoid show a variable degree of aeration.

Normally, five pneumatized regions are seen on imaging studies:

- The middle ear (Fig. 4.**1**).
- The mastoid (Fig. 4.**4**).
- The perilabyrinthine region.
- The petrous apex (Fig. 4.**5**).
- Accessory regions.

It should be noted that the mesotympanum can only be indirectly differentiated from the epitympanum and hypotympanum on CT scans.

The mastoid consists of the mastoid antrum, a space that communicates with the epitympanum through the aditus ad antrum, the central mastoid tract, and the peripheral portions of the mastoid. The peripheral portions are differentiated into various systems of air cells. The perilabyrinthine cells may occupy a supralabyrinthine or infralabyrinthine position, depending on their relation to the labyrinth. The petrous apex is pneumatized in 30–35% of all temporal bones. While the pneumatization of the temporal bone is variable in its extent, it is generally symmetric. A partial or complete absence of pneumatization on one side is usually a result of chronic otitis media.

Neurovascular Compartments of the Temporal Bone

The jugular foramen (Table 4.**2**) is anterior, lateral, and inferior in relation to the temporal bone and lies between the petrous portion of the temporal bone and the occipital bone. A fibrous or bony septum divides the jugular foramen into a smaller anteromedial part called the pars nervosa and a larger posterolateral part called the pars vascularis (Fig. 4.**7**). The pars nervosa transmits the inferior petrosal sinus and the glossopharyngeal nerve, which gives origin to a tympanic branch (Jacobson nerve) (Fig. 4.**7**) that supplies the middle ear along with the inferior tympanic artery. The inferior petrosal sinus drains the cavernous sinus. The pars vascularis of the jugular foramen contains the jugular bulb, which links the intracranial sigmoid sinus with the extracranial jugular vein; it also transmits the vagus nerve and accessory nerve (Fig. 4.**7**).

The vagus nerve gives off an accessory auricular branch called the Arnold nerve (Fig. 4.**7**), which supplies the skin of the external ear. The main significance of the Arnold and Jacobson nerves (Fig. 4.**7**) is that they may contain glomus structures.

The jugular foramen is extremely variable in its size and morphology (Figs. 4.**7** and 4.**8**) but is generally outlined by smooth cortical bone, which provides an important imaging criterion. Enlargement of the jugular foramen may occur as a normal variation. Tumor masses (Fig. 4.**9**) or large arteriovenous malformations cause sharp erosive expansion of the cortical margins of the foramen.

The jugular bulb (Figs. 4.**27** and 4.**28**) is also variable in position due to variations in the bony structure separating the jugular bulb from the hypotympanic area. A high jugular bulb may project posterosuperiorly into the region of the internal auditory canal and may mimic a tumor mass at otoscopic examination.

Table 4.2 Contents of the jugular foramen (Figs. 4.**7**–4.**9**)
Pars nervosa (anteromedial part): ➤ Inferior petrosal sinus (Fig. 4.**7**) ➤ Glossopharyngeal nerve (Fig. 4.**7**) ➤ Tympanic branch (Jacob nerve) (Fig. 4.**7**)
Pars vascularis (posterolateral part): ➤ Jugular bulb (Figs. 4.**27**, 4.**28**) ➤ Vagus nerve ➤ Auricular branch (Arnold nerve) (Fig. 4.**7**) ➤ Accessory nerve

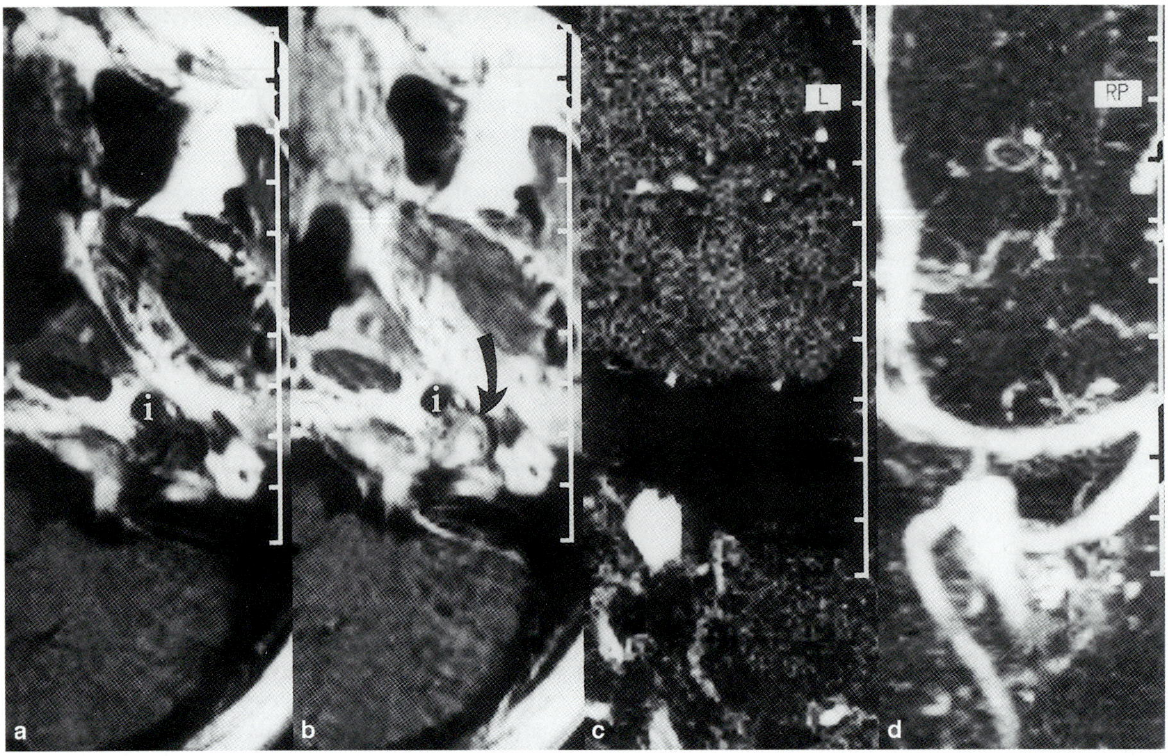

△
Figs. 4.**8 a–d** **Normal appearance of the jugular foramen and jugular bulb.**
(**a**) Noncontrast MR image documents the normal anatomic relationships in a T1-weighted SE sequence. The image shows intermediate signal intensity in the jugular foramen and sigmoid sinus.
(**b**) Gadolinium(Gd)-enhanced MR image shows high signal intensity in the jugular foramen and sigmoid sinus.
i = internal carotid artery
Arrow = jugular foramen
(**c**) MRA (2-D FLASH sequence, TR/TE = 36/10 ms, flip angle = 60°) documents the relative positions of the jugular foramen and jugular bulb, which display high signal intensity in the coronal plane.
(**d**) 3-D reconstruction of the MR angiogram.

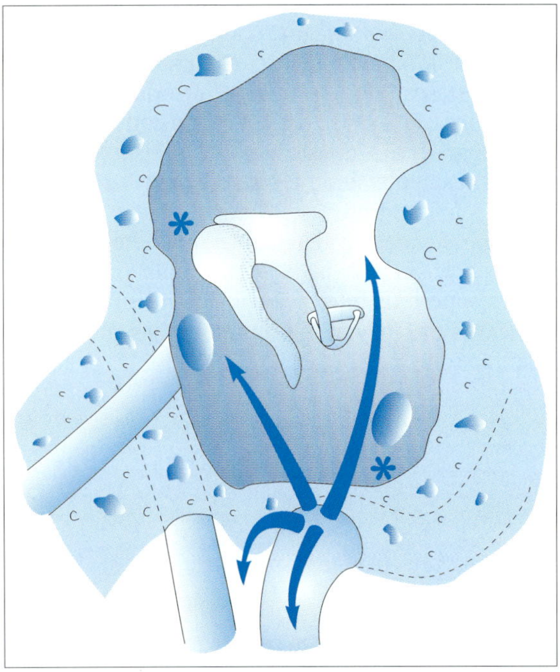

Fig. 4.**9** **Potential routes of spread of glomus jugulare tumors** (after Spector).

Carotid Canal

The internal carotid artery enters the cranium through the carotid canal and leaves the petrous apex above the foramen lacerum on its way to the cavernous sinus. This portion of the artery is accompanied by a sympathetic plexus that gives rise to the deep petrosal nerve. The carotid canal consists of a vertical and horizontal segment. The vertical segment lies below the cochlea, anterior to the jugular foramen and medial to the tympanic cavity. The horizontal segment runs parallel to the eustachian tube and to the canal of the tensor tympani muscle. The carotid canal is subject to far less variation than the jugular foramen. An aberrant internal carotid artery can critically influence the differential diagnosis of vascular masses in the middle ear. If an abnormal soft-tissue density is detected in the middle ear and the normal vertical segment of the carotid canal cannot be visualized, the differential diagnosis should include an aberrant internal carotid artery. Persistence of the stapedial artery is a very rare anomaly.

Hypoglossal Canal

The hypoglossal canal, though technically part of the occipital bone, lies closely adjacent to the jugular foramen. The hypoglossal nerve, a medial branch of the ascending pharyngeal artery, and a venous plexus can be identified within the canal. Rarely, a persistent hypoglossal artery may also be identified.

Table 4.**3** Overview of clinical differential diagnosis in general clinical otology

Otalgia	External ear Inner ear Internal auditory canal Neuralgias (Fig. 4.**24**)
Dysesthesia	External ear Middle ear (Fig. 4.14) Inner ear (Fig. 5.13)
Aural discharge (otorrhea)	External ear (Fig. 4.**10**) Middle ear (Fig. 4.**13**)
Morphologic change	Swelling (Figs. 4.**13**, 4.**36**) Mass lesion (Fig. 4.**10**) Otologic malformations Aural skin changes Otogenic facial paralysis (Fig. 4.**25**) Intracranial otogenic complications

Clinical Signs and Symptoms

This section reviews the main clinical manifestations that are associated with diseases of the middle-ear (Figs. 4.**13** and 4.**23**), external auditory canal, and mastoid, including disorders of the auditory apparatus, balance disorders, and the symptoms associated with facial nerve pathology (Fig. 4.**26**).

Clinical Differential Diagnosis of Hearing Disorders

The clinical differential diagnosis in general clinical otology covers the range of signs and symptoms listed in Table 4.**3**.

The two broad categories in the differential diagnosis of hearing disorders are conductive hearing loss due to middle ear pathology and sensorineural hearing loss due to inner ear pathology. The following discussions include middle ear disorders such as acute or chronic conductive hearing loss.

Clinical Symptoms

Acute hearing loss:
- Conductive hearing loss.
- Sensorineural hearing loss.
- Traumatic.

Chronic hearing loss:
- Tinnitus.
- Fluctuant hearing loss.
- Pediatric hearing loss.

Differential Diagnosis of Lesions Causing Peripheral Facial Nerve Palsy (Bell Palsy) (Fig. 4.**24**)

The clinical manifestations of idiopathic facial nerve palsy (Bell palsy) (Fig. 4.**24** and Table 4.**4**) are characterized by an abrupt onset followed by spontaneous recovery within 6 to 8 weeks. Most cases have a viral cause based on inflammation of the geniculate ganglion leading to swelling and nerve compression in noncompliant portions of the fallopian canal.

The clinical manifestations of sensory and motor dysfunction indicate the site of the facial nerve lesion. Lesions outside the stylomastoid foramen cause paralysis of the mimetic muscles. With more proximal lesions of the facial nerve trunk, this paralysis is often accompanied by hypoacusis and loss of taste sensation. Lesions of the motor roots and geniculate ganglion cause decreased lacrimation in addition to the above symptoms.

Table 4.**4** Clinical differential diagnosis of idiopathic facial nerve palsy

- Inflammatory/toxic-allergic (Fig. 4.**24**)
- Ramsay-Hunt syndrome: associated with herpes zoster of geniculate ganglion (Fig. 4.**25**)
- Millard–Gubler syndrome
- Crossed paralysis due to pontine lesion
- Direct trauma to facial nerve (Fig. 4.**38**)
- Facial nerve tumor (Fig. 4.**26**)

Imaging Evaluation and Differential Diagnosis

Conventional Radiography

The initial imaging procedure is conventional radiography (Fig. 5.**12 a**). The basic study is usually the Schüller view, which can quickly document the extent of inflammatory or neoplastic involvement, especially in the regions of the tympanic cavity and mastoid. While plain radiographs do not provide very high diagnostic accuracy, they will quickly disclose any middle ear effusion, destruction due to cholesteatoma, or mastoiditis-associated changes and direct the planning of further imaging procedures.

Computed Tomography (CT)

The primary imaging modality at present is HRCT using a 1-mm slice thickness in axial and coronal sections (Figs. 5.**11 a, b**). The primary acquisition of the data set should be supplemented by isolated digital enlargement of the bilateral structures (Fig. 5.**11 b**). If noncontrast CT does not show significant infiltration of adjacent structures such as the inner ear, middle cranial fossa, or sigmoid sinus, generally there is no need to proceed with contrast-enhanced scans. Intravenous contrast is essential, however, to confirm suspicion of a primary hypervascular mass lesion or to detect accompanying neoplastic or inflammatory changes in the adjacent structures of the middle skull base.

Magnetic Resonance Imaging (MRI)

The indications for the primary or secondary use of MRI should be considered separately. The primary use of MRI may be justified in the differential diagnosis of a suspected hypervascular mass lesion of the tympanic cavity, depending on the treatment modality being considered. A classic example is a bluish mass noted behind the tympanic membrane during the clinical examination. These cases should be investigated by high-resolution MRI (256 x 512 matrix, 3-mm slice thickness) using T1- and T2-weighted spin-echo (SE) sequences.

The intravenous administration of a paramagnetic contrast agent such as gadolinium (Gd)-DTPA is essential. The recommended study for differentiating a hemangioma from a glomus tumor is a dynamic turbo-FLASH T1-weighted MR sequence following a high-dose injection of paramagnetic contrast (0.3 mmol/kg bw). This study can be supplemented by arterial MR angiography (MRA) and venous angiography to define the relation of tumor masses to key arterial and venous structures and disclose any variations in the arterial and venous system (Figs. 4.**7** and 4.**8**).

Imaging Findings

Congenital Variations and Malformations

The occurrence and morphologic features of malformation syndromes of the middle ear, external auditory canal, and mastoid have changed markedly relative to cases seen during the past 30 years, especially in Europe. The typical clinical and radiologic anomalies induced by thalidomide use during early pregnancy have now given way to a variety of spontaneously occurring malformation syndromes.

Malformation of the Temporal Bone

In exploring the differential diagnosis of petrous malformations (Figs. 5.**7** – 5.**10**), we shall follow the classification in Table 4.**5**, which lists the anomalies in the order of their frequency and differentiates them into anomalies of the sound conduction system, membranous labyrinth, internal auditory canal, facial nerve, and vascular anomalies. The brief review in this section will be expanded upon in subsequent chapters.

HRCT is the primary imaging study for diagnosing anomalies of the sound conduction system. High-resolution MRI is best for detecting anomalies of the membranous labyrinth, inner ear, and internal auditory canal.

The basic approach to the diagnosis of temporal bone anomalies is to identify all possible affected spaces along with their contents and key structures and to describe and document the morphologic changes (Table 4.**6**).

Dysplasias of the external auditory canal are based on a failure of canalization of the epithelial cells. These deformities are more common in males and are bilateral in 29% of cases. Atresia of the external ear canal may occur as an isolated phenomenon but is commonly associated with various genetic syndromes including mandibulofacial dysostosis (Treacher–Collins syndrome), craniofacial dysostosis (Crouzon syndrome), and Goldenhar dysplasia (Fig. 5.**10**). The atresia may be bony or membranous, complete or incomplete. Cases with bony overgrowth and temporal bone deformity usually involve a bony atresia plate (Table 4.**7**).

Malformations and Variations of the Middle Ear

The cardinal symptom of middle ear anomalies and variations is conductive hearing loss. Fenestral otosclerosis is an important differential diagnosis in patients with this type of hearing impairment. Lack of progression of the hearing loss is considered pathognomonic for ossicular dysplasia.

Clinically, the most common ossicular deformity is fusion of the malleus and incus within the attic, resulting in absence of a normal incudomalleolar joint. Axial CT in these cases will demonstrate a normal ossicular configuration (Fig. 4.**5**), with close analysis revealing absence of an incudomalleolar joint line. In patients with an atresia plate, the manubrium of the malleus may be absent or deformed. A great variety of ossicular anomalies are described in the literature, and malformations of the auditory ossicles and round window tend to show varied and unique patterns in different individuals. Detailed visualization of the stapes is essential from a clinical and surgical standpoint. Overlapping axial scans at the level of the oval window should provide the necessary delineation.

Incudostapedial discontinuities are the most common congenital ossicular anomalies. In most cases the long process of the incus is absent or set too far posteriorly. Isolated congenital malformations of the oval window are rare and may be bilateral. When present, they are usually associated with ossicular anomalies.

The most common variations of the middle ear are disturbances of pneumatization, which are usually detected incidentally on CT or MRI (Figs. 4.**11** and 4.**12**).

Table 4.5 Anomalies of the temporal bone: general classification

Anomalies of the sound conduction system
- External auditory canal:
  - Stenosis
  - Agenesis
  - Bony or membranous atresia plate
- Auricle:
  - Microtia, possibly combined with other malformations
- Mastoid:
  - Hypoplasia
  - Atresia
- Middle ear:
  - Hypoplasia
  - Atresia

Anomalies of the membranous labyrinth (Fig. 5.**9**) or cochlea (Fig. 5.**7 b**)

Anomalies of the internal auditory canal (Fig. 5.**11**)

Anomalies of the facial nerve (Fig. 4.**6**):
- Ectopia
- Abnormal course
- Hypoplasia

Congenital vascular anomalies:
- High jugular bulb (Figs. 4.**27, 4.29**)
- Intratympanic jugular bulb
- Ectopic intratemporal course of internal carotid artery
- Persistent stapedial artery
- Aberrant middle meningeal artery

Rare lesions:
- Congenital obliterative labyrinthitis
- Dilated aqueduct

Table 4.6 Types of malformation syndromes

External auditory canal:
- Stenosis
- Atresia plate
- Atresia

Tympanic cavity:
- Agenesis
- Aplasia
- Deformation of epitympanic, tympanic, and hypotympanic space
- Ossicular malformations

Table 4.7 Evaluation of dysplasias of the external auditory canal, tympanic bone, and mastoid

Type of dysplasia:
- Bony
- Membranous
- Mixed
- Stenosis

Status of atresia plate:
- Complete
- Incomplete (determine thickness)

Pneumatization (Figs. 4.**11, 4.12**)

Size of middle ear cleft (Fig. 4.**1**)

Status of ossicular chain (Figs. 4.**2, 4.5**):
- Incudemalledar articulation
- Malleus
- Incus
- Stapes

Status of labyrinthine windows:
- Round window
- Oval window

Status of inner ear structures:
- Cochlea (Fig. 5.**7 b**)
- Vestibule (Fig. 5.**9**)
- Semicircular canals (Fig. 5.**9**)
- Internal auditory canal (Fig. 5.**11**)
- Aqueduct

Position of sigmoid sinus (Figs. 4.**4, 4.8 b**)

Position of jugular bulb (Fig. 4.**28**)

Location of mandibular condyle (Fig. 11.**7**)

Identification of facial nerve (Fig. 4.**6**)

Tumors

External Auditory Canal

Benign Tumors

The terms *keratosis obturans* and *cholesteatoma of the external auditory canal* are often used synonymously for a process involving an accumulation of keratin debris in the bony portions of the external auditory canal. Keratosis obturans mainly affects patients under 40 years of age and is associated with significant otalgia and conductive hearing loss. Otorrhea is uncommon. Imaging demonstrates widening of the bony external auditory canal. Cholesteatoma of the external auditory canal occurs in patients from 40 to 75 years of age and tends to be unilateral. Most patients have chronic pain and persistent otorrhea, and hearing loss is rare. The tympanic membrane usually appears normal.

Exostoses of the external auditory canal most commonly affect males. The lesions consist of fixed, multinodular bony outgrowths, which generally are induced by prolonged irritation of the canal, often by excessive contact with cold seawater ("surfer's ear"). The lesions are frequently bilateral and may cause conductive hearing loss. Rare cases present with complete occlusion of the ear canal.

Osteomas are solitary, unilateral, pedunculated bony growths occurring lateral to the isthmus. Osteomas are far less common than exostoses and may occur in extracanalicular portions of the temporal bone and in the mastoid. CT is the primary tool for diagnostic evaluation.

Malignant Tumors

A number of malignant tumors originate in, or adjacent to, the external auditory canal. The most common neoplasms are *squamous cell carcinoma, basal cell carcinoma*, and *tumors arising from the parotid gland. Malignant melanoma, sarcoma, glioma*, and *metastatic lesions* also occur but are generally far less common. Basal cell carcinoma usually arises on the auricle and involves the external auditory canal secondarily, whereas squamous cell carcinoma tends to involve the external meatus and canal directly. These tumors may also originate in the middle ear of patients with a long history of chronic otitis media (Fig. 4.**13**). Salivary gland tumors may arise within the canal of the middle ear (from the lesser salivary glands) or may arise directly from the parotid gland (Fig. 4.**10**). Besides the clinical examination, diagnosis relies mainly on CT, which guides the planning of an appropriate treatment strategy such as surgery or radiotherapy. Other adenomatous tumors of the external auditory canal are:

- Adenoma.
- Adenocarcinoma.
- Adenoid cystic carcinoma.
- Pleomorphic adenoma.

CT findings are generally nonspecific but can define the extent of the tumor for planning therapeutic intervention (Fig. 4.**10**).

Middle Ear

Facial Nerve Neuroma (Fig. 4.**26**)

The clinical manifestations of facial nerve neuroma depend on the location and size of the tumor. Generally there is a loss of facial nerve function, often associated with mixed conductive and sensorineural hearing loss. The CT appearance is that of a *tubular mass* expanding the facial nerve canal. A *schwannoma* may occur in the cerebellopontine angle–internal carotid artery area and mimic the morphology of an acoustic neuroma (Figs. 5.**17** – 5.**20**). T1-weighted MRI demonstrates an enhancing tubular mass causing expansion of the facial nerve canal.

Facial neuroma in younger patients may be mistaken for *congenital cholesteatoma*, which also occasionally grows along the facial nerve canal. When a mass is found in the internal auditory canal–cerebellopontine angle area, the facial nerve canal should be closely inspected for involvement of the first genu, which is a distinctive feature of facial nerve neuroma.

Hemangioma (and Ossifying Hemangioma)

Clinically, a hemangioma of the middle ear is often associated with *progressive peripheral facial nerve palsy* and sometimes with *pulsatile tinnitus*. CT shows an intensely enhancing mass with a spiculated appearance and intratumoral calcifications that may represent bone flecks. The most common site of involvement is the labyrinthine segment of the facial nerve. MRI shows an intensely enhancing, invasive mass tracking along the facial nerve canal. Focal masses are also found in the geniculate fossa or the labyrinthine segment of the facial nerve. The main lesions requiring differentiation in this area are facial nerve neuroma and idiopathic facial nerve palsy (Bell palsy).

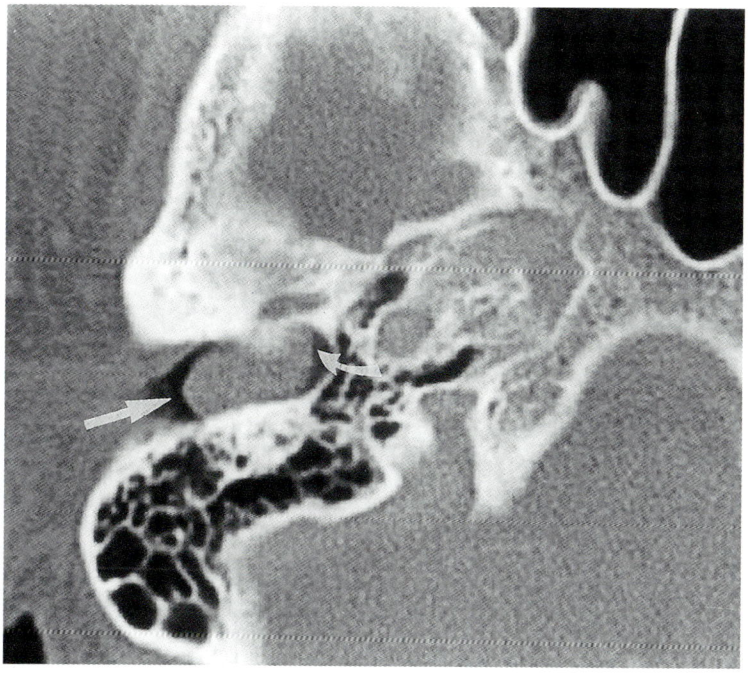

Fig. 4.**10** **Polyp in the external auditory canal.** Axial noncontrast CT scan demonstrates a well-circumscribed polypous mass in the internal auditory canal with a density of 70 HU. There is no evidence of bone destruction.

Arrow	Lateral margin of mass
Curved arrow	Tympanic margin of mass

Paragangliomas

Paragangliomas of the middle ear (glomus tympanicum tumors) (Fig. 4.**16**) are the most common primary tumor of the middle ear cavity and the second most common tumor of the temporal bone. Paragangliomas are an important differential diagnosis in evaluations of the jugular foramen.

The following main types of paraganglioma (glomus tumor) are recognized:

- Glomus tympanicum.
- Glomus hypotympanicum.
- Glomus jugulare (Fig. 4.**29**).
- Glomus parapharyngeale (Fig. 4.**30 a**).

Radiologic studies are of key importance, as glomus tumors are highly vascular lesions with a complex pattern of infiltration and spread. The glomus jugulare tumor (Figs. 4.**29** and 4.**30**) is characterized by asymmetric dilatation of the jugular foramen on the plain skull radiograph. Because the tumor must attain considerable size before producing this sign, contrast-enhanced CT has largely replaced plain films in diagnosis. The rich vascularity of the tumor is evident on CT angiography (CTA), which demonstrates rapid, intense enhancement over the position of the glomus jugulare tumor followed by a gradual washout phase.

On MRI, T2-weighted SE sequences of glomus tumors show significantly prolonged T2 relaxation times with a high signal intensity, while T1-weighted SE sequences show a low signal intensity based on the shortened T1 relaxation times (Fig. 4.**30 b**). Another criterion is the granular signal structure produced by flow voids within the mass.

Dynamic contrast-enhanced MRI shows a rapid rise of signal intensity within the tumor. When a triple dosage of paramagnetic contrast is administered, a specific dropout effect is reproducibly observed. Venous MRA should also be performed to confirm a glomus tumor and exclude a variation of the jugular bulb (Figs. 4.**27**, 4.**28**, 4.**30 c**). Generally this study will demonstrate the tumor as a soft-tissue mass devoid of flow phenomena.

Congenital Cholesteatoma

Primary cholesteatoma (Figs. 4.**18** and 4.**19**), known also as *epidermoid*, accounts for just 2% of all cholesteatomas of the middle ear cavity. They are thought to arise from aberrant embryonic epithelial rests and thus are identical to other intracranial or intradiploetic epidermoid lesions. The principal intracranial sites are the cerebellopontine angle and suprasellar cistern. Intradiploetic lesions occur primarily at the junction of the calvaria and skull base.

Congenital cholesteatomas have been described at the following sites within the temporal bone:

- Petrous apex.
- Mastoid.
- Middle ear cavity (Figs. 4.**18**, 4.**19**).
- External auditory canal.

A cholesteatoma that occurs behind an intact tympanic membrane in a patient with no history of otitis media is termed a congenital cholesteatoma. The most common site of origin in the middle ear cavity is the epitympanum (Fig. 4.**18**) near the incudostapedial joint.

Primary Carcinoma

Primary malignant tumors of the middle ear are rare in adult patients. They consist of *squamous cell carcinoma*, various types of *adenocarcinoma*, and *adenoid cystic carcinoma*. Squamous cell carcinomas are more common in males, while adenocarcinomas are documented with equal frequency in both sexes. The most common radiologic change is bone destruction, more extensive than that associated with simple chronic otitis media (Fig. 4.**13**).

Metastases

Most metastatic lesions infiltrate the middle ear and mastoid from the petrous apex (Figs. 4.**33** and 4.**35**). The *most common primary tumors* are:

- Breast carcinoma.
- Bronchial carcinoma.
- Renal carcinoma.
- Prostatic tumors.
- Head and neck tumors.
- Gastric carcinoma.

Diffuse metastases can develop at other sites through hematogenous dissemination, which most commonly results from bone marrow infiltration. CT may demonstrate either an osteoplastic or osteolytic type of growth.

Rhabdomyosarcoma

Rhabdomyosarcoma is a highly malignant but rare mesenchymal neoplasm of childhood (below 5 years of age). The tumors are classified pathologically as *embryonic*, *alveolar*, or *pleomorphic*, the embryonic type being the most common. While 50% of rhabdomyosarcomas occur in the head and neck region, only 7% involve the middle ear. The clinical features include painless bloody otorrhea, facial nerve palsy, and symptoms referable to concomitant cranial neuropathies. Imaging studies usually reveal significant bone destruction.

Although this tumor is rare, it is the most common primary middle ear tumor in the pediatric age group.

Histiocytosis X

While histiocytosis X is not a neoplasm in the true sense, it may occur as an infiltrative mass lesion of the middle ear. Two principal forms have been described:

- Infantile form (Abt–Letterer–Siwe disease, Hand–Schüller–Christian disease).
- Eosinophilic granuloma in older children.

Involvement of the tympanic bone is most common in Hand–Schüller–Christian disease. This involvement is unknown in Abt–Letterer–Siwe disease and is extremely rare with eosinophilic granuloma. Sixty-eight percent of patients are less than 10 years old and present clinically with otitis media or otitis externa. Typically there is extensive osteolysis with no clinical evidence of cranial nerve involvement.

Other Neoplasms

Certain neoplasms of the middle ear are known only from isolated reports. It is not too unusual to find middle ear involvement by *lymphoma*, *giant-cell tumor*, *meningioma* (Fig. 4.**17**), *multiple myeloma* (Fig. 4.**33**), and *osteoblastoma*. Because of their generally low incidence, however, specific imaging characteristics have not been established for these neoplasms (Figs. 4.**14** and 4.**16**).

Inflammatory Lesions

Inflammatory Diseases of the External Auditory Canal

Simple inflammation of the external ear canal is a common condition that does not require imaging evaluation. *Malignant otitis externa*, however, is a severe infectious process that is common in older patients with insulin-dependent diabetes, and in immunosuppressed patients. The principal causative organism is the gram-negative bacterium *Pseudomonas aeruginosa*. Inadequately treated, the infection can destroy cartilage, bone and soft tissues. The disease begins at the chondro-osseous junction of the external auditory canal. CT is best for evaluating the precise extent of the disease and the involvement of the skull base.

Manifestations of Inflammatory Middle Ear Disease

Eustachian tube dysfunction is the primary cause of nearly all types of inflammatory middle ear disease. The manifestations discussed below are middle ear effusion (Fig. 4.**13**), acute otitis media (Fig. 4.**13**), granulation tissue formation (Fig. 4.**16**), noncholesteatomatous ossicular erosion, and acquired cholesteatoma (Figs. 4.**18** and 4.**19**).

Acute Otitis Media

Acute otitis media (Fig. 4.**13**) is not an indication for primary diagnostic imaging, although middle ear effusion is often detected incidentally in imaging studies. While common in children, its presence in adults warrants exclusion of a nasopharyngeal neoplasm. Middle ear effusion is also seen in patients with deficient pneumatization of the middle ear spaces. CT demonstrates a horizontal fluid level, depending on the patient's position, and MRI shows the fluid effusion as an area of increased T2-weighted signal intensity (Figs. 4.**23 b, c**).

Granulation Tissue in the Tympanic Cavity

Granulation tissue frequently develops as an isolated phenomenon (Fig. 4.**16**) but may also form in association with effusions and cholesteatomas. CT shows an area of increased density that is without a fluid level unless bleeding is present. Cholesterol granuloma, a postinflammatory granulation tissue composed of cholesterol crystals, is an important entity requiring differentiation from cholesteatoma (Figs. 4.**18** and 4.**19**).

Retraction of the tympanic membrane may occur after prolonged middle ear disease. This phenomenon appears on CT scans as a medial retraction of the tympanic membrane and may be associated with ossicular erosions.

Noncholesteatomatous Ossicular Erosion

Ossicular erosion may be detected in the setting of various tumotympanic diseases. It may be seen in chronic otitis media (Fig. 4.**13**) without a cholesteatoma or in association with a retracted tympanic membrane. Stapedial erosions are common, while the head of the malleus and body of the incus are affected much less frequently. Isolated cases of incudomalleolar discontinuity may occur.

Table 4.**8** Complications of cholesteatomas of the middle skull base: intracranial complications

- Meningitis
- Abscess formation
- Venous sinus thrombosis
- Cerebrospinal fluid (CSF) fistula
- Temporal bone:
  - –Labyrinthine fistula
  - –Facial nerve palsy (Figs. 4.**24**, 4.**25**)
  - –Cochlear involvement
  - –Ossicular destruction

Acquired Cholesteatoma

By definition, cholesteatoma (Figs. 4.**18** and 4.**19**) is a saccular accumulation of squamous and keratin debris occurring in the middle ear and other pneumatized portions of the temporal bone. Acquired cholesteatoma may originate from the pars flaccida or pars tensa of the tympanic membrane, and it may be caused by any form of acute or chronic otitis media (Fig. 4.**13**). Pars flaccida cholesteatoma originates in the Prussak space, which opens posteriorly into the epitympanum.

The imaging procedure of choice is CT scanning in the axial and coronal planes. These scans will demonstrate the cholesteatomatous tissue as a primary low-density area and will define areas of bony and cartilaginous erosion. All cases should be scrutinized for possible involvement of vascular spaces and portions of the middle skull base. An important imaging issue is the detection of complications, which are listed in Table 4.**8**.

Imaging Criteria and Their Differential Diagnosis

Tumor Mass in the External Auditory Canal (Table 4.**9**)

A tumor mass in the external auditory canal should be diagnosed clinically, hence the role of diagnostic imaging is not so much detection of the lesion as aiding in its benign-malignant differentiation. The most common external auditory canal mass is a benign polyp (Fig. 4.**10**), which always requires histologic evaluation.

Increased Pneumatization of the Temporal Bone (Table 4.**10**)

Increased pneumatization is usually first noted on conventional radiographs (Schüller view), appearing as a collection of well-circumscribed lucent areas within a normal or pathologically enlarged mastoid bone. CT shows areas of approximately zero attenuation commonly located in the petrous apex (Fig. 4.**11**). On MRI, increased pneumatization produces low signal intensity in both T1- and T2-weighted sequences (Fig. 4.**12 b**). By contrast, decreased pneumatization appears as geometric zones of increased signal intensity in T1-weighted SE sequences (Fig. 4.**12**).

Liquid Lesions in the Tympanic Cavity and Mastoid (Table 4.**11**)

A conspicuous fluid collection can usually be detected even on conventional Schüller radiographs, but most liquid lesions are identified by their fluid-equivalent attenuation values on CT scans (Fig. 4.**13 a**) or by their increased signal intensity on T2-weighted MR images (Fig. 4.**13 b**).

Faintly Enhancing Solid Tumor Mass in the Tympanic Cavity (Table 4.**12**)

Whenever a tumor mass is visualized with CT or MRI, contrast-enhanced scans should be obtained to differentiate between lesions with high and low perfusion. Table 4.**12** lists the middle ear masses—adenoma being the most common (Fig. 4.**14**)—that show minimal contrast enhancement and the criteria that are useful in their differential diagnosis.

Table 4.**9** Tumor mass in the external auditory canal

Findings	**Differential diagnostic criteria**
Common:	
➤ Carcinoma	
—Squamous cell carcinoma	Destruction
—Basal cell carcinoma	Invasion
➤ Melanoma	Signal characteristics
➤ Metastasis	Destruction
➤ Exostosis	Density, signal
➤ Polyp (Fig. 4.**10**)	Density, absence of destruction
Rare:	
➤ Tumor	
➤ Fibroma (Fig. 4.**20 a**)	Margins
➤ Adenoma	Homogeneity

Table 4.**10** Etiology of increased pneumatization of the temporal bone

Common finding in:
- ➤ Acromegaly
- ➤ Adrenogenital syndrome
- ➤ Dyke–Davidoff–Masson syndrome
- ➤ Lipodystrophy

Table 4.**11** Fluid collections in the tympanic cavity or mastoid

Findings	**Differential diagnostic criteria**
Serous fluid in the middle ear (Fig. 4.**13**):	Density
➤ Irritative effusion	
➤ Inflammatory cause	
Hemorrhagic fluid:	
➤ Trauma (Figs. 4.**38**, 4.**40**)	Density, bone
Fluid isodense to CSF:	
➤ Traumatic dural leak	Density

Table 4.**12** Faintly enhancing tumor mass in the tympanic cavity

Findings	**Differential diagnostic criteria**
Variation:	
➤ Cyst	Density, margins, rim enhancement
Tumor:	
➤ Adenoma (Fig. 4.**14**) (degree of differentiation)	Margins
➤ Cholesterol granuloma	
➤ Rare benign tumors	
Inflammation:	
➤ Inflammatory polyp	Morphology, contrast enhancement

Intensely Enhancing (Hypervascular) Solid Tumor Mass in the Tympanic Cavity (Table 4.**13**)

Whenever an intensely enhancing mass is detected in the tympanic cavity, the primary diagnosis to be considered is hemangioma or paraganglioma. Extensions of a meningioma may also show intense contrast enhancement (Fig. 4.**17**), as may any acute or subacute inflammatory process. Glomus tympanicum tumor is the most common intensely enhancing middle ear mass (Fig. 4.**15**), followed by hypervascular granulation tissue (Fig. 4.**16**). Rare lesions include infiltrating neuromatous tissue or infiltration by a heavily vascularized meningioma (Fig. 4.**17**).

Erosion or Destruction of the Temporal Bone (Tympanic Cavity, Middle Ear, Mastoid) (Table 4.**14**)

Erosion or destruction of the temporal bone is a finding that can generally be verified by HRCT or, in severe cases, by conventional radiography (Figs. 4.**13 a**, 4.**18**–4.**20**, 4.**33 a**).

Clinical studies most commonly reveal primary or acquired cholesteatoma (Figs. 4.**18** and 4.**19**), acute or chronic otitis media (Fig. 4.**13**), or chronic mastoiditis (Fig. 4.**36**).

Table 4.**13** Intensity enhancing tumor mass in the tympanic cavity

Findings	**Differential diagnostic criteria**
Variation:	
➤ Dehiscent jugular bulb (Figs. 4.**27**, 4.**28**)	Topography
➤ Aberrant internal carotid artery	Vascular
➤ Stapedial artery	
Tumor:	
➤ Paraganglioma (Fig. 4.**15**)	Vascularity
➤ Neuroma (Fig. 4.**26**)	Morphology
➤ Meningioma (Fig. 4.**17**)	Contrast enhancement
➤ Cholesterol granuloma	Signal intensity, density
Inflammation:	
➤ Hypervascularized granulation tissue (Fig. 4.**16**)	Contrast enhancement

Table 4.**14** Erosion or destruction of the temporal bone

Findings	**Differential diagnostic criteria**
Common:	
➤ Cholesteatoma (Figs. 4.**18, 4.19**)	Destruction
➤ Mastoiditis, acute or chronic (Fig. 4.**36**)	Fluid
➤ Chronic otitis (Fig. 4.**13**)	Topography
➤ Postsurgical defects (Fig. 4.**23**)	
➤ Mastoidectomy (Fig. 4.**34**)	
➤ Squelae to trauma (Figs. 4.**38**, 4.**40**)	
➤ Cholesterol granuloma	Density
Rare:	
➤ Tumor:	Morphology
–Primary osseous: benign, malignant	
–Neurogenic: neuroma (Fig. 4.**26**)	Morphology
histiocytosis X	Density
dermoid cyst	
carcinoma: external auditory canal	
–Secondary: metastasis (Figs. 4.**35**, 5.**14**)	
Nasopharynx: carcinoma (Fig. 5.**24**)	
➤ Inflammation:	
➤ External otitis media	
➤ Granuloma (tuberculosis)	

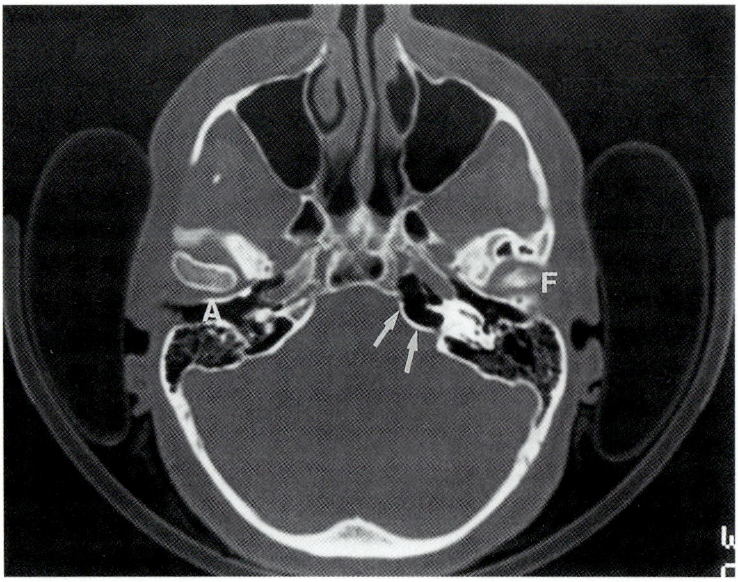

Fig. 4.**11** **Normal variant of petrous apex pneumatization.** Bone-algorithm CT scan at the level of the mandibular condyles shows increased pneumatization of the petrous apex (arrows), particularly on the left side.
A External auditory canal
F Mandibular fossa

Osteosclerotic Process of the Temporal Bone (Table 4.**15**)

The imaging appearance of an osteosclerotic process of the temporal bone is usually based on CT findings and less commonly on MRI (Figs. 4.**20**, 4.**21**), which is superior for demonstrating concomitant soft-tissue changes. Frequent causes are fibrous dysplasia, Paget disease, osteogenesis imperfecta, and other metabolic or neoplastic diseases. Osteosclerotic processes of the temporal bone include obliterative fenestral otosclerosis with oval window involvement (Figs. 4.**21** and 4.**22**) and artificial implants (Fig. 4.**23**).

Table 4.**15** Osteosclerotic process of the temporal bone

Findings	Differential diagnostic criteria
Common:	
➤ Fibrous dysplasia	Morphology
➤ Osteogenesis imperfecta	
➤ Paget disease	Morphology
➤ Obliterative fenestral otosclerosis (Fig. 4.**21**)	Topography
➤ Metallic implants (Fig. 4.**23**)	Density
➤ Tumor: —Osteogenic —Chondrogenic —Metastatic (Fig. 4.**35**)	Morphology
Rare:	
➤ Cleidocranial dysplasia	
➤ Hurler syndrome	
➤ Osteopetrosis	

Enhancing Facial Nerve Lesion with No Mass Effect (Tables 4.**16** and 4.**17**)

The radiologic evaluation of facial nerve lesions (Fig. 4.**6**) should include the following differential diagnoses. Most common are idiopathic (infectious, Fig. 4.**24**), posttraumatic, and postoperative lesions; involvement by erosive cholesteatoma; anomalies; and primary (Fig. 4.**26**) or secondary tumors. Differentiation relies on the analysis of morphology, topography, and destructive changes as in malignant otitis externa. Herpes zoster infection (Fig. 4.**25**) generally shows a distinctive pattern of contrast enhancement along multiple segments of the facial nerve (Fig. 4.**25**).

Tumor Mass of the Facial Nerve

(Table 4.**18**)

A common facial nerve tumor is the *schwannoma* that may occur anywhere along the course of the nerve (Fig. 4.**27**). *Meningioma*, on the other hand, tends to affect the proximal segment of the fallopian canal. *Hemangiomas* and *hamartomas* most commonly involve the mastoid and are identified by their specific signal characteristics or attenuation values.

a

b

c

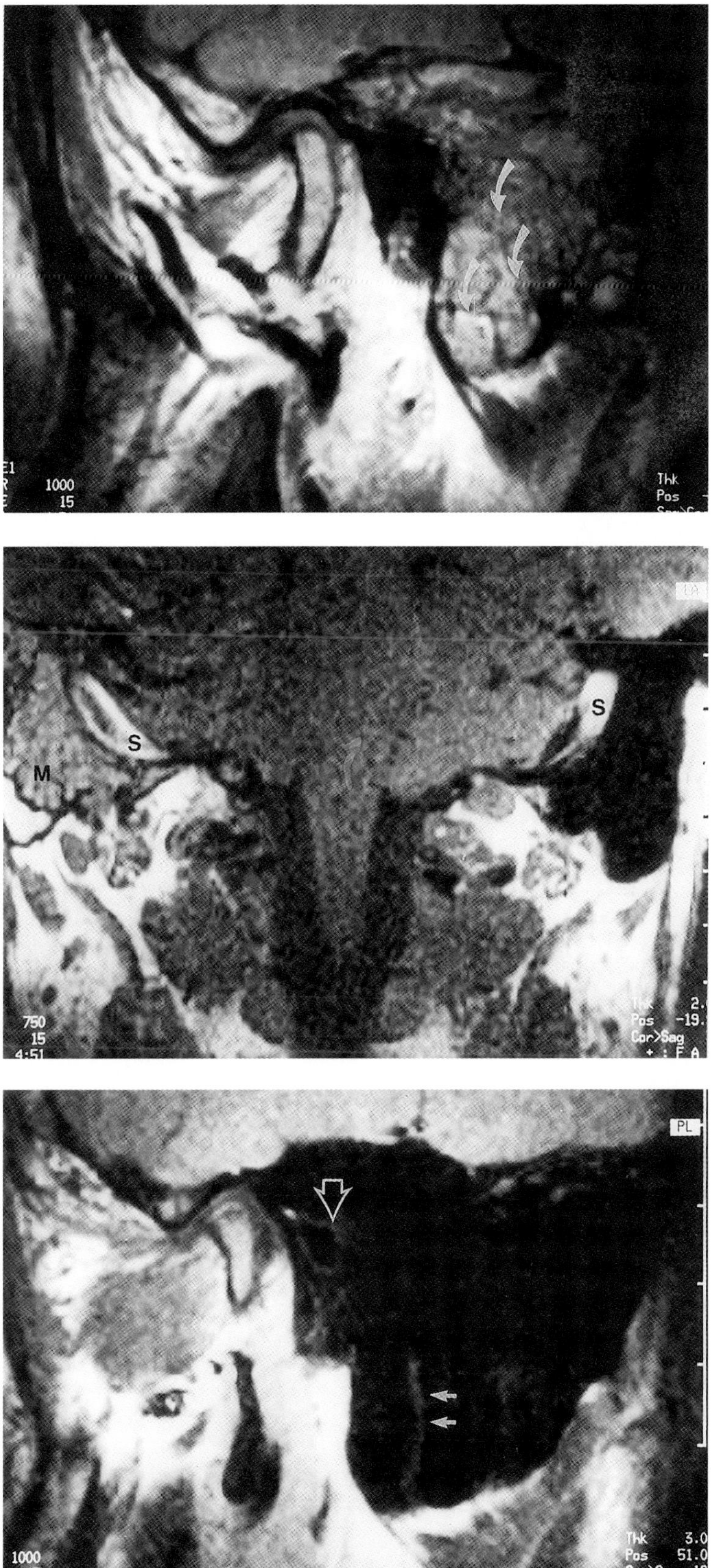

Figs. 4.**12 a – c** **Side-to-side comparison of MR images showing unilateral underaeration of the mastoid.**
(**a**) Sagittal T1-weighted MR image (TR/TE = 1000/15 ms) on the right side shows multiple lobulated areas of high signal intensity representing nonaerated portions of the mastoid (arrows). The image shows normal aeration of the middle ear and a temporomandibular joint of normal appearance.
(**b**) Coronal T1-weighted MR image (TR/TE = 700/15 ms) documents the underaeration of the right mastoid relative to the left side. High flow is visible in the sigmoid sinus.
M Mastoid
S Sigmoid sinus
(**c**) Sagittal T1-weighted MR image (TR/TE = 1000/15 ms) on the left side shows normal low signal intensity of the aerated mastoid and middle ear spaces. The mucosa of the external auditory canal shows moderately increased signal intensity (open arrow).
Note the intramastoid segment of the facial nerve (arrows).

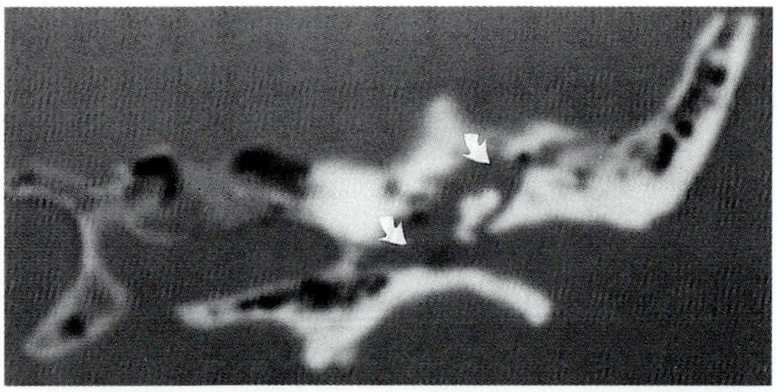

a

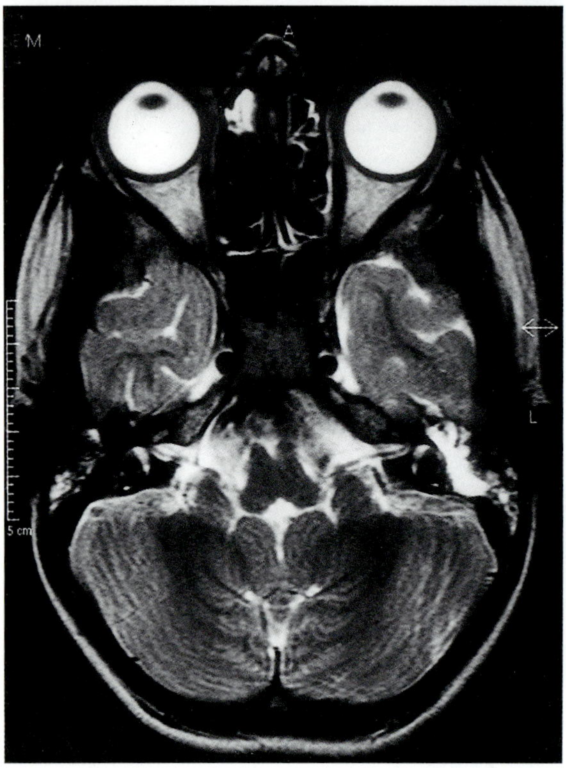

b

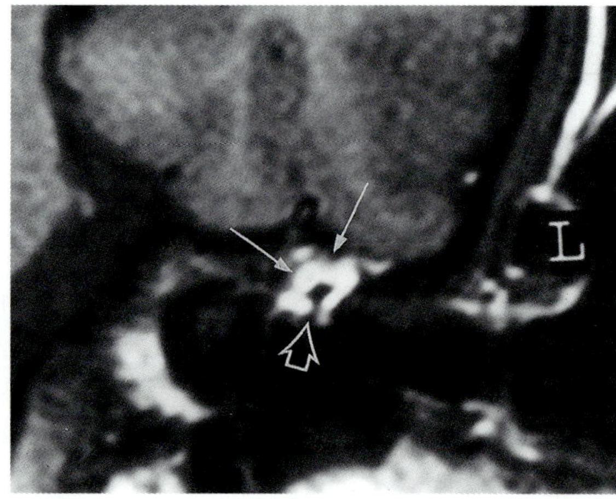

c

Figs. 4.**13 a – c** **Serous middle ear effusion in acute otitis media (acute exacerbation of chronic otitis media).**
(**a**) Unenhanced coronal CT scan shows structures of fluid attenuation (arrows) in the mesotympanum and epitympanum with a moderate caudal position of the ossicular chain.
(**b**) Axial MR image turbo spin-echo (, TR/TE = 2843/120 ms) shows a moderate fluid collection in the right mastoid and tympanic cavity with a prominent serous middle ear effusion on the left side. The structures of the internal auditory canal and vestibule appear normal.
(**c**) Unenhanced T1-weighted MRI (SE, TR/TE = 700/15 ms). Without contrast enhancement, the serosanguineous fluid in the middle ear displays high signal intensity (arrows). The malleus (open arrow) is clearly visualized relative to the hyperintense fluid collection in this T1-weighted sequence.

Table 4.**16** Small, focally enhancing lesion of the facial nerve

Findings	Differential diagnostic criteria
Common:	
➤ Idiopathic facial nerve palsy (Fig. 4.**24**)	Topography
➤ Posttraumatic/ postsurgical	Morphology, clinical features
➤ Herpes zoster (Fig. 4.**25**)	Topography
Rare:	
➤ Cholesteatoma: congenital, acquired	Destruction
➤ Malignant otitis externa (pseudomonas)	Destruction
➤ Neoplastic processes (Fig. 4.**26**)	Morphology
➤ Lymphoma	

Table 4.**17** Contrast enhancement of a long facial nerve segment

Findings	Differential diagnostic criteria
Idiopathic facial nerve palsy (Fig. 4.**24**)	Topography
Inflammation: ➤ Herpes zoster ➤ Varicella ➤ Sarcoidosis	Contrast enhancement
Tumor: ➤ Lymphoma	

Table 4.**18** Tumor mass of the facial nerve

Findings	Differential diagnostic criteria
Tumor:	
➤ Primary:	
–Neuroma (Fig. 4.**26**)	Topography
–Hemangioma	Signal characteristics
➤ Secondary:	
–Fxtratemporal tumors	Morphology
–Meningioma	Contrast enhancement
–Parotid gland tumors	Topography
–Metastases	
–Leukemic deposits	Long segmental involvment
–Chordoma	Signal intensity, density
Inflammation:	
➤ Sarcoidosis	Contrast enhancement
➤ Syphilis	

Table 4.**19** Erosive or destructive lesion of the jugular foramen

Findings	Differential diagnostic criteria
Variation:	
➤ High jugular bulb	Flow in MRA
➤ Asymmetric dilatation (Fig. 4.**28**)	MRA criteria
Tumor:	
➤ Common:	
–Paraganglioma (Fig. 4.**29**)	Enhancement dynamics
–Neuroma	Morphology
–Meningioma (Fig. 4.**31**)	
➤ Rare:	
–Chordoma	
–Neuromas of cranial nerves IX, XI, XII	Topography
–Chondrosarcoma	
–Metastasis	Destruction
–AV malformation	Vascular structures
–Cholesteatoma: primary (epidermoid) or secondary	Vascular tumor
–Internal carotid aneurysm (Fig. 4.**32**)	Morphology, vascular signal

Hypoplasia of the Jugular Foramen

Unilateral hypoplasia of the jugular foramen (Fig. 4.**27**) is a common finding in diagnostic radiology. It is a congenital variation that affects the left side slightly more often than the right. CT, or preferably MRI and MRA, can furnish an accurate morphologic analysis of key anatomic structures. Attention should be given to any contralateral changes such as paraganglioma.

Erosive and Destructive Lesions of the Jugular Foramen (Table 4.19)

The evaluation of an erosive or destructive mass lesion of the jugular foramen in patients with diverse clinical symptoms is a frequent clinical challenge. Generally it is necessary to differentiate a congenital variation (Figs. 4.**27** and 4.**28c**) from a tumor mass such as a paraganglioma (Figs. 4.**29** and 4.**30**), meningioma (Fig. 4.**31**), or neuroma. Any tumor mass that is detected by conventional radiography, CT, or unenhanced MRI should always be investigated further by contrast-enhanced MRI and venous MRA (Figs. 4.**28**–4.**30**).

By assessing the vascularity of the mass, the radiologist can differentiate among the three types of tumor listed above. The best approach is to analyze the enhancement dynamics of the mass in fast gradient-echo sequences. The "dropout effect" measured over the jugular vein or a paraganglioma reliably differentiates that structure or lesion from other, less vascular masses that may be encountered in this region. The dropout effect is defined as a rapid rise in signal intensity after the bolus injection of 0.3 mmol/kg contrast agent, followed by a temporary fall in signal intensity due to paramagnetic phenomena. Numerous studies have shown that the "dropout effect" is unique to highly vascular tumors such as paraganglioma (Figs. 4.**29**, 4.**30**), regardless of the primary location of the mass.

Venous MRA with arterial saturation (e.g., a FLASH 2-D sequence, Fig. 4.**30c**) can then be performed to differentiate a paraganglioma from a jugular bulb having an atypical position or configuration (Figs. 4.**28** and 4.**29**) or from an internal carotid aneurysm (Fig. 4.**32**). An atypical jugular bulb will exhibit venous flow on individual images and in the maximum intensity projection (MIP) reconstruction of the MRA, whereas glomus tumors at the jugular foramen will have no discernible venous flow (Fig. 4.**29**). The combination of contrast-enhanced MRI and MRA is also useful for making the therapeutically important differentiation of glomus jugulare (Fig. 4.**29**) and glomus jugulotympanicum tumors from glomus vagale tumors (Fig. 4.**30**).

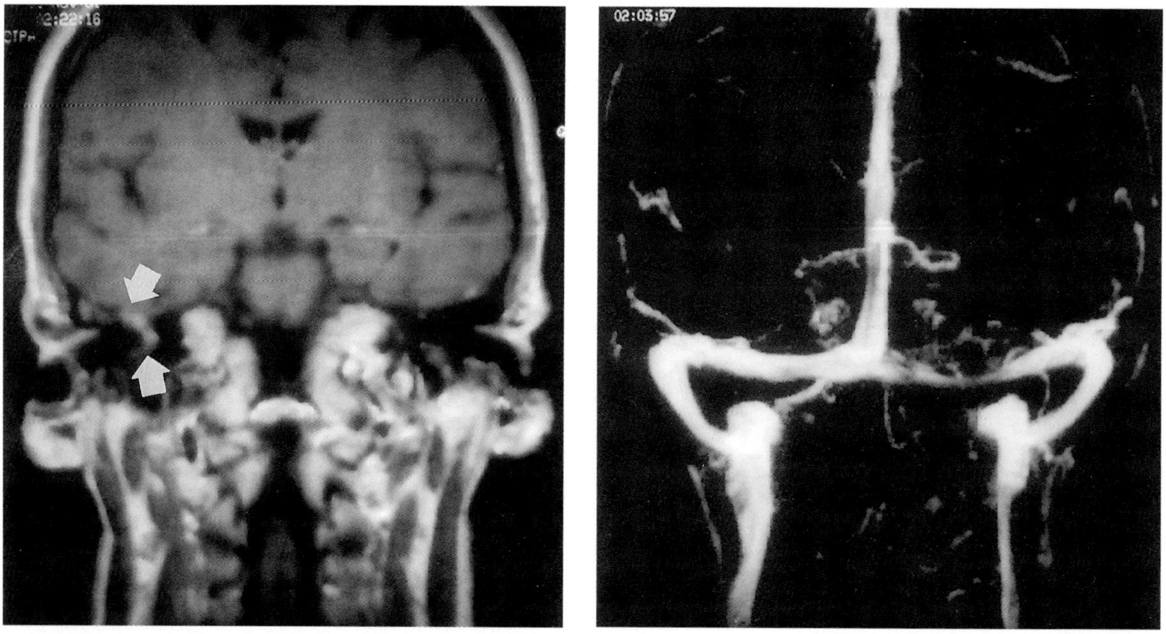

a b

Figs. 4.**14 a, b** **Middle ear adenoma appearing as a solid, moderately enhancing mass in the tympanic cavity.**
(**a**) Coronal Gd-enhanced MRI (SE, TR/TE = 700/15 ms) shows a moderately enhancing intratympanic mass (arrows) not associated with significant destructive changes. The degree of contrast enhancement (as a percentage) is markedly less than that seen with hypervascular glomus tumors or hemangiomas.

(**b**) Coronal reconstruction of venous MRA (TR/TE = 36/10 ms, flip angle = 60°) using MIP technique documents normal perfusion of the sigmoid sinus, transverse sinus, and jugular bulb with no obvious secondary compression signs. The normal appearance of the jugular fossa excludes concomitant jugular involvement.

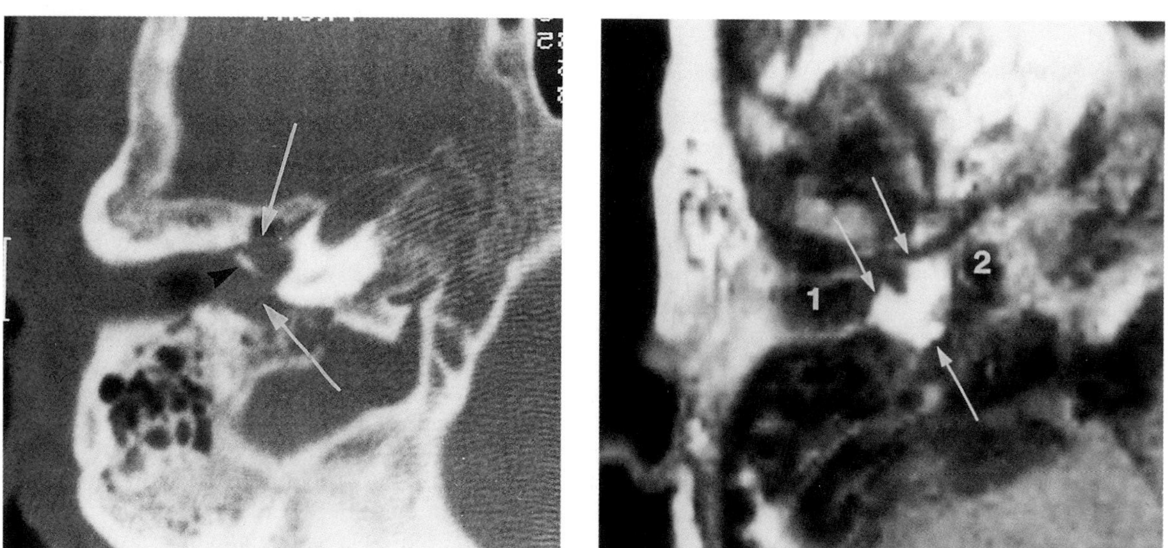

a b

Figs. 4.**15 a, b** **Differential diagnosis of an intensely enhancing middle ear mass. Documentation of a glomus tympanicum tumor (presenting clinically as a bluish retrotympanic mass).**
(**a**) High-resolution CT scan with a bone window shows a mass of soft-tissue density in the tympanic cavity (arrows) causing moderate ossicular displacement (arrowhead). There are no other definite signs of bone destruction.

(**b**) Gd-enhanced T1-weighted image (TR/TE = 500/15 ms) shows an intensely enhancing, geometric mass conforming to the boundaries of the epitympanum and mesotympanum (arrows). The external auditory canal and carotid artery segments appear normal. This appearance is typical of a glomus tympanicum tumor.
1 External auditory canal
2 Internal carotid artery

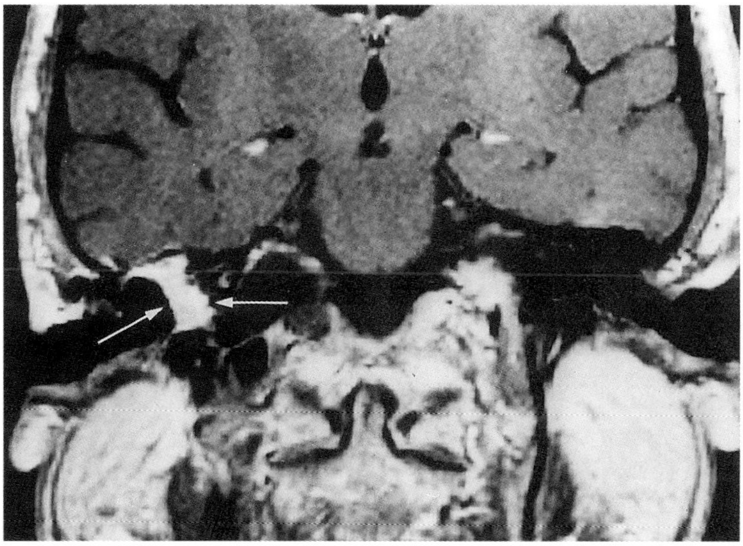

Fig. 4.**16** **Hypervascular middle ear mass, illustrated here by postoperative hypervascular granulation tissue.** Gd-enhanced coronal T1-weighted SE sequence (TR/TE = 500/15 ms) shows an intensely enhancing mass uniformly filling the tympanic cavity (arrows) and showing no extension into surrounding structures. Histology disclosed hypervascular granulation tissue secondary to previous surgery.

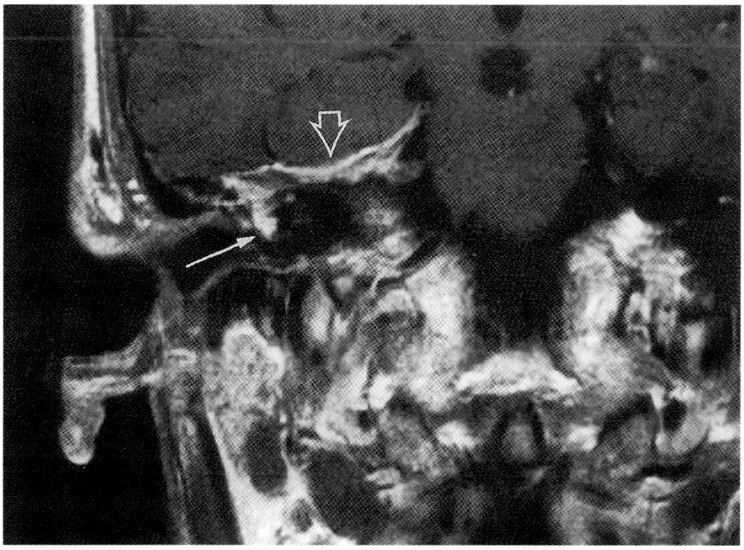

a

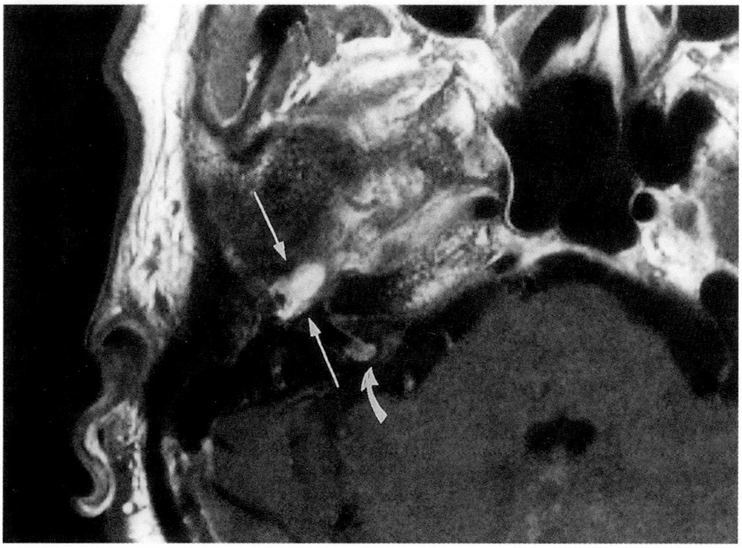

b

Figs. 4.**17 a, b** **Differential diagnosis of an intensely enhancing middle ear mass. A meningioma has grown along the petrous ridge and infiltrated the tympanic cavity.**
(**a**) Gd-enhanced coronal T1-weighted SE sequence (TR/TE = 50/15 ms) documents the relative position and growth direction of a petrous meningioma that has invaded the middle ear cavity (thin arrow). The differential diagnostic assessment is based on the relation of the mass to the line of meningeal contrast enhancement (open arrow).
(**b**) Gd-enhanced axial T1-weighted SE sequence (TR/TE = 500/15 ms) shows a smoothly marginated, intensely enhancing mass with nodular extension into the epitympanum (arrows). Moderate dural contrast enhancement is also seen in the internal auditory canal (curved arrow).

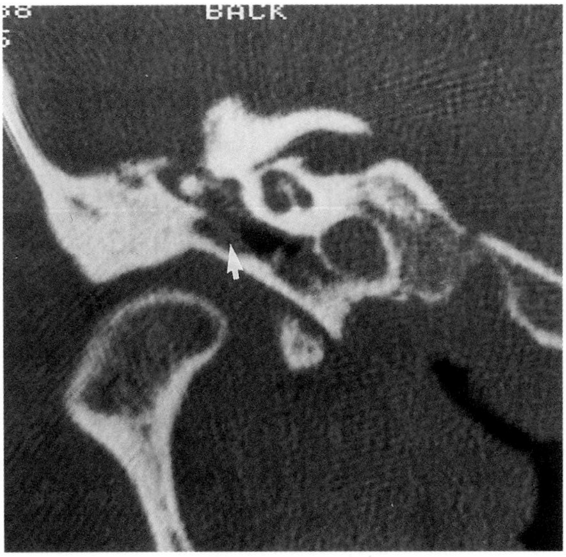

△
Fig. 4.**18** **Small, erosive cholesteatoma (arrow) in the mesotympanum and epitympanum.** Coronal CT scan shows a mass of soft-tissue density in the mesotympanum and epitympanum eroding the medial and apical bony walls of the middle ear cavity (arrow).

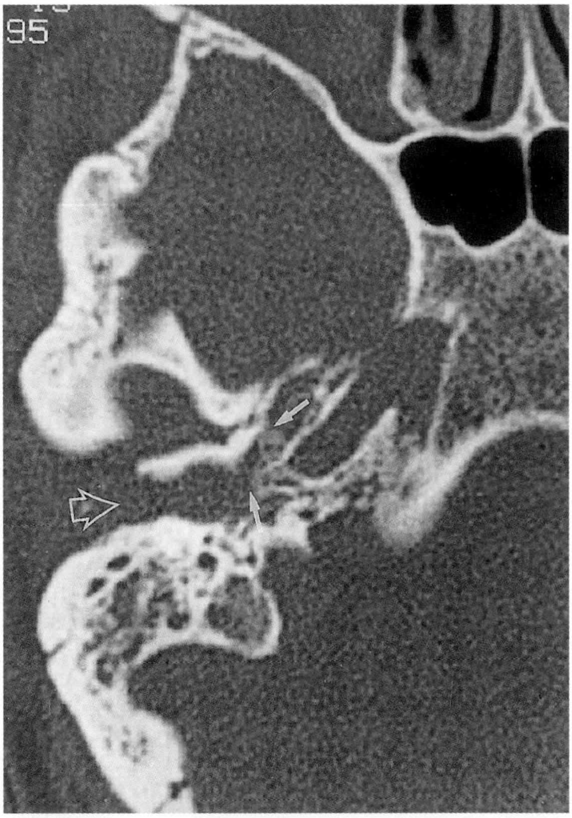

a

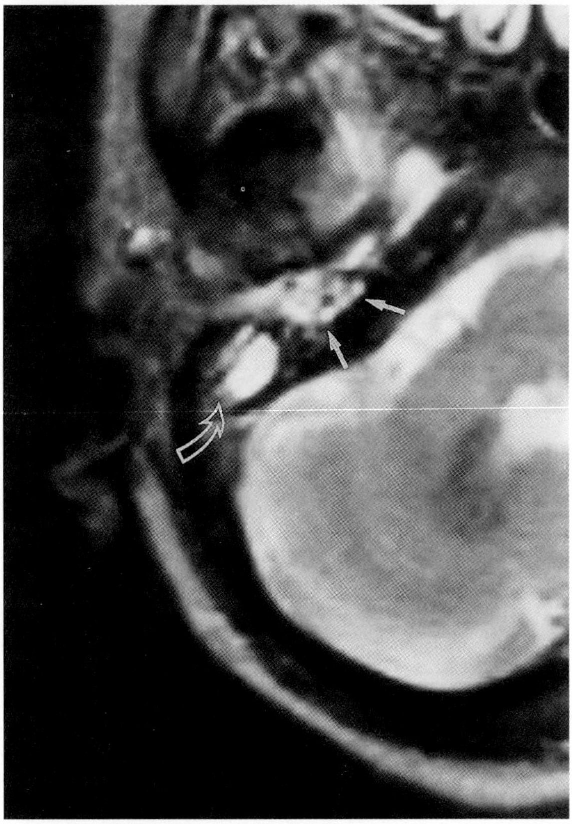

b

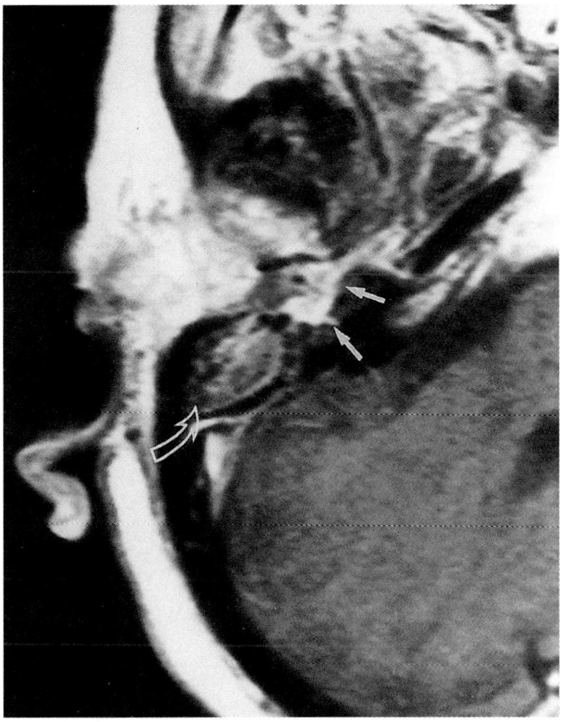

c

△

◁ Figs. 4.**19 a – c** **Differential diagnosis of a soft-tissue mass in the middle ear: cholesteatoma with bony sequestra.**
(**a**) Axial noncontrast HRCT scan documents hypodense but still nondelineated bone sequestra and cholesteatomatous debris (arrows) in the middle ear spaces. The scan also shows soft-tissue opacity in the region of the external auditory canal (open arrow) and a marked increase of soft-tissue density in portions of the mastoid.
(**b**) Axial T2-weighted MR image (TR/TE = 2500/90 ms) shows increased hyperintense fluid in the mastoid region (open arrow). Cholesteatomatous tissue completely fills the tympanic cavity and shows a moderately increased T2 relaxation time (arrows).
(**c**) Gd-enhanced T1-weighted SE sequence (TR/TE = 500/15 ms) on the same plane documents the nonenhancing inflammatory mastoid changes (open arrow) and the markedly enhancing cholesteatomatous tissue and adjacent granulation tissue filling the complex interior of the tympanic cavity (arrows).

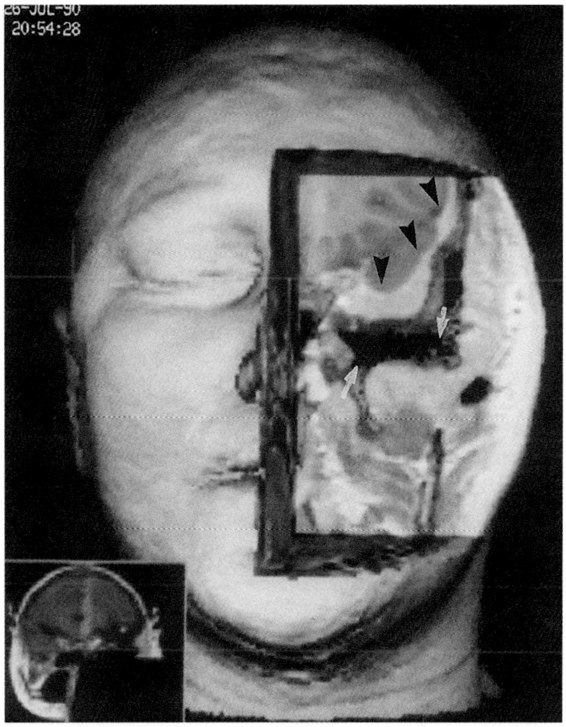

a

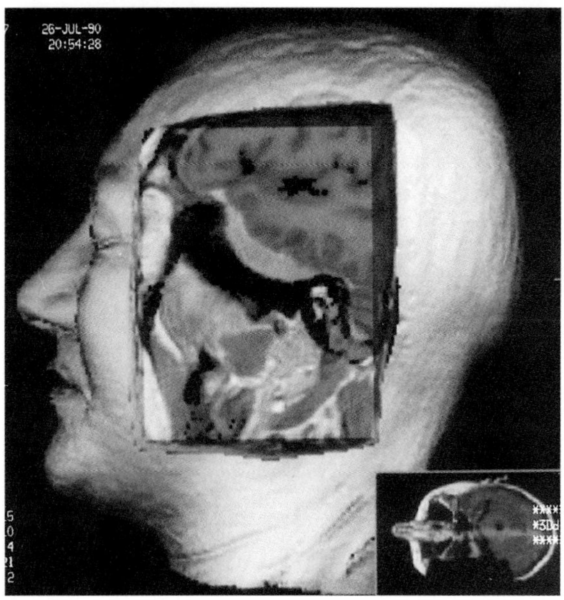

b

Figs. 4.**20 a, b** **Ossifying fibroma illustrating an osteosclerotic process of the temporal bone with significant dural and infratemporal soft-tissue involvement.**
(**a**) 3-D MP RAGE (magnetization-prepared rapid-acquisition gradient-echo) sequence with Gd-DTPA enhancement. The osteosclerotic portions of the temporal bone appear as areas of low signal intensity in the frontal surface-rendered 3-D reconstruction (arrows). Soft-tissue components of the ossifying fibroma are clearly visible along the dura (arrowheads) and in the infratemporal region.
(**b**) Sagittal view confirms the hypointense osteosclerotic components and the brightly enhancing soft-tissue elements of the tumor.

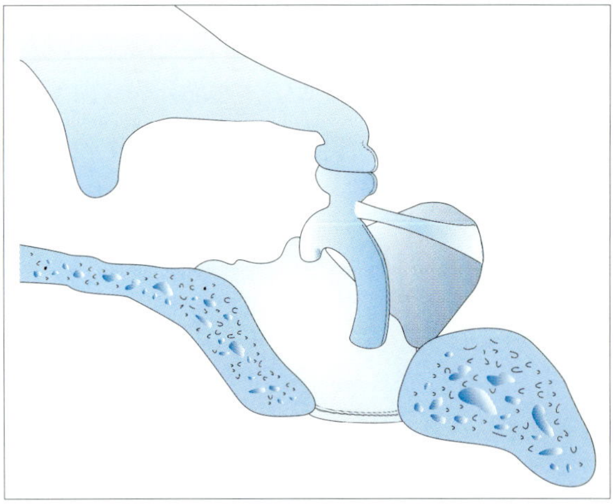

Fig. 4.**21** **Obliterative fenestral otosclerosis. Structures of bone intensity line the oval window** (after Swarts).

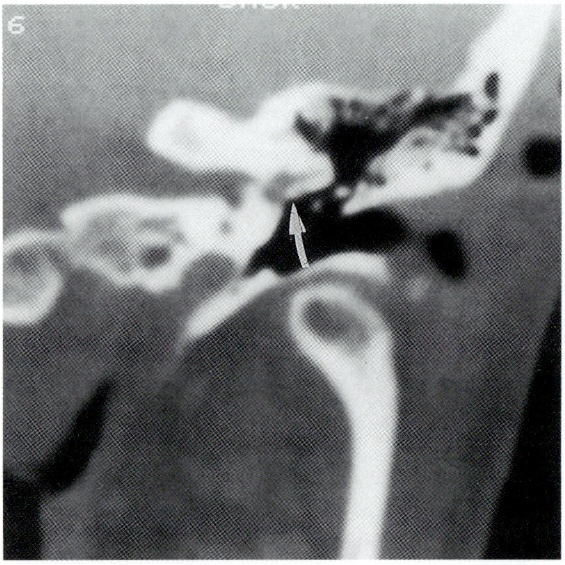

Fig. 4.**22** **Fenestral otosclerosis of the oval window, appearing on CT as a thickened area of bone density in the apical portion of the oval window** (arrow).

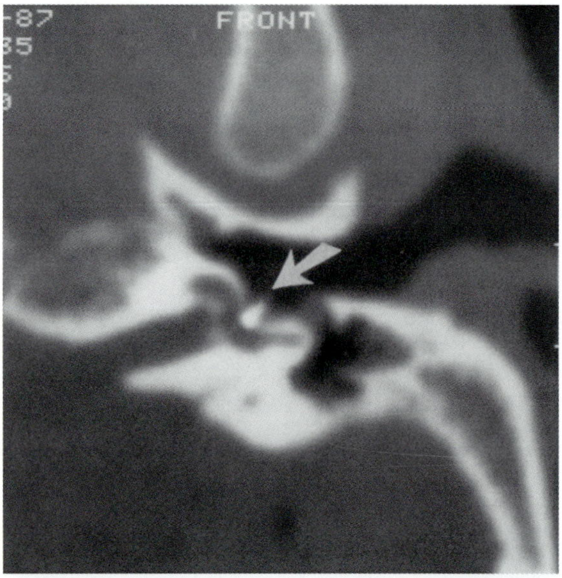

a

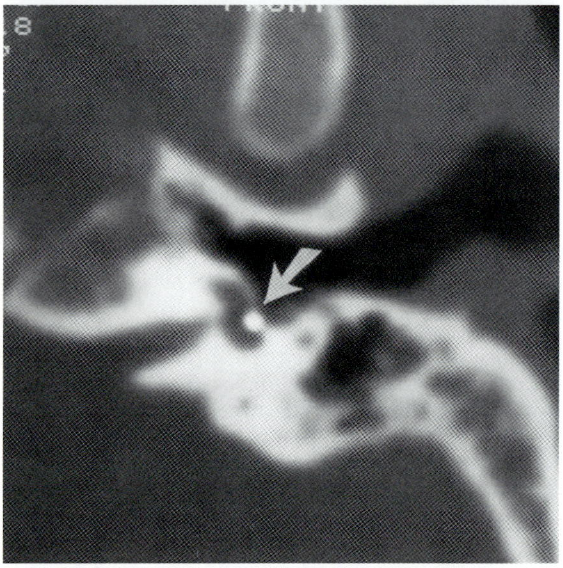

b

Figs. 4.**23 a, b** **Hyperdense structures in the temporal bone following stapes reconstruction, with protrusion of the metal prosthesis into the membranous labyrinth.**
(**a**) Coronal HRCT shows the relative position of the stapes' prosthesis within the membranous labyrinth (arrow).
(**b**) Scan documenting medial protrusion of the bony stapes (arrow).

Table 4.**20** Destructive lesion of the petrous apex

Findings	Differential diagnostic criteria
Common:	
➤ Variation: Fat inclusions	Signal intensity, density
➤ Tumor:	
–Metastasis (Fig. 4.**35**)	Morphology, destruction
–Cholesterol granuloma	Signal intensity, density
–Epidermoid	Density, morphology
–Plasmacytoma (Fig. 4.**33**)	
➤ Inflammation:	
–Bacterial, viral	
–Sarcoidosis	Contrast enhancement
Rare:	
➤ Tumor:	
–Chordoma	Morphology
–Chondrosarcoma	

Table 4.**21** Destructive mastoid mass

Findings	Differential diagnostic criteria
Tumor:	Topography
➤ Squamous cell carcinoma	
➤ Metastasis (Fig. 4.**35**)	
➤ Osteogenic sarcoma	Morphology
➤ Chondrosarcoma	Tumor matrix
Inflammation:	
➤ Cholesteatoma (Figs. 4.**18**, 4.**19**)	Topography
➤ Mastoiditis (Fig. 4.**36**)	Signal intensity, density
➤ Sarcoiditis, syphilis	Contrast enhancement

Table 4.**22** Nondestructive mastoid mass

- ➤ Postoperative sequelae (Fig. 4.**34**)
- ➤ Seroma cavity (Fig. 4.**34**)
- ➤ Benign tumors, lipoma (Fig. 4.**37**)

Destructive Petrous Apex Lesion

(Table 4.**20**)

Primary or secondary destructive lesions of the petrous apex (Fig. 4.**33**) are usually associated with obvious clinical manifestations. The emphasis in radiology is in making a specific diagnosis and evaluating primary incidental findings that may be associated with changes in MRI signal intensity. Contrast-enhanced CT (Fig. 4.**33**) and MRI (Figs. 4.**33 b–d**) are definitely indicated to evaluate the vascularity of a possible lesion. It is common to find variations such as increased pneumatization of the petrous apex (Fig. 4.**11**) or the presence of atypical fatty inclusions in the petrous cancellous bone. Plasmacytomas (Fig. 4.**33**) or metastases from various primary tumors, especially breast carcinoma, may also occur in this region.

Mass Lesion in the Mastoid

When the presence of a primary or secondary mastoid mass is verified (Figs. 4.**34**– 4.**36**), it should be determined whether the lesion is destructive or nondestructive (Tables 4.**21** and 4.**22**). If the lesion has been localized to the facial nerve (Fig. 4.**26**), the differential diagnoses in Table 4.**20** should be applied. It is important in these cases to distinguish between primary and secondary tumor infiltration of the nerve.

Traumatic Lesions of the Temporal Bone

In evaluating traumatic lesions of the temporal bone (Figs. 4.**38** – 4.**40**), a specific search should be made for primary osseous lesions such as *longitudinal and transverse fractures* of the petrous pyramid and *comminuted fractures.* When circumscribed soft-tissue changes are found, a *primary variation* or *inflammatory disease* should be considered in the differential diagnosis (Fig. 4.**36**). Trauma-related conditions of the inner ear are discussed in Chapter 5 (Figs. 4.**38** and 4.**39**).

Focal Enhancing Facial Nerve Lesion Showing Remission at Follow-Up

An inflammatory cause should always be considered first in the differential diagnosis of focal facial nerve lesions that enhance on post-gadolinium MR images (Fig. 4.**26 b**). Once it has been established that the lesion has regressed in size and enhancement intensity, the following causes should be investigated:

- ➤ Idiopathic facial nerve palsy (Bell palsy).
- ➤ Herpes zoster oticus (Fig. 4.**25**).
- ➤ Lymphocytic meningitis.

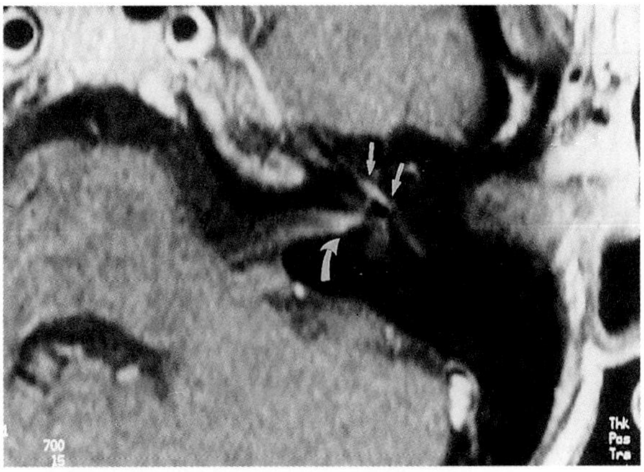

a

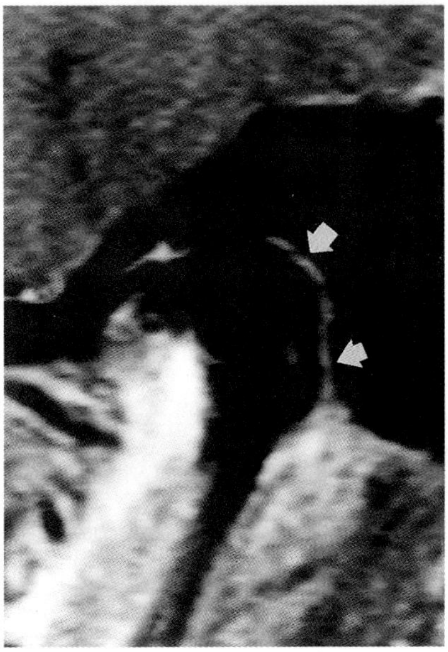

b

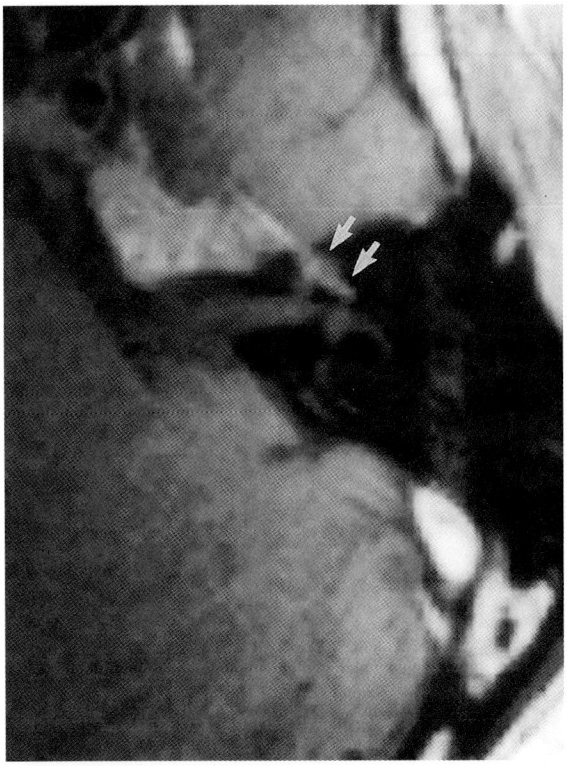

a

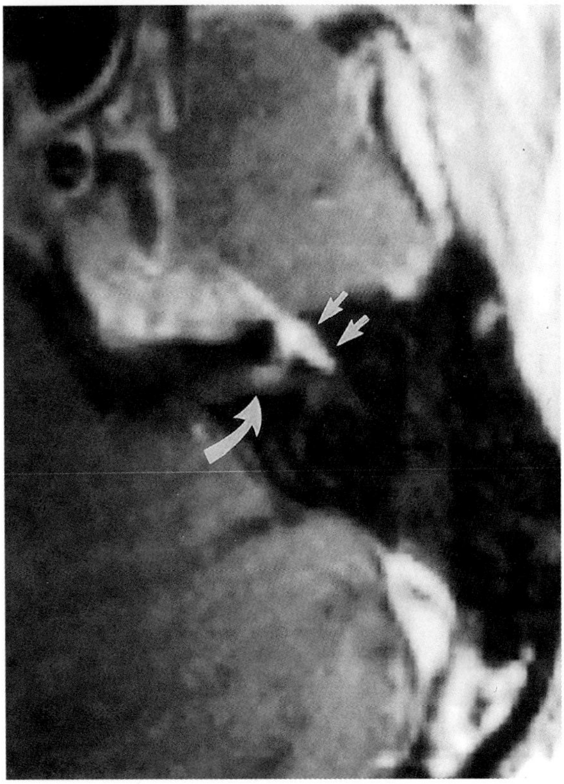

b

◁ Figs. 4.**24 a, b** **Focal neuritis involving the intrameatal segment and anterior genu of the facial nerve in a patient with peripheral facial-nerve palsy.**

(**a**) Axial unenhanced T1-weighted MR image (SE, TR/TE = 500/15 ms) shows soft-tissue structures of normal appearance in the internal auditory canal and moderate hyperintensity of the anterior genu of the facial nerve (arrows).

(**b**) Axial Gd-enhanced T1-weighted MR image (SE, TR/TE = 700/15 ms) shows significant enhancement of the intrameatal facial nerve segment (curved arrow) and greater-than-normal enhancement of the anterior genu (arrows). Follow-up MRI after 3 months' therapy showed a complete cessation of abnormal contrast enhancement in both facial nerve segments.

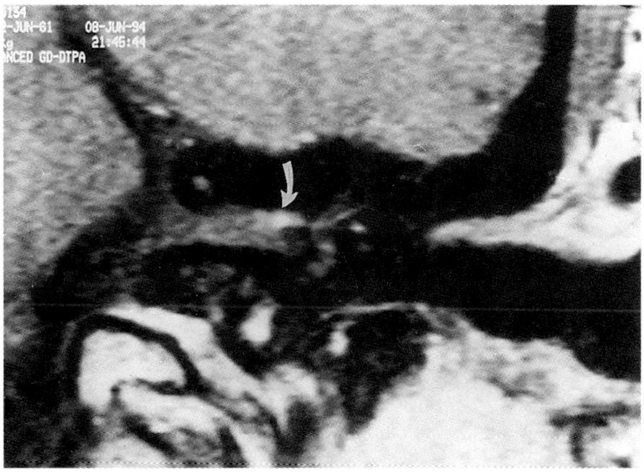

c

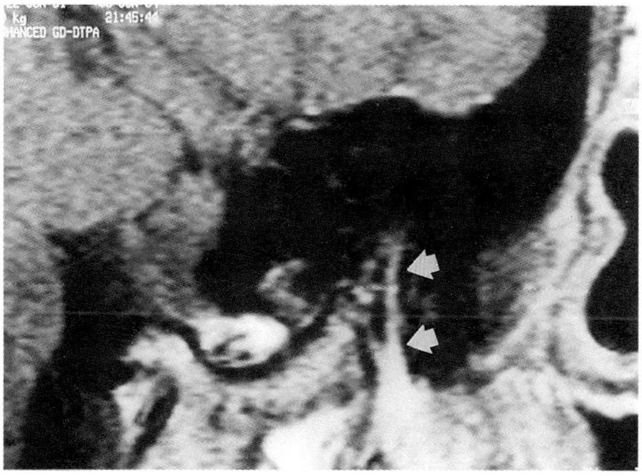

d

△

◁ Figs. 4.**25 a – d** **Isolated enhancement of the intrameatal and mastoid facial nerve segments in a patient with herpes zoster-induced facial nerve palsy, with normal enhancement of the anterior genu.**

(**a**) Axial Gd-enhanced T1-weighted SE sequence (TR/TE = 700/15 ms) documents marked enhancement of the intrameatal segment of the facial nerve (curved arrow). Enhancement of the nondistended anterior genu (arrows) is within normal limits.

(**b**) Parasagittal Gd-enhanced T1-weighted SE sequence (TR/TE = 700/15 ms) angled along the mastoid portion of the facial nerve shows enhancement of a long, nondistended segment of the nerve (arrows).

(**c**) Image on the coronal plane clearly documents the contrast enhancement, localizing it to the intrameatal segment of the facial nerve (curved arrow).

(**d**) Frontal image documents the enhancing facial nerve segment (arrows).

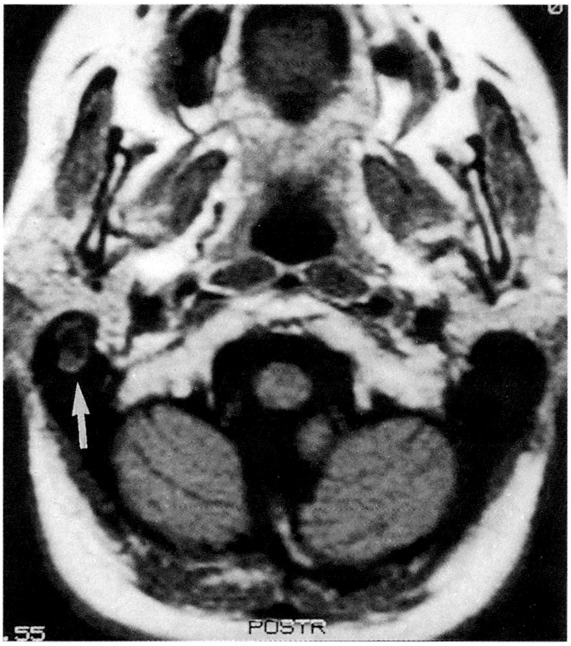

a

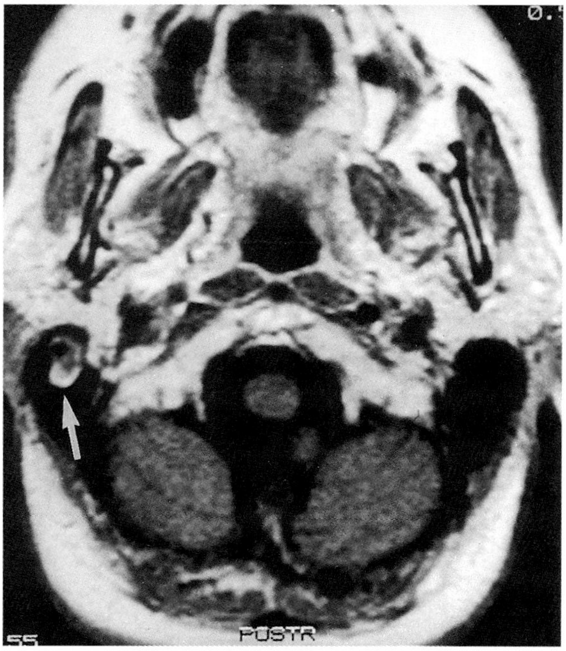

b

Figs. 4.**26 a, b** **Facial nerve neuroma of the mastoid segment.**

(**a**) Axial unenhanced T1-weighted SE sequence (TR/TE = 600/20 ms) shows a soft-tissue mass in the right mastoid (arrow) bordering directly on the mastoid segment of the facial nerve. The main diagnostic considerations are neuroma and hemangioma.

(**b**) Axial Gd-enhanced T1-weighted SE sequence (TR/TE = 600/20 ms) demonstrates intense enhancement of the facial neuroma. This image documents the marked contrast enhancement of a neural tumor occurring at a typical location (arrow).

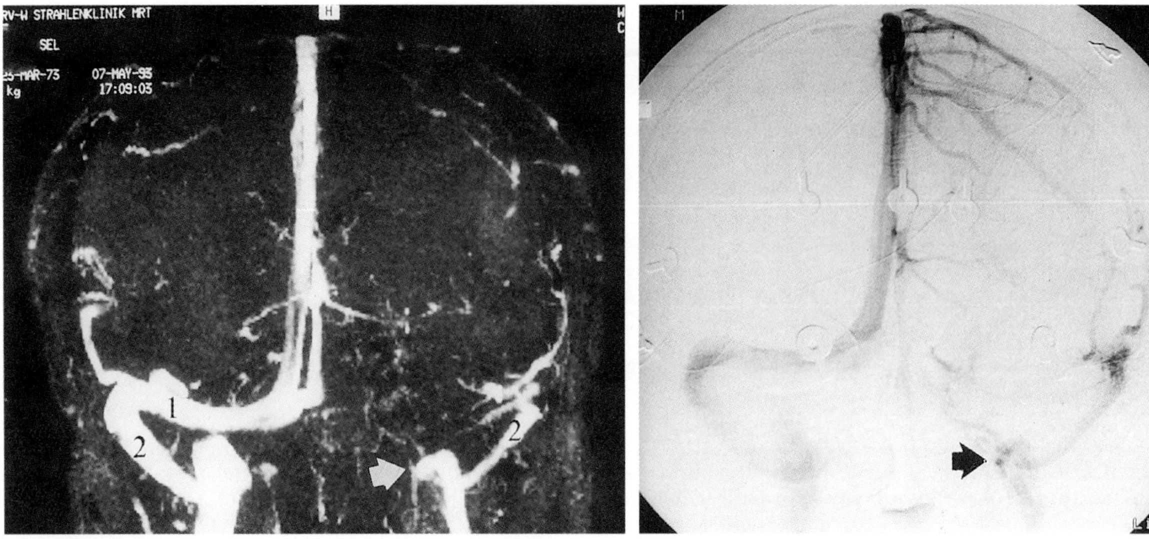

a b

Figs. 4.27

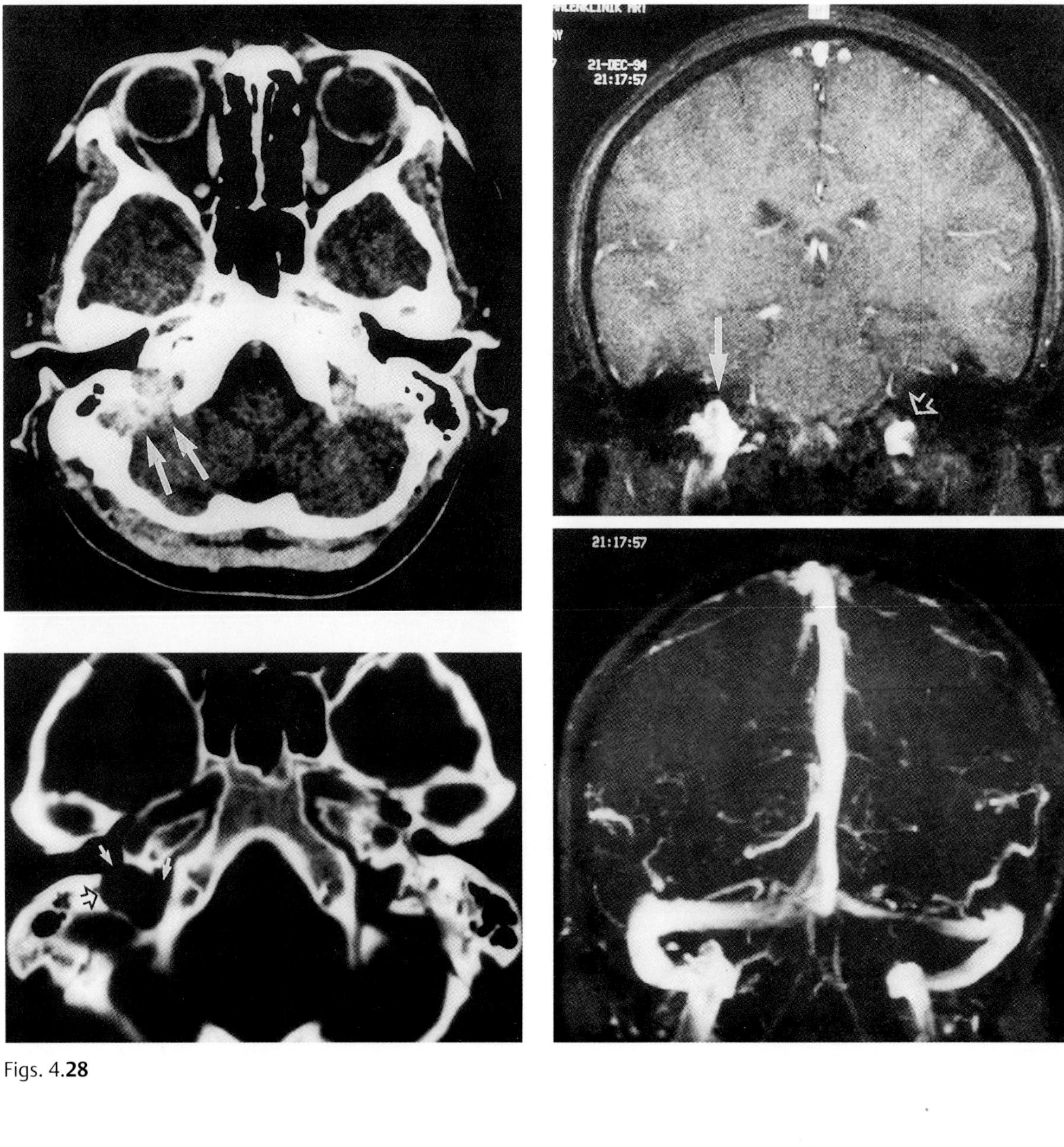

a b c d

Figs. 4.28

◁ Figs. 4.**27 a, b** **Hypoplasia of the jugular bulb.**
(**a**) Venous MRA (2-D FLASH sequence, TR/TE = 36/10 ms, flip angle = 60°) clearly demonstrates the hypoplastic left jugular bulb (arrow) with compensatory collateral flow through the sigmoid sinus and jugular bulb on the right side.
1 Transverse sinus
2 Sigmoid sinus
(**b**) Correlative DSA in the venous phase verifies the aplastic left transverse sinus and the hypoplastic sigmoid sinus and jugular bulb on the left side (arrow) with a compensatory flow increase on the right side.

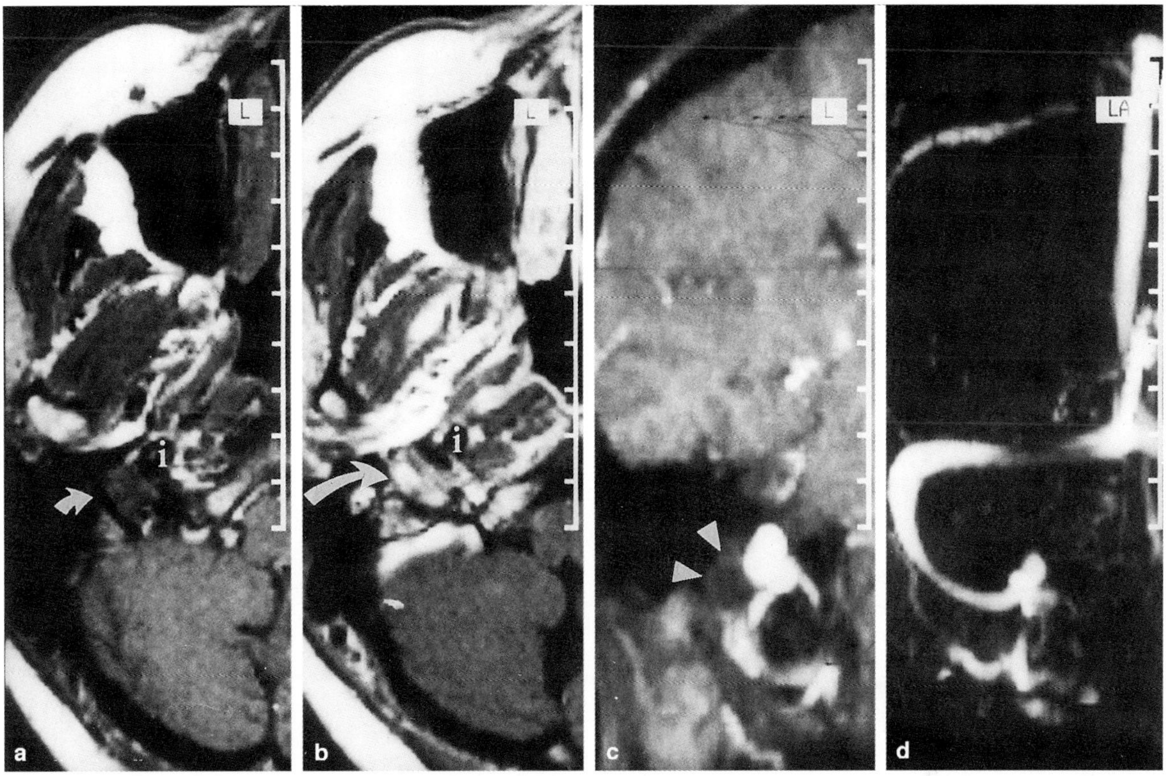

Figs. 4.**29 a – d** **Paraganglioma of the jugular foramen: type C glomus jugulare tumor. Comparison of unenhanced and contrast-enhanced T1-weighted MR images and venous MRA.**
(**a**) Unenhanced axial T1-weighted SE sequence (TR/TE = 500/15 ms) shows a hypointense soft-tissue mass in the jugular foramen (arrow) posterior to the internal carotid artery. Localization is difficult in the noncontrast T1-weighted image.
i Internal carotid artery
(**b**) Gd-enhanced axial T1-weighted SE sequence (TR/TE = 500/15 ms) shows intense enhancement of the jugular foramen mass (curved arrow) and the still-perfused portions of the jugular foramen and sigmoid sinus. It is unclear whether the enhancing mass represents a hyperperfused jugular foramen, bulbar ectasia, or a glomus tumor.
i Internal carotid artery
(**c**) Venous MRA (2-D FLASH sequence, TR/TE = 36/10 ms, flip angle = 60°). Without contrast enhancement, the mass appears as a hypointense area (arrowheads) in the jugular foramen causing medial displacement of the perfused portions of the jugular vein and jugular bulb.
(**d**) 3-D MIP reconstruction clearly documents the hypoperfused transverse sinus and the displaced jugular bulb. The tumor displacing the jugular bulb is not accurately delineated in the 3-D reconstruction.

◁ Figs. 4.**28 a – d** **Bizarre configuration of the right jugular bulb. Comparative evaluation by CT and MRA.**
(**a**) Contrast-enhanced CT scan of the middle skull base (100 mL contrast medium) shows an intensely enhancing structure with a bizarre configuration in the jugular foramen on the right side. The soft-tissue window does not permit exclusion of an infiltrative lesion.
(**b**) CT scan with a bone window defines an asymmetric right jugular foramen (arrows) with a thin posterior wall on the mastoid side.
(**c**) Venous MRA (2-D FLASH sequence, TR/TE = 36/10 ms) documents the location and unusual shape of the right jugular foramen (arrow). The left jugular foramen (open arrow) is hypoplastic. MRA definitively excludes a mass lesion in the jugular foramen.

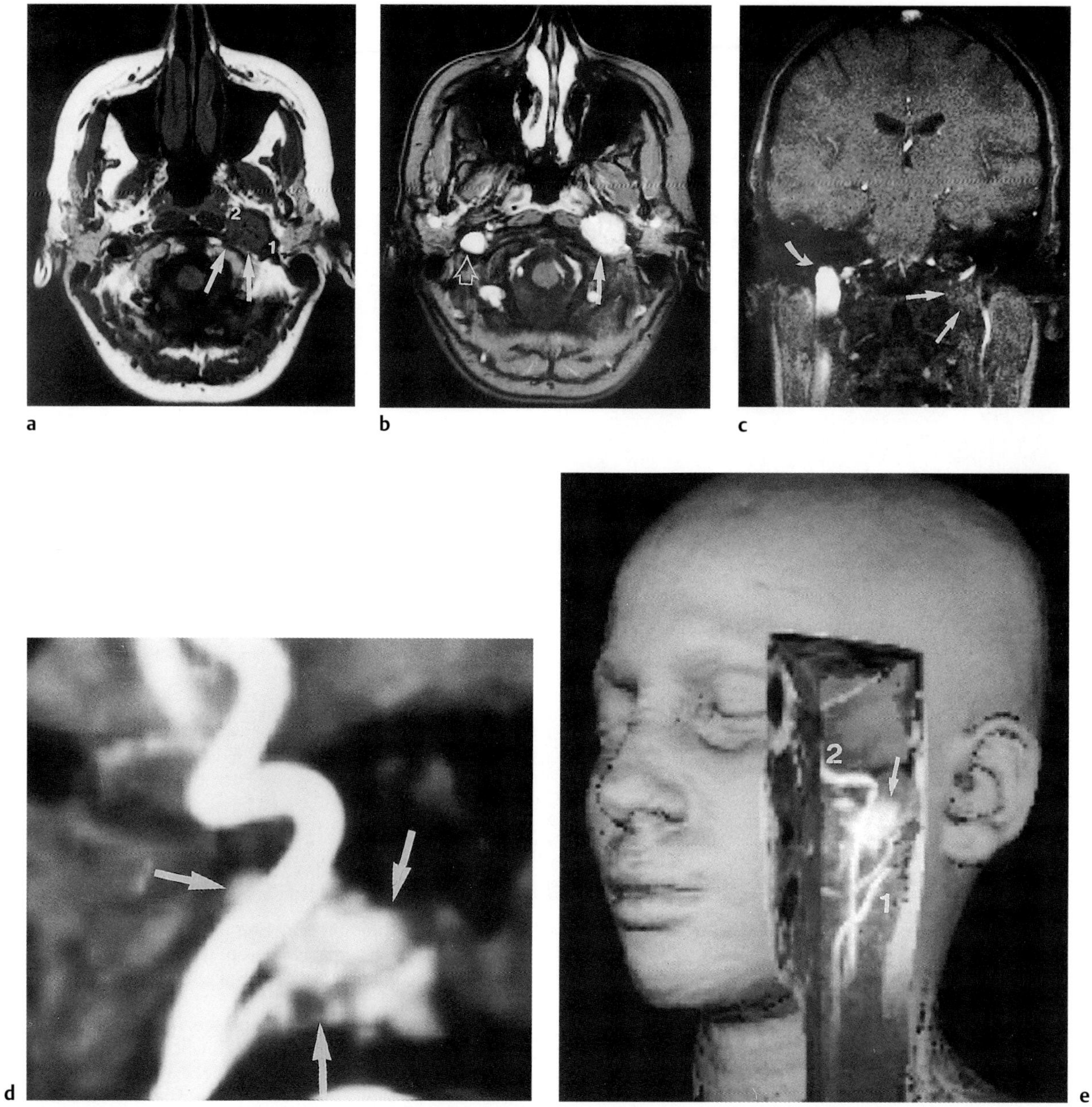

Figs. 4.**30a–e** **Infrajugular mass located below the jugular foramen and involving the parapharyngeal space on the left side: glomus vagale tumor.**
(**a**) Axial T1-weighted SE sequence (TR/TE = 500/15 ms) on a plane below the jugular foramen documents a soft-tissue mass of the parapharyngeal space (arrows) causing lateral displacement of the jugular vein and medial displacement of the internal carotid artery.
1 Jugular vein
2 Internal carotid artery
(**b**) Fat-saturated Gd-enhanced T1-weighted SE sequence (TR/TE = 500/15 ms) documents the hypervascularity of the left-sided glomus vagale tumor (arrow). High signal intensity in the right jugular vein (open arrow) is due to compensatory hyperperfusion of the vein.
(**c**) Venous MRA (2-D FLASH sequence, TR/TE = 36/10 ms, flip angle = 60°) with arterial saturation shows hypoperfusion of the jugular bulb and vein on the left side. The mass shows mixed, nonhomogeneous signal intensity on the unenhanced scan (arrows). The high signal intensity on the right side indicates hyperperfusion of the jugular bulb and vein (curved arrow).
(**d**) Arterial MRA (3-D FISP sequence, TR/TE = 40/7 ms, flip angle = 20°) vividly defines the perfused infrapetrosal segment of the internal carotid artery and the hyperperfused left-sided glomus vagale tumor (arrows) supplied by the external carotid artery.
(**e**) 3-D MP-RAGE sequence with Gd-DTPA enhancement verifies the relation of the glomus vagale tumor (arrow) to the branches of the internal and external carotid arteries.
1 External carotid artery
2 Internal carotid artery

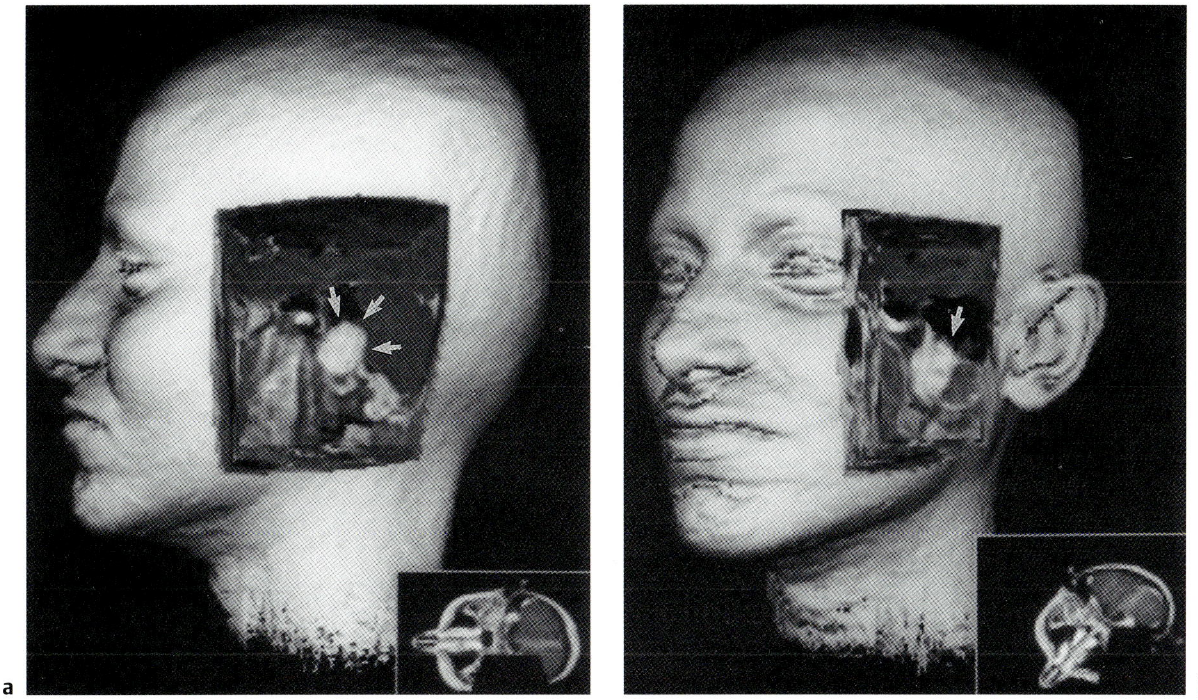

Figs. 4.**31 a, b** **Comparative 3-D MRI views of a meningioma of the jugular foramen.**
(**a**) Sagittal Gd-enhanced 3-D MP-RAGE sequence (TR/TE/TI = 11.5/5/150 ms, flip angle = 10°) documents a uniformly enhancing meningioma in the jugular foramen. The tumor shows no septations and is causing moderate displacement of adjacent structures (arrows).
(**b**) The parasagittal view shows the relative location of the homogeneous, hypervascular jugular foramen meningioma (arrow), which lies posterior to the internal carotid artery.

A regression of enhancement intensity and segmental involvement in a patient with facial nerve palsy excludes a facial nerve tumor such as hemangioma and schwannoma (Fig. 4.**26**) with a high degree of confidence.

Summary and Diagnostic Strategy

The strategy for evaluating diseases of the external auditory canal (Fig. 4.**4**), middle ear (Fig. 4.**1**), and jugular fossa (Figs. 4.**8 a, b**) is directed by the clinical manifestations. If clinical signs raise suspicion of a malformation, inflammatory disease, or traumatic lesion, the primary imaging study should be thin-section HRCT, supplemented as needed by contrast-enhanced scans. If clinical signs are consistent with a vascular lesion, anomaly, or tumor mass, especially in the jugular fossa, the imaging procedure of choice is MRI combined with MRA (Fig. 4.**29**).

In patients with the typical clinical presentation of facial nerve palsy, the consensus in the current literature is that there is no need for a primary imaging evaluation. However, primary contrast-enhanced MRI is warranted in cases where clinical symptoms are atypical and persist for longer than 2 months. Primary MRI is particularly important in patients who manifest a slowly progressive palsy, facial spasms, a remitting-relapsing course, pain, and multiple cranial neuropathies, and it should continue to be used during follow-up (Fig. 4.**26**).

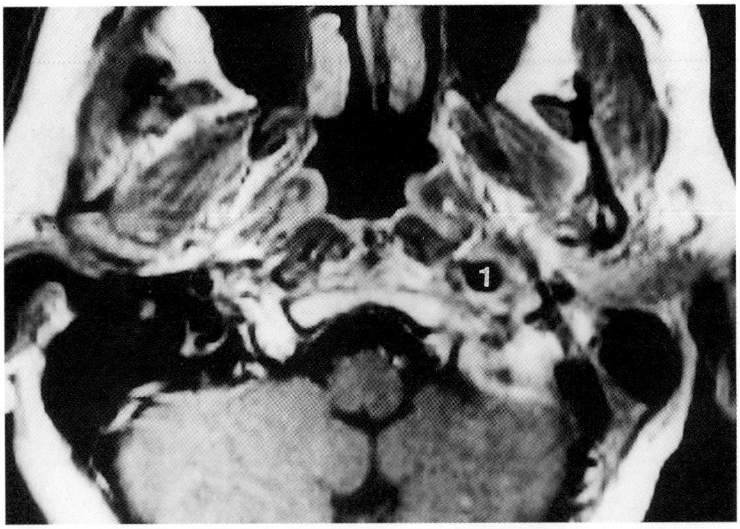

a

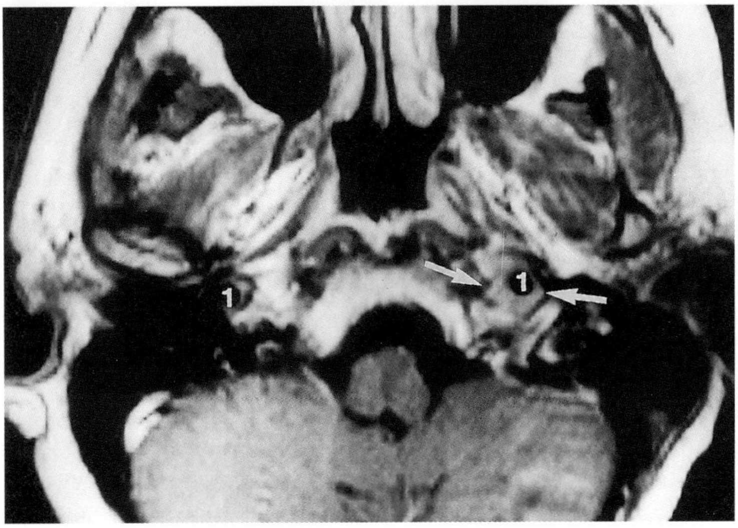

b

Figs. 4.**32 a, b** **Mass of mixed signal intensity located below the skull base and causing poor delineation of the jugular vein: internal carotid artery aneurysm penetrating into surrounding structures.**
(**a**) Axial Gd-enhanced T1-weighted SE sequence (TR/TE = 500/15 ms) on a plane 8 mm caudal to the section in **b**.
1 Internal carotid artery
(**b**) Axial Gd-enhanced T1-weighted SE sequence (TR/TE = 500/15 ms). The two adjacent images demonstrate a hypointense area representing the still-perfused portion of the internal carotid artery. The higher slice (**b**) shows the aneurysmatic dilatation of the internal carotid artery with a circumferential soft-tissue mantle caused by the partially thrombosed aneurysm (arrows).
1 Internal carotid artery

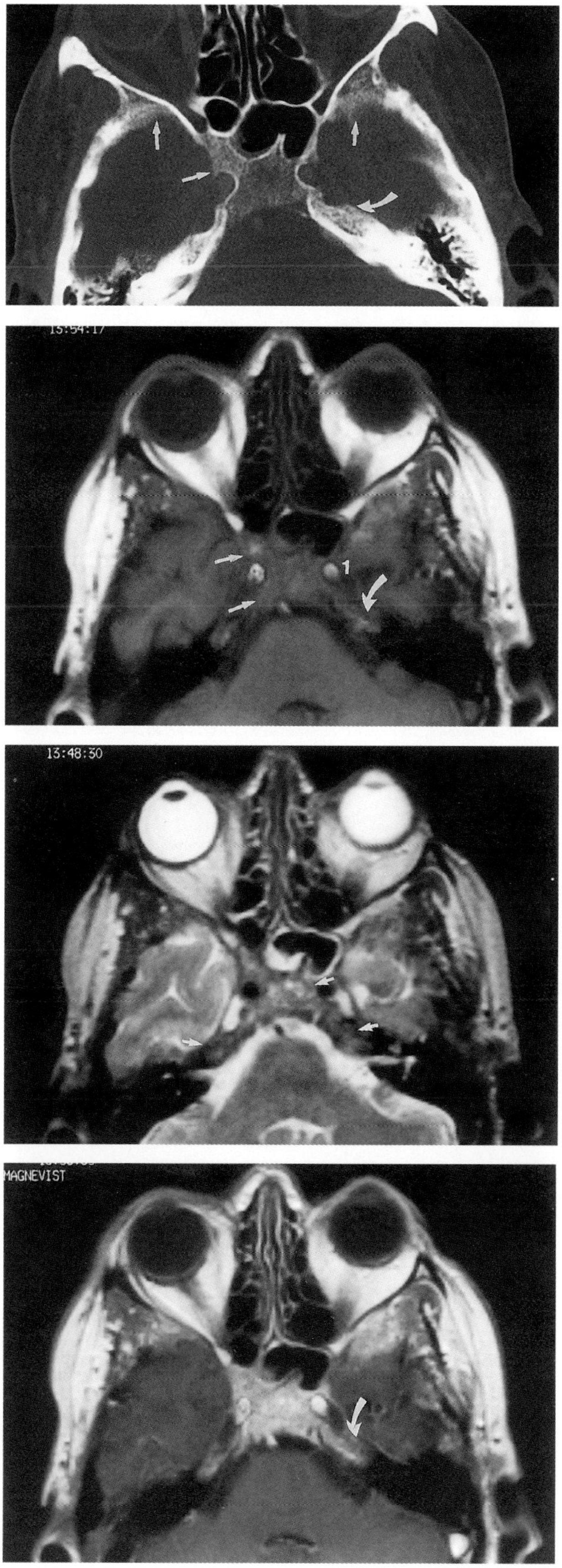

a b c d

Figs. 4.**33 a – d** **Plasmacytoma infiltrating the left petrous apex and the body of the sphenoid bone.**
(**a**) Axial CT scan parallel to the orbitomeatal line shows decreased structural density of the sphenoid body and greater and lesser sphenoid wings (arrows). Rarefaction is also seen in the direction of the left petrous apex (curved arrow).
(**b**) Unenhanced axial T1-weighted SE sequence (TR/TE = 500/15 ms) confirms hypointense infiltration by plasmacytoma tissue (arrows). Note the increased signal intensity caused by flow effects in both internal carotid arteries and the basal artery.
1 Internal carotid artery
(**c**) Unenhanced T2-weighted SE sequence (TR/TE = 2500/90 ms). With T2-weighting, the tumor shows intermediate signal intensity with a mixed, nonhomogeneous signal pattern (arrows). The sigmoid sinus shows moderate inflammatory change.
(**d**) Gd-enhanced T1-weighted SE sequence (TR/TE = 500/15 ms) shows nonhomogeneous contrast enhancement of the infiltrating plasmacytoma (curved arrow). Tumor extension is visible within the sphenoid bone and in the petrous apex.

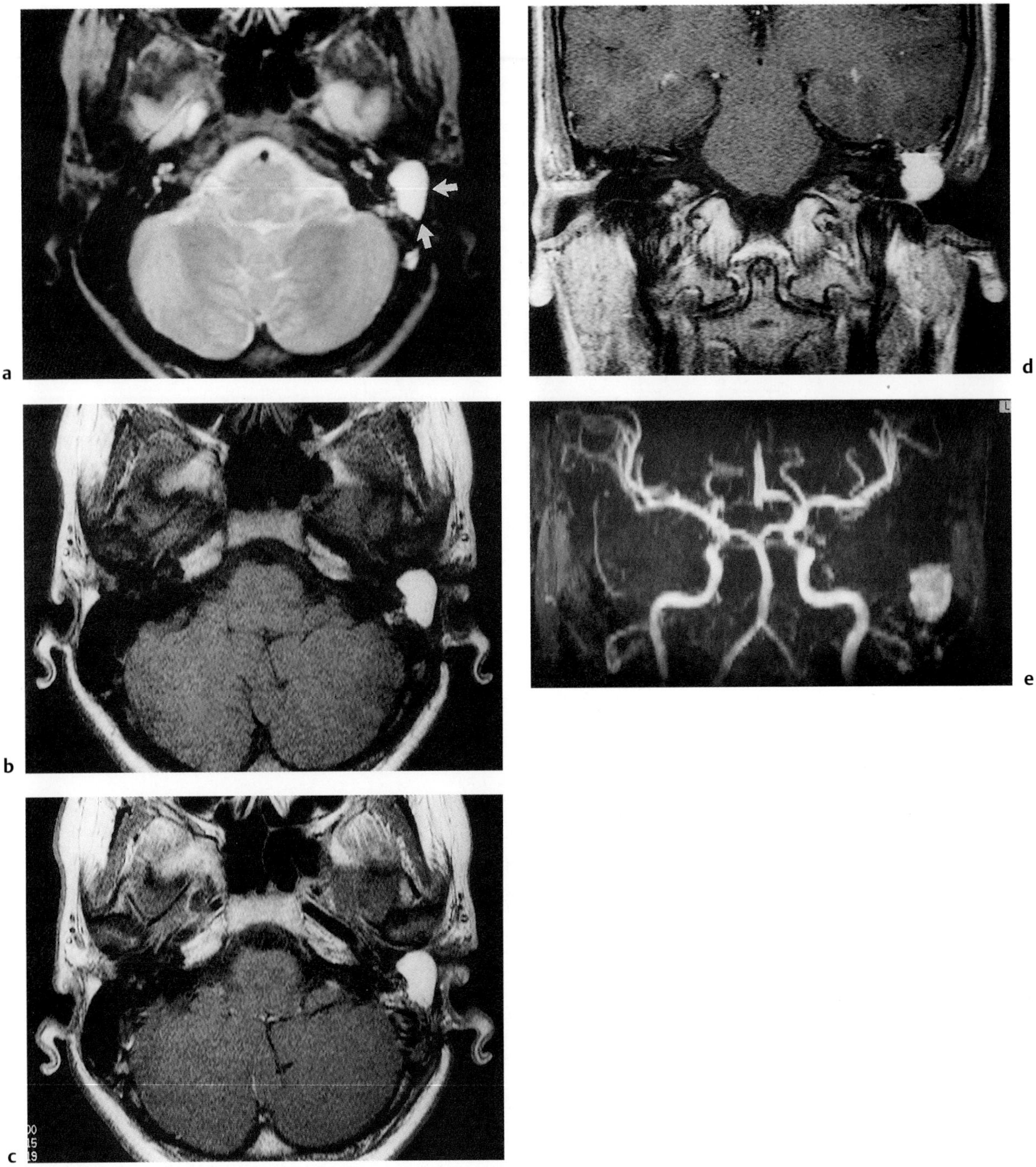

Figs. 4.**34 a–e Liquid mastoid mass: hemorrhagic seroma cavity with methemoglobin (post-partial mastoidectomy).**
(**a**) Unenhanced axial T2-weighted sequence (TR/TE = 2500/90 ms) shows a smooth-walled cavity in the mastoid filled with fluid of high signal intensity (arrows).
(**b**) Axial T1-weighted SE sequence (TR/TE = 500/15 ms) demonstrates high signal intensity based on the shortened T1 relaxation time.
(**c, d**) The post-contrast sequences show an absence of enhancement in and around the lesion, except for slight enhancement of posterior mastoid cells due to inflammatory change:
(**c**) Axial Gd-enhanced T1-weighted SE sequence (TR/TE = 500/15 ms).
(**d**) Coronal Gd-enhanced T1-weighted SE sequence (TR/TE = 500/15 ms).
(**e**) Arterial TOF MRA (TR/TE = 43/8 ms, flip angle = 20°) shows high signal intensity based on the inherent methemoglobin signal of the collection, distinguishing it from an aneurysm.

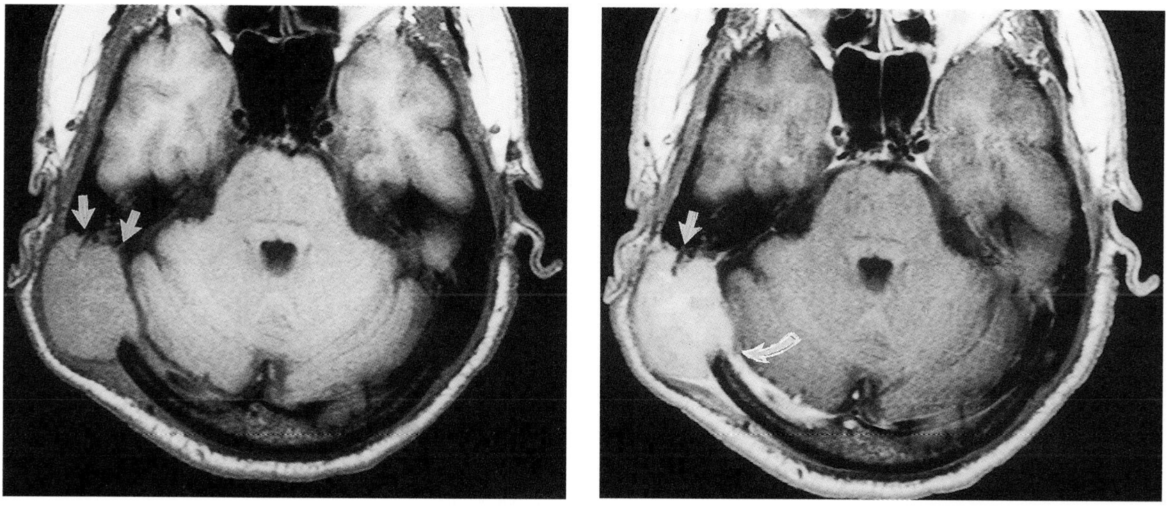

a b

Figs. 4.**35 a, b** **Mastoid mass: destructive metastatic adenocarcinoma in the right mastoid.**
(**a**) Axial T1-weighted sequence (TR/TE = 690/15 ms) without contrast enhancement shows a hyperintense mass with destruction of the calvaria and infiltration of the posterior mastoid (arrows).
(**b**) Gd-enhanced axial T1-weighted sequence (TR/TE = 690/15 ms) shows the intensely enhancing tumor, a metastatic adenocarcinoma (arrow), infiltrating the transverse sinus and central calvarial structures (curved arrow).

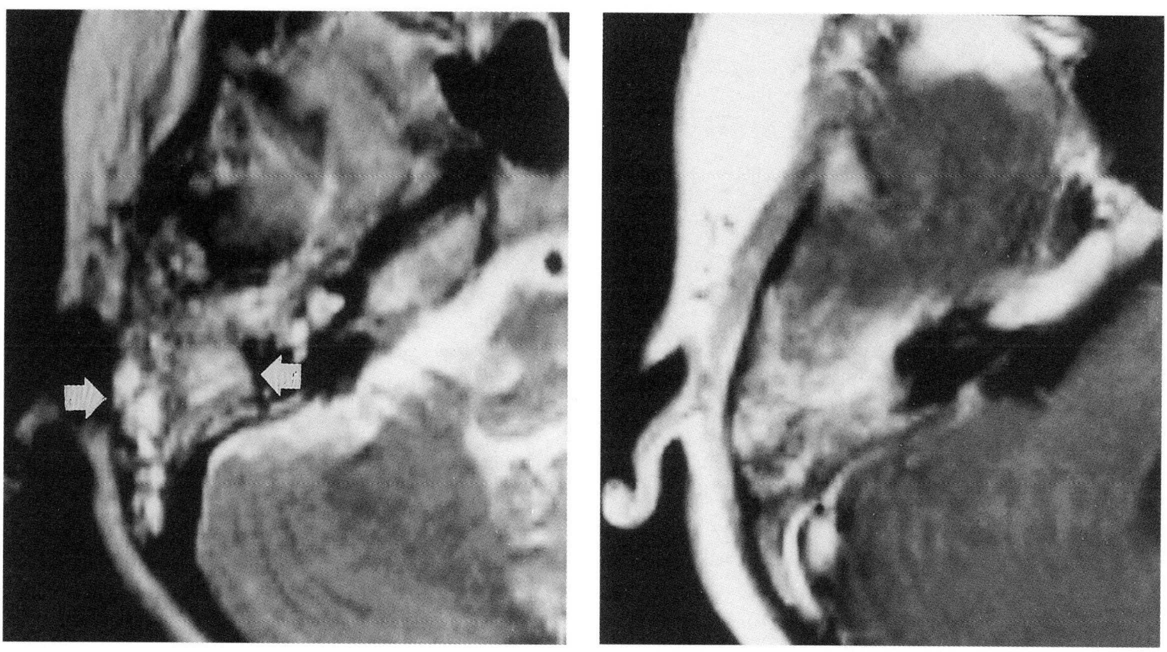

a b

Figs. 4.**36 a, b** **Acute liquefying mastoiditis, presenting as a mastoid mass.**
(**a**) Unenhanced T2-weighted SE sequence (TR/TE = 2500/90 ms) shows a partially confluent mass of high signal intensity (arrows).
(**b**) Gd-enhanced T1-weighted SE sequence (TR/TE = 500/15 ms) shows marked, nonhomogeneous enhancement throughout the mastoid region consistent with clinically verified liquefying mastoiditis.

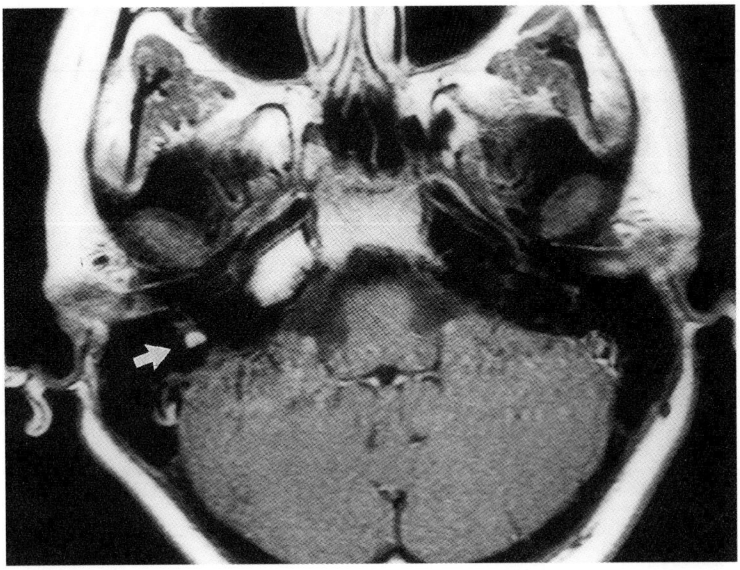

Fig. 4.**37** **Primary hyperintense mass in the aditus ad antrum with high T1-weighted signal intensity: intracancellous lipoma.** Axial Gd-enhanced T1-weighted sequence (TR/TE = 700/15 ms) documents a homogeneous mass with smooth borders within the cancellous bone of the aditus ad antrum (arrow). The high signal intensity and lack of contrast enhancement are consistent with the fatty tissue of a lipoma.

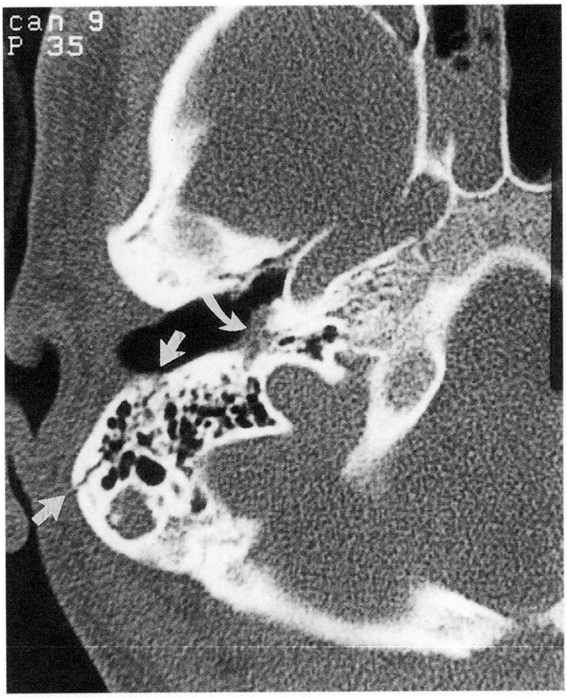

a

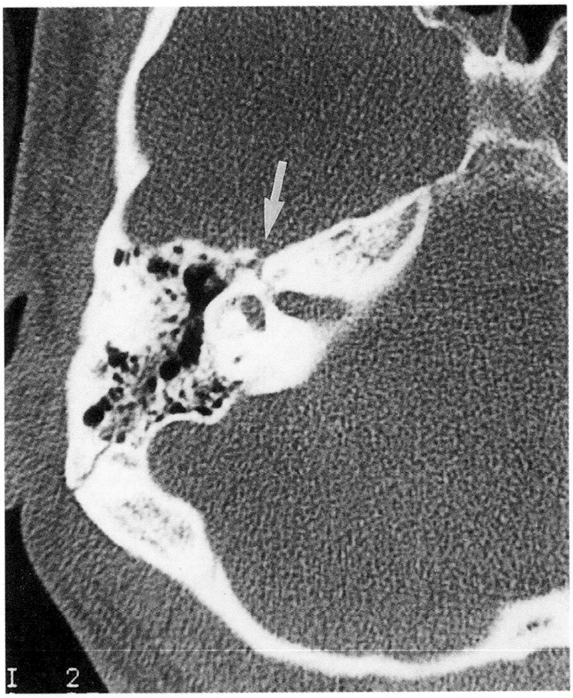

b

Figs. 4.**38 a, b** **Petrous bone fracture.**
(**a**) Axial HRCT scan demonstrates a fracture line through the mastoid (arrows) associated with a small intratympanic hemorrhage (curved arrow).

(**b**) This scan shows bleeding into the posterior part of the middle cranial fossa (arrow) and fracture extensions.

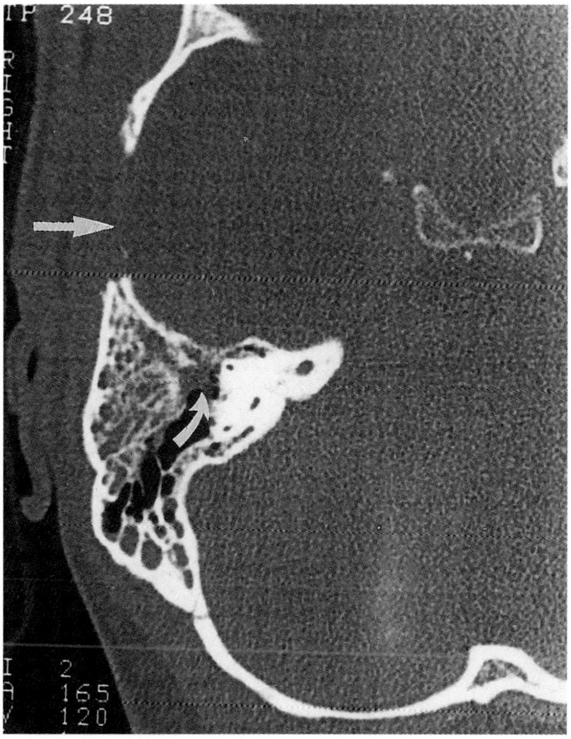

a

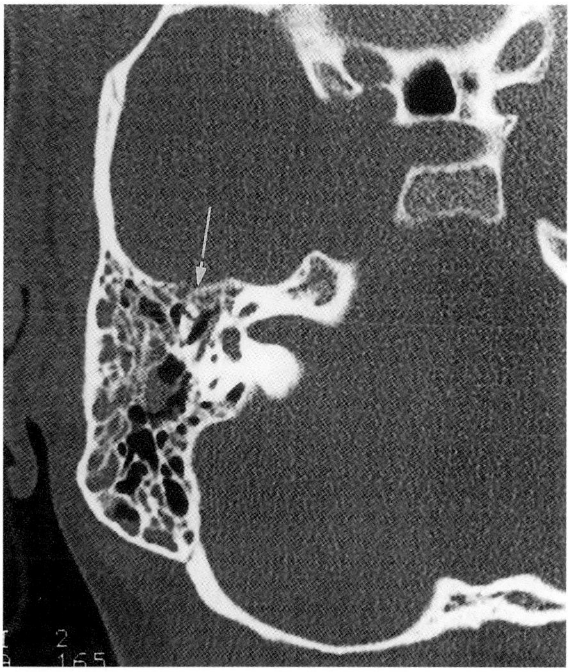

b

Figs. 4.**39 a, b** **Gunshot injury with prolapse of cerebral structures into the brain and middle ear.**
(**a**) Axial CT scan with a bone window shows defects in the anterior temporal bone (arrow), diffuse bleeding into the mastoid cells, and soft-tissue structures in the epitympanum (curved arrow) identified at operation as prolapsed cerebral structures.
(**b**) The ossicular chain is intact and undisplaced (arrow).

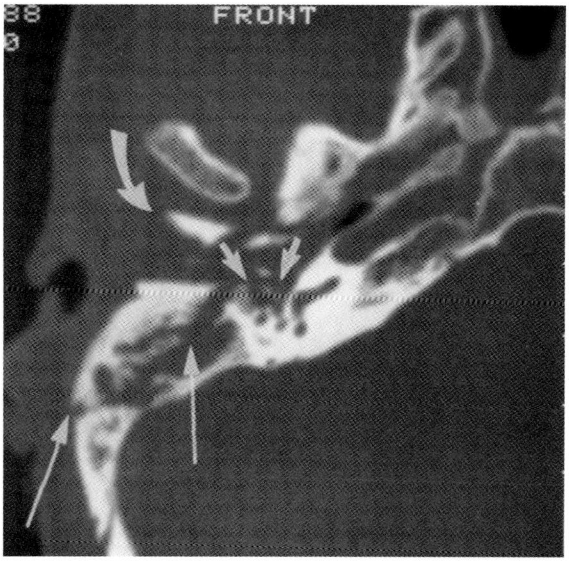

Fig. 4.**40** **Comminuted petrous bone fracture.** Axial CT scan with a bone window demonstrates a comminuted fracture of the right petrous bone with small fragments in the mastoid (long arrows) and displaced fragments of the external auditory canal (curved arrow). There is a concomitant fracture-dislocation of the incudomalleolar joint (short arrows).

References

1 Austin, J. R., D. R. Maceri: Anterior communicating artery aneurysm presenting as pulsatile tinnitus. J. Otolaryngol. 55 (1993) 54–57
2 Bradley, W. G., V. Waluch, K. Lai: The appearance of rapidly flowing blood on magnetic resonance imaging. AJR 143 (1984) 1167–1174
3 Bryant, R. G., K. Marill, C. Blackmore, C. Francis: Magnetic relaxation in blood and blood clots. Magn Reson Med. 13 (1990) 133–144
4 Fisch, U., D. Mattox: Classification of glomus temporale tumors. In: Microsurgery of the Skull Base. Thieme, Stuttgart 1988 (pp. 149–153)
5 Gebarski, S. S., S. A. Telian, J. K. Niparko: Enhancement along the normal facial nerve in the facial canal: MR Imaging and anatomic correlation. Radiology 183 (1992) 391–394
6 Glassock, M. E., J. R. Dickens, C. G. Jackson: Vascular anomalies of the middle ear. Laryngoscope 90 (1980) 77–88
7 Gomori, J. M., R. I. Grossmann, C. Yu-Ip, T. Asakura: NMR relaxation times of blood: dependence on field strength, oxidation state, and cell integrity. J Comput Assist Tomogr. 11 (1987) 684–690
8 Guild, S. R.: The glomus jugulare, a nonchromaffin paraganglion, in man. Ann Otol. 62 (1953) 1045–1071
9 Janick, P. A., D. B. Hackeney, R. I. Grossmann, T. Asakura: MR Imaging of various oxidation states of intracellular and extracellular hemoglobin. AJNR 12 (1991) 891–897
10 Kohsyu, H., M. Aoyagi, H. Tojima, et al.: Facial nerve enhancement in Gd-MRI in patients with Bell's palsy. Acta otolaryngol. Suppl 511 (1994) 165–169
11 Levine, S. B., J. B. Snow: Pulsatile tinnitus. Laryngoscope 97 (1987) 401–406
12 Lo, W. W. M., L. G. Solti-Bohman, J. T. McElveen Jr: Aberrant carotid artery: radiologic diagnosis with emphasis on high-resolution computed tomography. Radiographics 5 (1985) 985–993
13 Maasen, M. M., T. Lenarz, P. Ruck, S. Bien, D. Overkamp, E. Kaiserling: An active endocrine glomus tumor (paraganglioma) as cause of tinnitus and hypertension. HNO 41 (1993) 215–221
14 Mafee, M. F., M. Campos, S. Raju, et al.: Head and neck: high field magnetic resonance imaging versus computed tomography Otolaryngol Clin North Am. 21 (1988) 513–546
15 Mattle, H. P., K. U. Wentz, R. R. Edelman, et al.: Cerebral venography with MR. Radiology 178 (1991) 453–458
16 MJ, O. L., C. Shelton, N. A. Giddings, J. Kwartler, D. E. Brackmann: Glomus tympanicum tumors: a clinical perspective. Laryngoscope 101 (1991) 1038–1043
17 Naumann, H.-H.: Differentialdiagnostik in der Hals-Nasen-Ohren-Heilkunde. Symptome, Grenzgebiete. Thieme, Stuttgart 1990
18 Som, P. M., D. L. Reede, R. T. Bergeron, S. C. Parisier, J. M. A. Shugar, N. L. Cohen: Computed tomography of glomus tympanicum tumors. J Comput Assist Tomogr. 7 (1983) 14–17
19 Swartz, J. D., M. L. Bazarnic, T. P. Naidich, L. D. Lowry, H. T. Doan: Aberrant internal carotid artery lying within the middle ear: high resolution CT diagnosis and differential diagnosis. Neuroradiology 27 (1985) 322–326
20 Vogl, T. J., J. Ballhaus, S. Dresel, K. Kang: Gichttophus der Schädelbasis. Fortschr. Röntgenstr. 150 (1988) 613–614
21 Vogl, T. J., M. Bauer, H. Schedel, R. Brüning, K. Mees, J. Lissner: Kernspintomographische Untersuchungen von Paragangliomen des Glomus caroticum und Glomus jugulare mit Gd-DTPA. Fortschr. Röntgenstr. 148 (1988) 38–46
22 Vogl, T. J., R. Brüning, H. Schedel, G. Grevers, K. Kang, D. Hahn, J. Lissner: Paragangliomas of the jugular bulb and carotid body: MR imaging with short sequences and Gd-DTPA enhancemant. AJNR 10 (1989) 823–827
23 Vogl, T. J., M. G. Mack, M. Juergens, et al.: Skullbase glomus tumors: gadodiamide injection-enhanced MR Imaging-drop out effect in the early enhancemant pattern of paragangliomas versus different tumors. Radiology 188 (1993) 339–346
24 Wiet, R. J., S. A. Harvey, O. C., CA: Recent advances in surgery of the temporal bone and skull base. South Med J. 86 (1993) 5–12

5 Internal Auditory Canal, Cerebellopontine Angle, and Labyrinth

The clinical manifestations of diseases of the internal auditory canal, cerebellopontine angle, and labyrinth are based on the concomitant involvement of key bony, neural, and vascular structures by various types of pathology. Issues in diagnostic radiology center on the evaluation of mass lesions and inflammatory processes and their complications.

Once the clinical problem is known, an imaging procedure must be selected that is optimum for primary detection of the pathologic process. Some cases will require further investigation by an adjunctive procedure in order to make a precise differential diagnosis.

Normal Anatomy

As noted in Chapter 4, the temporal bone consists of *five bony parts*:

- Mastoid part.
- Squamous part.
- Petrous part.
- Tympanic part.
- Styloid process.

This section deals specifically with the petrous part of the temporal bone. The structures of the inner ear (Fig. 5.**1**) are contained within the petrous bone, which is often referred to as the petrous pyramid.

Two important structures on the *anterior surface* of the petrous pyramid are the tegmen tympani, which forms the roof of the tympanic cavity, and the arcuate eminence, the bony prominence over the semicircular canal that provides an important surgical landmark.

The *posterior surface* of the petrous pyramid contains the porus acusticus (Fig. 5.**2**), which is the opening of the internal auditory canal. Important bony structures in the internal auditory canal are the modiolus, or entrance to the cochlea, and the falciform crest, a bony septum in the lateral 3 mm of the internal auditory canal.

The *inferior surface* of the pyramid forms the carotid canal and jugular fossa. It is separated from the clivus by the petro-occipital fissure and foramen lacerum.

The complex anatomy of the internal auditory canal can be demonstrated by CT pneumocisternography and by MRI (Fig. 5.**3**). With high-resolution techniques, however, the imager must possess a detailed knowledge of the anatomic landmarks that are encountered. The lateral part of the canal, or fundus, is divided by a horizontal ridge (the falciform crest) and a vertical plate into four quadrants that characterize the anatomy and structure of the internal auditory canal. The facial nerve and adjacent nervus intermedius traverse the anterior superior quadrant of the fundus. The cochlear nerve occupies the anterior inferior quadrant, the superior vestibular nerve occupies the posterior superior quadrant, and the inferior vestibular nerve occupies the posterior inferior quadrant (Fig. 5.**4**).

The posterior ampullary nerve can sometimes be identified in the most posterior part of the fundus. The superior vestibular nerve supplies the utricle and the superior and lateral semicircular canals. The inferior vestibular nerve supplies the saccule, and the posterior ampullary nerve supplies the posterior semicircular canal. It is common for the anterior inferior cerebellar artery to form a vascular loop near the porus acusticus, but the relative position of this loop is highly variable.

Inner ear. The inner ear essentially contains the membranous labyrinth, which is contained within the bony labyrinth. The membranous labyrinth consists of the *vestibule* with the utricle and saccule, the *semicircular canals*, endolymphatic duct, *cochlear duct*, and multiple communicating channels (Fig. 5.**5**).

These anatomic details form the basis for the applications of imaging modalities in the inner ear. Thus, computed tomography (CT) is best for evaluating the bony structures of the labyrinth while heavily T2-weighted MR images can depict the fluid-containing structures of the membranous labyrinth (Fig. 5.**4**).

Cochlea. The cochlea usually makes two and one-half turns (Fig. 5.**5**), which can generally be visualized with CT and Magnetic resonance imaging (MRI). The basal turn opens posteriorly into the round window. The turns are directed about a central bony axis called the modiolus. The cochlear nerve enters the cochlea through the modiolus on its way to the multiple spiral ganglia.

Vestibule. The vestibule is the largest part of the membranous labyrinth (Fig. 5.**4 c**). Its subunits are the

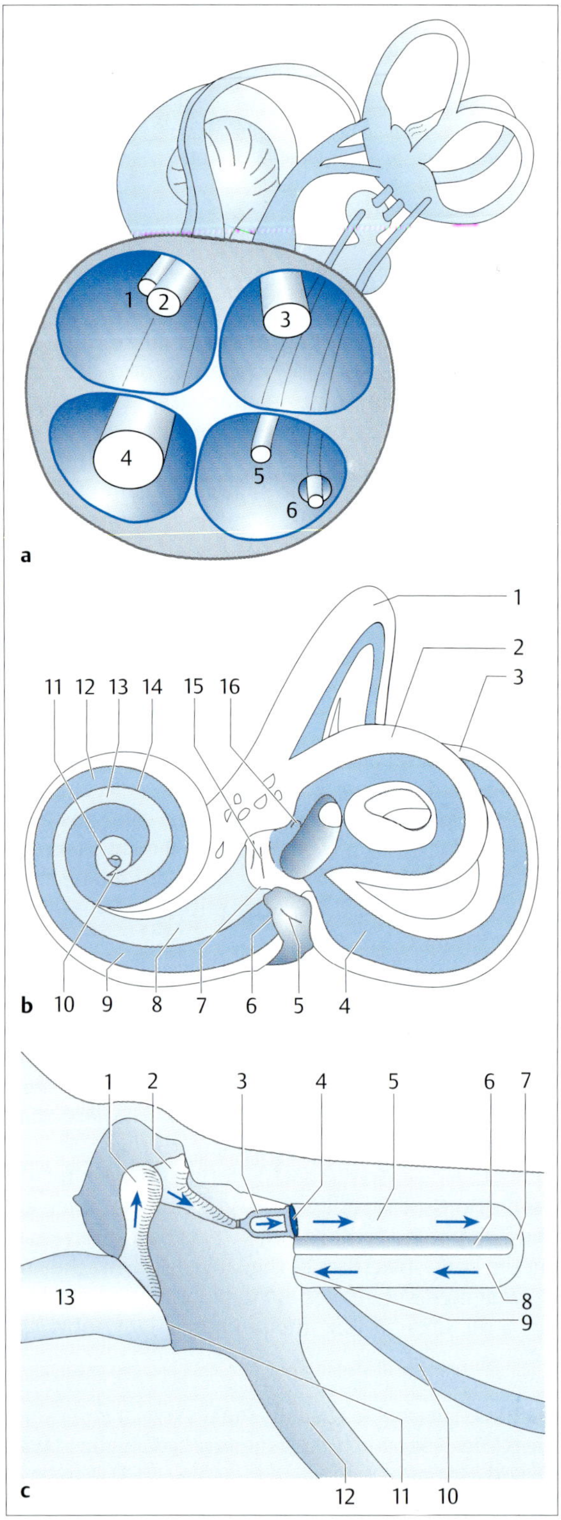

Figs. 5.**1 a–c** **(a)** Schematic representation of the neural anatomy of the inner ear (after Proctor).

1 Nervus intermedius (of Wrisberg)
2 Facial nerve
3 Superior vestibular nerve
4 Cochlear nerve
5 Inferior vestibular nerve
6 Posterior ampullary nerve

(**b**) Schematic cutaway view of the bony labyrinth, cochlea, and membranous labyrinth.

1 Superior semicircular canal
2 Lateral semicircular canal
3 Posterior semicircular canal
4 Posterior bony ampulla
5 Bony fossa of cochlear round window
6 Bony ridge of cochlear round window
7 Elliptical recess of vestibule
8 Bony spiral lamina
9 Hamulus of spiral lamina
10 Modiolus
11 Scala tympani
12 Bony spiral lamina
13 Scala vestibuli
14 Bony ridge of scala vestibuli
15 Inner orifice of vestibular aqueduct
16 Common bony crus

(**c**) Perilympathic and endolymphatic spaces in the cochlea. Sound vibrations from the tympanic membrane are transmitted by the malleus, incus, stapes, and footplate to the oval window and thence to the perilymph within the scala vestibuli. The wave motion induced in the perilymph rounds the helicotrema, travels back through the scale tympani to the base of the cochlea, and expends itself at the membrane of the round window. The cochlear duct is a blindly terminating membranous channel that contains the endolymph and is surrounded by the perilymphatic space (after Charletta).

1 Malleus
2 Incus
3 Stapes
4 Oval window
5 Scala vestibuli
6 Cochlear duct
7 Helicotrema
8 Scala tympani
9 Round window
10 Vestibular aqueduct
11 Tympanic membrane
12 Semicanal of eustachian tube
13 External auditory canal

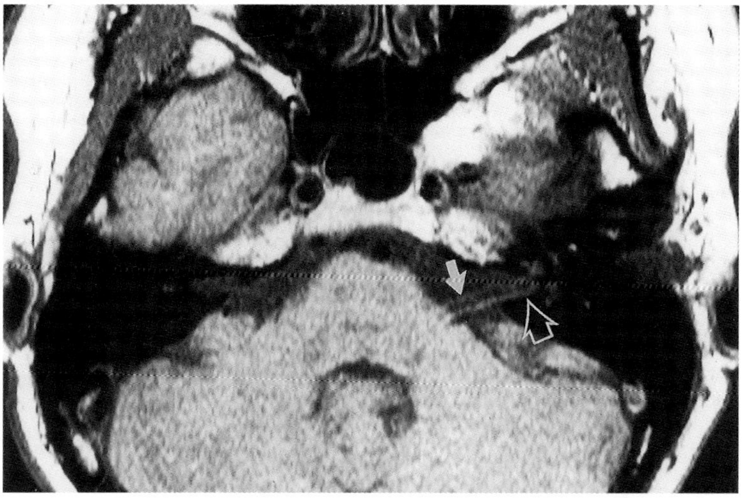

a

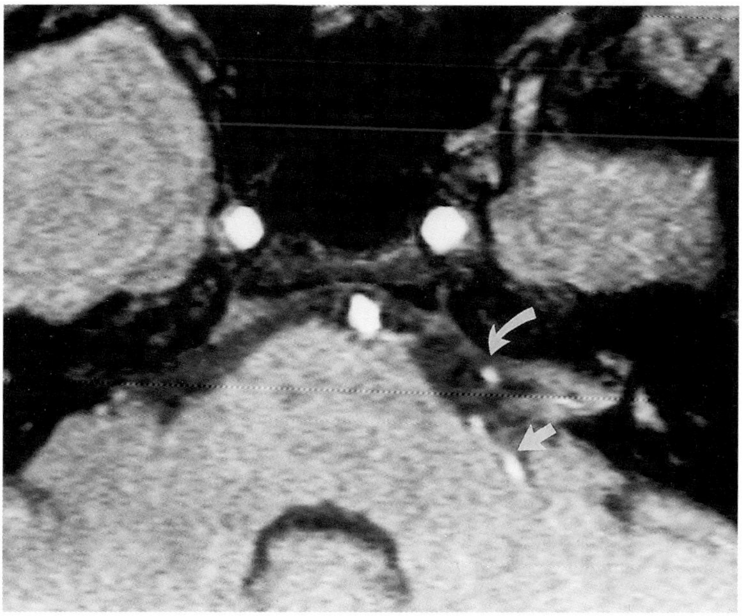

b

Figs. 5.**2 a, b** **Normal appearance of the internal auditory canal on MR images.**
(**a**) Axial MR image (1.5 T, TR/TE = 500/17 ms) demonstrates the double cranial nerve bundle in the internal auditory canal on the left side.
Arrow Facial nerve
Open arrow Superior vestibular nerve
(**b**) Axial MRA (3-D FISP sequence, TR/ TE = 40/7 ms, flip angle = 20°) defines the terminal branches of the labyrinthine artery (curved arrow) arising from the terminal portion of the anterior inferior cerebellar artery (arrow) on the left side.

utricle and saccule (Fig. 5.**5**), the utricle forming the more superior part of the vestibule and the saccule the inferior part. The vestibule is separated from the middle ear cavity by the oval window. It communicates superiorly with the superior semicircular canal.

Semicircular canals. These structures are termed the superior, posterior, and lateral semicircular canals. The upper border of the *superior* semicircular canal forms the arcuate eminence. The *posterior* semicircular canal is directed posteriorly along the petrous ridge (Fig. 5.**1 a**). The *lateral* semicircular canal, known also as the horizontal semicircular canal, relates very closely to the epitympanum. This explains the tendency of epitympanic cholesteatomas to fistulize the membranous labyrinth by eroding the lateral semicircular canal.

Cochlear aqueduct. The cochlear aqueduct contains the perilymphatic duct (Fig. 5.**4 c**). Approximately 8 mm long, the aqueduct connects the basal turn of the cochlea with the lateral border of the jugular foramen (Fig. 5.**5**). Because the cochlear aqueduct is parallel to the internal auditory canal and may be mistaken for it, the aqueduct requires careful differentiation on axial CT and MR images.

The vestibular aqueduct accompanies the cochlear aqueduct, extending from the vestibule and running approximately 1 cm posteroinferiorly to the endolymphatic sac (Fig. 5.**5**). The function of the endolymphatic sac and duct is to equilibrate endolymphatic fluid pressures.

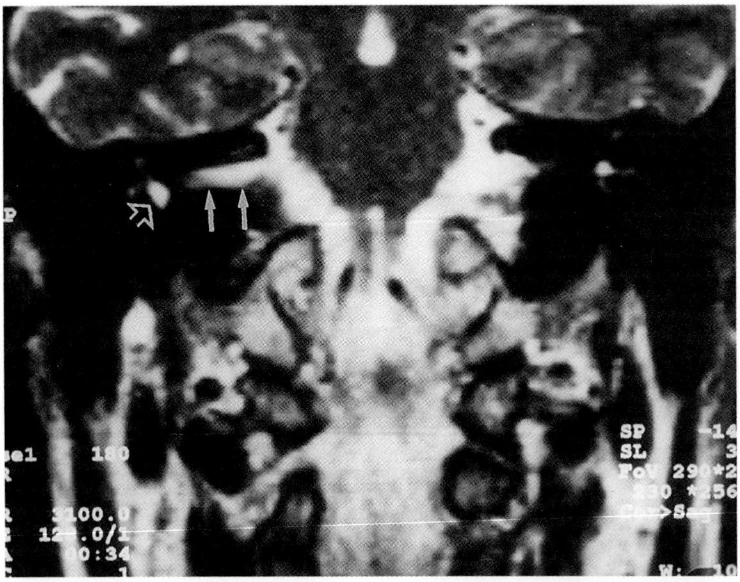

a

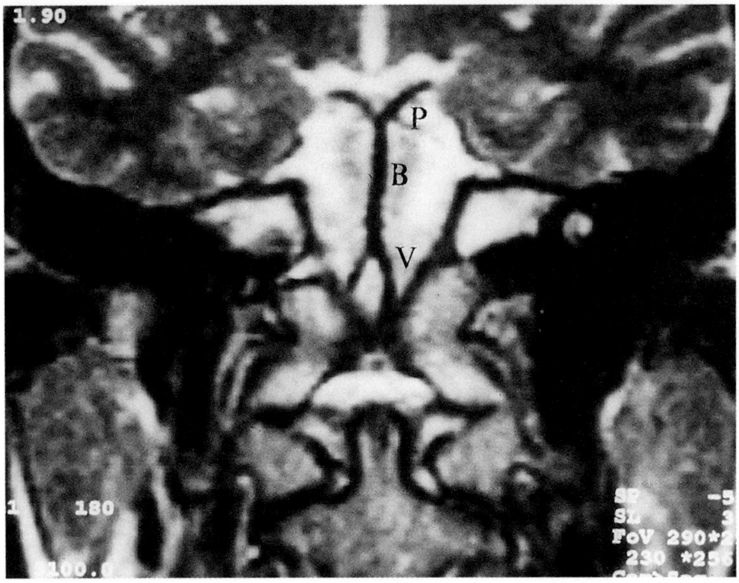

b

Figs. 5.3 **a, b Evaluation of the normal structures of the internal auditory canal in coronal TSE sequences.**
(**a**) TSE sequence (TR/TE = 3100/120 ms) defines the vestibular labyrinth (open arrow) and the hyperintense CSF-containing portions of the internal auditory canal (arrows). The pons displays a normal homogeneous texture.
(**b**) TSE sequence (TR/TE = 3100/120 ms) defines the course of both vertebral arteries, the basilar artery, and the posterior cerebral artery.

B Basilar artery
P Posterior cerebral artery
V Vertebral arteries

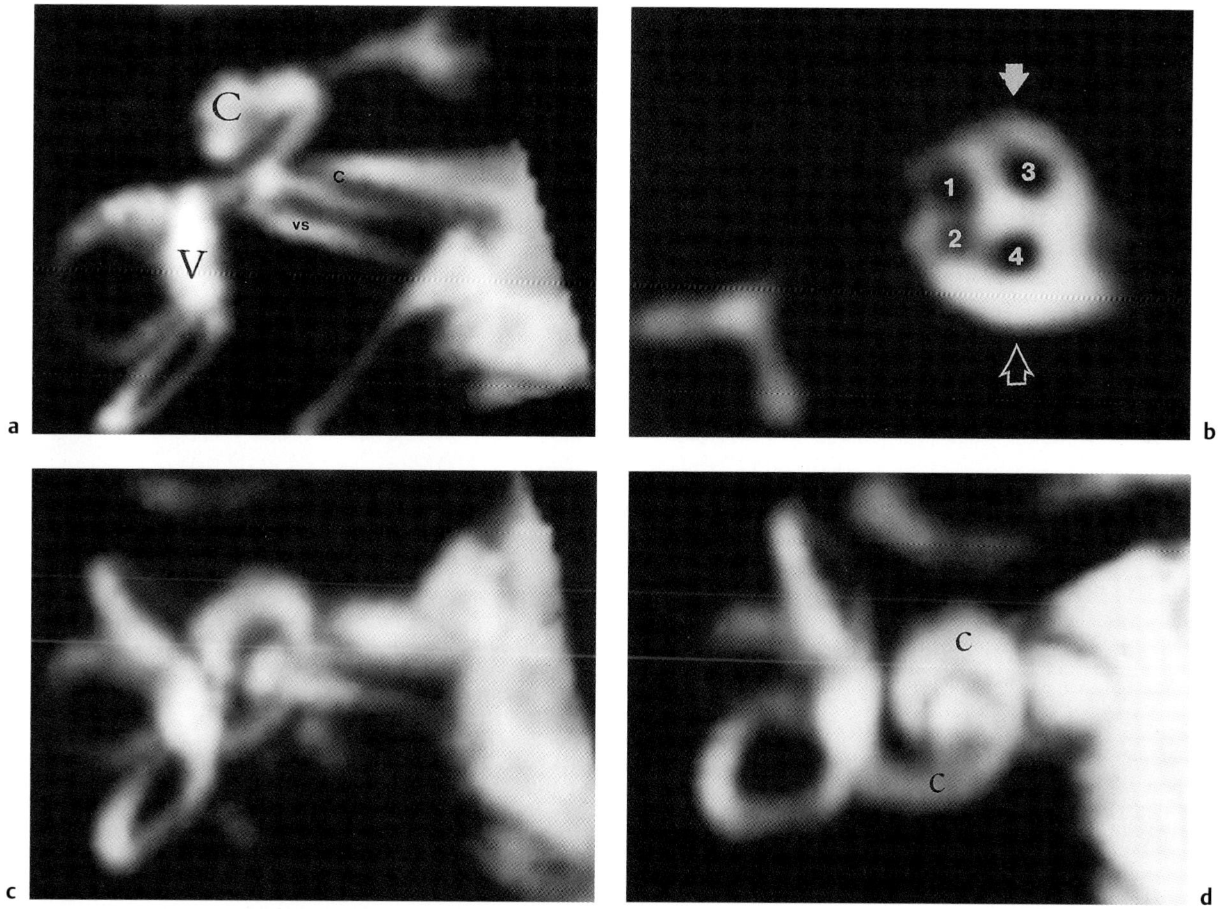

Figs. 5.**4 a – d** **Normal anatomic relationships in the internal auditory canal and inner ear.** High-resolution MRI using a T2-weighted SE sequence (TR/TE = 4797/400 ms):
(**a**) Maximum intensity projection (MIP) reconstruction from the 3-D data set vividly defines the fluid-containing structures in the internal auditory canal, cochlea, vestibule, semicircular canals, and associated neural structures (cochlear and superior vestibular nerves).
C Cochlea
c Cochlear nerve
V Vestibule
vs Superior vestibular nerve

(**b**) Sagittal reconstruction of the neural structures traversing the internal auditory canal. Fluid in the internal auditory canal gives a high signal intensity in the sagittal section. Anterior is left, posterior right. The white arrow points to the superior border of the canal, the open arrow to the inferior border.
1 Facial nerve
2 Cochlear nerve
3 Superior vestibular nerve
4 Inferior vestibular nerve

(**c**) MIP reconstruction defines the membranous labyrinth and other structures from a different viewing angle, giving particularly fine definition of the cochlear turns **(d)**.

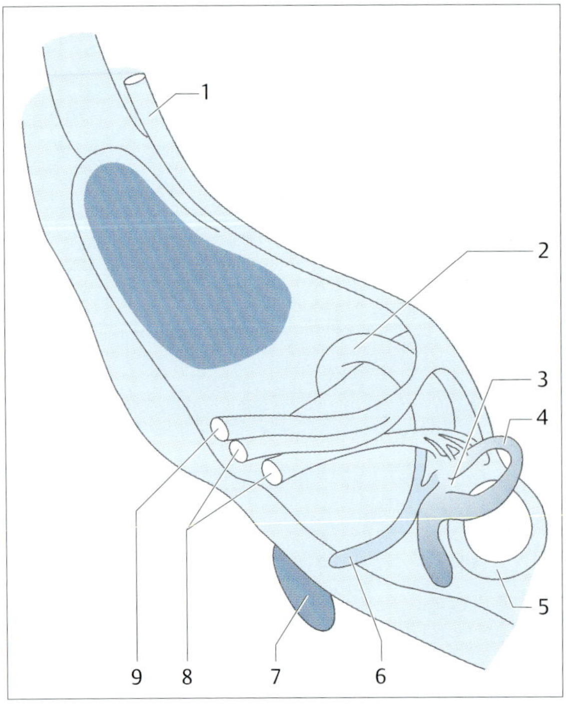

Fig. 5.**5** **Schematic diagram of the relationships of the cochlea, vestibule, semicircular canals, and jugular foramen.**

1 Petrosal nerve
2 Cochlea
3 Vestibule
4 Superior semicircular canal
5 Lateral semicircular canal
6 Posterior semicircular canal
7 Jugular foramen
8 Vestibulocochlear nerve
9 Facial nerve

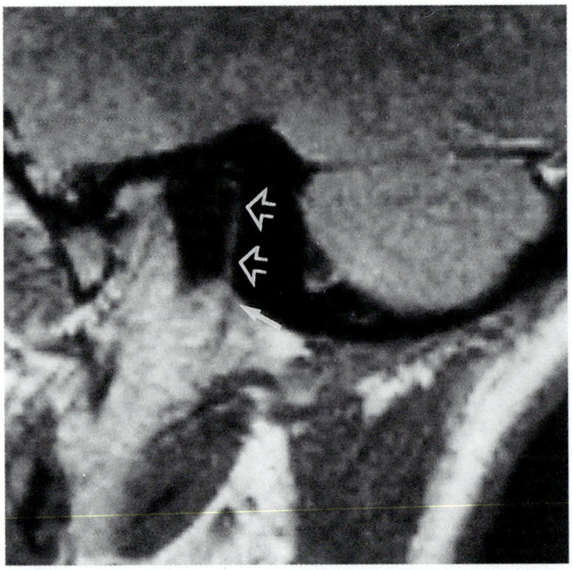

Fig. 5.**6** **Normal anatomy.** Unenhanced T1-weighted SE sequence (TR/TE = 500/15 ms). The mastoid segment of the facial nerve (open arrows) appears hyperintense relative to the low signal intensity of the mastoid. The intraparotid facial nerve branches appear hypointense (arrow).

Clinical Signs and Symptoms

The clinical manifestations of diseases of the internal auditory canal, inner ear, and cerebellopontine angle consist primarily of *sensorineural hearing loss, tinnitus*, and *vertiginous symptoms. Acute sensorineural hearing loss*, while a descriptive term for just one symptom, encompasses many disorders that fall under the heading of sudden hearing loss. Clinically it would include acute traumatic sensorineural hearing loss resulting from shock-wave trauma (gunshot, explosion), a transverse temporal bone fracture, a rupture of the round or oval window, or a high-energy electric shock or lightning strike. Acute toxic-infectious sensorineural hearing loss is often the result of viral infections such as herpes zoster oticus and other forms of meningoencephalitis. Ototoxic causes of sensorineural hearing loss include the use of ototoxic drugs such as aminoglycoside antibiotics, local anesthetics, and salicylates.

Chronic sensorineural hearing loss is most commonly due to chronic acoustic trauma, presbycusis, neuromas, and other conditions such as central mesencephalic hearing disorders.

The differential diagnosis of tinnitus is based on its locus of origin: middle ear tinnitus, cochlear tinnitus, or cervical tinnitus. Combined cochlear-neural forms and central tinnitus have also been described.

Clinical manifestations of vertigo. Vertigo, defined as the illusion of rotary or linear motion, can occur physiologically as "dizziness" or "motion sickness" in response to physical movement, or may occur pathologically. Pathologic vertigo may be continuous, paroxysmal, or induced by certain movements or body positions. Continuous vertigo may be subclassified as rotary vertigo, elevation vertigo, unsteady vertigo, and phobic vertigo.

The symptom of vertigo presents clinically with a great variety of causes and forms. The main considerations in differential diagnosis are Meniere disease, paroxysmal vertigo, postural vertigo, and vertiginous symptoms due to multiple sclerosis, vertebrobasilar insufficiency, vestibular neuritis, or acoustic neuroma.

Imaging Evaluation and Differential Diagnosis

Conventional Radiography

Conventional radiographic projections such as the Stenvers view (Fig. 5.**12a**) and the Schüller and Mayer views have become less important as primary investigations and as aids to differential diagnosis. Today they are used mainly for making side-to-side comparisons, the Stenvers view being particularly useful for this purpose.

Computed Tomography (CT)

High-resolution CT (HRCT) is considered the primary imaging study for evaluating the most common clinical symptoms such as conductive hearing loss (Figs. 5.**12c, d**). Axial scans are performed parallel to the orbitomeatal line, a slice thickness of 1 – 1.5 mm yielding optimum diagnostic results. For challenging diagnostic problems such as otospongiosis or otosclerosis, the axial CT scans should be supplemented by coronal scans or coronal reconstructions. Conventional scan techniques have been recommended in the past, but conventional spiral CT scanning of the petrous bone may compromise image quality due to kilovoltage limitations.

Magnetic Resonance Imaging (MRI)

High-resolution MRI yields outstanding results in the investigation of sensorineural hearing loss (Figs. 5.**12e**, 5.**14**, 5.**15**). The protocol for the MRI examination should always include heavily T1- and T2-weighted sequences, each providing high spatial resolution. Use of the new turbo spin-echo (TSE) sequences in this region can significantly improve the diagnostic results. It is essential to obtain both axial and coronal images, which may be supplemented by sagittal images if detailed topographic information is needed on the structures in the cerebellopontine cistern and internal auditory canal. Identical T1-weighted sequences obtained after the administration of an extracellular contrast agent (gadolinium[Gd]-DTPA, gadodiamide, or gadobutrol) will provide accurate delineation of structures showing normal or pathologic contrast enhancement (Fig. 5.**13c**).

With the advent of contrast-enhanced MRI as well as new 3-D techniques and high-resolution T2-weighted sequences using inversion-recovery techniques, MRI is also gaining increased clinical acceptance for the investigation of cochlear lesions and lesions of the vestibular apparatus (Table 5.**1**).

Table 5.**1** Diagnostic criteria in MR imaging

Precise topographic information in at least two planes.

Typical signal characteristics:
- Unenhanced T1-, T2-, and heavily T2-weighted SE sequences

Contrast-enhanced studies:
- Use of dynamic sequence protocols to improve the differential diagnosis of mass lesions and appreciate levels of contrast enhancement, homogeneity, margination, and accompanying perifocal changes.

Detection of the relative position of vascular processes and accompanying changes:
- Use of criteria such as displacement, thrombosis, and infiltration.

Findings at follow-up MRI:
- With small enhancing lesions and intense linear enhancement along neural structures: determination of cause by contrast-enhanced follow-up; regression of an enhancing mass or declining enhancement intensity are important indicators of a primary inflammatory or reactive process. Always to be interpreted within the clinical context.

Analysis of internal structures:
- Cyst containing cystic fluid (Fig. 5.**27**)
- Necrosis
- Calcifications
- Central vascular structures

Documentation of the fluid status of structures in the cochlea, vestibule, and semicircular canals to evaluate for primary malformations, degenerative inflammatory processes, or sites of tumor-related destruction (Figs. 5.**4c, d**).

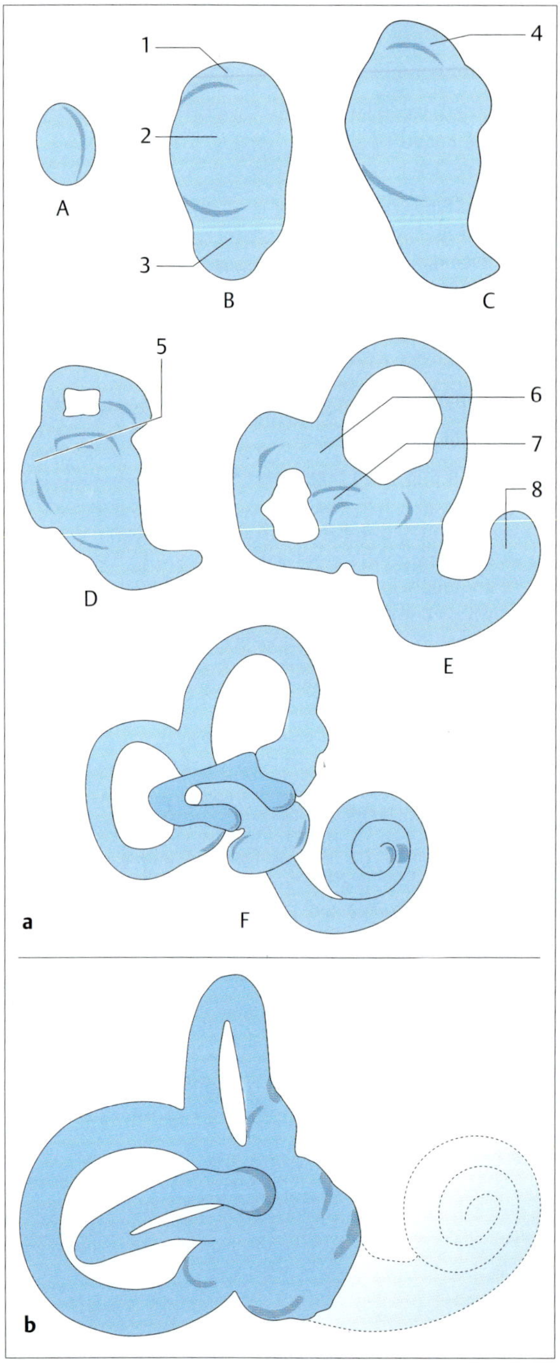

Figs. 5.**7 a, b** **Inner ear development and cochlear aplasia.**
(**a**) Development of the inner ear.
A Otocyst (day 26)
B Day 33
C Day 36
D Day 44
E Day 47
F Day 70
1 Endolymphatic process
2 Vestibular process
3 Cochleosaccular process
4 Process for superior semicircular canal
5 Process for posterior semicircular canal
6 Ampullary process
7 Process for lateral semicircular canal
8 Cochlear duct
(**b**) Cochlear aplasia. The cochlea is absent, presumably due to failure of the saccular part of the auditory vesicle to form a cochlear duct (at approximately 5 weeks' development).

Imaging Findings

Congenital Variations and Malformations

The detection of morphologic changes relating to malformations of the inner ear has assumed major importance in the diagnosis of patients with sensorineural hearing loss (Fig. 5.**11**). Labyrinthine anomalies are classified according to the stage of development of the otic capsule between the 5th and 7th weeks of fetal development (Figs. 5.**7** – 5.**10**).

HRCT has been the primary imaging tool in the past, with high-resolution MRI in "steady-state" protocols offering a new and promising data source. Today, with new MRI protocols such as GRASS, CISS, and TSE inversion-recovery sequences, it is possible to generate 3-D reconstructed images of these

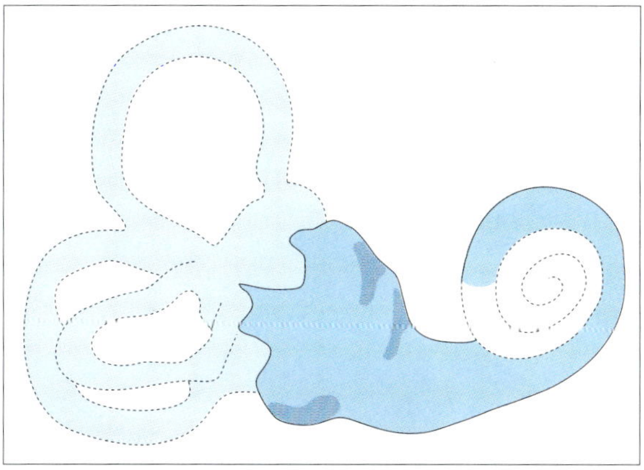

Fig. 5.**8** **Noonan syndrome.** Mondini deformity and bilateral aplasia of the semicircular canal. Cochlear development is incomplete due to deficient development of the cochlear duct (around week 7). Aplasia of the semicircular canals (around week 5 or 6).

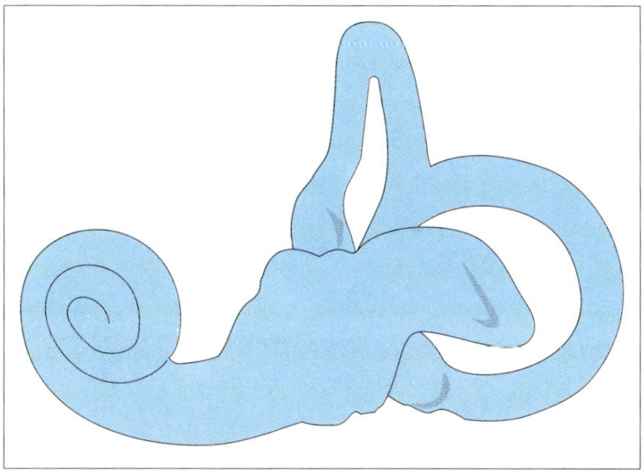

Fig. 5.**9** **Dysplasia of the lateral semicircular canal and vestibule** (around day 47).

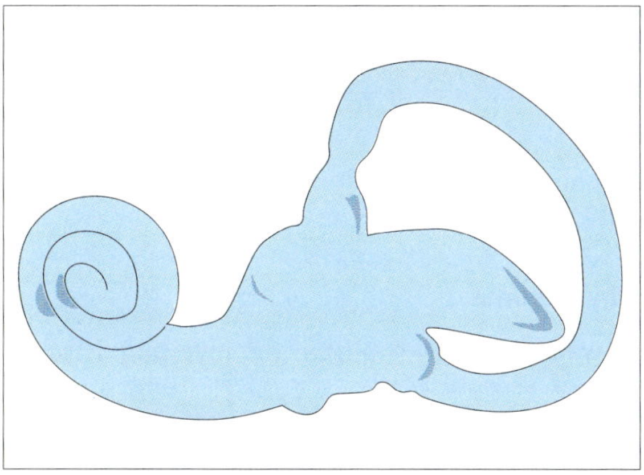

Fig. 5.**10** **Goldenhar syndrome.** Single posterior superior semicircular canal plus dysplasia of the lateral semicircular canal and vestibule (around day 45–47).

structures from various viewing angles (Figs. 5.**4 c, d**).

Malformations of the Inner Ear

An accurate knowledge of the embryologic development of the inner ear and associated neural structures (Fig. 5.**11**) enables us to assign potential malformations to specific developmental stages.

Cochlear Aplasia with or without Aplasia of the Cochlear Nerve (Fig. 5.**7 b**)

This anomaly is characterized by complete absence of the cochlea due to failure of the saccular part of the auditory vesicle to form a cochlear duct at the end of 5 weeks' development.

Noonan Syndrome (Fig. 5.**8**)

- Bilateral deafness.
- Facial, skeletal, and cardiac anomalies.

Mondini malformation. This term has various definitions in the literature but generally refers to incomplete partitioning of the cochlea with an abnormal number of cochlear turns.

Mondini deformity and bilateral aplasia of the semicircular canal. This refers to incomplete cochlear development due to deficient development of the cochlear duct (in the 7th week) plus aplasia of the semicircular canal in the 5th or 6th week (Fig. 5.**9**).

Goldenhar Syndrome (Fig. 5.**10**)

This syndrome, known also as oculoauriculovestibular dysplasia, is characterized by a single posterior superior semicircular canal with dysplasia of the lateral semicircular canal and vestibule (45th to 47th day) (Fig. 5.**7**).

- Enlarged lymphatic duct, bilateral aplasia of the semicircular canals.

Dysplasia of the lateral semicircular canal and vestibule (Fig. 5.**9**). High-resolution sub-millimeter-thick T2-weighted spin-echo (SE) sequences or gradient-echo sequences can resolve subtle anatomic details and provide high precision in the visualization of fluid-containing endolymphatic and perilymphatic spaces (Fig. 5.**4 c**).

Vestibular Aqueduct Syndrome

This malformation is generally associated with enlargement of the endolymphatic sac and may be accompanied by enlargement of the upper vestibule. The anomaly may be unilateral or bilateral.

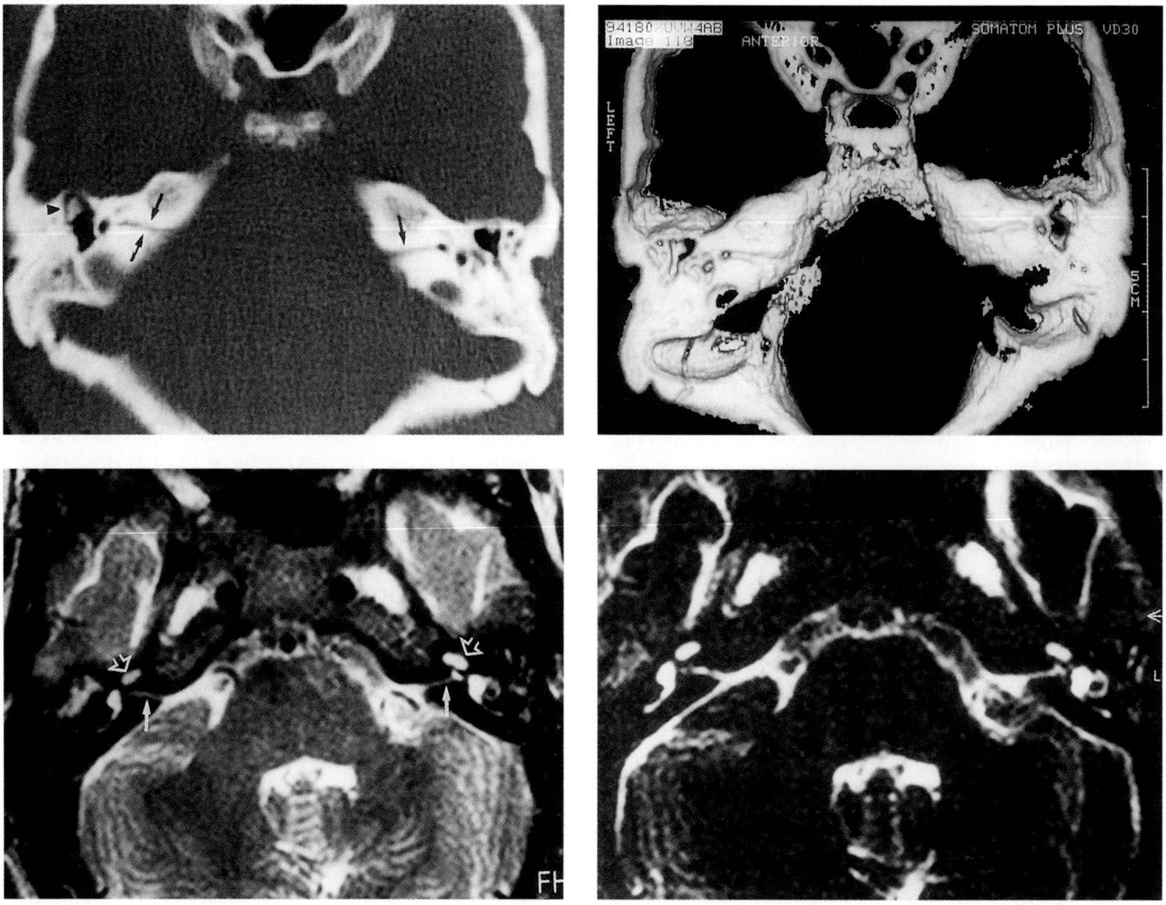

a b c d

Figs. 5.**11 a – d** **Malformation of the internal auditory canal with bilateral hypoplasia and aplasia of the vestibulocochlear nerve.**
(**a**) Axial HRCT shows bilateral hypoplasia of the internal auditory canal, which has a luminal diameter of 2 mm (arrows). The scan shows normal aeration of the tympanic cavity, in which the malleus can be seen (arrowhead).
(**b**) 3-D bilateral surface reconstruction of the petrous pyramids shows normal anatomic relationships including the relation of the pyramid to the clivus.
(**c**) Axial SE sequence with heavy T2 weighting (TR/TE = 2500/90 ms) confirms hypoplasia of the internal auditory canal and defines a linear CSF-filled channel about 1 mm in diameter (arrows). Normal signal intensity is noted in the anterior cochlea (open arrows) and vestibular labyrinth on each side.
(**d**) T2-weighted TSE sequence (TR/TE = 4797/400 ms) gives a superior view of fluid-containing structures in the region of the hypoplastic internal auditory canal. The high-resolution image confirms the CSF-intense structures in the hypoplastic canal and shows normally developed cochlear and vestibular structures.

Michel Deformity

This is an extremely rare dysplasia involving a complete lack of development of the inner ear.

Tumors

The diagnostic evaluation of tumor masses of the inner ear, internal auditory canal, and cerebellopontine angle is based on localizing the lesion to a specific site and establishing its identity (Table 5.**2**).

The analysis of large pathologic series documents the predominance of benign tumors, the most common of which is acoustic neuroma (Figs. 5.**18** – 5.**21**).

Schwannoma

Schwannomas develop from the investing Schwann cells of sensory nerves (Fig. 5.**29**). These cells are homologous to oligodendrocytes, as they are responsible for maintenance of the myelin sheath. This accounts for the variations in terminology: neuroma, neurinoma, neurilemoma.

Neuroma and *neurinoma* refer to a proliferation of nerve-cell fibers, while *neurilemoma* denotes a neoplastic transformation of the neural membrane.

Table 5.2 Differential diagnosis of tumor masses in the temporal bone

Benign tumors:
- Acoustic neuroma (Figs. 5.**17** – 5.**22**)
- Neuromas of cranial nerves V, VII, IX, X, XI, XII (Figs. 5.**33**, 5.**34**)
- Epidermoid
- Glomus jugulare tumor (Fig. 4.**29**)
- Adenoma: external auditory canal
- Meningioma (Fig. 5.**37**)
- Osteogenic tumors: osteoma, giant cell tumor, exostosis of external auditory canal
- Hemangioma
- Cholesterol granuloma (Fig. 5.**28**)

Malignant tumors:
- Carcinoma: external auditory canal (common), middle ear (rare)
- Lymphoma, leukemia
- Metastasis: breast, lung, kidney, prostate, melanoma (Fig. 5.**14**)
- Local infiltration: parotid gland carcinoma
- Myeloma
- Sarcoma: rhabdomyosarcoma, fibrosarcoma, lymphosarcoma, osteosarcoma, chondrosarcoma, undifferentiated sarcoma

All these terms are somewhat imprecise, however, and should be replaced by the term *schwannoma*.

Cranial nerve VII arises in the brainstem (Fig. 5.**4 b**), followed by cranial nerve VIII (the vestibulocochlear or acoustic nerve). The vestibular part of cranial nerve VIII reaches the brainstem before the cochlear part. The migration of the glial cells along the vestibular nerve structures during embryonic development explains why most schwannomas arise from the vestibular portion of cranial nerve VIII. The specific site of origin is the region of the Scarpa ganglion at the leptomeningeal junction, an area located between glial and Schwann cells.

Schwannomas of cranial nerve VIII (Fig. 5.**29**) account for 8 – 10% of all intracranial tumors and 80 – 90% of all cerebellopontine tumors. The average age at diagnosis is 45 years. Most of these tumors are homogeneous and encapsulated, but some may show central hemorrhage, edema, or cyst formation. The presence of cystic changes signifies a more aggressive tumor.

The predominant clinical symptoms are tinnitus and a sudden or slowly progressive sensorineural hearing loss. Larger tumors may also cause symptoms due to adjacent cranial nerve involvement. Bilateral neoplasms of the same histologic type should raise suspicion of Recklinghausen disease. It should be considered that bilateral expansion of the internal auditory canal may occur in patients with Recklinghausen disease in the absence of a tumor mass.

On CT scans, acoustic schwannoma appears as an enhancing lesion in or adjacent to the internal auditory canal (Figs. 5.**29**, 5.**34**, 5.**35**). Most tumors show uniform enhancement, but nonhomogeneous or rim enhancement is sometimes seen. Large schwannomas that arise directly from the canal may cause bony erosion. More extensive bone destruction is unusual and should suggest other diagnostic possibilities. Calcifications are rarely seen.

It should be noted that isolated expansion of the internal auditory canal may occur as a congenital variation. Also, vessels that take an aberrant course in the internal auditory canal may be a source of marked contrast enhancement. Pneumocisternography (radiography following the intrathecal injection of air) has been abandoned in favor of MRI, which permits the accurate diagnosis and differential diagnosis of schwannomas in the region of the internal auditory canal and cerebellopontine angle.

Schwannomas of Other Cranial Nerves (Figs. 5.**34** and 5.**35**)

Schwannomas may involve various cranial nerves in the cerebellopontine angle region. After the vestibulocochlear nerve, the facial nerve is the most commonly affected. In cases where a facial neuroma has not enlarged the labyrinthine segment of the nerve, producing characteristic CT and MR findings, it can be difficult to recognize the tumor even at operation. In these cases the clinical manifestations of facial nerve dysfunction are the most helpful diagnostic sign.

Neuromas of the trigeminal nerve (cranial nerve V) can also be identified in the cerebellopontine angle even though they arise near Meckel's cavity, a dural recess lying at the junction of the posterior and middle cranial fossae at the petrous apex. Generally these tumors have a more anterior location than tumors of cranial nerve VIII. Schwannomas of the four lower cranial nerves usually cause expansion of the jugular foramen or hypoglossal canal (Fig. 5.**34**).

Meningioma (Fig. 5.**37**)

Meningiomas of the cerebellopontine angle are less common than schwannomas but may be indistinguishable from them by their enhancement features alone. Meningiomas are more likely to show increased density on noncontrast CT scans, and they are more frequently associated with calcifications. Because meningiomas arise from arachnoid villi in the cerebellopontine angle, they occupy a more anterior site in relation to the petrous apex. Expansion of the internal auditory canal may occur but is an uncommon finding.

Meningiomas that do cause bony expansion of the internal auditory canal will display a broader base than schwannomas and will show greater involvement of nearby structures.

Epidermoid (Congenital Cholesteatoma) (Fig. 5.**26**)

Epidermoid or congenital cholesteatoma is, according to various sources, the second or third most common cerebellopontine angle tumor. Most are uniformly hypodense on CT scans, and some display rim enhancement on postcontrast CT and MR images. There may be scalloping or displacement of adjacent bony structures. Clinical manifestations are generally mild and less pronounced than radiologic findings would suggest.

Arachnoid Cyst (Fig. 5.**27**)

A number of causes have been proposed for arachnoid cysts, including trauma, infection, and duplication of the arachnoid membrane. The lesions appear as uniformly low-attenuation masses on CT scans and show typical relaxation characteristics on MR images. Arachnoid cysts are generally associated with little or no bony changes and display a smooth inner wall.

Glomus Tumors

See Chapter 4.

Astrocytoma, Medulloblastoma, and Ependymoma (Fig. 5.**23**)

Astrocytomas, medulloblastomas, and ependymomas may arise in the cerebellar hemisphere or fourth ventricle and extend toward the cerebellopontine angle. Most have an intra-axial origin, making them easy to differentiate from schwannomas, but the occasional presence of extra-axial exophytic components may cause diagnostic uncertainty. The absence of demonstrable bone erosion can aid in the evaluation of these cases. Very rarely, choroid plexus papillomas may be found in the cerebellopontine angle region or in the lateral recess if the latter contains a prolongation of choroid plexus.

Endolymphatic Sac Tumors

Tumors of the endolymphatic sac often present clinically with sensorineural hearing loss, tinnitus, facial weakness, or adenomatous tumors of the petrous pyramid.

CT and MRI depict an erosive tumor on the posterior wall of the petrous apex. The tumor has cystic contents and may contain methemoglobin. Angiography usually demonstrates a hypervascular mass.

Differential Diagnosis

The principal benign and malignant tumor masses of the temporal bone are listed in order of frequency in Table 5.**2**. A number of other lesions have been described in the region of the cerebellopontine angle and internal auditory canal including *mucoceles, osteotomas, cholesterol granulomas* (Fig. 5.**28**), *cholesterol cysts, chondrogenic tumors*, and *giant cell tumors*. The differential diagnosis of these lesions can be quite challenging, and we refer the reader to journal articles that detail the features of individual cases.

The differential diagnosis should also include invasive malignant neoplasms that spread from the nasopharynx or external auditory canal to involve the inner ear, internal auditory canal, or cerebellopontine angle.

The differential diagnosis of *cerebellopontine-angle tumors* should include the full spectrum of mass lesions that may arise from brainstem structures or from adjacent areas such as the subarachnoid space. *Acoustic neuroma* is by far the most common cerebellopontine angle mass (Figs. 5.**17**–5.**22**), followed by *arachnoid cysts, epidermoid (primary cholesteatoma)* (Fig. 5.**26**), and *meningioma* (Fig. 5.**37**). *Vascular masses* such as vertebral or basilar artery ectasia and intracranial aneurysms may also present in the cerebellopontine angle.

Primary brainstem tumors include *pons glioma, tumors of the fourth ventricle*, and lateral extensions of *cerebellar neoplasms* such as astrocytoma or hemangioblastoma.

Rare mass lesion of this region include *arteriovenous angioma, chordoma, metastases, rhabdomyosarcoma*, and *neuromas* of other cranial nerve groups (VII, X, XI, XII) (Fig. 5.**35**). Other masses may originate from the jugular fossa, such as glomus tumors or rhabdomyosarcomas with extension to the cerebellopontine angle. In principle, *parasellar masses* such as chromophobic adenoma, optic glioma, craniopharyngioma, or nasopharyngeal carcinoma also may involve the cerebellopontine angle secondarily.

A common *congenital tumor* of this region is congenital cholesteatoma. Common inflammatory lesions are cholesterol granuloma and petrous apicitis (Gradenigo syndrome). True tumor masses may consist of primary or secondary tumors such as neuroma, hemangioma, meningioma, metastases, secondary infiltrative lesions, and paraganglioma.

Inflammatory Lesions

Various inflammatory diseases may originate in the region of the inner ear or adjacent structures:

Ossifying Labyrinthitis

Ossifying labyrinthitis presents clinically with progressive deafness, often prompting an evaluation for cochlear implantation. The most frequent cause is postinflammatory ossification of the membranous labyrinth. Tympanogenic, posttraumatic, postoperative, and postmeningitic causes have also been implicated.

CT usually demonstrates a normal membranous labyrinth compromised by scattered foci of bony deposition. A tympanogenic cause has been postulated for unilateral cases and a postmeningitic cause for bilateral cases.

Petrous Apicitis (Gradenigo Syndrome)

This condition is marked clinically by retro-orbital pain, abducens nerve palsy, and otorrhea. CT shows a destructive osteomyelitic lesion of the petrous apex, often combined with fluid in the ipsilateral middle ear and mastoid. T2-weighted MRI shows a patchy hyperintense area with ill-defined borders.

Facial Nerve Palsy

The dominant clinical entity is primary facial nerve palsy (Bell palsy), which often requires differentiation from secondary forms of facial palsy.

Whereas primary facial nerve palsy is considered to have a viral or idiopathic cause, secondary forms can have various causes as listed in Table 5.**3**.

It is normal for high-resolution contrast-enhanced T1-weighted MR images of the facial nerve to demonstrate linear or focal enhancement in the anterior genu and horizontal segment of the nerve. This does not constitute a pathologic finding—unlike the contrast enhancement of the labyrinthine and/or descending facial nerve segment that signifies an inflammatory, traumatic, or neoplastic process.

Accordingly, the diagnostic imaging of facial nerve palsy is warranted only in cases that manifest one or more of the indications listed in Table 5.**4**.

Table 5.3 Secondary causes of facial nerve palsy

Neoplastic:
- Neuroma: acoustic neuroma (Figs. 5.**17**–5.**22**), facial neuroma, brainstem neuroma, parotid gland neuroma

Inflammatory:
- Sarcoidosis, Lyme disease, cholesteatoma, trauma (Figs. 5.**31**, 5.**32**), multiple sclerosis

Table 5.4 Indications for diagnostic imaging (MRI, CT) in facial nerve palsy

- Persistence of facial nerve palsy for more than 2 months
- Gradual progression of palsy
- Facial spasm
- Recurrence of facial nerve palsy
- Significant pain
- Multiple cranial neuropathies
- Clinical suspicion of vascular compression syndrome: coiling/kinking of posterior inferior cerebellar artery, vertebral artery, labyrinthine artery

Osteodystrophic Diseases of the Temporal Bone (Otosclerosis, Otospongiosis)

Several clinical forms are recognized:

The *fenestral type* is associated with conductive hearing loss and normal otoscopic findings. Early *tinnitus* develops in two-thirds of patients and is bilateral in 85%. The *cochlear type* presents clinically with sensorineural hearing loss, and *combined forms* present with mixed sensorineural and conductive hearing loss.

The pathogenesis involves the early replacement of enchondral bone by foci of spongy new bone. Later the foci recalcify into a dense, ossified plaque.

Fenestral Otosclerosis

This most common type of otosclerosis (80–90% of cases) begins in the fissula antefenestrum on the anterior margin of the oval window. CT may demonstrate new bone formation in the fissular area. Occasionally plaque is also found on the posterior oval window margin and the round window. In the early lytic phase, the oval window appears too wide as a result of osteoclastic resorption.

Cochlear Otosclerosis (Retrofenestral Type)

Cochlear otosclerosis is much less common than the fenestral type, but both forms may be combined. Sensorineural hearing loss is generally present.

CT usually shows focal lucencies in the otic capsule, which may appear as a "third turn" of the cochlea on axial scans. Subtle forms of cochlear otosclerosis may produce no CT abnormalities, however.

MRI demonstrates focal areas of punctate contrast enhancement in the otic capsule on T1-weighted SE sequences.

Paget Disease

Paget disease (osteitis deformans) is an inherited, progressive bone disease that predominantly affects the axial skeleton. It may occur in the *monostotic form* or the more common *polyostotic form*. The skull is frequently involved, showing features of circumscribed osteoporosis; the temporal bone is less commonly affected. Infiltration of the membranous labyrinth by adjacent pagetic bone results in sensorineural or mixed hearing loss.

CT findings are characteristic, consisting of diffuse demineralization and foci of increased density with ill-defined borders and a cotton-wool appearance.

Fibrous Dysplasia (Figs. 7.**21 b**, **c**)

Fibrous dysplasia is a slowly progressive, inherited bone disease that is generally monostotic when it involves the temporal bone. Its pathogenesis, while still obscure, involves the development of fibro-osseous tissue in the interior of the affected bone. The clinical presentation usually consists of conductive hearing loss with bony stenosis of the external ear canal.

CT generally permits an accurate diagnosis of fibrous dysplasia. The affected bone usually appears hyperdense, although cystic components have been reported. A bony prominence is seen in the external ear canal. Generally the membranous labyrinth, facial nerve, and internal auditory canal are spared. A cholesteatoma may develop medial to the stenotic external ear canal.

Osteogenesis Imperfecta

The delayed form of osteogenesis imperfecta has the same pathogenesis as otosclerosis, and it has been suggested that both conditions have a common genetic cause. Osteogenesis imperfecta is marked clinically by the occurrence of painless spontaneous fractures in response to minor trauma. When the temporal bone is involved, the clinical manifestations of osteogenesis imperfecta are identical to those of otosclerosis, and the CT findings are the same as in fenestral and cochlear otosclerosis. The combination of osteogenesis imperfecta, otosclerosis, and blue sclera is termed *Hoeve syndrome*.

Temporal Bone Trauma

(Figs. 5.**31** and 5.**32**)

The following areas are of central concern in evaluations for temporal bone trauma:

- The carotid canal: fractures in this area may cause occlusion of the internal carotid artery.
- The bony labyrinth: a fracture through the bony labyrinth may cause acute labyrinthine dysfunction including vertigo and immediate deafness.
- The facial nerve: involvement of the facial nerve canal may cause immediate and complete facial nerve palsy.

Imaging Criteria and Their Differential Diagnosis

This section deals with the main criteria that are used to analyze radiologic findings in the inner ear, internal auditory canal, and cerebellopontine angle. High-resolution, contrast-enhanced MRI is becoming an increasingly important imaging tool compared with CT, depending on the clinical presentation.

Asymmetric Expansion of the Internal Auditory Canal on Conventional Radiography and CT

Before the advent of CT and MRI, the search for head and neck tumors relied on conventional X-ray studies such as the Stenvers projection (Fig. 5.**12**) or motion-controlled tomography. A comparative analysis of bilateral Stenvers views can provide a gross impression as to the presence of a unilateral or bilateral mass lesion.

But the detection rate and differential diagnostic results with this approach are highly questionable due to the low sensitivity and specificity of conventional X-ray films. Thus, any asymmetric dilatation of the internal auditory canal that is noted on a Stenvers film should always be investigated by contrast-enhanced MRI.

The most common cause for an asymmetric dilatation of the internal auditory canal is an anatomic variant that is not associated with any definite pathology. In patients with marked bilateral dilatation of the internal auditory canal, the differential diagnosis should include Recklinghausen disease, which is often not accompanied by a visible tumor mass. All the other usual considerations apply to the differential diagnosis of internal auditory canal expansion.

Solid Enhancing Mass Larger than 5 mm in the Internal Auditory Canal on CT or MRI

A mass lesion in the internal auditory canal larger than 5 mm in diameter can be accurately evaluated by CT or preferably by contrast-enhanced MRI. The various neuromas and meningiomas can be differentiated by their location in the great majority of cases (Fig. 5.**13**). Signs of meningeal carcinomatosis should be sought in patients with metastatic disease (Fig. 5.**14 a** and Table 5.**5**).

Table 5.**5** Solid enhancing mass larger than 5 mm in the internal auditory canal on CT or MRI

Findings	**Differential diagnostic criteria**
Common:	
➤ Tumor:	
–Acoustic neuroma (schwannoma) (Figs. 5.**13**, 5.**14**, 5.**17**)	Topography
–Facial nerve neuroma	Topography
–Meningioma (Fig. 5.**5**)	Topography
–Osseous hemangioma	Signal characteristics
➤ Vascular lesion:	
–Arteriovenous malformation (Fig. 5.**18**)	Vascular structures
➤ Inflammation:	
–Focal arachnoiditis	Follow-up
–Sarcoidosis	Focal enhancement
–Meningitis (Fig. 5.**16**)	
Rare:	
➤ Tumor:	
–Metastasis	Destruction
–Other neuromas (Figs. 5.**33**–5.**36**)	Topography
–Arachnoid cyst (Fig. 5.**27**)	Signal characteristics
➤ Inflammation	

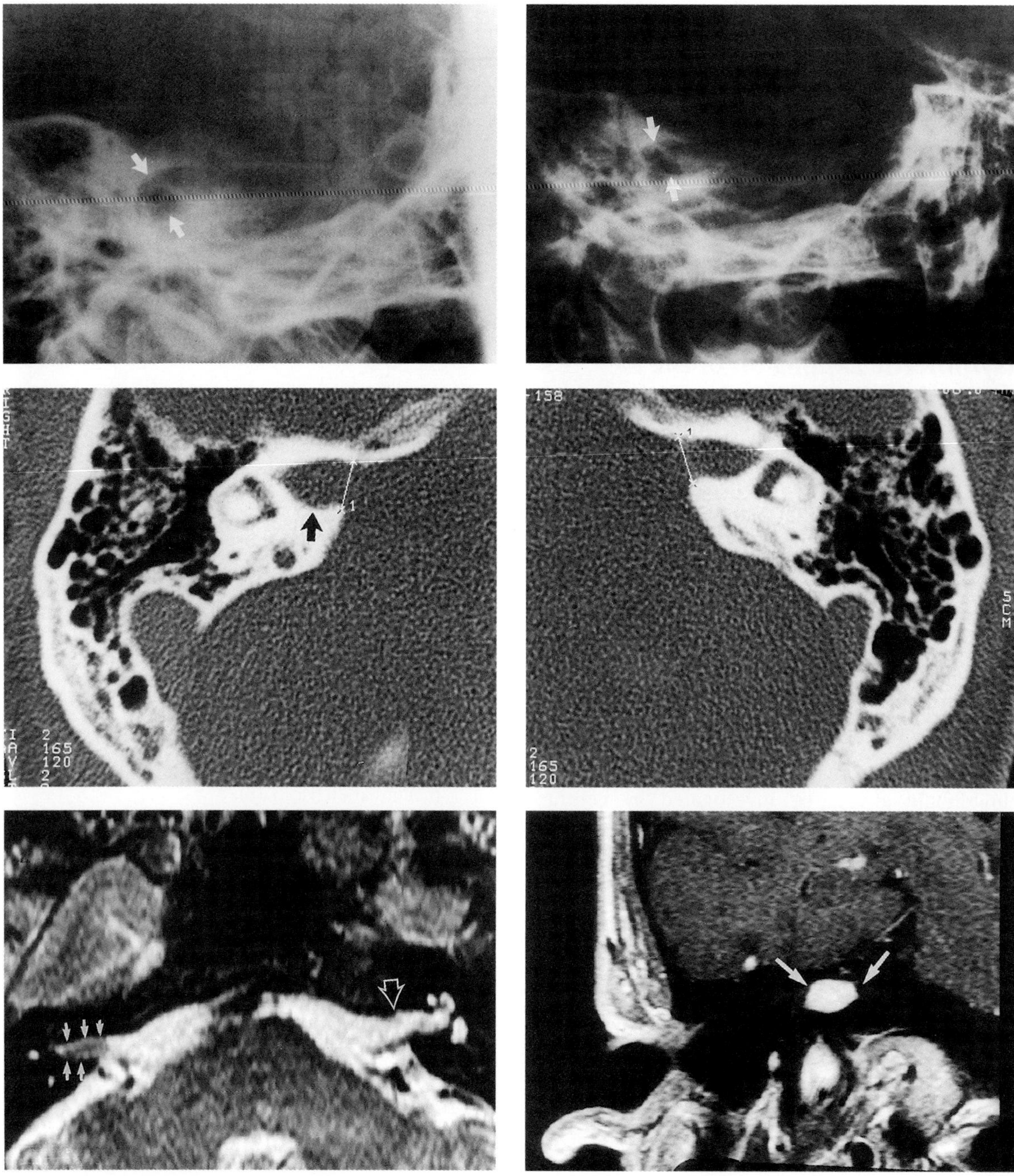

a b c d e f

Figs. 5.**12 a – f** **Asymmetric expansion of the right internal auditory canal by acoustic neuroma: comparison of conventional radiographs, CT, and MRI.**
(**a**) Stenvers radiograph shows club-like expansion of the right porus acusticus extending to Bill's bar (arrows).
(**b**) Contralateral scan shows normal size and configuration of the internal auditory canal (arrows) on the left side.
(**c**) HRCT scan with a 2-mm slice thickness documents the club-like deformation of the internal auditory canal and rounded posterior wall of the porus acusticus (arrow).
(**d**) Comparative evaluation of the normal left internal auditory canal.
(**e**) T2-weighted SE sequence (TR/TE = 2500/90 ms) shows a hypointense soft-tissue mass (arrows) in the right internal auditory canal. Compare with the normal hyperintense CSF in the left internal auditory canal (open arrow).
(**f**) Coronal image documents the club-like intrameatal acoustic neuroma. The size and shape of the lesion show good agreement with the bony expansion documented by radiographic studies.

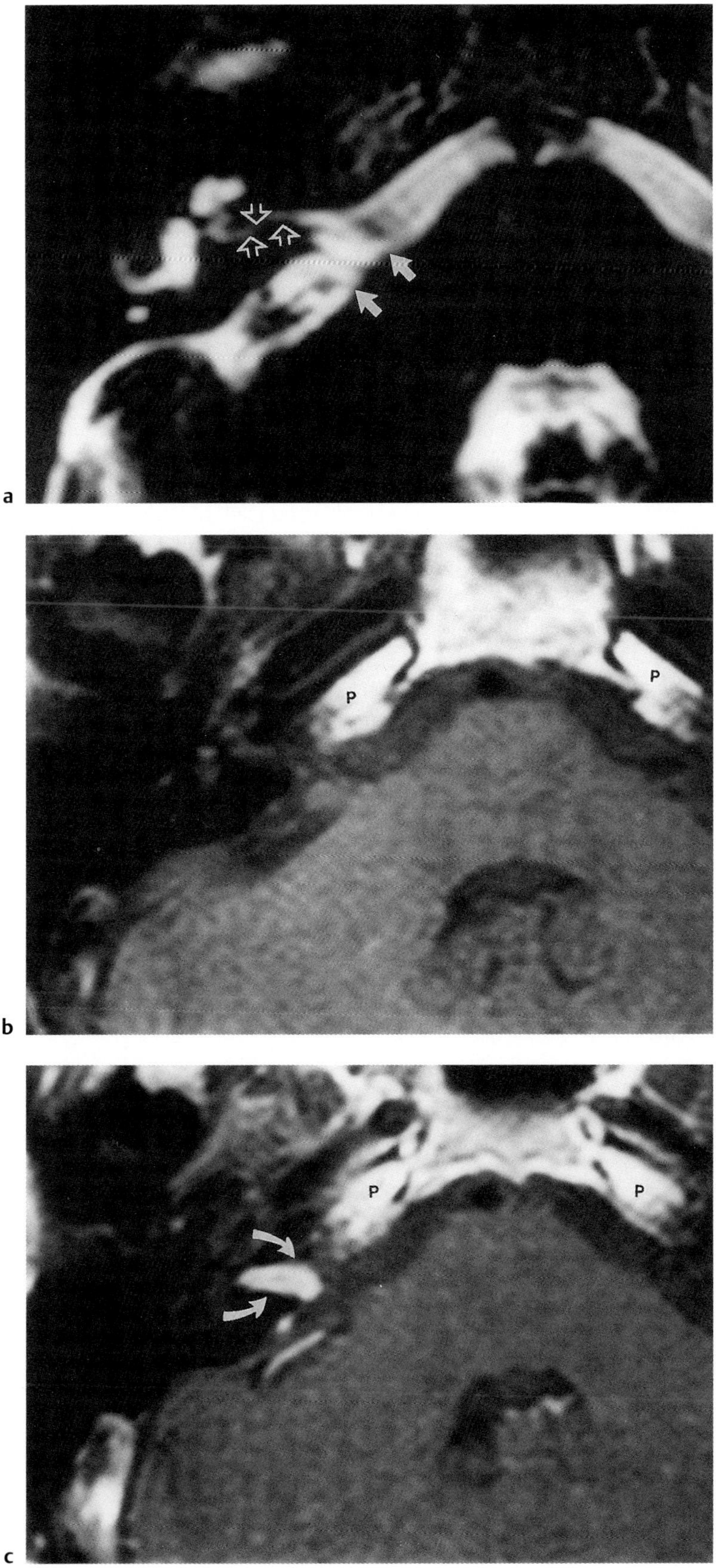

Figs. 5.**13 a – c** **Intrameatal acoustic neuroma extending into the cerebellopontine cistern: comparison of different MR imaging sequences.**

(**a**) TSE sequence (TR/TE = 4797/400 ms) demonstrates hyperintense CSF in the prepontine and cerebellopontine cisterns (arrows). The fluid in the internal auditory canal is displaced by a mass of low signal intensity (open arrows). The cochlea and vestibule display normal signal intensity. Scattered linear structures within the CSF are pulsation artifacts.

(**b**) Gd-enhanced T1-weighted SE sequence (TR/TE = 500/15 ms).

(**c**) Gd-enhanced T1-weighted SE sequence (TR/TE = 500/15 ms) demonstrates the intrameatal form of the acoustic neuroma (curved arrows), which is confined to the internal auditory canal.

P High primary signal intensity of the petrous apex due to the presence of fatty tissue (without contrast enhancement).

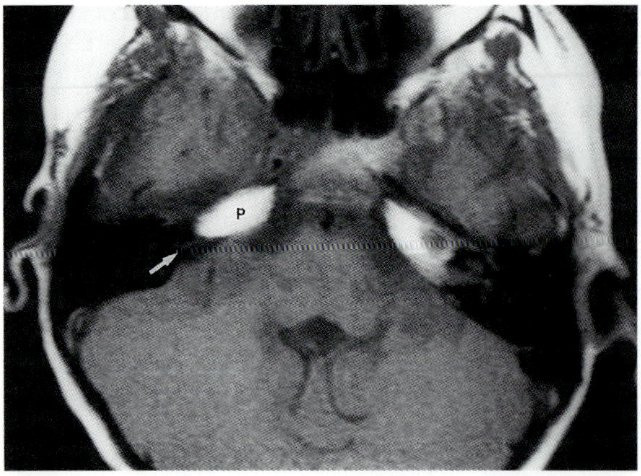

a

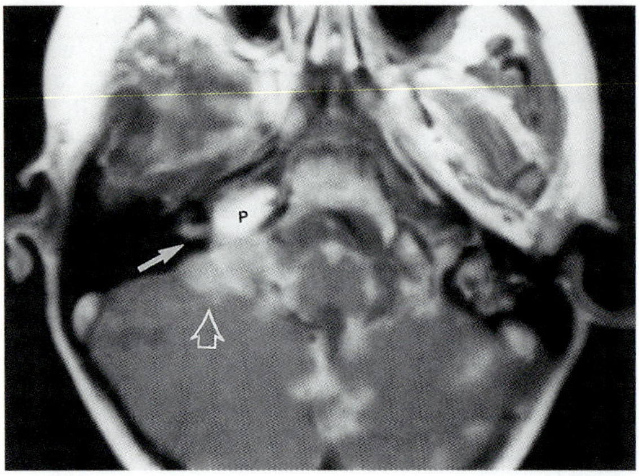

b

Figs. 5.**14** a, b **Infiltration of the right internal auditory canal with involvement of the cerebellopontine angle and other cerebellar structures by a metastasis from a primitive neuroectodermal malignant tumor in a pediatric patient.**

(**a**) Axial T1-weighted SE sequence (TR/TE = 500/15 ms) shows low signal intensity in the right internal auditory canal (arrow), a hypointense mass in the cerebellopontine angle, and nonhomogeneous intensities throughout the brainstem.

P Petrous apex

(**b**) Gd-enhanced axial T1-weighted SE sequence (TR/TE = 500/15 ms) shows signs of meningeal carcinomatosis with infiltration of the meninges in the region of the right internal auditory canal (arrow), cerebellopontine angle, and the entire subarachnoid space (open arrow). The high primary signal intensity of the petrous pyramid does not change significantly after the administration of Gd-DTPA, indicating that the pyramid is not infiltrated by tumor.

P Petrous apex

Solid Enhancing Mass Smaller than 5 mm in the Internal Auditory Canal (on MRI Only)

Because hemorrhage is a primary accompaniment of certain lesions, the location of a hemorrhage showing high signal intensity on noncontrast T1-weighted MR images provides a useful criterion for the precise localization of an enhancing lesion. This underscores the importance of obtaining unenhanced T1- and T2-weighted SE sequences supplemented by T1-weighted sequences following the intravenous administration of a paramagnetic contrast agent. All enhancing lesions 5 mm or less in diameter should raise suspicion of an inflammatory process such as focal arachnoiditis (Fig. 5.**15**) or meningitis (Fig. 5.**16**), which should undergo a standard follow-up program consisting of contrast-enhanced MRI examinations performed at 3-month intervals. An inflammatory lesion will generally show a change in morphology or enhancement intensity with the passage of time (Table 5.**6**).

Table 5.**6** Solid enhancing mass smaller than 5 mm in the internal auditory canal on MRI

Findings	Differential diagnostic criteria
Common:	
➤ Inflammation:	
—Arachnoiditis (Fig. 5.**15**)	Focal enhancement
—Sarcoidosis	Focal enhancement
—Meningitis (Fig. 5.**16**)	Follow-up
➤ Tumor:	
—Acoustic neuroma (schwannoma) (Figs. 5.**17** – 5.**22**)	Topography
—Facial neuroma	Topography
—Meningioma (Fig. 5.**37**)	Topography
➤ Vascular lesion:	
—Arteriovenous malformation	Vascular structures
Rare:	
➤ Tumor:	
—Metastasis (Fig. 5.**14**)	
—Other neuromas (Figs. 5.**33** – 5.**35**)	
—Arachnoid cyst (Fig. 5.**27**)	

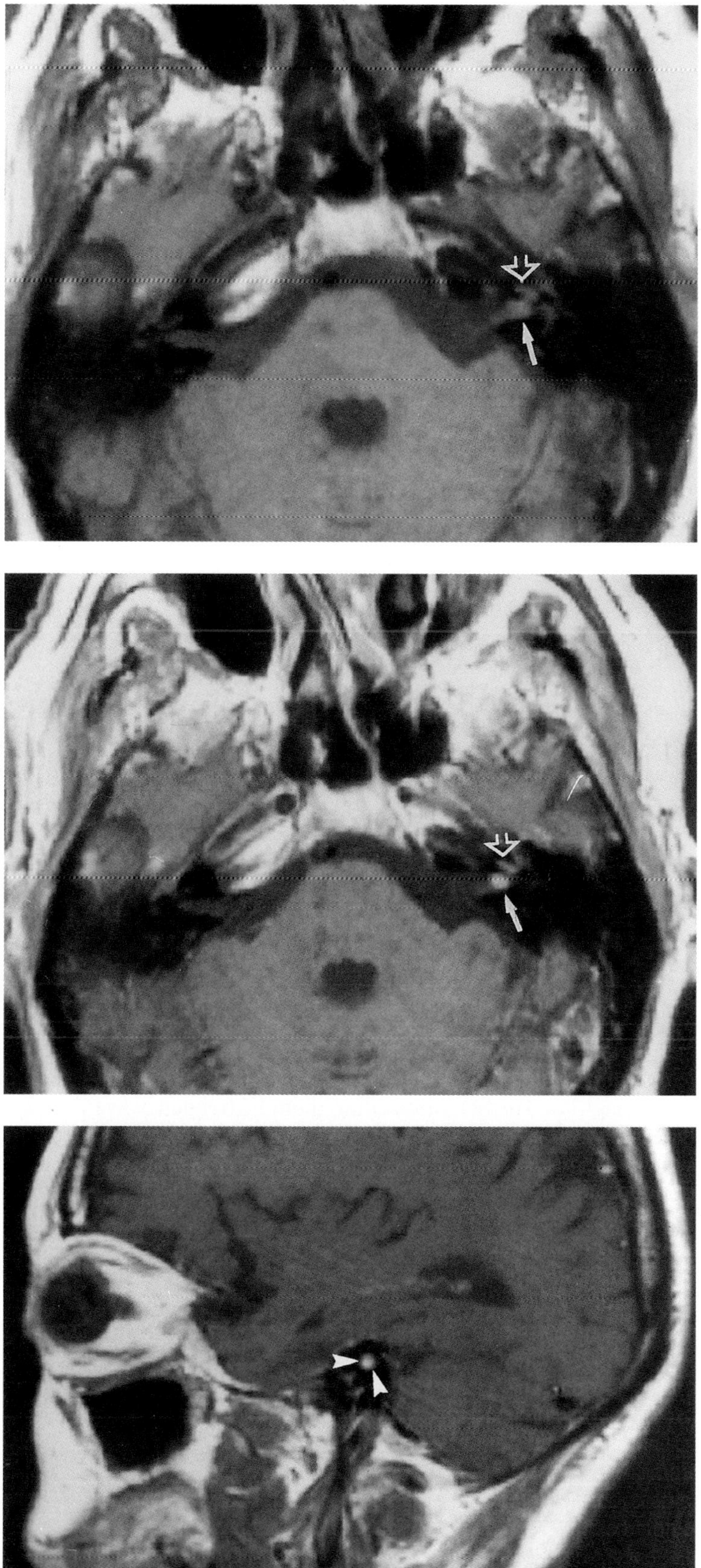

a

b

c

Figs. 5.**15 a – c Focal arachnoiditis and cochlear involvement of unspecified cause.** Documentation of focal arachnoiditis by contrast-enhanced MRI. A complete absence of contrast enhancement was noted at 3-month follow-up, establishing the lesion as an inflammatory process.

(**a**) Unenhanced axial T1-weighted SE sequence (TR/TE = 500/15 ms) shows normal appearance of the inner ear, membranous labyrinth, and cerebellopontine angle on the right side. The left side shows a moderate, focal increase of signal intensity in the central portions of the internal auditory canal (arrow) and in the cochlea (open arrow).

(**b**) The Gd-enhanced image demonstrates marked punctate enhancement of the intrameatal lesion (arrow) and enhancement at the basal cochlear orifice (open arrow). This lesion cannot be positively distinguished from an intrameatal acoustic neuroma by its primary morphologic features, but the linear enhancement suggests an inflammatory process.

(**c**) Image in the sagittal plane shows an ill-defined, nonhomogeneous enhancement pattern that is confirmatory of intrameatal focal arachnoiditis (arrowheads).

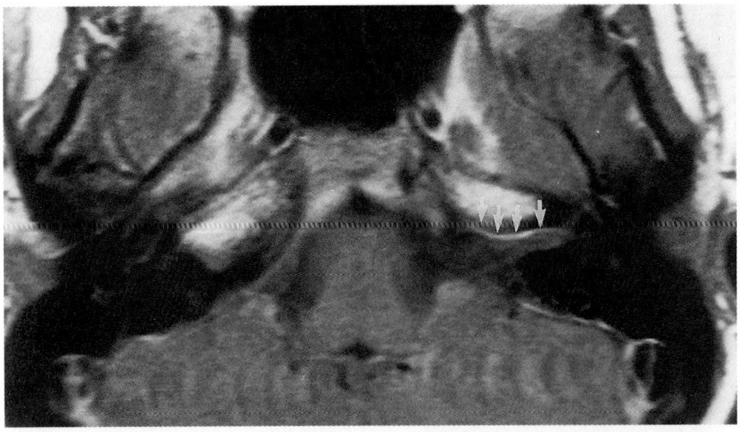

a

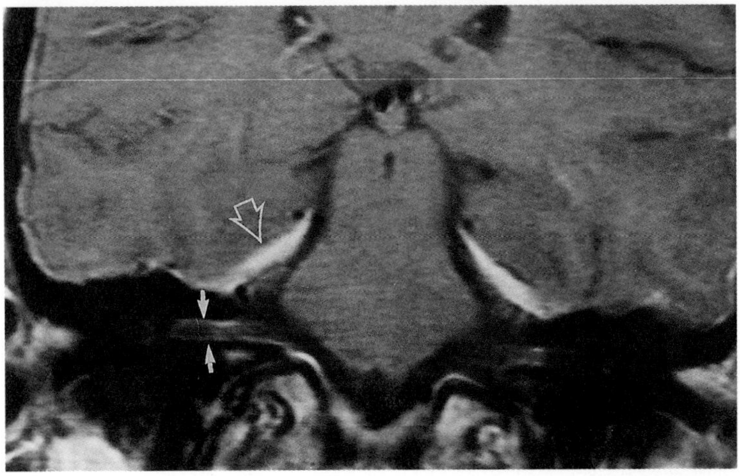

b

Figs. 5.**16 a, b** **Tuberculous meningitis.**
(**a**) Axial Gd-enhanced T1-weighted SE sequence (TR/TE = 500/25 ms) shows linear enhancement along the left internal auditory canal (arrows) involving the anterior meningeal structures. The solid neural structures do not show circumscribed enhancement.
(**b**) Coronal Gd-enhanced T1-weighted SE sequence (TR/TE = 500/25 ms) accurately defines the meningeal enhancement along the internal auditory canal on each side (arrows). Note also the marked enhancement of the basal meninges over the medial temporal pole (open arrow). The overall morphology of the meningeal enhancement is nonspecific but is fully consistent with the known presence of tuberculous meningitis.

Linear Enhancement in the Internal Auditory Canal (on MRI)

Only a select group of causes can produce discernible linear contrast enhancement in the internal auditory canal on MR images—most notably meningitis (Fig. 5.**16**) and vascular structures (Fig. 5.**18**). Linear forms of acoustic neuroma should also be considered in the differential diagnosis (Table 5.**7**).

Solid Enhancing Mass in the Cerebellopontine Angle on CT or MRI

Cerebellopontine angle masses are classified clinically and radiologically as *primary* or *secondary*. Further subdividing them by frequency, we find that the majority consist of primary tumors. A combined intrameatal-extrameatal mass is most likely a neuroma or schwannoma (Figs. 5.**19** – 5.**21**) and rarely a meningioma (Fig. 5.**22**). The coexistence of neuromas and meningiomas should be considered in patients with Recklinghausen disease (Figs. 5.**21** and 5.**22**). In rare cases, primary cerebral tumors (Fig. 5.**23**) or nasopharyngeal processes that infiltrate the skull base may show concomitant involvement of the cerebellopontine angle (Fig. 5.**24**) or meningeal carcinomatosis (Fig. 5.**25** and Table 5.**8**).

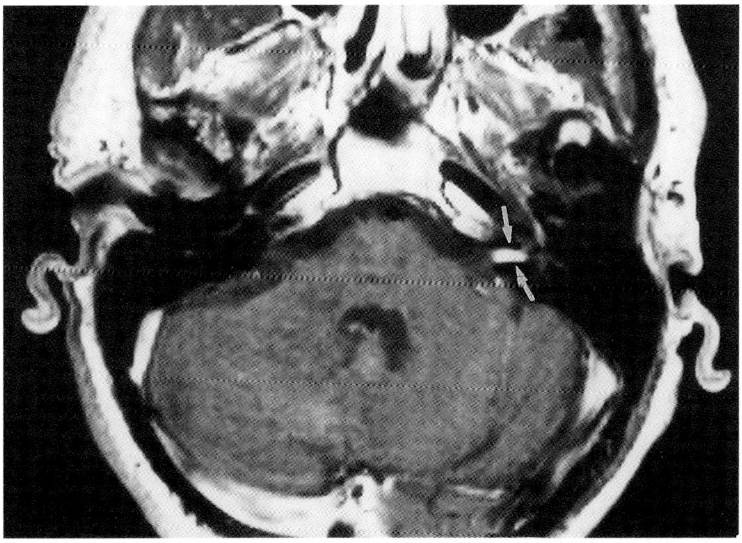

Fig. 5.**17** **Acoustic neuroma.** Gd-enhanced T1-weighted SE sequence (TR/TE = 500/15 ms) demonstrates the linear shape of the acoustic neuroma (arrows), which is strictly confined to the internal auditory canal.

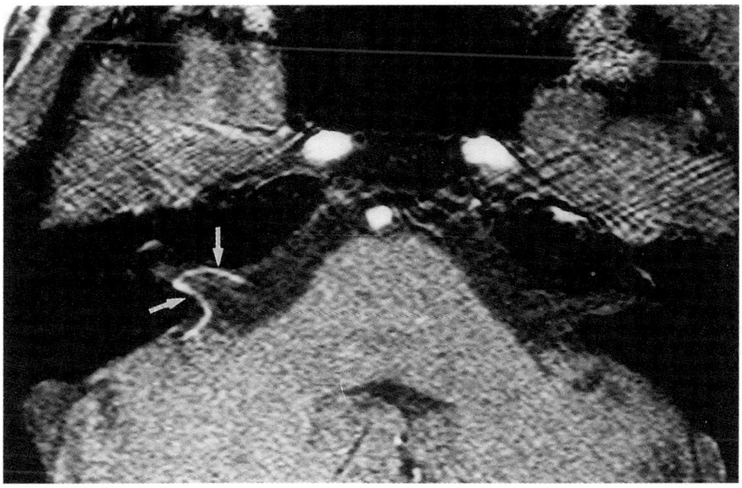

Fig. 5.**18** **Vascular loop appearing as a linear hyperintense structure on contrast-enhanced MRI.** Gd-enhanced arterial MRA (TR/TE = 40/8 ms, flip angle = 60°) documents the morphologic changes caused by a loop of the labyrinthine artery arising from the anterior inferior cerebellar artery on the right side (arrows). Given the absence of clinical manifestations in this patient (no tinnitus), this finding represents a normal variant.

Cystic Mass in the Cerebellopontine Angle, Internal Auditory Canal, or Inner Ear

The diagnosis of a liquid mass in this region is based largely on information derived from CT scans showing fluid-equivalent attenuation values between 0 and 30 HU. On MRI, fluid-containing masses in this region display prolonged T2 and T1 relaxation times. Generally these lesions have low primary signal intensities and do not enhance after the administration of 0.1 mmol Gd-DTPA, gadodiamide, or gadobutrol.

The most common cause is an arachnoid cyst in the cerebellopontine angle (Figs. 5.**26** and 5.**27**) or internal auditory canal. Moreover, any tumor that is accompanied by central or complete necrosis may present as a primary cystic mass. Today an important diagnostic criterion is expansile growth, which is a specific feature of primary epidermoid cysts (Fig. 5.**26**). Useful adjuncts in these cases are arterial and venous magnetic resonance angiography (MRA) protocols to evaluate for displacement, compression, and collateralization (Table 5.**9**).

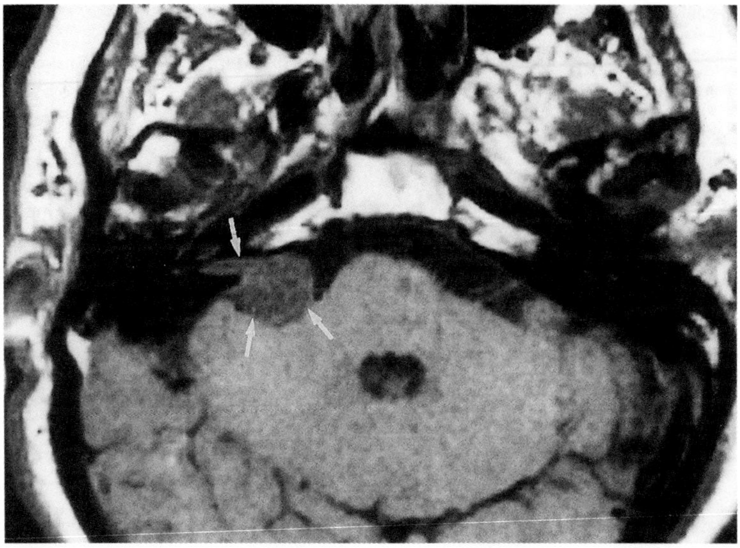

a

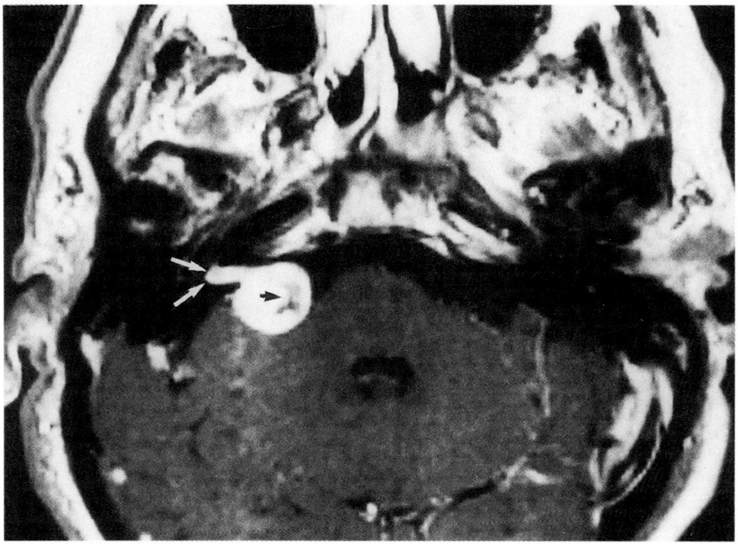

b

Figs. 5.**19 a, b** **Solid enhancing mass in the cerebellopontine angle**.
(**a**) Unenhanced T1-weighted SE sequence (TR/TE = 500/15 ms) demonstrates an intrameatal and extrameatal acoustic neuroma on the right side with a small necrotic area in the extrameatal portion. The tumor appears as a soft-tissue mass of intermediate signal intensity (arrows) in the right internal auditory canal. The extrameatal component is compressing the brainstem.
(**b**) Contrast-enhanced T1-weighted SE sequence (TR/TE = 500/15 ms) after the intravenous administration of 0.1 mmol/kg Gd-DTPA demonstrates the intrameatal and extrameatal tumor extension with a solid component in the internal auditory canal (white arrows) and a small necrotic area in the extrameatal portion (black arrow).

Air in the Cerebellopontine Angle and Internal Auditory Canal

Air-containing spaces are an uncommon finding in the differential diagnosis of internal auditory canal–cerebellopontine angle masses. They may result from *liquefying inflammatory processes* that become superinfected by gas-forming organisms. Another possible cause is *iatrogenic changes* following myelography, pneumocisternography, or other intracranial neurosurgical procedures. It is extremely rare for primary or secondary tumors in this region to display air-containing spaces on imaging studies.

Hyperintense Lesion on Unenhanced T1-Weighted SE MRI

Table 5.**10** lists the diagnostic possibilities that should be considered for lesions that show high signal intensity on unenhanced MR images.

The confident diagnosis of a lipoma in the internal auditory canal–cerebellopontine angle region is based on unenhanced T1- or T2-weighted MR images to demonstrate the inherent high signal intensity of the tumor. The specific use of a fat suppression sequence can further substantiate the diagnosis.

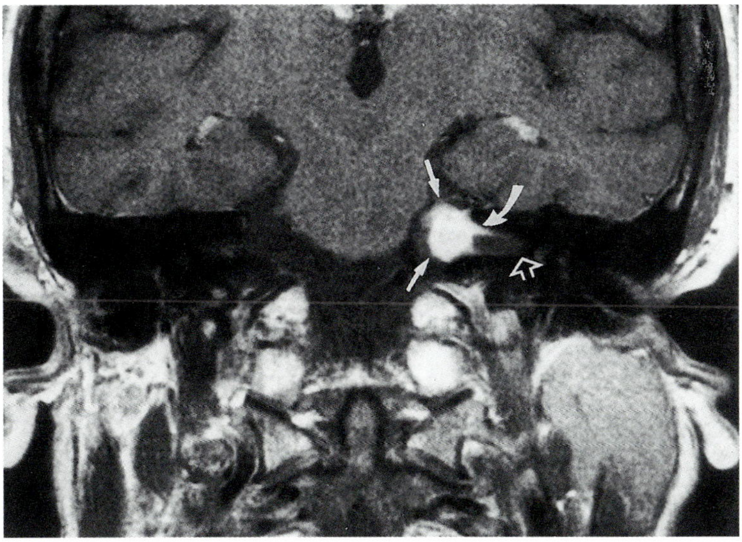

Fig. 5.**20** **Intrameatal and extrameatal acoustic neuroma with an almost completely necrotic intrameatal portion: an important differentiating criterion.** Gd-enhanced coronal T1-weighted SE sequence (TR/TE = 500/15 ms) demonstrates the hyperintense extrameatal component of the acoustic neuroma (arrows). Note the tapered extension (curved arrow) from the upper part of the extrameatal component to the internal auditory canal. Definite enhancement is not visible in the canal itself (open arrow). This finding signifies necrosis of the intrameatal tumor component, which requires surgical removal.

Table 5.**7** Linear contrast enhancement in the internal auditory canal

Findings	Differential diagnostic criteria
Common:	
➤ Variation:	
–Vascular loop (Fig. 5.**18**)	Vascular structure
➤ Inflammation:	
–Specific meningitis (Fig. 5.**16**)	
–Nonspecific meningitis	Morphology Contrast enhancement
Rare:	
➤ Tumor:	
–Hemangioma	Topography
–Intracanalicular meningioma	Topography
–Lymphoma	
–Carcinomatosis	
–Arteriovenous malformation	Morphology
–Lipoma	Signal characteristics
➤ Inflammation:	
–Neuritis	
–Labyrinthitis	

Table 5.**8** Solid enhancing mass in the cerebellopontine angle

Findings	Differential diagnostic criteria
Common:	
➤ Tumor:	
–Acoustic neuroma (Figs. 5.**19**–5.**21**)	Topography
–Meningioma (Fig. 5.**37**)	Topography
–Pontine glioma	Morphology
–Cerebellar neoplasm (Fig. 5.**26**)	Topography
–Tumors of the fourth ventricle	Topography
➤ Vascular:	
–Ectasia or aneurysm of basilar or vertebral artery	Vascular structures
Rare:	
➤ Tumor:	
–Chordoma	Signal characteristics
–Metastasis (Fig. 5.**14**)	Contrast enhancement
–Neuroma of cranial nerves VII, X, XI, XII (Figs. 5.**33**, 5.**35**)	Topography
–Rhabdomyosarcoma	Nonspecific
–Parasellar neoplasms	Topography
–Glomus jugulare tumor	Vascularity
–Meningeal carcinomatosis	Contrast enhancement
➤ Vascular:	
–Arteriovenous malformation	Vascular structures

Enhancing Labyrinthine Structures

Contrast enhancement of the membranous labyrinthine structures is a rare imaging finding. Usually this criterion is seen in contrast-enhanced T1-weighted SE sequences and is accompanied by clinical manifestations.

Nearly all patients with cochlear or vestibular enhancement on MRI have corresponding clinical symptoms, which are usually a result of pronounced reactive changes. As the symptoms subside, imaging will usually show concomitant regression in the volume of the lesion and its enhancement intensity. With enhancing cochlear lesions, the level of contrast enhancement in the basal turns of the cochlea corre-

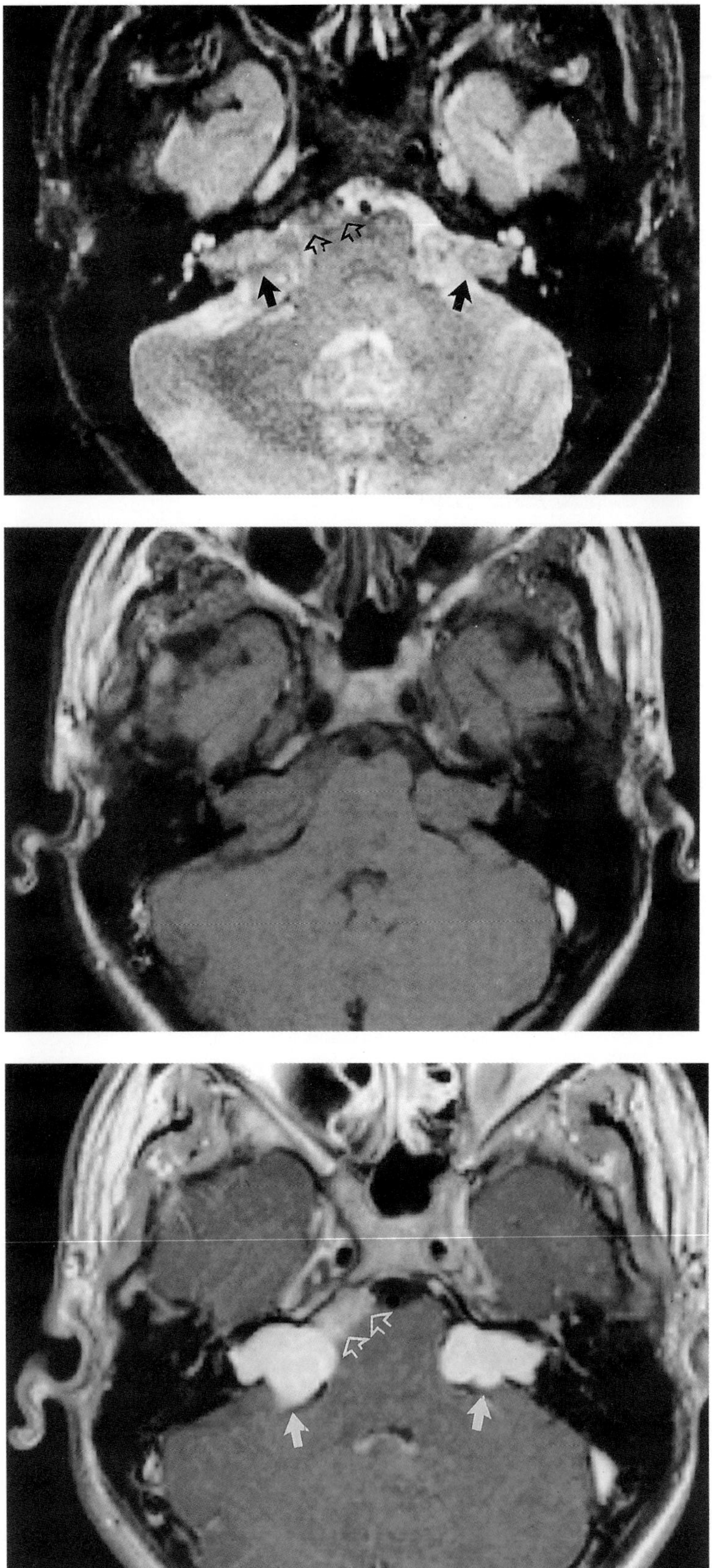

a

b

c

Fig. 5.**21** **Bilateral acoustic neuromas and meningioma in Recklinghausen disease.** Comparison of MR imaging criteria for neuroma versus meningioma.
(**a**) Axial T2-weighted SE sequence (TR/TE = 2500/90 ms) shows a large bilateral mass in the internal auditory canal and cerebellopontine angle on both sides (black arrows) and a moderately hyperintense mass in the prepontine cistern on the right side (open arrows).
(**b**) The bilateral mass is isointense to adjacent brain, with no visible line of demarcation. Note the slightly increased signal intensity of the clivus due to the presence of fat.
(**c**) Gd-enhanced T1-weighted SE sequence (TR/TE = 500/17 ms). The bilateral intrameatal and extrameatal acoustic neuromas (arrows) show intense, uniform enhancement following contrast administration. The image also shows a prepontine meningioma relating to the right cerebellopontine angle (open arrows). The contrast-enhanced view is essential for delineating the isointense mass from clivus structures. Histologic examination confirmed the imaging findings.

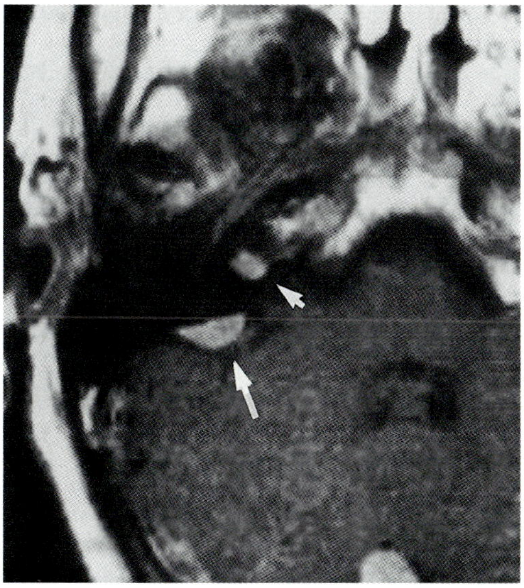

Fig. 5.22 **Intrameatal acoustic neuroma combined with a petrous ridge meningioma in a patient with Recklinghausen disease.** Gd-enhanced axial T1-weighted SE sequence (TR/TE = 500/15 ms) shows an intensely enhancing nodular mass (long arrow) in the internal auditory canal–cerebellopontine-angle area representing an intrameatal acoustic neuroma. An adjacent, topographically distinct mass in the right cerebellopontine angle (short arrow) is a petrous ridge meningioma on the right side. The differentiating criteria for these lesions are their relative locations, signal intensity, and enhancement characteristics. Both lesions are isointense.

Table 5.**9** Cystic mass in the cerebellopontine angle and internal auditory canal

Findings	Differential diagnostic criteria
Tumor:	
➤ Arachnoid cyst (Fig. 5.**27**)	Smooth margins, no rim enhancement
➤ Epidermoid cyst (Fig. 5.**26**)	Smooth margins, expansile, slight rim enhancement
➤ Cystic acoustic neuroma	
➤ Cystic meningioma	
Inflammation:	
➤ Abscess, granulations	
Vascular:	
➤ Arterial aneurysm: AICA, PICA	Vascular structures

AICA Anterior inferior cerebellar artery
PICA Posterior inferior cerebellar artery

lates with the clinical symptom of hearing loss in the high-frequency range. Apical cochlear lesions are associated with hearing loss at lower frequencies.

The final stage of an inflammatory process is usually characterized by obliteration of the membranous labyrinth with an absence of contrast enhancement and an absence of signal in T2-weighted SE or TSE sequences.

Perilymphatic fistula, defined as an abnormal communication between the inner ear and middle ear, is usually based on pathology of the membranous structures of the round or oval window or both. MRI demonstrates abnormal contrast enhancement.

Labyrinthine neoplasms are characterized histopathologiclly as benign or malignant. The most common tumor is labyrinthine schwannoma (Fig. 5.**29**), which is analogous to schwannomas of the internal auditory canal. The cardinal imaging feature is a mass that enhances more intensely than labyrinthitis. Other criteria for a neoplasm are the persistence of contrast enhancement for several months and an expansile type of growth. Labyrinthitis-associated enhancement usually regresses with time, while a tumor shows persistent constant enhancement that may or may not be accompanied by a change in clinical symptoms (Fig. 5.**29**).

Rare malignant tumors of the cochlea include squamous cell carcinoma and rhabdomyosarcoma with infiltration of the labyrinth. Metastatic tumors tend to exhibit perineural growth along the cochlear nerve. Cholesteatomas may invade the labyrinth in rare cases and are associated with characteristic clinical symptoms.

Diffuse contrast enhancement involving large portions of the cochlea provides a subtle but verifiable criterion for the diagnosis of otospongiosis (Fig. 5.**30**).

Bleeding into the Labyrinth

This is most common in patients with coagulopathies or lymphomatous diseases or following trauma (Figs. 5.**31** and 5.**32**, Table 5.**11**).

Table 5.**10** High T1-weighted signal intensity

Bleeding:
➤ Hemangioma
➤ Arteriovenous malformation
➤ Lipoma: cholesterol granuloma (Fig. 5.**28**)
➤ Accompanying high T2-weighted signal intensity
Inflammation:
➤ Labyrinthitis

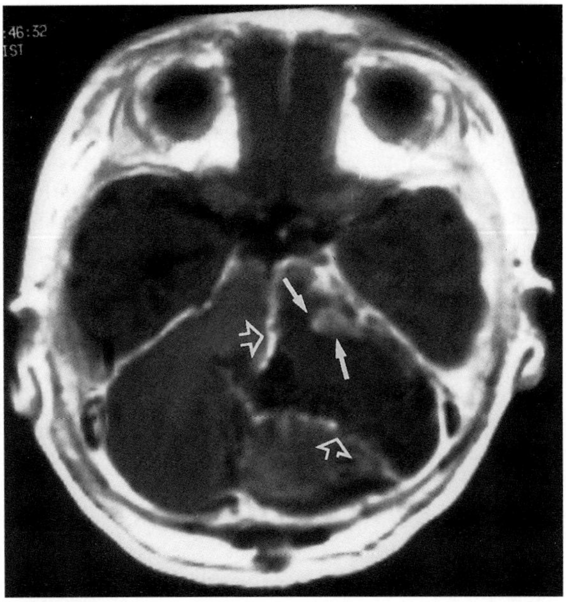

Fig. 5.**23** **Ependymoblastoma with a component in the cerebellopontine angle on the left side.** Gd-enhanced T1-weighted SE sequence (TR/TE = 500/15 ms) shows a cystic mass in the left cerebellar hemisphere extending past the midline and showing marked rim enhancement (open arrows). Concomitant enhancement in the cerebellopontine angle on the left side (arrows) suggests infiltration by ependymoblastoma as a possible interpretation of the cerebellopontine angle mass.

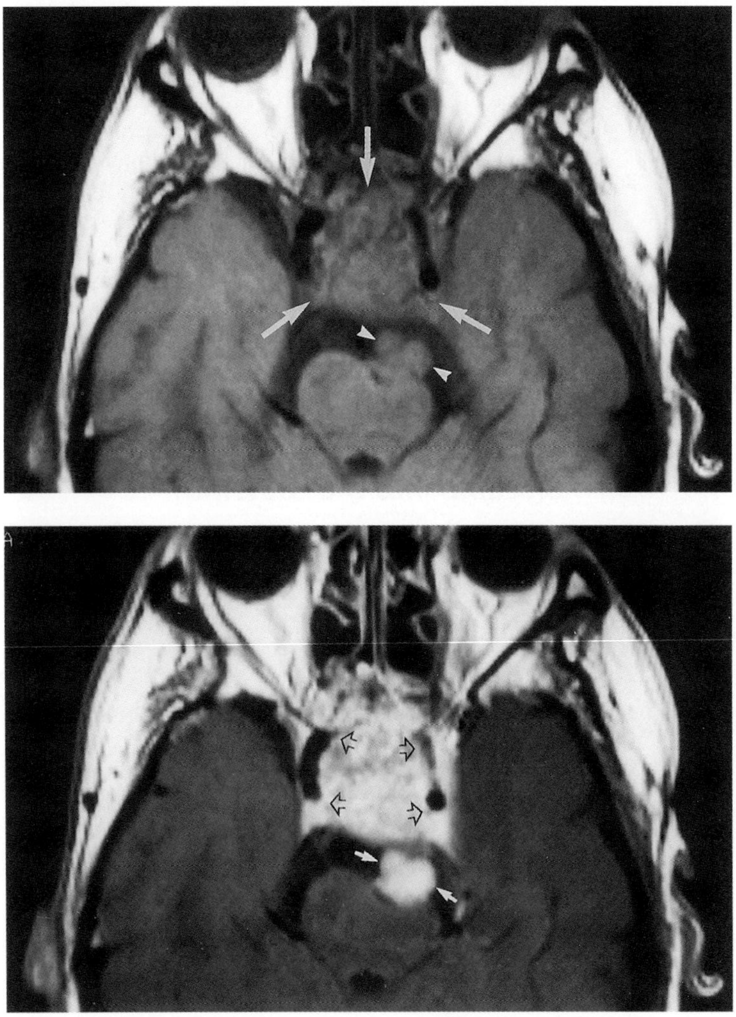

a

b

Figs. 5.**24** **a, b** **Secondary invasion of the skull base by nasopharyngeal carcinoma with involvement of the abducent nerve and vestibulocochlear nerve in the cerebellopontine angle.**
(**a**) Unenhanced T1-weighted SE sequence (TR/TE = 500/15 ms) shows an isointense mass in the middle skull base with extension into the prepontine cistern and cerebellopontine angle (arrowheads) and destructive changes (arrows).
(**b**) Gd-enhanced T1-weighted SE sequence (TR/TE = 500/15 ms) shows nonhomogeneous enhancement in the area of the skull base infiltrated by the nasopharyngeal carcinoma. Note the solid enhancing component in the prepontine cistern and cerebellopontine angle on the left side (arrows). There is marked displacement of the internal carotid artery in the area of the siphon (open arrows).

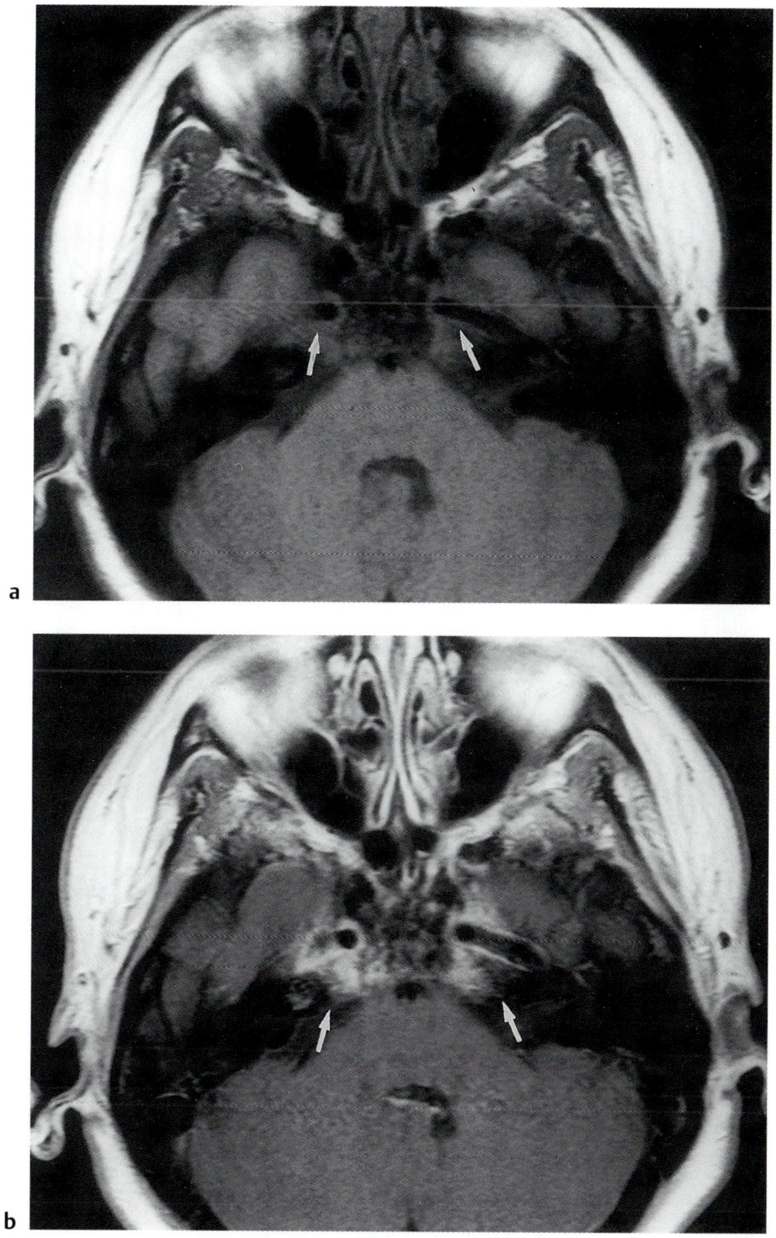

Figs. 5.**25** **a, b** **Meningeal carcinomatosis, marked by multiple sites of abnormal MRI enhancement in a patient with breast carcinoma.**
(**a**) Unenhanced T1-weighted SE sequence (TR/TE = 500/15 ms) shows bilateral hypointensity of the petrous apex and bilateral thickening of the internal carotid artery walls (arrows).
(**b**) Gd-enhanced T1-weighted SE sequence (TR/TE = 500/15 ms) shows marked abnormal enhancement of the petrous apices (intracancellous infiltration), paravascular space, anterior cerebellopontine angle, and the wall of the intrapetrosal segment of both internal carotid arteries (arrows).

Table 5.**11** Bleeding into the labyrinth

Findings
Tumor: ➤ Hemangioma ➤ Cholesterol granuloma (Fig. 5.**28**) ➤ Carcinoma of endolymphatic sac
Inflammation: ➤ Viral labyrinthitis (rubella, measles, mumps, herpes zoster)
Trauma

Absence of MRI Signal in the Labyrinth

In patients being evaluated for cochlear implantation, it is necessary to evaluate the fluid status of the membranous labyrinth by MRI. The imaging findings will direct the planning of the procedure and help identify the optimum side for placement of the implant.

If the membranous labyrinth appears as a signal void in the T2-weighted SE sequence, the entities listed in Table 5.**12** should be considered in the differential diagnosis.

Figs. 5.**26**

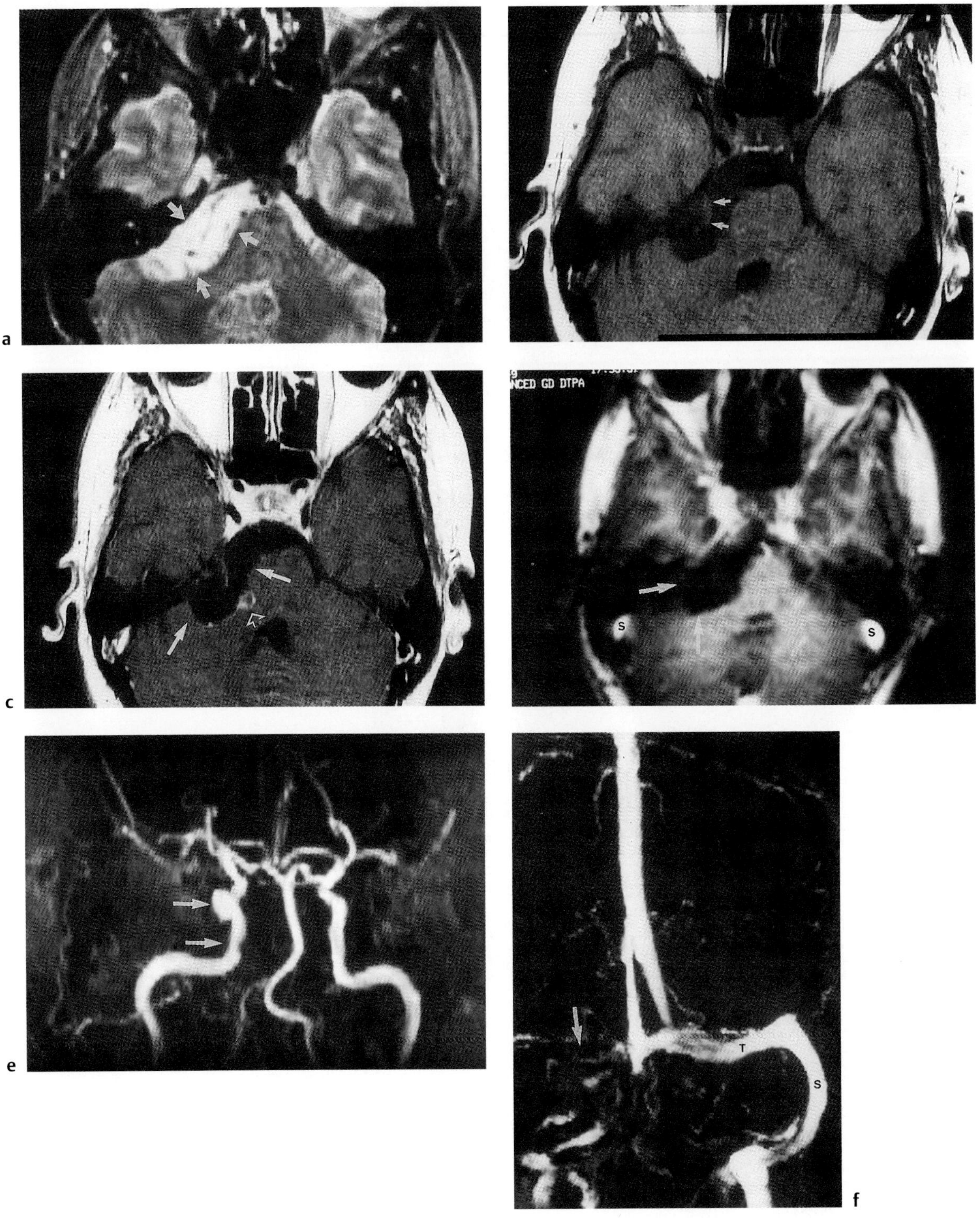

◁ Figs. 5.**26 a–f** **Epidermoid in the right cerebellopontine angle.**
(**a**) Axial T2-weighted SE sequence (TR/TE = 2500/90 ms) documents a hyperintense mass in the right cerebellopontine angle. Attention is directed to the lesion, which is isointense to CSF, by its mass effect on surrounding structures (arrows).
(**b**) In the unenhanced axial T1-weighted SE sequence (TR/TE = 500/15 ms), the mass is isointense to the CSF in the prepontine cistern and is manifested by secondary signs. Structures of moderately increased signal intensity are visible at the center of the mass (arrows).
(**c**) Gd-enhanced axial T1-weighted SE sequence (TR/TE = 500/15 ms) demonstrates subtle rim enhancement over much of the tumor (arrows). Lateral to the cerebral peduncle is a 3 x 3-mm area of ring enhancement (open arrow) marking a disruption of the blood-brain barrier. A conspicuous mass effect is also apparent.
(**d**) Axial turbo-FLASH image from a dynamic series (TR/TE = 6.5/3 ms) 60 seconds after contrast administration documents the mass but still does not show definite rim enhancement. Note the primary low signal intensity of the mass (arrows) and the high signal intensity of the enhancing sigmoid sinus (S).
(**e**) Arterial MRA (3-D FISP sequence, TR/TE = 40/7 ms, flip angle = 20°, MIP reconstruction) shows a mass effect evidenced by medial displacement and kinking of the right internal carotid artery (arrows).
(**f**) Venous MRA (2-D FLASH sequence, TR/TE = 36/10 ms, flip angle = 60°, MIP reconstruction). The transverse sinus (T) and sigmoid sinus (S) on the left side are prominent and heavily perfused, while the right transverse sinus is occluded and devoid of flow. Note the collateral flow directed toward the right jugular vein (arrow).

Table 5.**12** Absence of labyrinthine signal on MRI
Malformation
Tumor
Inflammation
Most commonly due to labyrinthitis, which has the following main causes: ➤ Viral: —Rubella —Mumps —Measles —Herpes zoster ➤ Bacterial: —Secondary: syphilis ➤ Primary autoimmune: —Cogan syndrome —Panarteritis nodosa —Wegener granulomatosis

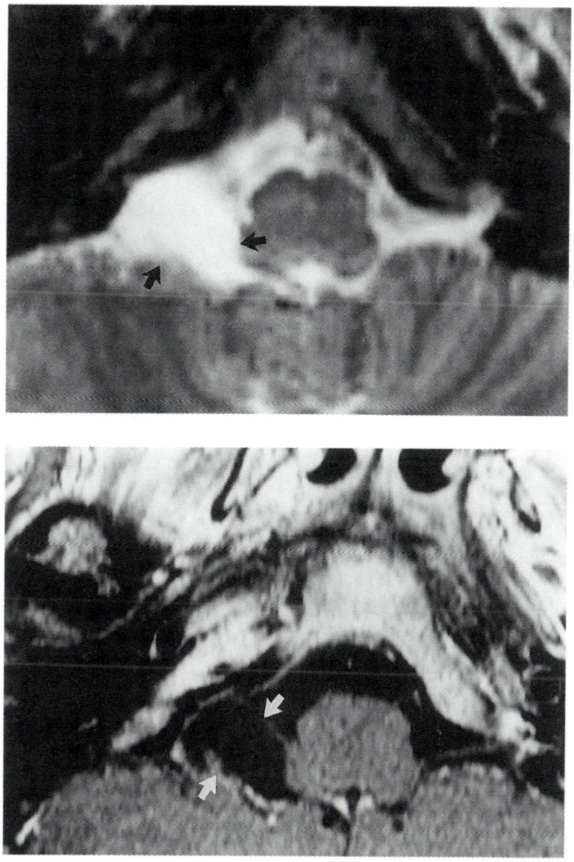

a

b

Figs. 5.**27 a, b** **Right-sided arachnoid cyst versus epidermoid** (Fig. 5.**26**). The arachnoid cyst is noninvasive, nonexpansile, and does not produce a mass effect.
(**a**) Axial T2-weighted SE sequence (TR/TE = 2500/90 ms) shows an area of high signal intensity starting at the lower border of the cerebellopontine angle (arrows). The area is isointense to CSF and expands the bordering spaces without showing definite signs of invasiveness or mass effect.
(**b**) Gd-enhanced axial T1-weighted SE sequence (TR/TE = 500/15 ms) shows a nonenhancing cystic mass (arrows) with fine linear enhancement along its right lateral wall corresponding to adjacent meninges.

Brainstem Mass

Brainstem masses should always be considered in the differential diagnosis of pathology in the internal auditory canal–cerebellopontine angle area, including low-attenuation masses that are detected on CT scans (Table 5.**13**).

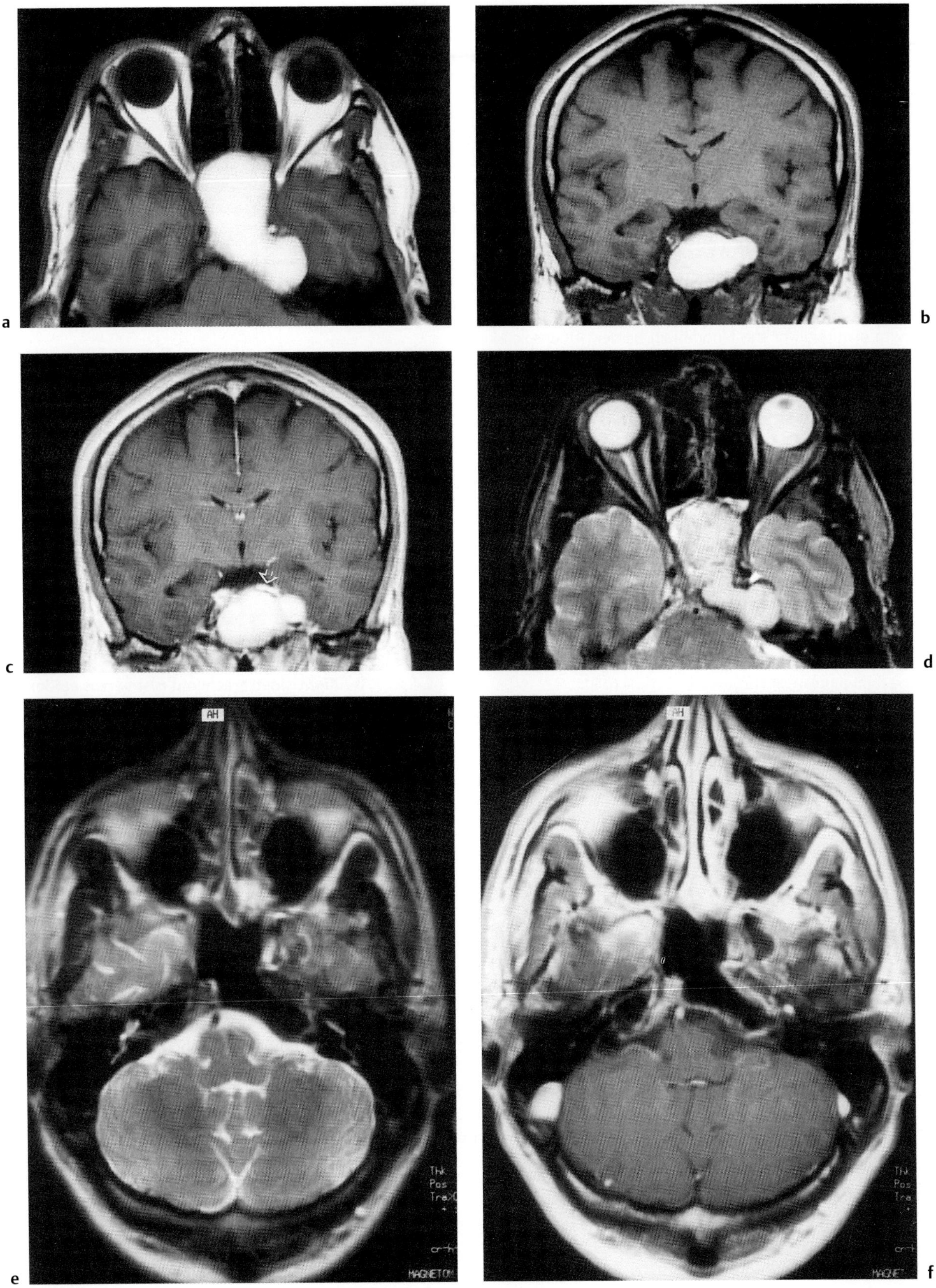

Figs. 5.**28**

◁ Figs. 5.**28 a–f** **Cholesterol granuloma, appearing as a hyperintense mass in the unenhanced T1-weighted SE sequence: comparison of pretherapeutic and posttherapeutic images.**
(**a**) Axial unenhanced T1-weighted SE sequence (TR/TE = 500/15 ms) demonstrates a uniformly hyperintense mass involving the sphenoid sinus and petrous apex. The expansile nature of the mass is an important differentiating criterion from pneumosinus dilatans with protein-rich fluid. Note the mass effect on the cerebellopontine angle.
(**b**) Coronal T1-weighted SE sequence (TR/TE = 500/15 ms) confirms the relative position of the mass, which shows no infiltrative signs.
(**c**) T1-weighted SE sequence (TR/TE = 500/15 ms) after the administration of Gd-DTPA shows no definite enhancement of the adjacent skull base, no obvious infiltrative signs, and no apparent disruption of the blood-brain barrier. There is marked enhancement of the superiorly displaced vascular structures (open arrow).
(**d**) Axial T2-weighted SE sequence (TR/TE = 2500/90 ms) shows high primary signal intensity of the mass with scattered foci of lower intensity. In themselves, the signal characteristics in the T2-weighted sequence are nonspecific and do not permit an accurate diagnostic classification.
(**e**) Axial T2-weighted SE sequence (TR/TE = 2500/90 ms) following operative removal of the cholesterol granuloma. The surgical cavity appears as a signal void.
(**f**) Gd-enhanced T1-weighted SE sequence (TR/TE = 500/15 ms) shows subtle peripheral enhancement around the surgical cavity. The now-communicating air spaces appear characteristically as areas of signal void.

Cystic or Necrotic Mass in the Posterior Cranial Fossa

Cystic masses in the posterior cranial fossa are radiologically indistinguishable from necrotic tumors. The differential diagnosis of both entities is considered jointly in Table 5.**14**.

Mass of the Clivus and Prepontine Cistern

In evaluations of the skull base, a careful search should be made for mass lesions of the clivus and/or prepontine cistern. The highest topographic resolution is obtained with high-resolution contrast-enhanced axial and coronal MR images. Sagittal images may also be helpful for the evaluation of midline lesions. Table 5.**15** lists common and rare entities that may be encountered in this region.

Table 5.**13** Brainstem mass

Findings	**Differential diagnostic criteria**
Common:	
➤ Tumor:	
—Glioma	Morphology
—Metastasis	Morphology
—Neuroma: accessory nerve, hypoglossal nerve (Fig. 5.**34**)	Topography
➤ Vascular:	
—Hemorrhage	Signal characteristics
—Large basilar artery (Fig. 5.**36**)	Vascular structure
➤ Variation:	
—Disseminated encephalitis	Morphology
—Infarction	
Rare:	
➤ Tumor:	
—Ependymoma	Morphology
—Lipoma, hamartoma, teratoma	
—Epidermoid (Fig. 5.**26**)	
—Lymphoma	Signal characteristics
—Hemangioblastoma	
—Medulloblastoma	
➤ Inflammation:	
—Abscess, encephalitis	
—Granulomatous inflammations: tuberculosis (Fig. 5.**16**), sarcoidosis	Focal contrast enhancement
➤ Syringobulbia	

Table 5.**14** Cystic or necrotic mass in the posterior cranial fossa

Malformation:
- ➤ Dandy–Walker cyst
- ➤ Extra-axial arachnoid cyst (Fig. 5.**27**)
- ➤ Enlarged cisterna magna

Tumor:
- ➤ Acoustic neuroma combined with arachnoid cyst (5%)
- ➤ Epidermoid (Fig. 5.**26**)
- ➤ Cystic astrocytoma
- ➤ Hemangioblastoma
- ➤ Metastases
- ➤ Medulloblastoma (rare)
- ➤ Brainstem glioma

Inflammation:
- ➤ Abscess
- ➤ Granulomatous inflammation (Fig. 5.**16**)
- ➤ Parasitism: cysticercosis, echinococcosis

Figs. 5.29

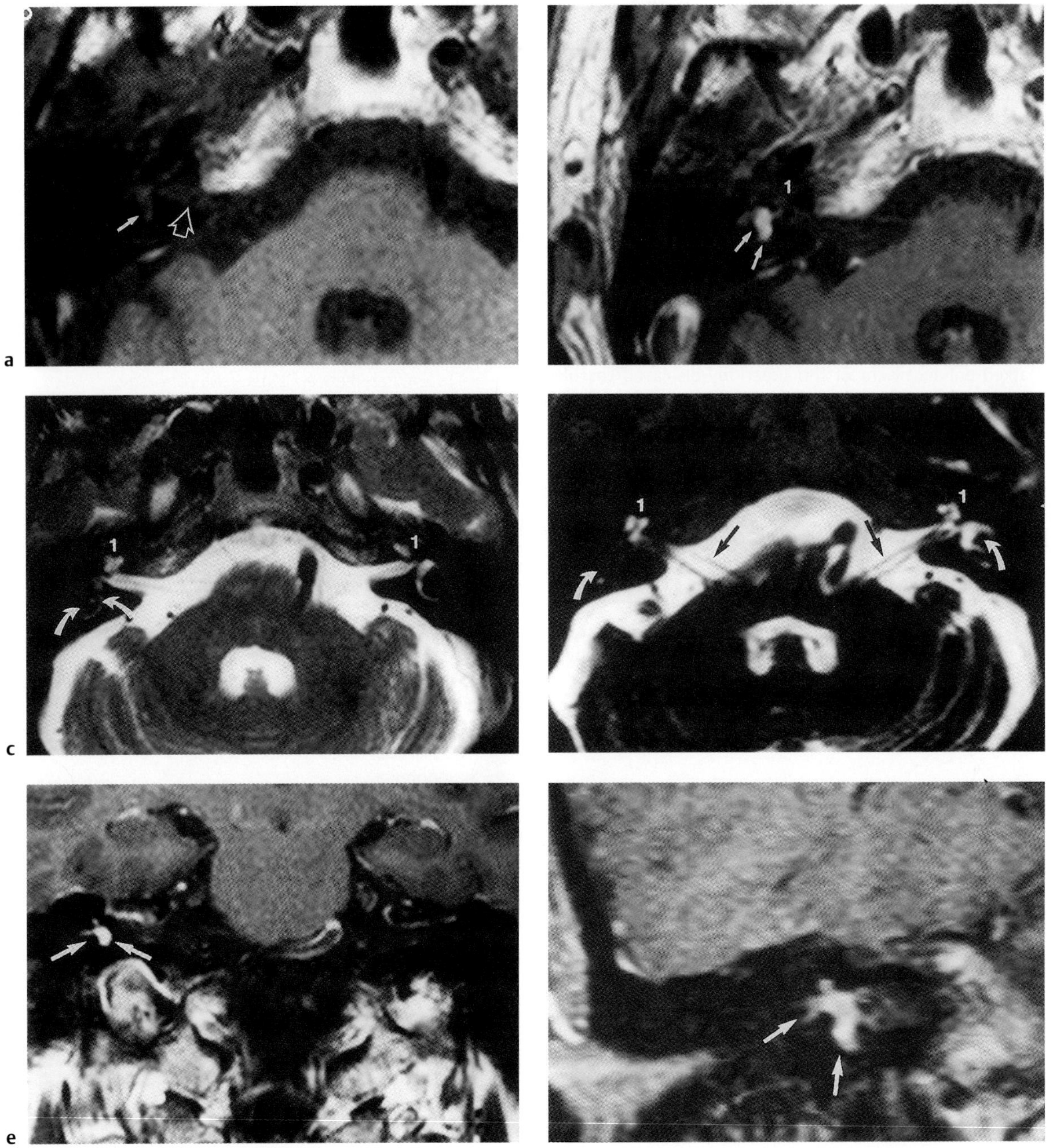

Ring Enhancement in the Posterior Cranial Fossa

Structures or masses in the posterior cranial fossa that show ring enhancement on post-contrast CT and MRI can be accurately identified in many cases based on their imaging topography, clinical presentation, and clinical course (Table 5.**16**).

Multiple Enhancing Masses in the Cerebellum and Bordering Spaces

The differential diagnosis of multiple enhancing cerebellar masses basically follows the criteria for supratentorial lesions (Fig. 5.**37**). The principal differential diagnoses are listed in order of frequency in Table 5.**17**.

◁ Figs. 5.**29a–f** **Vestibular nerve neuroma appearing as an enhancing labyrinthine lesion.**
(**a**) Unenhanced axial T1-weighted SE sequence (TR/TE = 500/15 ms) shows moderate prominence of vestibular labyrinthine structures on the right side (arrow). The internal auditory canal and its contents appear normal (open arrow).
(**b**) Gd-enhanced T1-weighted SE sequence (TR/TE = 500/15 ms) demonstrates a focal enhancing mass with smooth margins (arrows) in the right vestibular labyrinth with no signs of central necrosis.
1 Cochlea
Open arrow Right internal auditory canal
(**c**) Axial T2-weighted SE sequence (TR/TE = 2500/90 ms) shows labyrinthine structures of normal appearance on the left side. The vestibule on the right side contains a dark structure in place of the normal high signal intensity, providing indirect evidence of a mass. Suppression of signal intensity is also noted in the semicircular canals (curved arrows).
1 Cochlea
(**d**) T2-weighted TSE sequence (TR/TE = 4797/400 ms) gives a high-definition view of the nerve bundles (arrows) in the cerebellopontine angles. The cochlear structures on both sides display normal signal intensity. The absence of signal in the right vestibule contrasts with the hyperintensity of the contralateral vestibule (curved arrows).
1 Cochlear structures
(**e**) Gd-enhanced T1-weighted SE sequence (TR/TE = 500/15 ms) in the coronal plane permits an accurate side-to-side comparison and demonstrates the enhancing vestibular lesion with cranial extension toward the superior and lateral semicircular canals (arrows), which show enhancement relative to the nonenhancing opposite side.
(**f**) Gd-enhanced coronal T1-weighted SE sequence (TR/TE = 500/15 ms) at maximum magnification confirms tumor extensions from the vestibule into the membranous labyrinthine system (arrows) and establishes the diagnosis of a neuroma.

Table 5.**15** Masses of the clivus and prepontine cistern

Common:
- Tumor:
  - –Chordoma
  - –Meningioma
- Vascular:
  - –Aneurysm: basilar artery, vertebral artery

Rare:
- Tumor:
  - –Sarcomas: osteosarcoma, chondrosarcoma
  - –Epidermoid (Fig. 5.**26**)
  - –Metastasis
  - –Osteochondroma
  - –Nasopharyngeal neoplasm (Fig. 5.**24**)
  - –Parasellar tumors

Table 5.**16** Ring enhancement in the posterior cranial fossa

Common:
- Tumor:
  - –Glioblastoma
  - –Lymphoma (HIV, transplantation)
- Inflammation:
  - –Abscess
- Vascular:
  - –Subdural hematoma
  - –Intracerebral hematoma

Rare:
- Tumor:
  - –Craniopharyngioma
  - –Atypical meningioma (Fig. 5.**37**)
- Inflammation:
  - –Cysticercosis
  - –Echinococcosis
- Vascular:
  - –Aneurysm
- Therapeutically induced:
  - –Radiation-induced necrosis

Bony Erosion of the Petrous Apex

Inflammatory and neoplastic mass lesions are frequent causes of petrous apex erosion, which is generally verified by CT (Fig. 5.**14** and Table 5.**18**).

Bony Erosion of the Internal Auditory Canal

Erosion of the internal auditory canal is usually associated with expansion of the canal lumen. In rare cases imaging may demonstrate subtle erosion of the internal auditory canal as an isolated finding. The differential diagnoses are reviewed in Table 5.**19**.

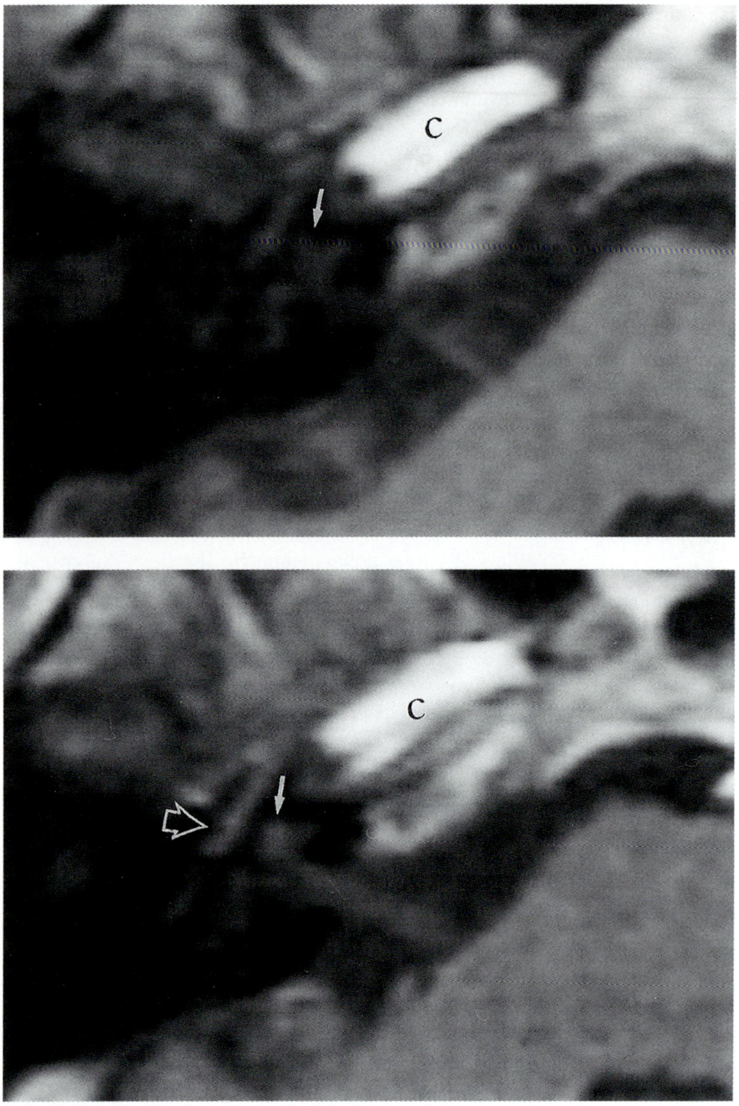

a

b

Figs. 5.**30** a, b **Subtle enhancing lesion in the right cochlea due to active otospongiosis.**
(**a**) Unenhanced axial T1-weighted SE sequence (TR/TE = 500/15 ms) defines the hypointense basal and first turns of the cochlea (arrow) next to the bright flow signal from the internal carotid artery.
C Internal carotid artery
(**b**) Gd-enhanced axial T1-weighted SE sequence (TR/TE = 500/15 ms) demonstrates nodular enhancement in the central turn of the cochlea (white arrow) and moderate enhancement along the horizontal segment of the facial nerve (open arrow).
C Internal carotid artery

Table 5.**17** Multiple enhancing masses in the posterior cranial fossa

Common:
- Tumor:
  - Metastases: lung, breast, colorectal carcinoma, kidney, melanoma
  - Inflammation: tuberculosis (Fig. 5.**16**), histoplasmosis
  - Parasitism: cysticercosis, toxoplasmosis
- Disseminated encephalitis

Rare:
- Tumor:
  - Lymphoma
- Inflammation:
  - Sarcoidosis (meningeal)
- Vascular:
  - Infarction, subacute, multifocal
  - Arterial: embolism, vasculitis
  - Venous: sinus vein thrombosis with intralesional hemorrhage

Erosion of Bony Structures in the Middle Cranial Fossa

In principle, any mass lesions or inflammatory processes arising from structures of the middle skull base may be associated with areas of bone destruction (Table 5.**20**).

Erosion of the Sphenoid Bone

Erosion of the sphenoid bone can generally be verified on bone-algorithm CT scans (Table 5.**21**).

Table 5.18 Erosion of the petrous apex

Common:
- Tumor:
  - —Acoustic neuroma (Figs. 5.**19**–5.**21**)
  - —Benign and malignant tumors: hemangioma, osteoblastoma, chondroma, chordoma, metastasis (Fig. 5.**14**)
- Inflammation:
  - —Cholesteatoma, primary, secondary
  - —Cholesterol granuloma (Fig. 5.**28**)

Rare:
- Tumor:
  - —Glioma
  - —Glomus jugulare tumor (Fig. 4.**9**)
  - —Histiocytosis X
  - —Leptomeningeal cyst
  - —Meningioma in the Meckel cavity
  - —Neuroma (Figs. 5.**19**–5.**21**)
  - —Nasopharyngeal malignancy (Fig. 5.**24**)
- Inflammation:
  - —Osteomyelitis, petrositis (Gradenigo syndrome)
- Vascular:
  - —Aneurysm of internal carotid artery
  - —Intracavernous or intrapetrosal segment

Table 5.19 Bony erosion of the internal auditory canal

Common:
- Normal variation
- Acoustic neuroma (Fig. 5.**13**)

Rare:
- Tumor:
  - —Glioma
  - —Metastasis (Fig. 5.**14**)
  - —Neuroma of cranial nerves V, VII; neurofibromatosis (Fig. 5.**21**)
  - —Meningioma
  - —Hydrocephalus
  - —Cyst
  - —Cholesteatoma, primary
- Vascular:
  - —Aneurysm of labyrinthine artery
  - —Arteriovenous malformation
  - —Hemangioma

Table 5.20 Bony erosion of the middle cranial fossa

Common:
- Tumor:
  - —Arachnoid cyst (Fig. 5.**27**)
  - —Chordoma
  - —Glomus jugulare tumor
  - —Meningioma (Fig. 5.**37**)
  - —Nasopharyngeal or paranasal sinus malignancy (Fig. 5.**24**)
- Vascular:
  - —Aneurysm of internal carotid artery
  - —Carotid-cavernous fistula

Rare:
- Tumor:
  - —Benign osseous tumors such as chondroma, giant-cell tumor
  - —Epidermoid (Fig. 5.**26**), cholesteatoma
  - —Histiocytosis X
  - —Metastasis (Figs. 5.**14**, 5.**25**)
  - —Neuroma of cranial nerve V (foramen ovale)
  - —Neurofibromatosis (Fig. 5.**21**)
  - —Temporal lobe glioma
- Vascular:
  - —Increased intracranial pressure
  - —Arterial aneurysms
- Iatrogenic:
  - —Postoperative defect

Table 5.21 Erosion of the sphenoid wing

Common:
- Congenital defect, isolated or combined with neurofibromatosis

Rare:
- Tumor:
  - —Benign osseous tumors
  - —Chordoma
  - —Craniopharyngioma
  - —Glioma
  - —Histiocytosis X
  - —Metastasis
  - —Parasellar aneurysm
  - —Sella tumors
  - —Plexiform neuroma

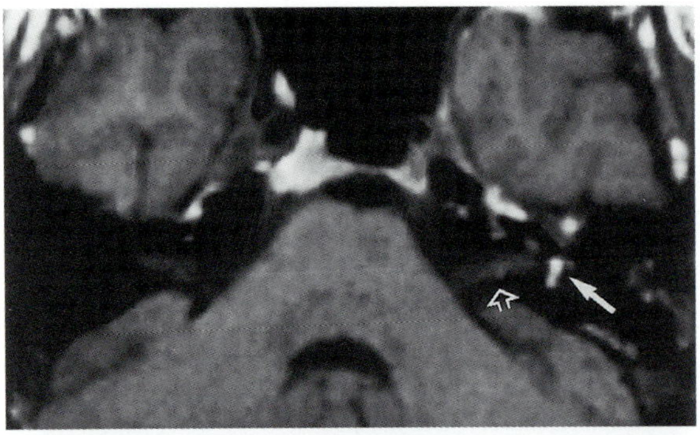
a

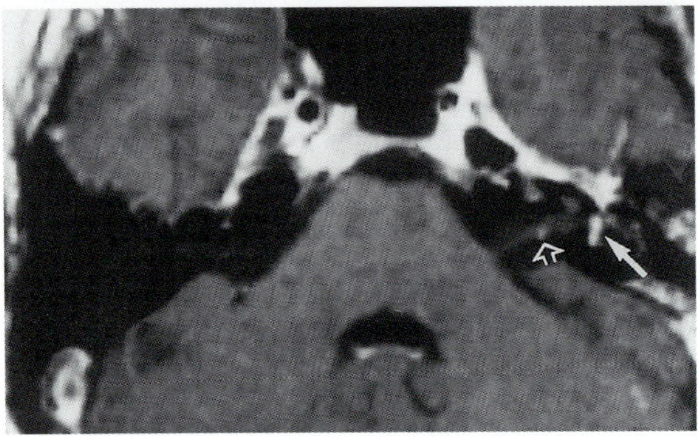
b

Figs. 5.**31 a, b** **Lesion of low T1-weighted signal intensity: bleeding in the vestibular labyrinth due to fracture and contusion of the petrous bone.**
(**a**) Unenhanced axial T1-weighted SE sequence (TR/TE = 500/15 ms) shows a linear, club–like area of increased signal intensity projected over the vestibular labyrinth on the left side (arrow). The focal zone of increased signal intensity projected onto the left superior vestibular nerve (open arrow) provides further evidence of hemorrhage.
(**b**) Gd-enhanced axial T1-weighted SE sequence (TR/TE = 500/15 ms) shows marked enhancement of the focal hemorrhagic area in the vestibule (arrow) accompanied by bleeding within the superior vestibular nerve (open arrow).

Figs. 5.**32 a–f** **Promontory fracture with trauma to the membranous labyrinth.** ▷
(**a**) Stenvers radiograph. Despite the known trauma history and clinical presentation, the Stenvers film is essentially negative, showing no abnormalities of the internal auditory canal or semicircular canals.
(**b**) HRCT scan of the right mastoid (1-mm slice thickness) demonstrates an intratympanic hemorrhage, displaced intratympanic bone fragments (arrows), and a chip fracture of the lateral border of the right promontory (open arrow).
(**c**) Axial TSE sequence (TR/TE = 4797/400 ms) shows hyperintense fluid-containing structures and hemorrhagic areas in the left mastoid (arrows) and tympanic cavity. The vestibular labyrinth appears normal. Only half of the basal turn of the cochlea is visualized, and fluid loss is apparent in the remaining cochlear structures.
2 Vestibular labyrinth
(**d**) Axial TSE sequence (TR/TE = 4797/400 ms) shows a membranous labyrinth of normal appearance on the left side and a hemorrhagic collection on the right side (arrows).
1 Cochlea
2 Vestibular labyrinth
(**e**) T1-weighted SE sequence shows pontine structures of normal appearance and petrous apices that contain hyperintense fat. The left cochlea shows intermediate signal intensity and appears normal. Air-containing structures are visible on the right side.
P Petrous apex
1 Cochlea
(**f**) Gd-enhanced T1-weighted SE sequence (TR/TE = 500/15 ms) shows contrast enhancement in the membranous labyrinth and cochlea on the right side (arrows).

Masses Associated with Increased Radiographic Density of the Temporal Bone

The differential diagnosis of increased temporal-bone density noted on conventional X-ray films or CT scans should follow the criteria in Table 5.**22**.

Table 5.**22** Mass associated with increased radiographic density of the temporal bone

Common:
- Fibrous dysplasia
- Chronic sclerosing mastoiditis

Rare:
- Malformation:
  —Craniometaphyseal dysplasia
- Tumor:
  —Ossifying fibroma
  —Osteoplastic metastasis
  —Osteosarcoma
- Metabolic abnormality:
  —Osteodystrophy
  —Paget disease
  —Osteopetrosis

Figs. 5.**32**

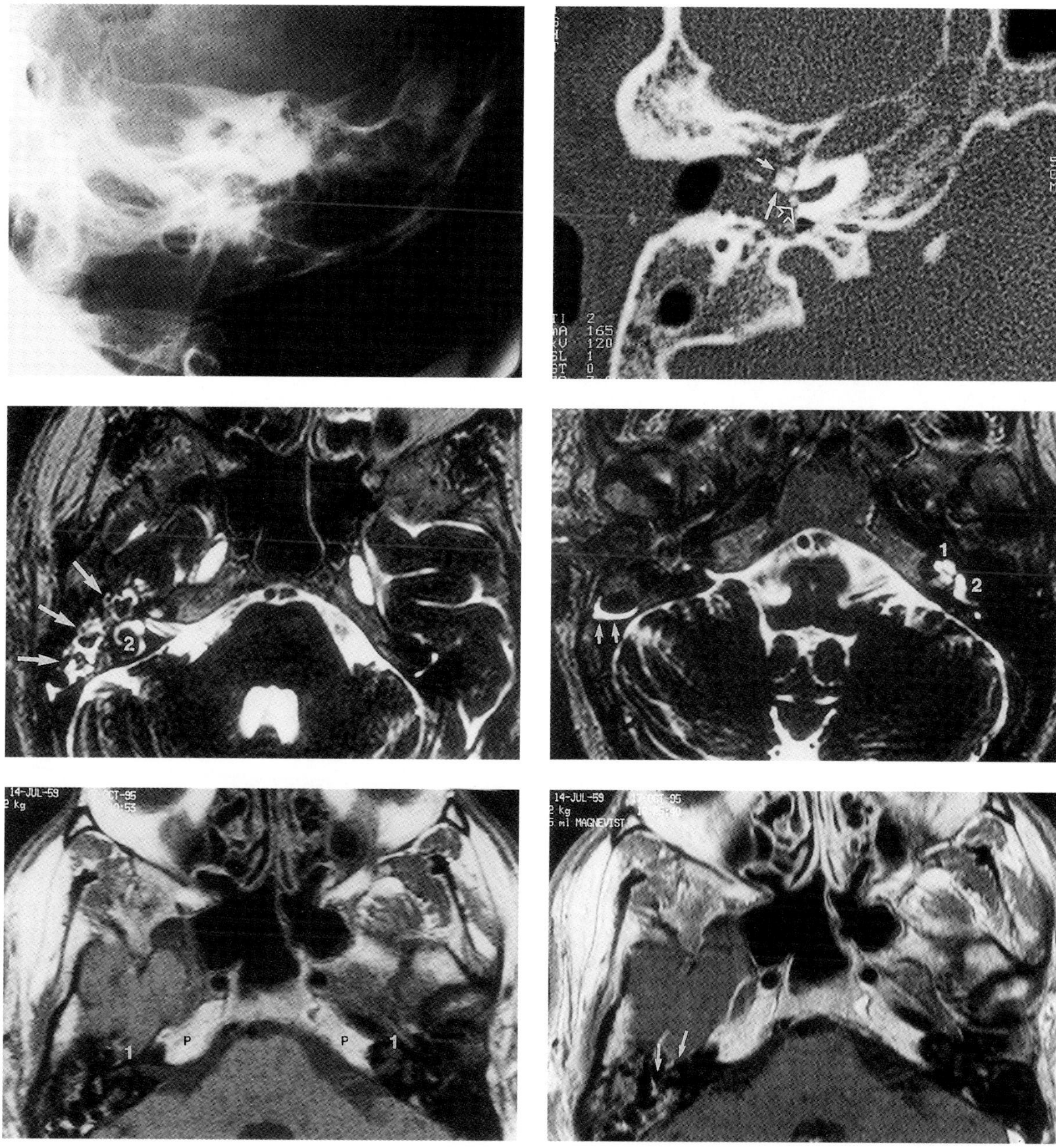

a b c d e f

Mass in the Foramen Ovale

Various imaging criteria are applied in the differential diagnosis of foramen ovale masses based on standard modalities such as contrast-enhanced CT and high-resolution MRI. The essential criteria are listed in Tables 5.**23** and 5.**24**.

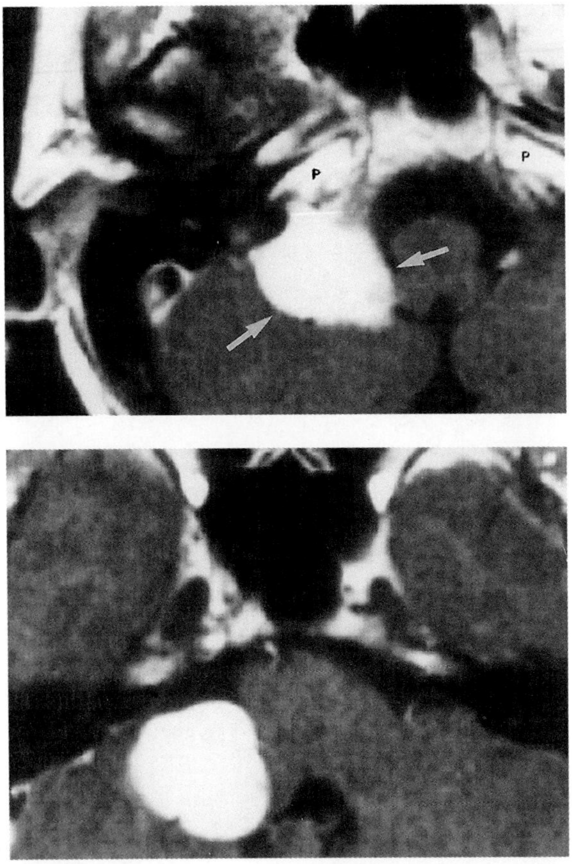

a

b

Figs. 5.**33 a, b** **Masses arising from brainstem structures or lower cranial nerves: accessory neuroma.**
(**a**) Gd-enhanced axial T1-weighted SE sequence (TR/TE = 500/15 ms) shows a mass extending from the lower precerebellar space lateral to the brainstem upward into the cerebellopontine angle (arrows). A high fat content is responsible for the high signal intensity in the petrous apex. The geometry of the mass is consistent with a neuroma of the lower cranial nerve group.
P Petrous apex
(**b**) Gd-enhanced T1-weighted SE sequence (TR/TE = 500/15 ms) 8 mm higher than in **(a)** defines the lobulated borders of the tumor, whose mass effect and growth characteristics are not consistent with a primary mass arising from cerebellopontine angle structures.

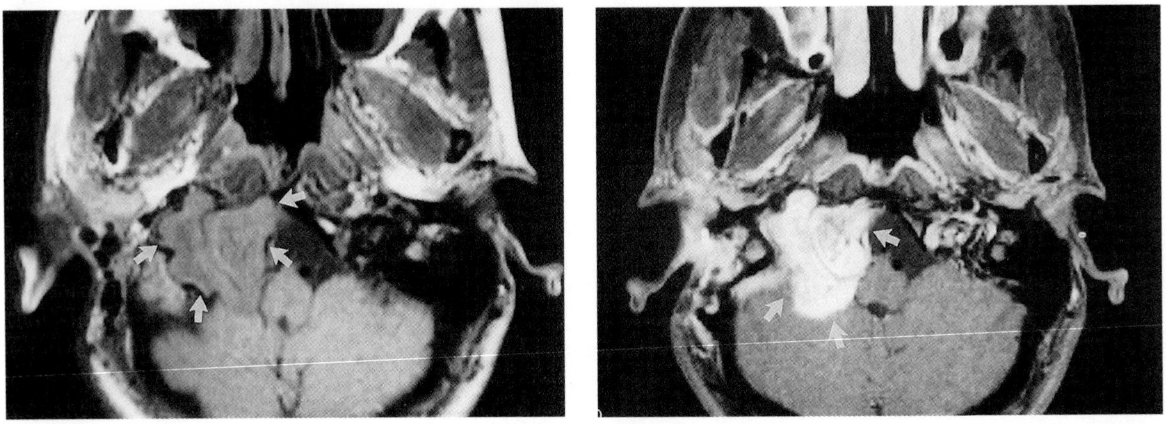

a b

Figs. 5.**34 a, b** **Hypoglossal neuroma.**
(**a**) Unenhanced axial T1-weighted SE sequence (TR/TE = 500/15 ms) demonstrates a mass that is approximately isointense to gray matter with extension into the hypoglossal nerve canal (arrows) and jugular foramen.
(**b**) Gd-enhanced axial T1-weighted SE sequence (TR/TE = 550/17 ms) shows an intensely enhancing mass that is well delineated by its relation to the foramina and brainstem and by its mass effect on surrounding structures. The morphologic criteria are characteristic of hypoglossal neuroma. The differential diagnosis would also include accessory meningioma or an atypical neuroma of the jugular foramen (arrows).

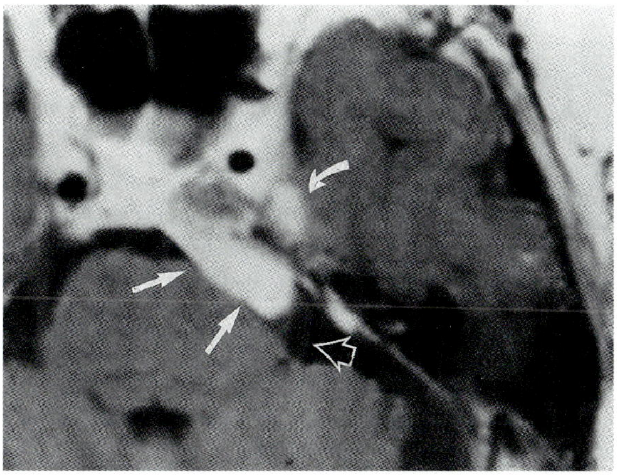
a

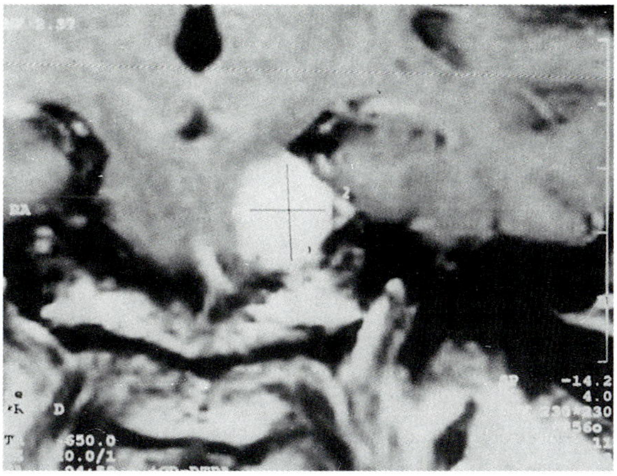
b

Figs. 5.**35 a, b** **Trigeminal neuroma.**

(**a**) Gd-enhanced axial T1-weighted SE sequence (TR/TE = 500/15 ms) shows a mass extending posteriorly into the cerebellopontine angle (arrows) and an adjacent mass in the Meckel cavity (curved arrow). The origin of the trigeminal nerve at the brainstem can be identified on the right and left sides (open arrow).

(**b**) Gd-enhanced coronal T1-weighted SE sequence (TR/TE = 500/15 ms) demonstrates the medial tumor component (crosshairs) compressing the brainstem and showing the morphologic and topographic characteristics of a trigeminal neuroma.

Table 5.**23** Mass in the foramen ovale: CT criteria
➤ Symmetric
➤ Asymmetric
➤ Marginal sclerosis
➤ Peripheral demineralization
➤ Intraforaminal contrast enhancement

Table 5.**24** Mass in the foramen ovale: MRI criteria
➤ Uniform thickening of the mandibular nerve (V_3)
➤ Concentric expansion of the foramen ovale, intermediate T1-weighted signal intensity
➤ Replacement of hypointense signal in trigeminal cistern by tumor tissue showing moderately high T1-weighted signal intensity
➤ Atrophy of masticatory muscles

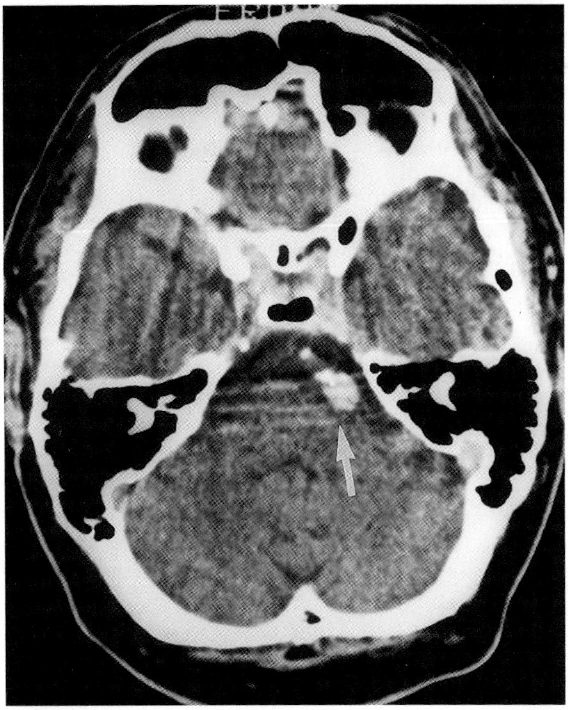
a

Figs. 5.**36 a – c** **Neurovascular compression syndrome in trigeminal neuralgia.**
(**a**) Contrast-enhanced axial CT shows a dense mass with a vascular appearance on the left side of the brainstem extending into the prepontine cistern (arrow). Pneumosinus dilatans is present as an incidental finding.
(**b**) Axial T1-weighted SE sequence (TR/TE = 500/15 ms) demonstrates a large basilar artery on the left side (arrows) with displacement of the right trigeminal nerve (open arrow).
(**c**) MRA (3-D FISP sequence). Sagittal MIP reconstruction confirms the large, high-riding basilar artery as the cause of the compression syndrome.

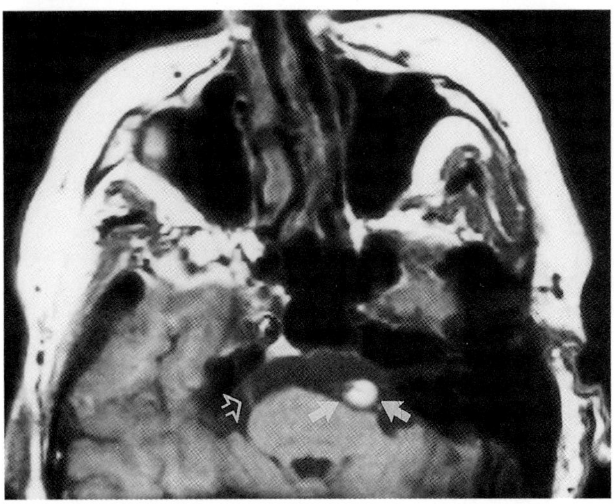
b

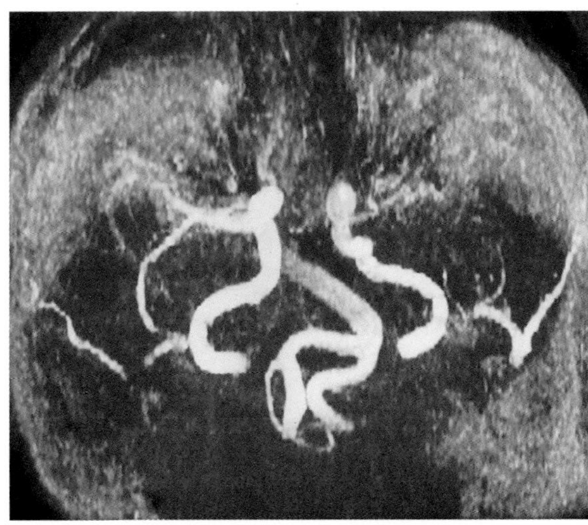
c

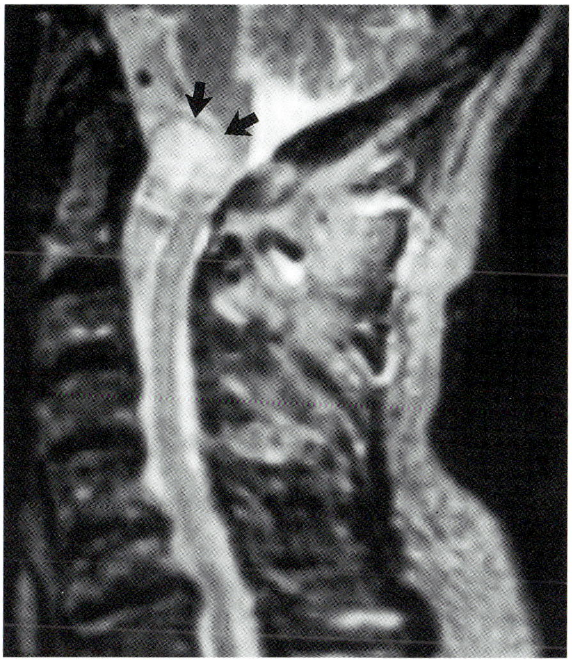

a

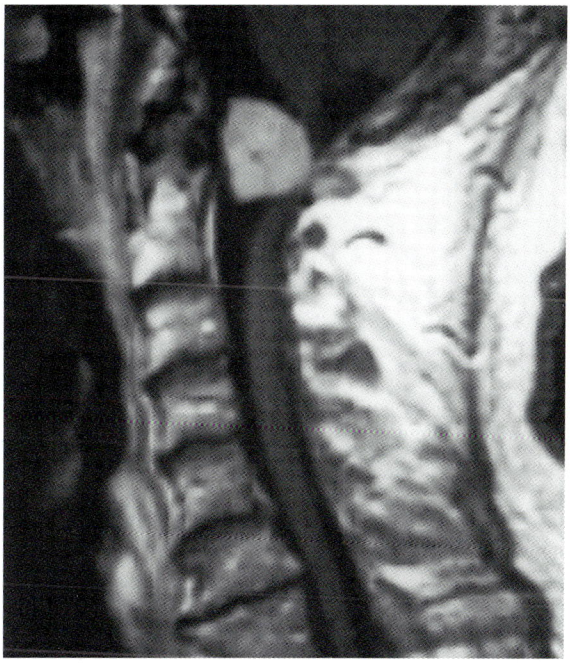

b

Figs. 5.**37 a, b** **Meningioma of the foramen magnum.**
(**a**) Sagittal T2-weighted SE sequence (TR/TE = 2500/90 ms) shows a mass approximately isointense to the pons (arrows) displacing the medulla oblongata posteriorly.

(**b**) Gd-enhanced sagittal T1-weighted SE sequence (TR/TE = 500/15 ms) shows intense, uniform enhancement of a geometric mass in the foramen magnum. The location, enhancement characteristics, and geometric outlines of the mass are pathognomonic for a foramen magnum meningioma.

Summary and Diagnostic Strategy

The strategy for investigating diseases of the inner ear, internal auditory canal, and cerebellopontine angle should be strictly standardized according to the nature of the clinical problem (Figs. 5.**38** – 5.**40**). High-resolution MRI using specific contrast techniques and high-resolution, heavily T2-weighted sequences is now considered the primary imaging procedure of choice for investigations of the inner ear and internal auditory canal. With the adjunctive use of MR angiographic protocols, invasive diagnostic DSA has become less important as a primary modality. Today, conventional angiographic techniques in the head and neck are mainly of value as a prelude to interventional therapeutic procedures.

The clinical presentation of progressive sensorineural hearing loss with abnormal inner ear function tests has become the most common indication for MR imaging of the inner ear and cerebellopontine angle. The next most common clinical indications are disequilibrium and tinnitus, followed by other nerve compression syndromes, especially those involving the facial or trigeminal nerve.

While the primary task of diagnostic imaging is the detection of a possible mass lesion, its secondary purpose is to assist in making an accurate differential diagnostic classification of the disease.

When MRI is used, the differential diagnostic considerations are based on the points summarized in Table 5.**1**.

Once an appropriate and comprehensive clinical evaluation has been completed, high-resolution MRI is the optimum primary imaging study for the cerebellopontine angle, internal auditory canal, and inner ear. In 90% of cases, high-resolution MRI alone can provide an accurate diagnosis and can exclude a lesion that is detectable within the limits of present-day capabilities. Today the detection and differential diagnosis of tumor masses are the most common findings that are verifiable by MRI.

The key to an accurate MRI evaluation is an optimum examination program that includes:

- The use of a head coil.
- Thin image slices separated by gaps of no more than 3 mm.
- High-resolution T2-weighted SE and TSE sequences.
- Adjunctive cerebrospinal fluid (CSF)-specific sequences such as special inversion-recovery or CISS techniques.

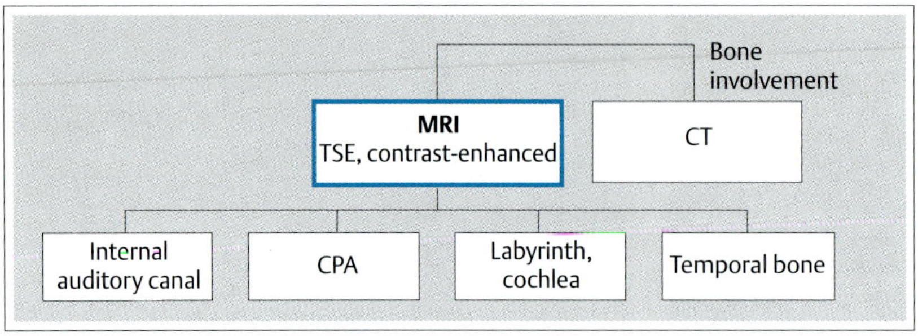

Fig. 5.**38** **Diagnostic strategy for neoplasms.**
CPA Cerebellopontine angle
TSE Turbo spin-echo

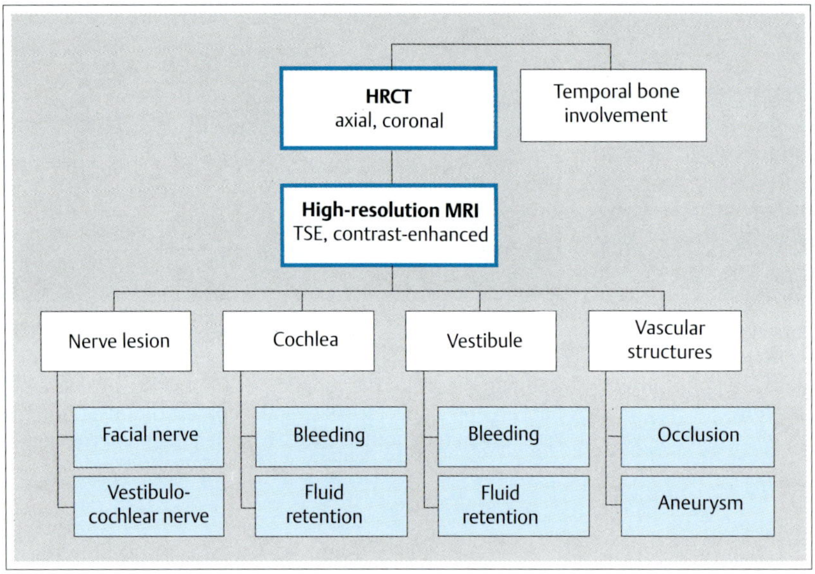

Fig. 5.**39** **Diagnostic strategy for trauma.**
TSE Turbo spin-echo

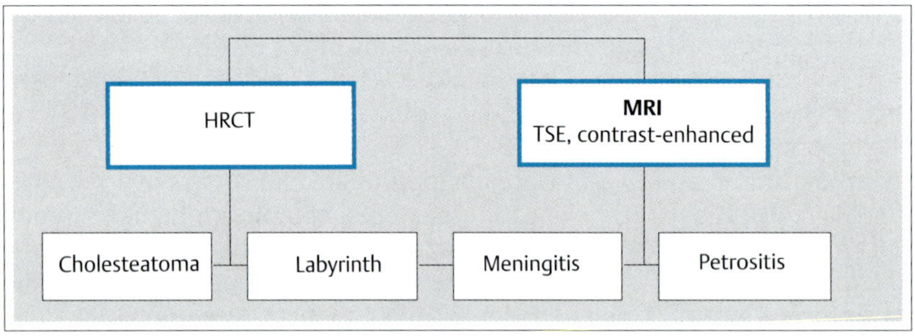

Fig. 5.**40** **Diagnostic strategy for inflammatory diseases.**
TSE Turbo spin-echo

This type of program can provide an accurate assessment of the inner ear and the relation of key neural structures to the internal auditory canal.

Despite recent controversy in the literature, we strongly recommend the combined use of plain and contrast-enhanced MRI sequences. While it is true that heavily T2-weighted imaging can accurately localize a small mass adherent to the superior vestibular nerve without contrast administration, this technique cannot evaluate vascularity—an important drawback in terms of follow-ups and especially in differentiating neoplastic from inflammatory disease.

The use of a high-dose paramagnetic contrast protocol is not currently recommended for routine examinations, as there is no proof that it improves sensitivity. But in cases where it is difficult to identify a cerebellopontine angle mass as a paraganglioma, meningioma, or neuroma, the differential diagnosis can be advanced by high-dose contrast administration in a dynamic protocol. The vascular information furnished by the contrast-enhanced scan will accurately differentiate a highly vascular paraganglioma from other mass lesions in this region.

Through the adjunctive use of arterial and venous MRA, the radiologist can also define the precise topographic relationship of the mass to key vascular structures. Venous images can provide a particularly high degree of diagnostic accuracy. In patients who have vascular masses or arteriovenous malformations, the next step in diagnosis and treatment is invasive DSA, which allows for preoperative or definitive interventional therapeutic procedures.

The strategies for applying the various imaging modalities in patients with neoplasms, traumatic lesions, or inflammatory diseases are reviewed in Figures 5.**38** to 5.**40**.

References

Albers, F. W., R. Van Weissenbruch, J. W. Casselman: 3 DFT-Magnetic Resonance Imaging of the inner ear in Meniere's disease. Acta Otolaryngol. 114 (1994) 595 - 600

Albers, F. W., K. M. Demuynck, J. W. Casselman: Three-dimensional Magnetic Resonance Imaging of the inner ear in idiopathic sudden sensorineural hearing loss. J Otolaryngol. 56 (1994) 1 - 4

Bauman, N. M., L. J. Kirby-Keyser, K. D. Dolan et al: Mondini dysplasia and congenital cytomegalovirus infection. J Pediatr. 124 (1994) 71 - 78

Casselman, J. W., M. H. Majoor, F. W. Albers: MR of the inner ear in patients with Cogan syndrome. AJNR 15 (1994) 131 - 138

Casselman, J. W., R. Kuhweide, I. Dehaene, W. Ampe, F. Devlies: Magnetic Resonance examination of the inner ear and cerebellopontine angle in patients with vertigo and/or abnormal findings at vestibular testing. Acta Otolaryngol. 513, Suppl. (1994) 15 - 27

Dimopoulos, P., C. Muren: Anatomic variations of the cochlea and relations to other temporal bone structures. Acta Radiol. 31 (1990) 439 - 444

Eisenberg, R. L.: Clinical Imaging: an Atlas of Differential Diagnosis, Aspen 1992

Jackler, R. K., W. M. Luxford, D. E. Brackmann, E. M. Monsell: Endolymphatic sac surgery in congenital malformations of the inner ear. Laryngoscope 98 (1988) 698 - 704

Lee, S. H., K. Rao: Cranial computed tomography and MRI. McGraw-Hill, New York 1987

Mark, A. S., D. Fitzgerald: MRI of the inner ear. Baillieres Clin Neurol. 3 (1994) 515 - 535

Vogl, T. J., M. Bauer, D. Hahn, R. Brüning, K. Mees, J. Lissner: Kernspintomographische Untersuchungen bei Verdacht auf Akustikusneurinom. Vorgehen und differentialdiagnostische Überlegungen. Fortschr. Röntgenstr. 145 (1986) 631 - 638

Vogl, T. J., M. Bauer, D. Hahn, K. Mees, R. Brüning, J. Lissner: MR-Imaging of acoustic neuroma: plain and contrast-enhanced studies. Magn Reson Imaging. 5 (1987) 573 - 577

Wilson, J. T., S. W. Leivy, R. A. Sofferman, S. L. Wald: Mondini dysplasia: spontaneous cerebrospinal fluid otorrhea. New perspectives in management. Pediatr. Neurosurg 16 (1990) 260 - 264

6 Nasopharynx and Nasal Cavity

The nasopharynx forms an important boundary zone between the anterior and middle skull base and the parapharyngeal space. Diagnostic imaging is used in this region for the morphologic evaluation, localization, and staging of primary lesions of the nasopharynx and nasal cavity. Because the clinical examination is limited to inspection by direct or fiberoptic techniques, supplemented in some cases by the sampling of biopsy material, radiologic procedures have a major role in the detection, diagnosis, and differential diagnosis of clinically occult disease. This chapter deals with the essential differential diagnostic aspects of nasal and nasopharyngeal lesions.

Normal Anatomy

Nasopharynx

The nasopharynx forms the upper portion of the pharynx and is continuous anteriorly with the nasal cavity. The roof of the nasopharynx is formed by the *sphenoid bone*, while its floor and junction with the oropharynx are at the level of the *soft palate*. These anatomic relationships are readily appreciated on sagittal and coronal sections. The *pharyngeal recess* (Rosenmüller fossa) is a pouch-like recess in the lateral wall of the nasopharynx directed toward the parapharyngeal space and lying directly adjacent to the eustachian tube orifice. This region is a common site of origination for nasopharyngeal malignancies. The *torus tubarius* is the posterior part of the cartilaginous eustachian tube. Lateral to the torus tubarius is the *levator veli palatini muscle*. The pharyngobasilar fascia, which runs between this muscle and the tensor veli palatini, combines with the levator veli palatini to define the boundary of the parapharyngeal space. The *pharyngobasilar fascia* is a tough connective-tissue structure that unites the pharynx with the skull base and is perforated bilaterally for passage of the eustachian tube. Infiltration of this fascia signifies the presence of an aggressive nasopharyngeal tumor.

Superficial structures like the pharyngeal recess and torus tubarius are readily identified on T1-weighted magnetic resonance (MR) images, as are the pterygoid muscles. Because the mucosa shows greater enhancement on post-contrast images than the surrounding tissues, gadolinium(Gd)-enhanced T1-weighted sequences are excellent for visualizing the levator and tensor veli palatini muscles, the pharyngobasilar fascia, the tubal orifices, and the pharyngeal recess (Figs. 6.**1** and 6.**2**, Table 6.**1**).

Even without contrast medium, magnetic resonance imaging (MRI) can demonstrate tumor infiltration or encasement of the internal carotid artery and jugular vein, and can define intratumoral blood vessels. If the blood supply to a mass lesion is not clearly defined on preoperative MR images, selective digital substraction angiography (DSA) should be performed as an adjunct.

With its multiplanar capabilities, MRI can demonstrate the extent of a mass in three dimensions and, most importantly, can define the relationship of the mass to cranial nerves V, IX, and X.

The administration of Gd-DTPA is advantageous for studies of the adjacent bony structures of the skull base, because this agent will enhance the marrow contained in the cancellous bone. Slow blood flow in the cavernous sinus and the veins traversing the skull base cause these structures to enhance brightly on post-contrast images, whereas arterial vessels carrying rapid flow appear hypointense.

A thick layer of lymphatic tissue lines the walls of the nasopharynx, particularly the roof and pharyngeal recess. Hypertrophy of this tissue can obstruct the tubal orifice and lead to hearing problems. The lymphatic tissue appears hyperintense to muscle and fascia on MRI.

Nasal Cavity

The nasal cavity is an air-filled space with thin bony walls. The nasal cavity and paranasal sinuses are bounded superiorly by the ethmoid bone and inferiorly by the hard palate, whose content of bone marrow causes it to display high signal intensity on MR images. Axial and coronal views are best for demonstrating the nasal cavity and surrounding structures. The thin bony walls of the nasal cavity itself are not visualized with MRI, and the surrounding fat and muscle tissue serve to define its boundaries. The thinnest portion of the bony walls, and the part most easily eroded by tumors, lies along the posteromedial wall of the antrum. Among the important structures that can be identified in this area are the infraorbital nerve and its accompanying vein and artery, which appear in the posterior portion of the antral roof.

Table 6.**1** Ability of various MR sequences to define anatomic structures in and around the nasopharynx

Structures	**T1-weighted, unenhanced**	**Proton-density**	**T2-weighted**	**T1-weighted, Gd-enhanced**
Superficial structures:				
➤ Pharyngeal recess	2	3	2	3
➤ Torus tubarius	2	3	2	2
Muscles:				
➤ Levator veli palatini	2	2	1	3
➤ Tensor veli palatini	2	2	1	3
➤ Medial/lateral pterygoid	2	3	1	2
➤ Longus colli	2	3	2	3
Deep structures:	3	3	2	3
➤ Parapharyngeal space				
➤ Infratemporal fossa	2	2	1	3
➤ Sphenoid bone	2	2	2	3
➤ Skull base	2	2	2	3
➤ Internal carotid artery	2	2	2	3
➤ Cavernous sinus	2	2	2	3
➤ Eustachian tube	2	2	1	2
➤ Pharyngobasilar fascia	1	1	1	2
➤ Walls of maxillary sinus	1	2	1	2

Key:
1 Satisfactory
2 Good
3 Excellent, optimal

An important structure bordering on the paranasal sinuses from an imaging standpoint is the retromaxillary space, which is bounded by the pterygopalatine and infratemporal fossae.

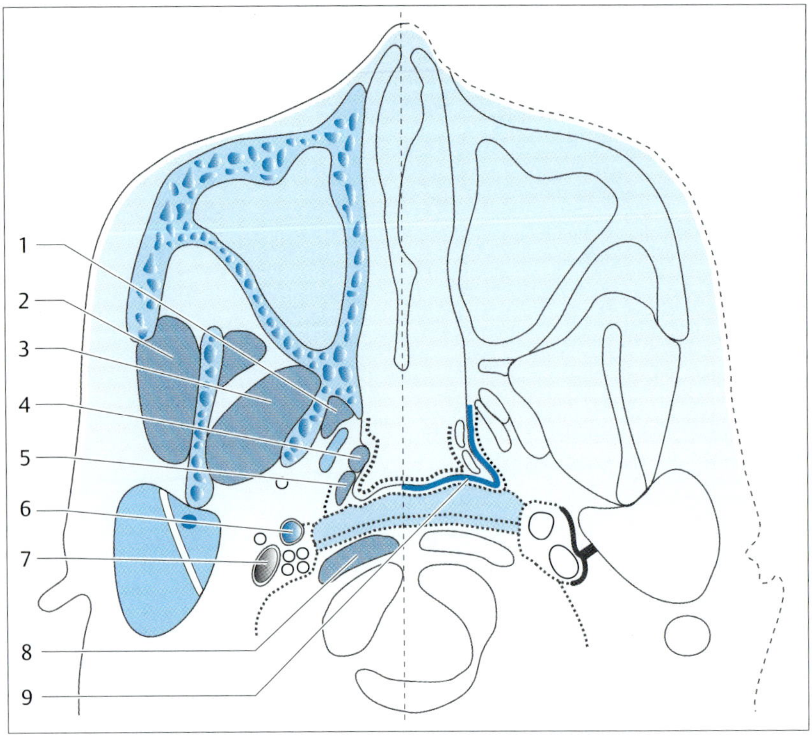

Fig. 6.**1** **Axial diagram of the principal anatomic structures about the nasopharynx.**
1 Medial pterygoid muscle
2 Masseter muscle
3 Lateral pterygoid muscle
4 Tensor veli palatini muscle
5 Levator veli palatini muscle
6 Internal carotid artery
7 Internal jugular vein
8 Longus colli muscle
9 Pharyngobasilar fascia

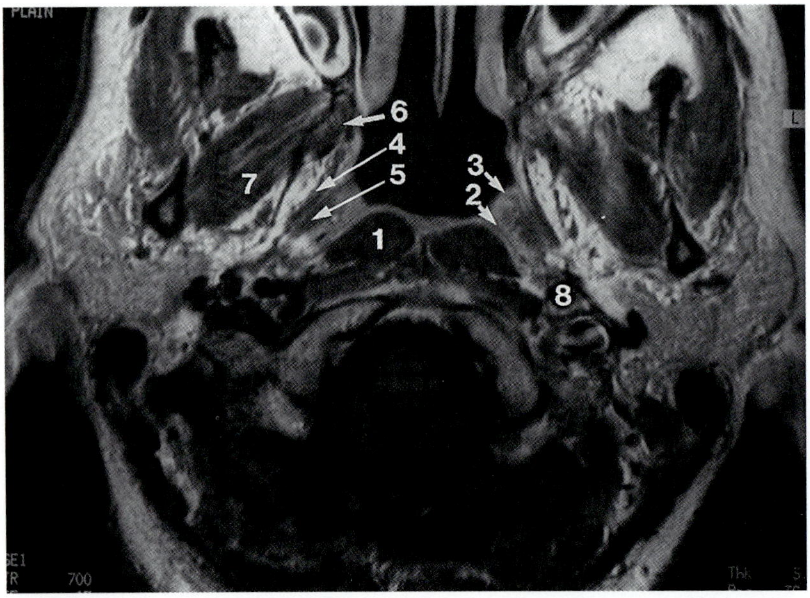

Fig. 6.**2** **Normal anatomy of the nasopharynx** as defined on a Gd-enhanced axial SE sequence (TR/TE = 700/15 ms).
1 Longus colli muscle
2 Lateral pharyngeal recess
3 Torus tubarius
4 Tensor veli palatini muscle
5 Levator veli palatini muscle
6 Medial pterygoid muscle
7 Lateral pterygoid muscle
8 Internal carotid artery

Table 6.2 Important clinical syndromes associated with lesions of the nasal cavity and nasopharynx

Syndrome	Symptom	Cause
Pterygopalatine fossa syndrome	Severe pain, restriction of jaw mobility	Relation of maxillary sinuses to nasopharyngeal tumors
Godtfredsen syndrome	Unilateral trigeminal neuralgia, abducens paralysis, subsequent paralysis of cranial nerves II–IV	Relation of maxillary sinuses to nasopharyngeal tumors
Lateral niche syndrome	Unilateral trigeminal neuralgia, eustachian tube obstruction, hearing loss, ipsilateral nodal metastasis in mandibular angle or neck	Topography of lateral nasopharyngeal tumors
Trotter syndrome	Unilateral neuralgiform pain in mandible, tongue, and ear; conductive hearing loss; ipsilateral bulge of soft palate; possible trismus; nasal airway obstruction	Topography of nasopharyngeal tumors

Table 6.3 Clinical symptoms associated with disorders of the nasopharynx and nasal cavity and their possible causes

Symptom	Cause	Example
Pain, dysesthesia	Inflammation, tumor, foreign body	Rhinitis, sinusitis, nasopharyngeal tumor, rhinolith
Rhinorrhea	Inflammation, trauma, tumor, foreign body	Rhinitis, frontobasal fracture, granulomatosis, nasopharyngeal tumor
Epistaxis	Idiopathic, inflammation, trauma, tumor, foreign body	Rhinitis, sore throat, frontobasal fracture, neoplasms (nasopharyngeal fibroma)
Nasal airway obstruction	Malformations, inflammation, trauma, foreign body	Rhinitis, acute sinusitis, edema, fracture
	Neoplasm	Nasal polyps, adenoids, nasopharyngeal fibroma, granulomatosis
Fetid nasal odor	Inflammation, tumor	Rhinitis, sinusitis, neoplasia
Morphologic change	Inflammation, tumor	Sinusitis, nasal tumors, nasopharyngeal tumors
Malformation	Anomaly, inflammation, tumor	Cephalocele, deviated septum, craniofacial dysplasias, rhinitis, rhinophyma, sinusitis, nasal or nasopharyngeal tumor
Olfactory impairment	Inflammation, trauma, tumor	Rhinitis, sinusitis, frontobasal fracture, neoplasia

Clinical Signs and Symptoms

The *most common clinical symptoms* observed in patients with tumors of the nasopharynx or nasal cavity are:

- Unilateral nasal obstruction (48%).
- Swelling of the face or palate (41%).
- Facial pain (41%).
- Rhinorrhea (37%).
- Epistaxis (35%).

Additionally, tumors of the nasopharynx are frequently associated with *hearing loss* and *cervical lymphadenopathy*. Hearing loss in these cases is secondary to eustachian tube dysfunction.

Nasal obstruction and epistaxis may be clinical manifestations of *nasopharyngeal carcinoma* but are observed in only approximately 30% of these patients.

Patients with problems involving the nasopharynx and nasal cavity may be examined by indirect or direct rhinoscopy or by direct flexible or rigid endoscopy. The use of endoscopic techniques has greatly simplified the early diagnosis of small nasopharyngeal tumors. Careful endoscopic evaluation of the nasopharynx is essential in patients with unilateral eustachian tube dysfunction or serous otitis media of undetermined cause (Tables 6.**2** and 6.**3**).

Imaging Evaluation and Differential Diagnosis

Sound treatment planning depends on establishing the precise location and extent of malignant nasopharyngeal tumors, as well as of certain benign tumors, prior to therapy. Rhinoscopy and even endoscopy may be unable to detect lesions located in the nasopharyngeal space or spreading at the submucosal level. The early detection of such neoplasms, however, will critically affect the prognosis.

In the case of benign, highly vascularized lesions such as angiofibroma, moreover, it is important to determine the vascular supply of the tumor and its relations to other structures so that safe, effective surgical treatment can be planned.

A variety of therapeutic measures may be applied to tumors in this region, depending on the diagnosis. The primary treatment for benign and small malignant lesions is surgical, while primary radiotherapy is indicated for larger, infiltrative malignancies. Recurrent tumors are managed with a combined treatment regimen. A new treatment modality is MRI-guided laser-induced interstitial thermotherapy (LITT), which has yielded very encouraging initial results in this region.

Methods of clinical examination of the nasopharynx and nasal cavity include inspection, palpation, and indirect mirror examination. If clinical findings raise the suspicion of a tumor, the examiner should proceed with rigid or flexible endoscopic inspection. As a rule, imaging procedures are performed only after the endoscopic examination has been completed.

The imaging study of first choice in patients with a suspected nasal or nasopharyngeal mass based on clinical and endoscopic findings is MRI, which is superior to computed tomography (CT) both in defining normal anatomy and in delineating the various tumor masses that occur in this region. High-resolution CT (HRCT) is still important, however, in identifying osseous involvement or infiltration of the bony walls of the nasopharynx and nasal cavity.

Unenhanced MR images can accurately define superficial structures such as the pharyngeal recess, torus tubarius, and pterygoid muscles on T1-weighted sequences. The administration of a paramagnetic contrast agent will improve delineation of the levator and tensor veli palatini muscles, the pharyngobasilar fascia, the eustachian tube orifice, and the pharyngeal recess because these structures will enhance less intensely than the surrounding mucosa. Additionally, MRI and MRA (magnetic resonance angiography) can demonstrate infiltration and encasement of the internal carotid artery and internal jugular vein, and MRI can define the individual vessels supplying the tumor.

Another key advantage of MRI is its multiplanar capabilities, which can better demonstrate the precise extent of the tumor, its topographic relationships, and especially the involvement of cranial nerves.

The lateral and superior walls of the nasopharynx are lined with lymphatic tissue. This circumstance is particularly favorable for MR imaging, inasmuch as contrast-enhanced T1-weighted sequences can clearly differentiate lymphatic hyperplasia from lymphomatous involvement.

Conventional Radiography

Given the wide availability of CT scanners, conventional radiographs of the nasopharynx are of minor importance today, and conventional tomography has become obsolete. Conventional X-ray films can provide only indirect evidence of a nasopharyngeal soft-tissue mass, which is best appreciated on biplane skull films and paranasal sinus films in the occipitomental and occipitofrontal projections. The latter views are particularly useful in the diagnosis of chronic or acute sinusitis, with or without an air–fluid level. Destruction of the bony boundaries of the nasal cavity or nasopharynx is seen with stage T4 neoplasms and can be appreciated on conventional X-ray films.

Computed Tomography (CT)

CT examination of the nasopharyngeal region and nasal cavity is usually performed with a series of 2- to 5-mm axial scans during the intravenous administration of contrast medium. Either conventional or spiral CT technique may be used. Additional information can be obtained by supplementing the axial scans with coronal images reconstructed from thin axial slices. Axial scan coverage should extend from the frontal sinus to the level of the tracheal bifurcation.

The primary CT documentation should consist of both soft-tissue and bone-window images. If bony lesions are suspected, a high-resolution bone algorithm with a high window setting (approximately 4000 HU) should also be used.

Magnetic Resonance Imaging (MRI)

Nasopharyngeal MRI should always employ a head coil or, for tumors with marked cervical extension, a combined head-and-neck coil as used for MRA. Following a sagittal survey sequence with a short TR, contiguous axial scans are obtained with use of the head coil. Optimum contrast is provided by a long T2-weighted spin-echo (SE) sequence using double-echo technique, a TR of 3000 ms, and a TE of 25 and 90 ms. Turbo spin-echo (TSE) sequences or a short T1-weighted sequence (TR/TE = 700/15 ms) also may be used. With the advent of fast imaging sequences, enhancement dynamics can be accurately plotted over time as a means of narrowing the differential diagnosis. This is best accomplished with gradient-echo sequences using a flip angle of 30° (TR/TE = 30/12 ms). When this T1-weighted technique is used, an initial "plain view" is obtained, then the intensity of contrast enhancement in the lesion is documented in axial sections for a period of 5 to 6 minutes. The usual technique is to obtain contiguous slices of 4-mm thickness, taking two averages per slice. Lesions larger than 65 mm are imaged with a slice thickness of 6 mm. The total examination time averages between 40 and 60 minutes. Identical imaging parameters should be used for the precontrast and post-contrast T1-weighted images. The axial scans are usually supplemented by coronal T1-weighted sequences.

Special sequences may also be obtained if more information is needed. For example, arterial or venous MRA can document the vascular supply of a lesion, define its relationship to surrounding structures, and exclude vascular pathology. MRA should be performed without contrast medium, because the high affinity of the nasal and nasopharyngeal mucosae for Gd-DTPA can create a high signal intensity that will obscure vascular structures on subsequent projection angiograms.

A fat suppression sequence is useful for accurately defining the extent of tumor infiltration following contrast administration.

Imaging Findings

Five percent of all malignant tumors of the head and neck originate in the nasopharynx, and more than 90% of these are carcinomas. The most common nasopharyngeal malignancies in adults are *squamous cell carcinoma* and *lymphoepithelial neoplasms*. *Lymphomas* and *rhabdomyosarcomas* are more common in children and tend to undergo early, extensive lymphogenous spread.

Given the variety of cell types that occur normally in the nasopharyngeal region, many different lesions may originate in the nasopharynx, ranging from embryologic malformations to benign and malignant tumors. Carcinomas and lymphoepithelial tumors account for some 75% of all nasopharyngeal neoplasms in adults.

Benign nasopharyngeal tumors are rare, the most common being *juvenile nasopharyngeal fibroma* (skull base angioma). Although nasopharyngeal fibroma is histologically benign, it tends to show malignant clinical characteristics because of its expansile, locally aggressive growth.

Mesenchymal tumors are the most common benign tumors of the nose and paranasal sinuses. This group includes papillomas, hemangiomas, fibromas, and other rare tumors.

Malignant tumors of the nasal cavity and paranasal sinuses account for less than 1% of all malignant neoplasms. The histologic types are anaplastic carcinoma (59%), lymphoepithelial carcinoma (30%), squamous cell carcinoma, and mesenchymal tumors.

Congenital Variations and Malformations

Two well-known congenital variants and malformations of the nasopharynx are the *Tornwaldt cyst* (Fig. 6.**3**) and *hyperplasia of the torus tubarius*. They are often detected incidentally on MR images. A Thornwaldt cyst is readily identifiable as a midline cystic mass.

Tumors

It is important clinically to detect and differentiate *primary* and *secondary masses* in the nasopharynx. In the *TNM classification*, the following staging criteria are applied to nasopharyngeal carcinomas:

- T1: tumor confined to one subsite in the nasopharynx.
- T2: tumor invading more than one subsite.
- T3: tumor invading the nasal cavity, oropharynx, or both.
- T4: tumor invading the skull base, cranial nerves, or both.

Usually these tumors first infiltrate the levator and tensor veli palatini muscles and the pharyngobasilar fascia. Tumors arising from the nasal and paranasal sinus mucosae invade the parapharyngeal and retromaxillary space and infiltrate the pterygoid and longus colli muscles. Intracranial spread may occur directly by bony invasion of the skull base or by way of the sphenoid sinus and basal foramina. It is common to find invasion of the poststyloid compartment of the parapharyngeal space with encasement and compression of the internal carotid artery.

The *WHO* subdivides *nasopharyngeal carcinomas* into four main groups:

- The first group consists of all squamous cell carcinomas, which account for approximately 25% of all carcinomas in this region and are most common between 40 and 50 years of age. They show some association with the Epstein–Barr virus (19%), and the response to therapy depends greatly on tumor grade.
- Two other groups are undifferentiated and nonkeratinizing carcinomas, which respectively account for about 63% and 12% of all nasopharyngeal carcinomas. Both types show a high association with the Epstein-Barr virus (84% and 82%, respectively) and are most common between 40 and 50 years of age.
- The fourth group consists of all nasopharyngeal adenocarcinomas, which are somewhat rare and so far have not been associated with elevated titers of the Epstein–Barr virus.

Squamous Cell Carcinoma

Approximately 80% of squamous cell carcinomas of the nasopharynx arise from the lateral walls, especially the pharyngeal recess (Fig. 6.**4**). They almost always infiltrate the levator and tensor veli palatini muscles and destroy the pharyngobasilar fascia. Tumors arising from the nasopharyngeal mucosa invade the parapharyngeal space, nasal cavity, and paranasal sinuses and infiltrate the longus colli muscles posteriorly. They may invade the cranial cavity directly through the bony skull base or via the sphenoid sinus and basal foramina (Fig. 6.**5**). Subtle invasion of the thin bony walls of the paranasal sinuses is rare with these squamous cell cancers, which tend to spread superiorly and posteriorly or invade the nasal cavity by direct extension.

Radiologically, these tumors usually show indistinct margins and areas of necrosis (Fig. 6.**6**). Occasionally the tumor may extend into the parotid gland. Many tumors invade the poststyloid compartment of the parapharyngeal space, encasing and compressing the internal carotid artery. Involvement of cranial nerves IX to XII and extensive lymph node metastases are also common.

Conventional axial and lateral skull films may demonstrate opacities in the nasopharynx and/or sites of bone destruction in the skull base. However, CT and MRI, especially with contrast enhancement, are essential for diagnosing squamous cell carcinomas of the nasopharynx and identifying areas of soft-tissue infiltration. MRI, with its excellent soft-tissue contrast, is particularly useful for the accurate staging of these lesions.

MR images of these tumors will show an average 1.6-fold increase in signal intensity after the administration of contrast medium. Typically the tumors show a slightly nonhomogeneous signal pattern that includes less intense areas of intratumoral necrosis. Use of the paramagnetic contrast agent Gd-DTPA will yield additional diagnostic information in all cases. Many tumors are clearly delineated from adjacent structures only on contrast-enhanced images. It is common for tumors to infiltrate the eustachian tube and impair its ventilation, inciting a mastoiditis that is best appreciated on T2-weighted images. Relaxation-time calculations indicate decreased T1 times and intermediate T2 times.

Approximately 80% of *paranasal sinus tumors* are squamous cell carcinomas. Since chronic inflammatory sinus disease is a common antecedent, the early symptoms of a sinus malignancy are often overlooked, and many tumors are diagnosed only after they have caused destruction of the bony sinus walls.

The MRI characteristics of these tumors are similar to those of nasopharyngeal carcinomas. After destroying the thin bony walls of the maxillary sinus, the tumor may grow into the nasopharynx and retromaxillary space or may directly invade the nasal cavity by tracking along the mucosa. MRI demonstrates intermediate T1 times, moderately prolonged T2 times, and moderate enhancement after contrast administration. A comparison of different imaging parameters shows that a combination of T1- and T2-weighted sequences usually yields the best information in unenhanced studies. Because tumor tissue and inflammatory changes show similar T2 relaxation times in many cases, the administration of Gd-DTPA is definitely helpful for delineating muscle infiltration in the retromaxillary space. At present, CT is superior to MRI for detecting small erosions in the thin walls of the maxillary sinus and pterygoid process. MRI is better for defining the extent of paranasal sinus masses and distinguishing inflammatory sinus disease from neoplastic involvement.

Lymphoepithelial Carcinoma and Adenoid Cystic Carcinoma

Lymphoepithelial carcinoma (Fig. 6.**7**) and adenoid cystic carcinoma (Figs. 3.**19c–e**) are considerably more aggressive than squamous cell carcinomas of the nasopharynx, and they are quicker to infiltrate surrounding structures. Most of these tumors arise from the lateral or posterior wall of the nasopharynx and are still relatively small when diagnosed, having already eroded portions of the bony skull base and invaded the cranial cavity, usually by way of the sphenoid bone and petrous apex. Because of their greater vascular supply, these tumors enhance by an approximate factor of 2.0 on post-contrast images. Like squamous cell carcinomas, these tumors often contain necrotic areas of decreased signal intensity.

Lymphoepithelial and adenoid cystic carcinomas manifest slightly prolonged T1 times and intermediate or prolonged T2 times.

Juvenile Angiofibroma (Fig. 6.8)

Juvenile angiofibroma (known also as nasopharyngeal fibroma) is a rare tumor that predominantly affects adolescent males. While histologically benign, the tumor is locally invasive in approximately 60% of cases. From the roof of the nasopharynx, it grows along the mucosa into the nasal cavity. Even extensive tumors do not usually contain necrotic areas owing to their rich vascular supply. The margins are consistently well defined and heavily vascularized. A comparison of MRI and CT shows that MRI is superior to CT for tumor delineation, especially when T2-weighted sequences are used. Axial images can exclude intracranial extension, and coronal images will often document orbital invasion from the nasal cavity.

Data on the enhancement dynamics of nasopharyngeal fibromas confirm the rich vascularity of these tumors, which show more than a 2.3-fold increase in signal intensity after the administration of Gd-DTPA.

The value of combined T1- and T2-weighted imaging and the documentation of intense enhancement after contrast administration make MRI the optimum modality for the evaluation of these tumors.

Pretherapeutic imaging is essential for documenting anatomic variants and excluding arteriovenous fistulas and shunts between the internal and external carotid systems. Treatment for malignant tumors usually consists of radiotherapy to the primary tumor and affected nodal groups.

Lymphatic Hyperplasia and Lymphoma (Fig. 6.9)

The nasopharynx is second only to the tonsillar fossa as a site of occurrence of lymphatic hyperplasia in the head and neck. "Adenoids" are a well-known physiologic cause of respiratory problems in the pediatric age group. In adults, lymphatic hyperplasia can

Table 6.**4** Review of soft-tissue tumors of the nasopharynx

Lesion	CT morphology	MRI morphology
Meningioma	Isodense or hypodense on plain scans, homogeneous enhancement	Isointense on plain images; intense, homogeneous enhancement
Metastases	Bone destruction, nonhomogeneous enhancement	T2-weighted: isodense or hyperintense; intense enhancement
Craniopharyngioma	Calcifications, cysts, variable enhancement pattern	Cyst-equivalent signal intensity, rim enhancement
Chordoma	Bone destruction, calcifications, bone fragments	T2-weighted: hyperintense; marked enhancement
Esthesioneuroblastoma (Fig. 6.**16a**)	Bone destruction; rarely: calcifications, intense enhancement	Nonhomogeneous T1- and T2-weighted signal intensity; intense enhancement
Chondroma	Predominantly soft-tissue tumor with sites of calcification or ossification; moderate enhancement	Intermediate T1-weighted signal intensity, high T2-weighted signal intensity; marked enhancement, somewhat nonhomogeneous
Chondrosarcoma	Slightly hyperdense on plain scans; flocculent calcifications; moderate enhancement	High T2-weighted signal intensity; moderate enhancement

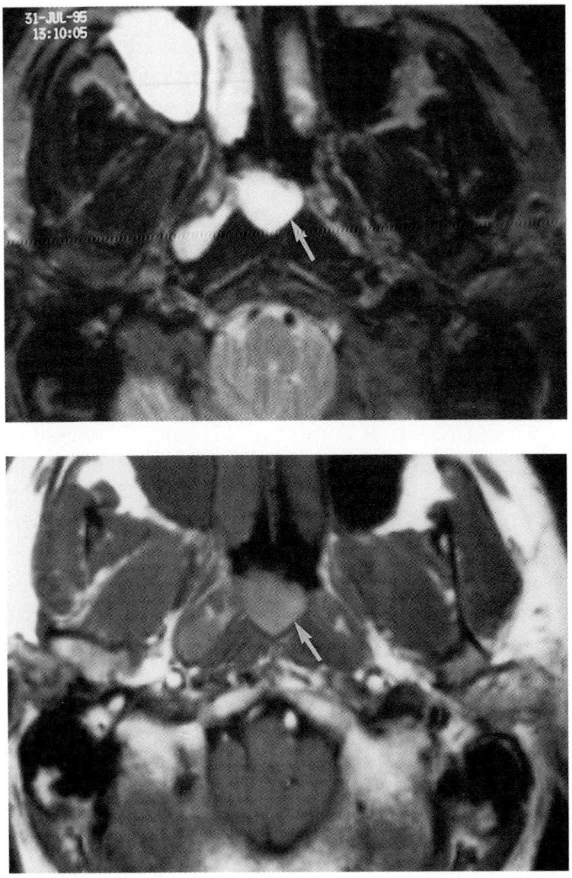

a

b

Figs. 6.3 a, b **Tornwaldt cyst.**
(**a**) Unenhanced axial T2-weighted SE sequence (TR/TE = 3000/90 ms) demonstrates the cyst as a well-circumscribed hyperintense lesion (arrow) in the sellar region.
(**b**) Gd-enhanced axial T1-weighted SE sequence (TR/TE = 700/15 ms) shows faint, uniform enhancement of the lesion (arrow), which is well demarcated from surrounding structures.

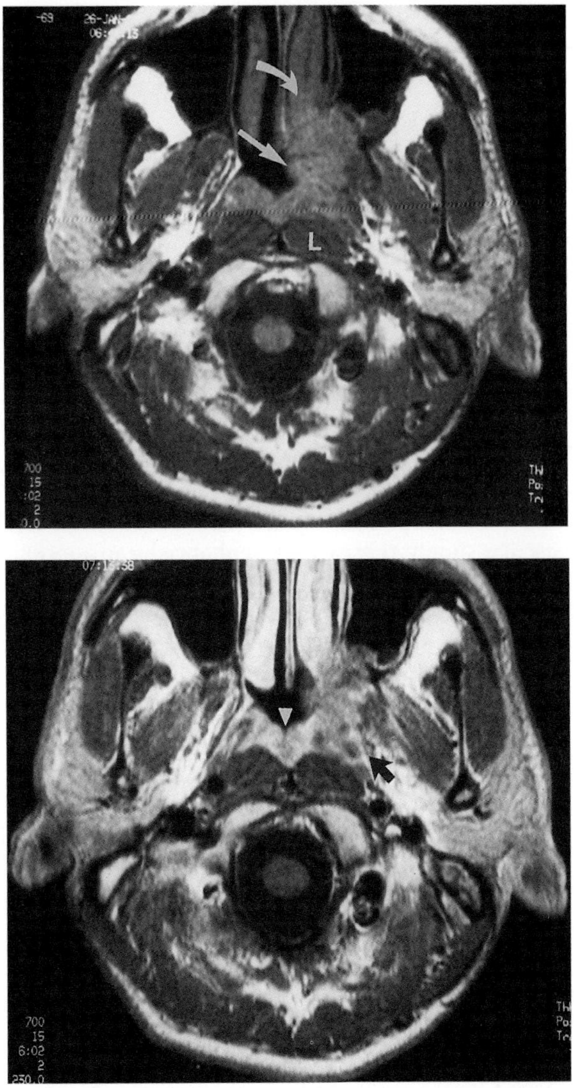

a

b

Figs. 6.4 a, b **Carcinoma of the lateral nasopharyngeal wall.**
(**a**) Unenhanced axial T1-weighted SE sequence (TR/TE = 700/15 ms) demonstrates a mass with indistinct margins (arrow) on the left lateral nasopharyngeal wall with extension into the left nasal cavity (curved arrow). The lesion extends posteriorly to the longus colli muscle (L).
(**b**) Gd-enhanced axial SE sequence (TR/TE = 700/15 ms) shows nonhomogeneous enhancement of the lesion and reveals extension toward the parapharyngeal space (arrow). The lesion does not transgress the midline (arrowhead).

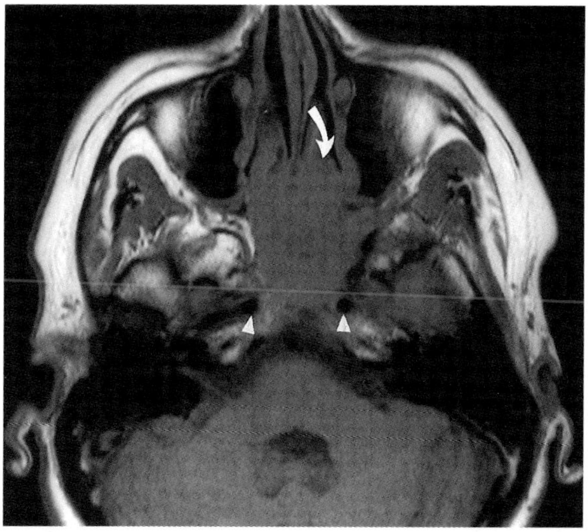

a

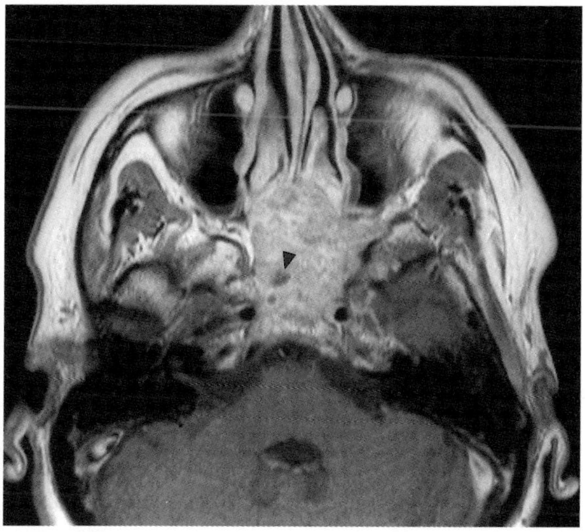

b

Figs. 6.**5 a, b** **Nasopharyngeal carcinoma infiltrating the skull base.**
(**a**) Unenhanced axial T1-weighted SE sequence (TR/TE = 700/15 ms) shows a large, homogeneous mass at the junction of the nasopharynx and anterior skull base. The mass extends anteriorly into the nasal cavity (curved arrow) and posteriorly to the internal carotid artery on each side (arrowheads).
(**b**) Gd-enhanced axial SE sequence (TR/TE = 700/15 ms). After contrast administration, the mass shows predominantly homogeneous enhancement with small hypointense foci representing areas of necrosis (arrowhead).

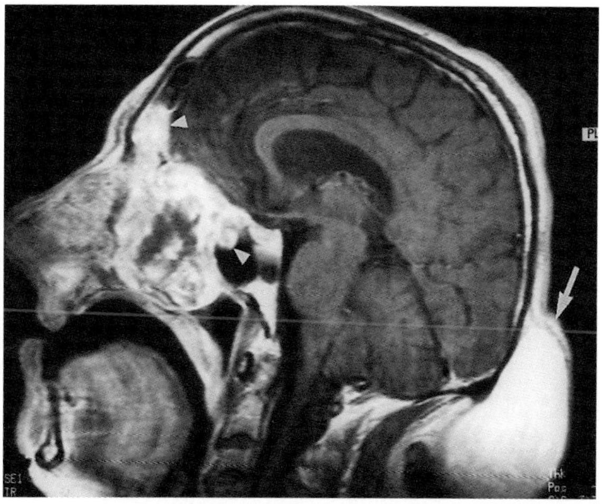

a

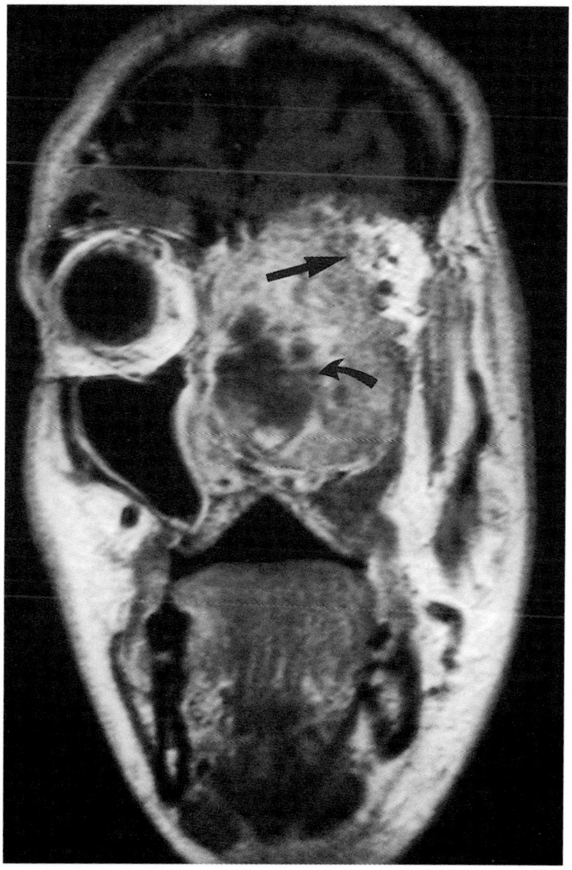

b

Figs. 6.**6 a, b** **Infiltration of the skull base by a nasopharyngeal carcinoma with a necrotic center.**
(**a**) Sagittal Gd-enhanced SE sequence (TR/TE = 700/15 ms) shows a centrally necrotic nasopharyngeal carcinoma invading the anterior skull base, paranasal sinuses (arrowheads), and nasal cavity. An occipital lipoma (arrow) is present as an incidental finding.
(**b**) Coronal Gd-enhanced SE sequence (TR/TE = 700/15 ms) defines the extent of the infiltration, with involvement of the left orbit (arrow) and both nasal cavities. An area of central necrosis (curved arrow) is also documented.

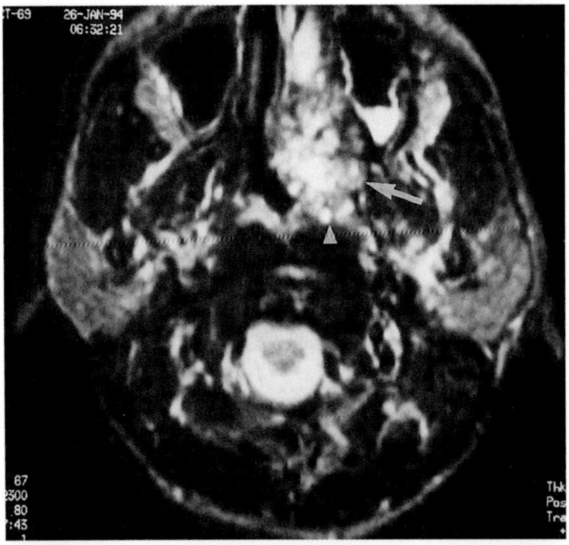

a

Figs. 6.**7 a–c** **Lymphoepithelial carcinoma of the nasopharynx.**

(**a**) Unenhanced axial T2-weighted SE sequence (TR/TE = 3000/90 ms) shows a nonhomogeneous, very hyperintense mass (arrow) on the left lateral nasopharyngeal wall with extension toward the nasal cavity. The mass is poorly demarcated from the posterior nasopharyngeal wall (arrowhead).

(**b**) In the axial T1-weighted SE sequence (TR/TE = 700/15 ms), the lesion appears isointense to the mucosa. There is slight medial displacement of the left nasopharyngeal mucosa (arrowhead) and marked displacement of the muscular structures of the lateral nasopharyngeal wall (arrows).

(**c**) Gd-enhanced axial SE sequence (TR/TE = 700/15 ms) shows that the lesion has transgressed the midline (arrowhead) and contains a central necrotic area (curved arrow). The overall boundaries of the mass are ill-defined.

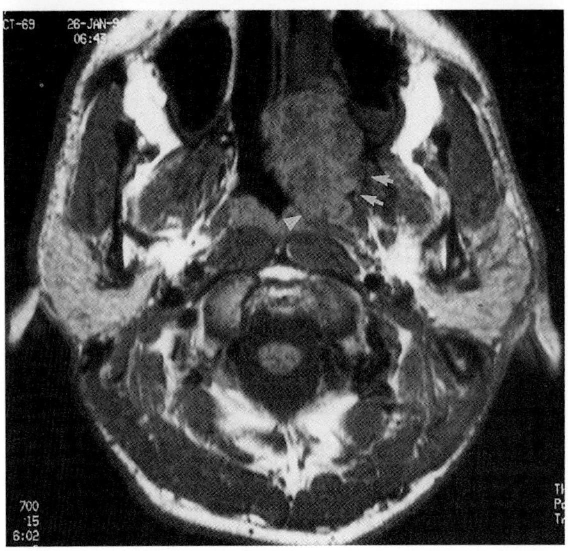

b

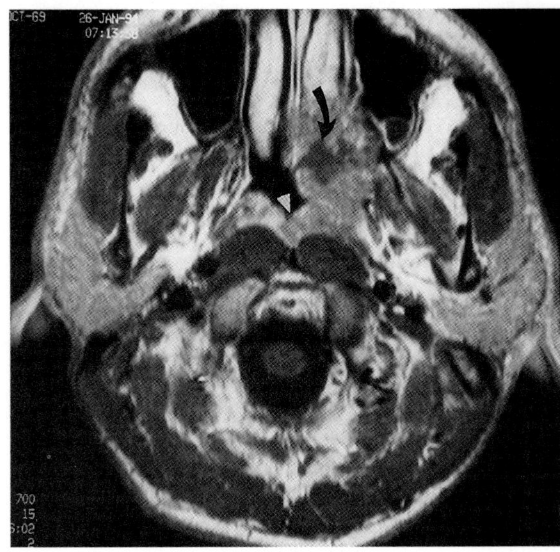

c

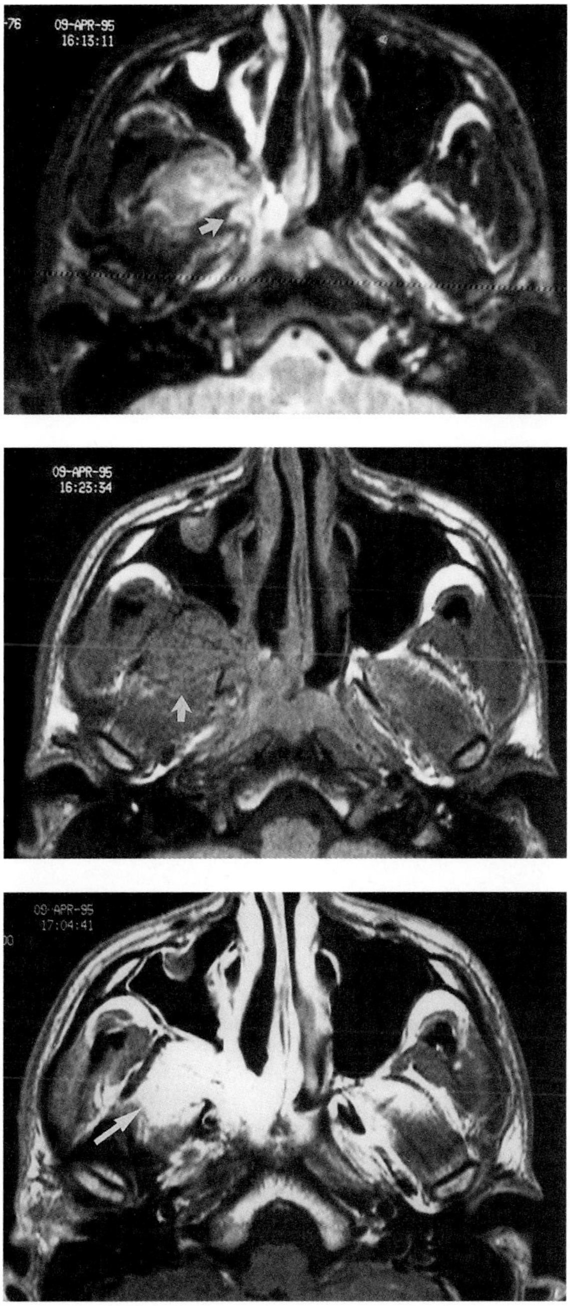

a

b

c

Figs. 6.**8 a – c** **Juvenile angiofibroma.**
(**a**) Unenhanced axial T2-weighted SE sequence (TR/TE = 3000/90 ms) demonstrates a patchy, ill-defined lesion (arrow) of high signal intensity extending into the right medial wall of the maxillary sinus.
(**b**) Unenhanced axial T1-weighted SE sequence (TR/TE = 700/15 ms) cannot delineate the lesion from surrounding structures because of its isointensity but does show marked asymmetry on the right side with structural nonhomogeneities (arrow).
(**c**) Gd-enhanced axial SE sequence (TR/TE = 700/15 ms) demonstrates intense, early enhancement of the lesion (arrow). The tumor extends to the midline but does not cross it.

occur in association with chronic infectious diseases and is particularly common in HIV-positive individuals. The peak incidence is between 20 and 30 years of age.

On MRI, lymphatic hyperplasia appears hyperintense in both T1- and T2-weighted sequences, showing symmetric extension into the nasopharyngeal lumen. Septa are usually present but are clearly defined only on contrast-enhanced T1-weighted images (Fig. 6.**9**). Fast sequences, plain or contrast-enhanced, do not demonstrate these characteristic internal structures.

The main condition requiring differentiation from lymphatic hyperplasia is lymphomatous involvement of the nasopharynx. The most common histologic type is the non-Hodgkin lymphoma, which mainly affects patients over the age of 40. Nasopharyngeal lymphomas show an asymmetric growth pattern and generally do not infiltrate surrounding structures.

While lymphatic hyperplasia and lymphoma have similar signal characteristics on T1- and T2-weighted MR images, lymphomas always show moderate, homogeneous contrast enhancement with a ground-glass appearance on T1-weighted images. None of the lymphomas in our patients displayed linear internal features. These differences provide a means of distinguishing lymphoma from hyperplasia on MR images (Figs. 6.**11** and 6.**12**).

This differentiation cannot be accomplished on CT scans, where both lymphatic hyperplasia and lymphoma appear as a symmetric mass without bone destruction (Fig. 6.**10**).

Rhabdomyoma and Rhabdomyosarcoma (Fig. 6.**13**)

Rhabdomyosarcoma is a tumor that most commonly affects children between 2 and 5 years of age. Infiltration of the anterior skull base occurs in approximately 35% of cases.

MRI depicts rhabdomyosarcoma as a solid, sharply marginated tumor that shows intermediate signal intensity on T1-weighted images and is slightly hyperintense on T2-weighted images. Following contrast administration, the tumor shows moderate enhancement with no other differential diagnostic clues. Imaging often documents growth through the anterior skull base and cavernous sinus, with associated clinical manifestations of cranial neuropathy. Rhabdomyosarcoma is relatively uncommon in the nasopharynx and nasal cavity compared with other malignant neoplasms of this region; involvement of the neck is more typical. The aggressive nature of this tumor can be appreciated on MR images by its asymmetric, indistinct margins and nonhomogeneous enhancement.

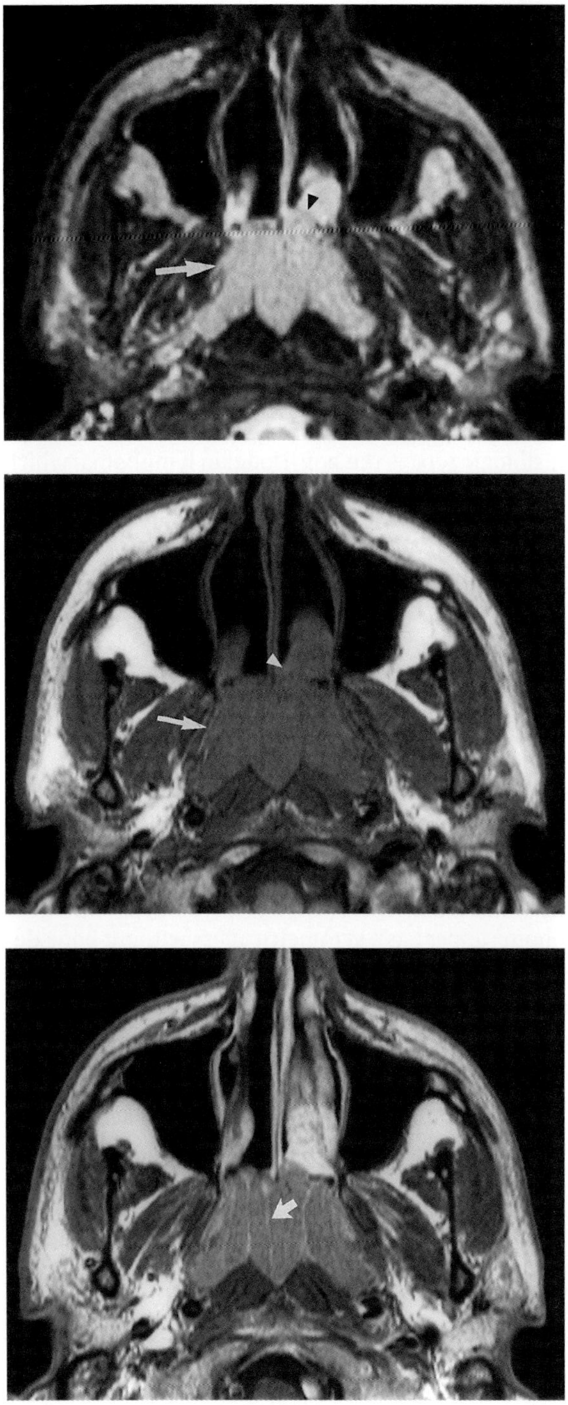

a

b

c

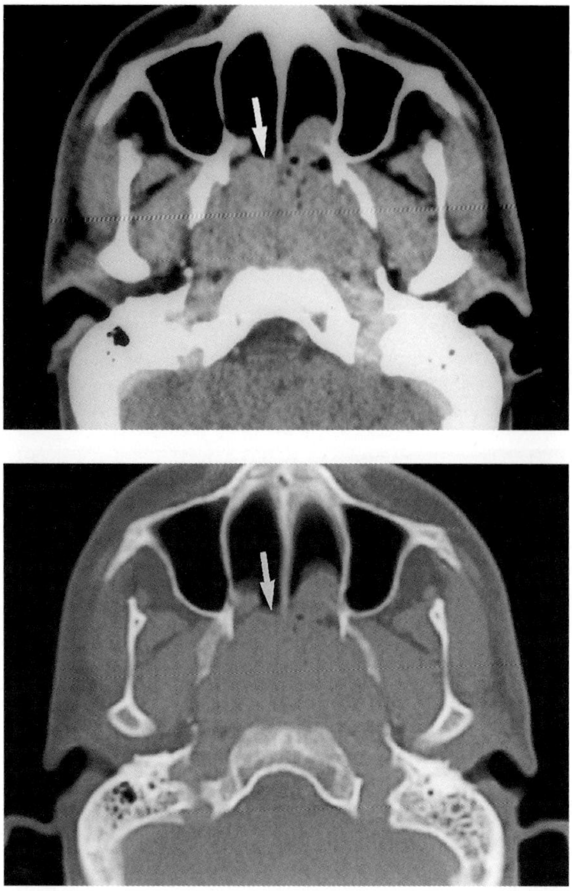

a

b

Figs. 6.**10 a, b** **Lymphatic hyperplasia of the nasopharynx.**
(**a**) Axial CT scan (5 mm) with a soft-tissue window following the intravenous administration of 100 mL Ultravist 370 demonstrates a uniformly isodense mass (arrow) completely occluding the nasopharyngeal lumen.
(**b**) Unenhanced axial CT scan (5 mm) with a bone window shows no peripheral bone destruction by the large mass (arrow), suggesting that the lesion is benign. The identity of the lesion cannot be established, however.

△
Figs. 6.**9 a – c** **Lymphatic hyperplasia.**
(**a**) Unenhanced axial T2-weighted SE sequence (TR/TE = 3000/90 ms) shows a uniformly hyperintense mass (arrow) occupying all of the nasopharynx and showing no infiltrative signs. The lesion extends anteriorly into the cranial nerve (arrowhead).
(**b**) Unenhanced axial T1-weighted SE sequence (TR/TE = 700/15 ms) shows a uniformly isointense lesion that is indistinguishable anteriorly from the nasal turbinate.
(**c**) Gd-enhanced axial SE sequence (TR/TE = 700/15 ms) demonstrates internal septations (arrow) that are pathognomonic for lymphatic hyperplasia. The moderate enhancement of the mass clearly differentiates it from the more intensely enhancing nasal turbinates. Like the previous views, the contrast-enhanced image shows no signs of infiltration.

Figs. 6.**11 a – c** **Nasopharyngeal lymphoma.**
(**a**) Unenhanced axial T2-weighted SE sequence (TR/TE = 3000/90 ms). Unlike lymphatic hyperplasia, the nasopharyngeal lymphoma shows markedly nonhomogeneous high signal intensity on the T2-weighted image along with slightly indistinct margins (arrowheads).
(**b**) Unenhanced axial T1-weighted SE sequence (TR/TE = 700/15 ms) defines the lymphoma as a slightly but uniformly hyperintense mass (arrow) with extensions toward the parapharyngeal space.
(**c**) Gd-enhanced axial SE sequence (TR/TE = 700/15 ms) shows intense, uniform enhancement that gives the lesion a ground-glass appearance (arrow). There is no sign of intratumoral septations.

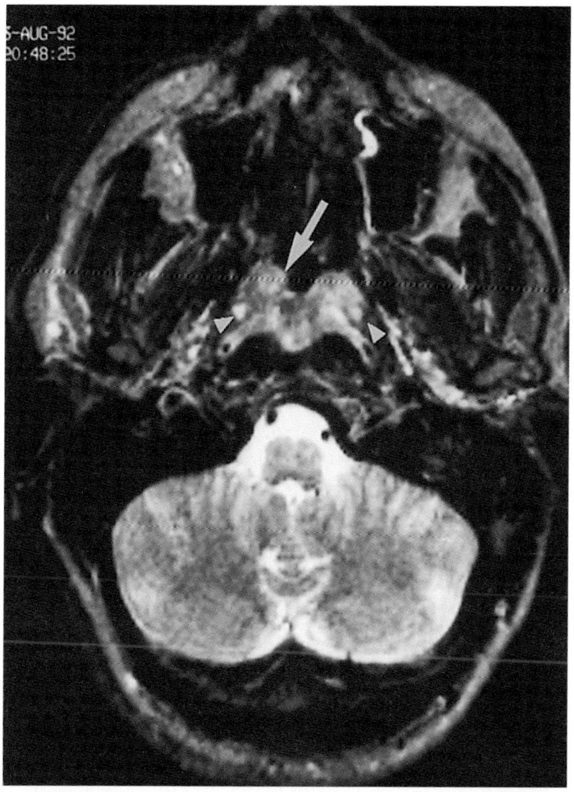

a

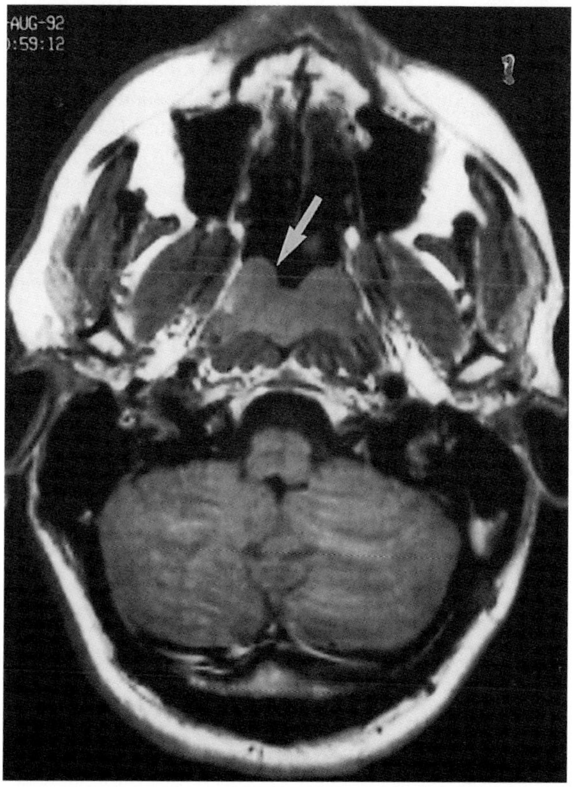

b

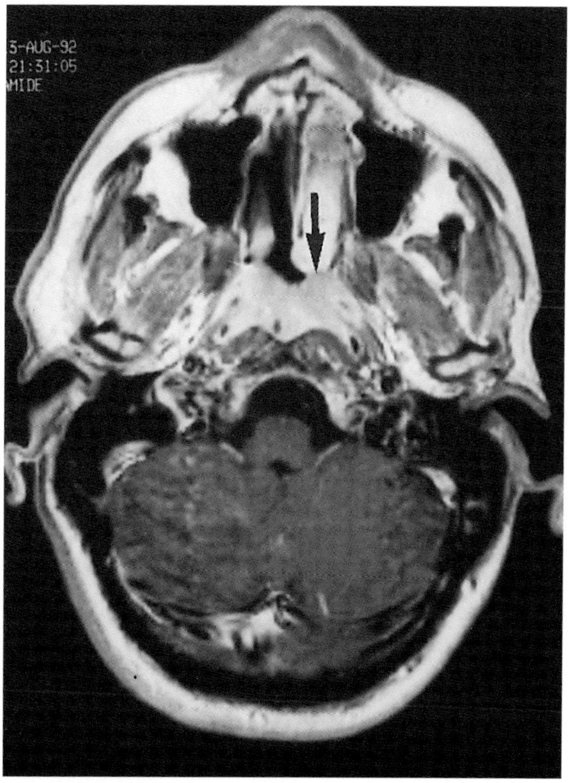

c

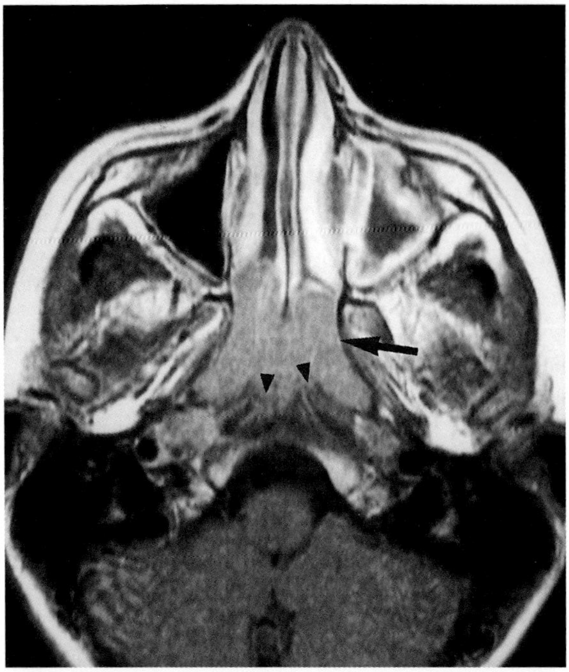

a

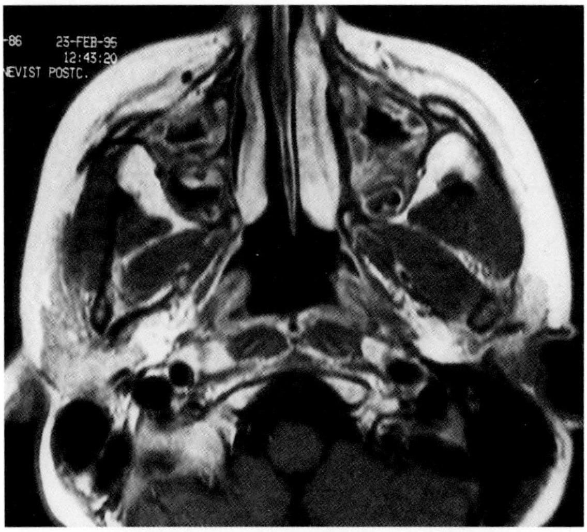

b

Figs. 6.**12 a, b** **Non-Hodgkin lymphoma of the nasopharynx before (a) and after (b) radiotherapy.**
(**a**) Gd-enhanced axial T1-weighted SE sequence (TR/TE = 700/15 ms) shows a uniformly enhancing mass (arrow) with no septations that completely fills the nasopharynx and extends into the nasal cavity. The indistinct posterior margins of the lesion (arrowheads) suggest infiltration.
(**b**) Gd-enhanced axial SE sequence (TR/TE = 700/15 ms) after the completion of radiotherapy shows no signs of tumor in the nasopharynx, indicating a complete remission.

Rhabdomyosarcoma is, however, indistinguishable from its benign form, *rhabdomyoma*, and thus histologic confirmation is still required.

While MRI is the modality of choice for detecting the tumor and defining its extent and is superior to CT for detecting intracranial tumor extension, CT still has a role in the detection of small osseous lesions.

Lipoma and Liposarcoma (Fig. 6.**14**)

Lipoma. This is the most common mesenchymal tumor and may occur anywhere in the body. The peak incidence is between 50 and 60 years of age, with a slight predilection for males. Multifocal occurrence is documented in approximately 5–7% of cases. Histologically, lipoma is composed of mature adipose cells in which depot fat cannot be metabolized.

The CT appearance is that of a smoothly marginated, homogeneous mass with attenuation values in the range of -65 to -120 HU.

On MRI, the above characteristics are frequently accompanied by intratumoral septa. The signal intensities on T1- and T2-weighted images are equivalent to those of subcutaneous fat. A fat suppression sequence can be helpful in identifying this tumor and differentiating it from other lesions.

Liposarcoma. This tumor is among the most common soft-tissue sarcomas, with approximately 6% occurring in the head and neck region. The peak incidence is the same as for lipomas: between 50 and 60 years of age. Histologically, a *well-differentiated form* of liposarcoma is distinguished from a *myxoid, round-cell,* and *pleomorphic form.* As the composition of the tumor varies, so do its manifestations on CT and MRI. While myxoid liposarcoma shows predominantly water-equivalent attenuation values and signal intensities, the well-differentiated form shows predominantly fat-equivalent densities. The typical tumor is nonhomogeneous, containing both fatty and soft-tissue components and enhancing after contrast administration. This helps differentiate the lesion from lipoma, which shows little or no contrast enhancement.

Papilloma and Inverted Papilloma (Fig. 6.**15**)

Papillomas of the nasal cavity and paranasal sinuses are benign mucosal neoplasms that fall into three categories based on their specific location and characteristics. *Fungiform papilloma* and *inverted papilloma* account for approximately 97% of all papillomas. The third type, *cylindrical papilloma*, is a very rare entity. Fungiform papilloma typically occurs as an exophytic growth involving the anterior nasal cavity and septum. Most inverted papillomas arise from the lateral wall of the nasal cavity, show a high rate of recurrence, and may undergo malignant transformation. An association of inverted papilloma and squamous cell carcinoma of the nasal cavity and paranasal sinuses with human papillomavirus infection has been postulated but is still unsettled. In contrast to inflammatory nasal polyps, which are a form of inflammatory hyperplasia, inverted papillomas are true neoplasms. They are more common in males than females and show a peak incidence between 40 and 60 years of age. The tumors have a firm consistency and a cauliflower–like surface. They spread by continuity and tend to cause local bone destruction. The papillary growths result from a reserve-cell hyperplasia of the excretory ducts of mucous glands, differentiating into masses composed of transitional cells or squamous epithelium. The tumors have a tendency to recur following incomplete excision. Most inverted papillomas are unilateral. Orbital involvement is usually a late development resulting from blockage of the nasolacrimal duct. Infiltration of the skull base is rare. Because inverted papillomas have a high rate of recurrence and a variable association with squamous cell carcinoma (2–50%), CT and/or MRI should be used for the accurate determination of tumor extent.

The CT appearance of inverted papilloma is variable and nonspecific. The diagnosis of inverted papilloma is likely if scans show a unilateral mass on the lateral nasal wall that is associated with benign bone changes, widening of the infundibulum, and centrifugal spread into the maxillary and ethmoid sinuses. Bony sclerosis is a nonspecific sign that, while common in patients with inverted papilloma, is also a feature of chronic sinusitis. Larger inverted papillomas may erode the medial sphenoid wing, cribriform plate, lamina papyracea, hard palate, or nasolacrimal duct. Inflammatory changes and fluid retention are indistinguishable on CT scans.

On MRI, the heterogeneous appearance of the tumor in all sequences and its nonhomogeneous pattern of contrast enhancement are the principal imaging criteria for paranasal sinus neoplasms. The ring enhancement of inverted papilloma serves to distinguish it from squamous cell carcinoma.

Contrast-enhanced MR images should be obtained to evaluate for skull-base infiltration. This is particularly important if there is invasion of the ethmoid cells, for it is then necessary to exclude orbital involvement and intracranial spread. Meningeal enhancement does not necessarily signify malignant infiltration of the skull base.

Secondary Masses

Esthesioneuroblastoma (Fig. 6.**16**) is a rare but important tumor from the standpoint of differential diagnosis. It arises from the olfactory epithelium and commonly spreads into the sphenoid and maxillary sinuses and through the cribriform plate into the anterior cranial fossa.

MRI typically shows a nonhomogeneous mass with prolonged T1 and T2 times that enhances intensely after the administration of Gd-DTPA (by a factor of 2.3).

These tumors are very similar to meningiomas of this region in their MRI signal characteristics and their capacity for intracranial spread. A *meningioma* arising in the cranium or skull base may extend secondarily into the frontal skull base and paranasal sinuses. Typically meningiomas are isointense to cerebral gray matter on MR images. Often they have a nonhomogeneous appearance with central calcifications or necrosis, but the majority have well-defined, noninfiltrative margins. Because meningiomas disrupt the blood-brain barrier, the administration of Gd-DTPA induces intense enhancement with more than a two-fold increase in signal intensity. Axial and coronal T1-weighted sequences are the best source of imaging information. Contrast-enhanced MRI and CT are equivalent in the preoperative detection of meningiomas, but MRI is superior for defining the relation of the tumor to surrounding structures.

A number of rare tumors should be considered in the differential diagnosis of sinonasal lesions. An analysis of topography, signal intensity, enhancement dynamics, and morphology can provide critical clues to the identity of the mass (hamartoma, lipoma, inverted papilloma, melanoma, pleomorphic adenoma [Fig. 6.**17**], etc.). Another rare lesion to be considered is meningoencephalocele, which should figure in the differential diagnosis of nasopharyngeal masses.

Rare Masses

Chordoma, chondroma, and chondrosarcoma were described in previous chapters but will be briefly reviewed here (Tables 6.**4** and 6.**5**).

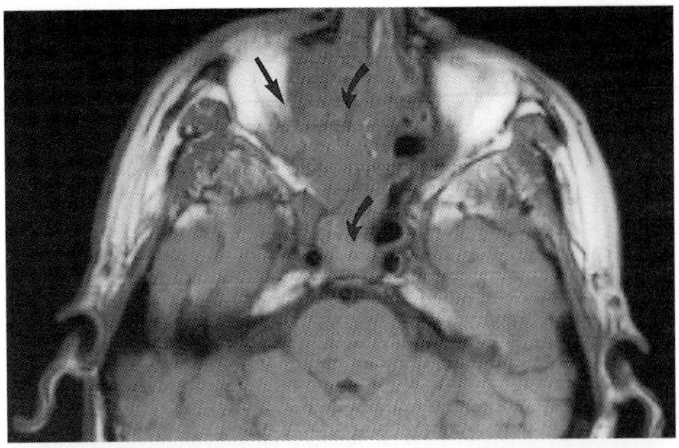
a

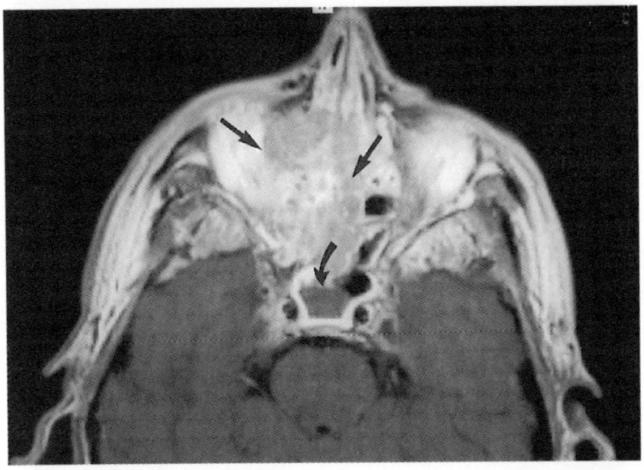
b

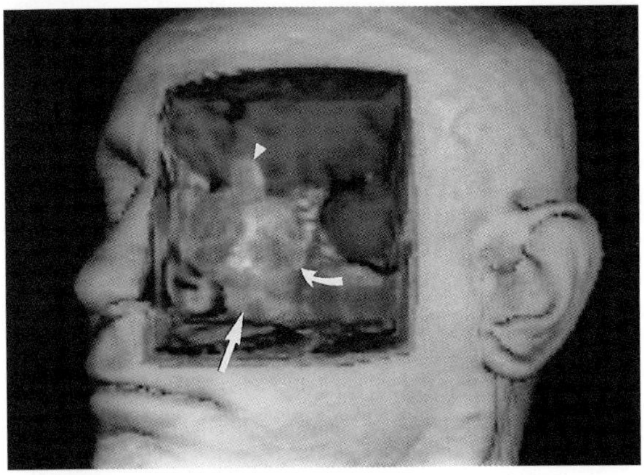
c

Figs. 6.**13 a–c** **Nasopharyngeal rhabdomyosarcoma infiltrating the anterior skull base.**
(**a**) Unenhanced axial T1-weighted SE sequence (TR/TE = 700/15 ms) shows a conspicuous lesion that appears to infiltrate the right orbit (arrow), ethmoid cells, and sphenoid sinus (curved arrows).
(**b**) Gd-enhanced axial SE sequence (TR/TE = 700/15 ms) shows intense but nonhomogeneous tumor enhancement with infiltration of the ethmoid cells and right orbit (arrows). A mucocele (curved arrow) in the region of the sphenoid sinus (secondary to impaired ventilation) is clearly demarcated from the areas of tumor involvement.
(**c**) Gd-enhanced sagittal 3-D magnetization-prepared rapid-acquisition gradient-echo (MP-RAGE) sequence (TR/TE = 10/4.5, flip angle α = 15°). Windowed 3-D magnetization-prepared rapid-acquisition gradient-echo reconstruction demonstrates the extent of the tumor (arrow) and simulates the route of surgical approach. Note the infiltration of the anterior skull base (arrowhead) and the complete obstruction of the nasopharynx (curved arrow).

Figs. 6.**14 a–d** **Liposarcoma of the nasopharynx and masticator space.** ▷
(**a**) Unenhanced axial T2-weighted SE sequence (TR/TE = 3000/90 ms) shows a large, nonhomogeneous mass (arrow) of fat-equivalent signal intensity in the right parapharyngeal space with extension to the nasopharyngeal submucosa. The right pterygoid muscle is obscured, and the tumor margins are poorly demarcated with respect to the nasopharyngeal roof (arrowhead).
(**b**) Gd-enhanced axial SE sequence (TR/TE = 700/15 ms) shows a nonhomogeneously enhancing mass that is poorly demarcated from the maxillary sinus wall (curved arrow) and nasal cavity (arrowhead).
(**c**) Gd-enhanced coronal SE sequence (TR/TE = 700/15 ms) defines the overall tumor extent and also shows that the roof of the nasal cavity (arrow) and the right orbit (curved arrow) have been infiltrated. The histologically confirmed liposarcoma extends high into the right temporal area (open arrow).
(**d**) Axial CT scan (5 mm) with a soft-tissue window after the intravenous administration of 100 mL Ultravist 370 reveals significant bone destruction by the liposarcoma, which shows a predominance of soft-tissue components.

Figs. 6.**14**

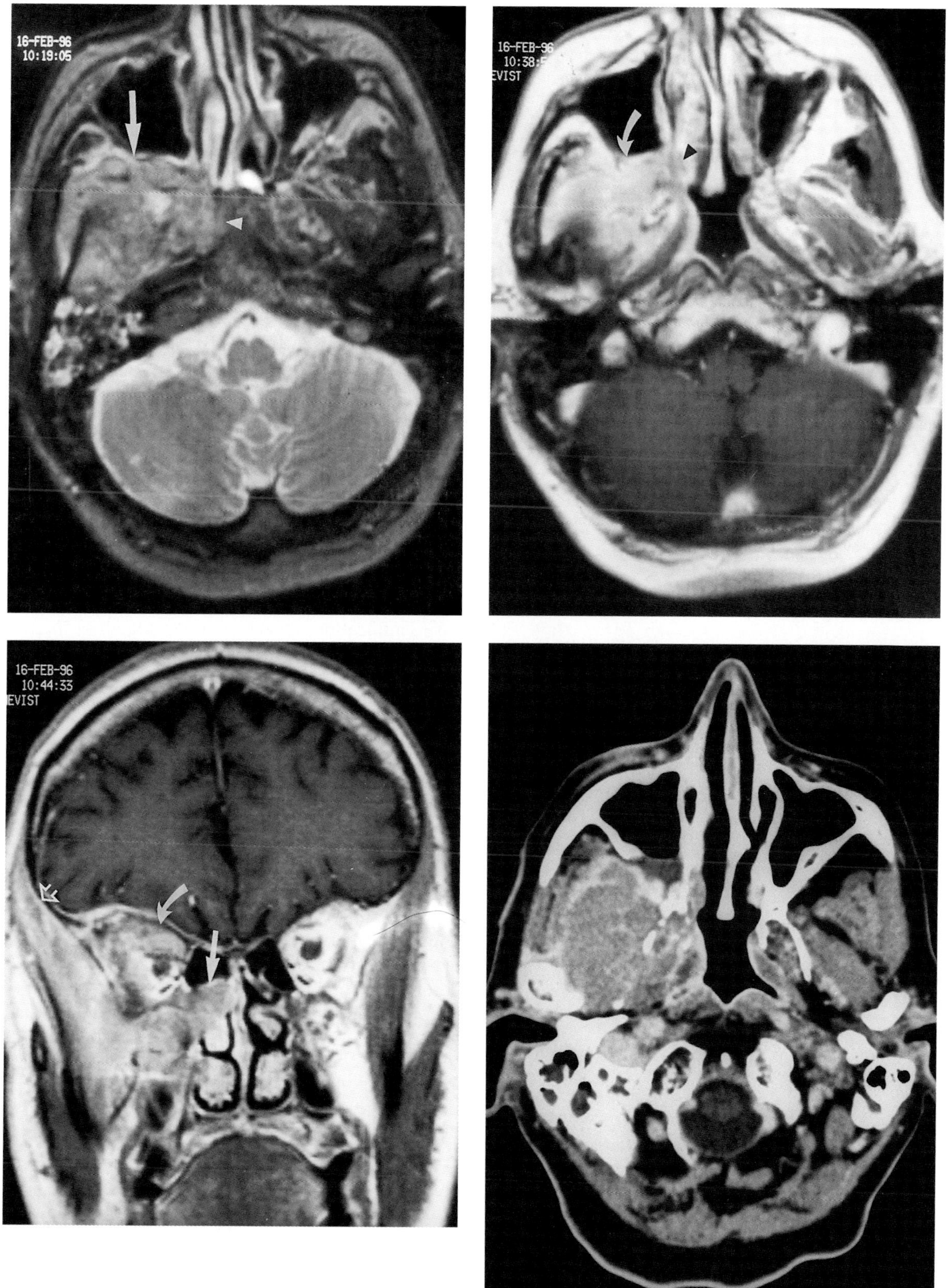

a b c d

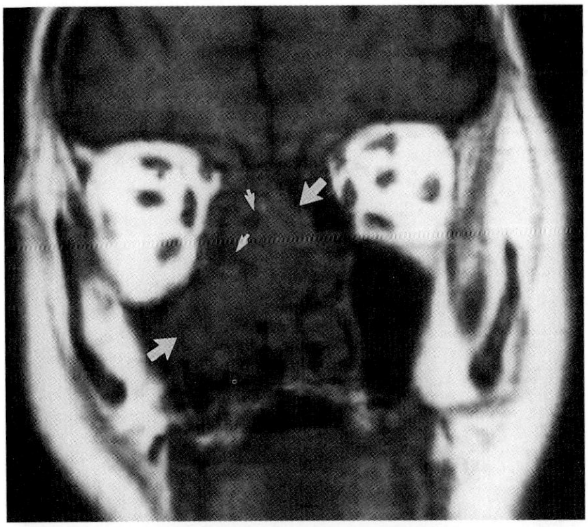
a

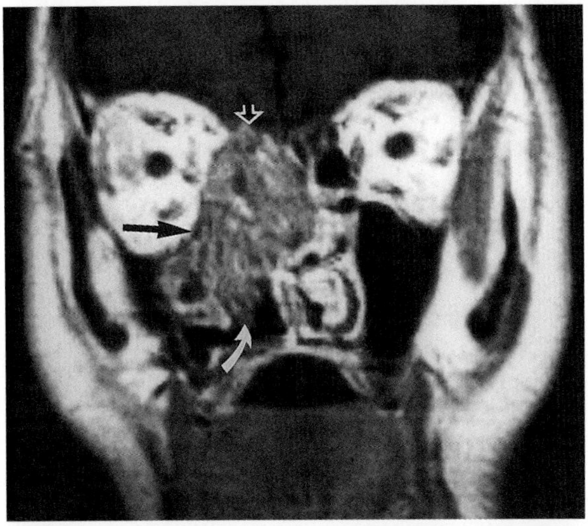
b

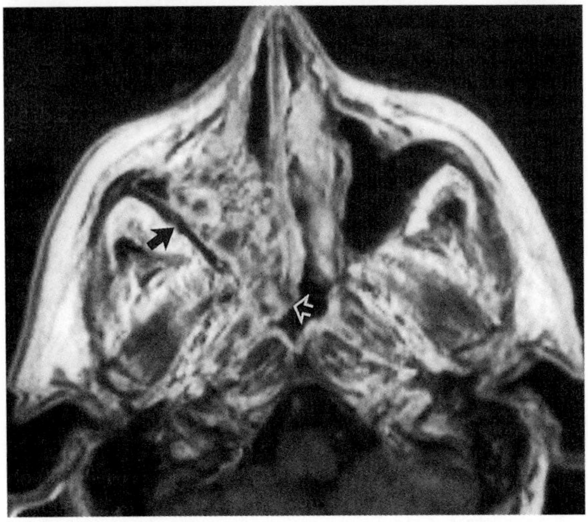
c

Figs. 6.**15 a – c Inverted papilloma of the nasal cavity and right maxillary and ethmoid sinuses.**
(**a**) In the unenhanced coronal SE sequence (TR/TE = 700/15 ms), the inverted papilloma (arrows) appears isointense to muscle and shows a nonhomogeneous internal pattern with hypointense areas (arrowheads) that represent calcifications.
(**b**) In the Gd-enhanced coronal SE sequence (TR/TE = 700/15 ms), the lesion (arrow) shows a nonhomogeneous, laminar pattern of enhancement. The tumor almost completely fills the right maxillary sinus (curved arrow) and right ethmoid sinus (open arrow) with no definite signs of bone destruction.
(**c**) Gd-enhanced axial T1-weighted SE sequence (TR/TE = 700/15 ms) shows the anteroposterior (AP) extent of this inverted papilloma, which extends into the nasopharynx (open arrow) and shows a characteristic enhancement pattern. The tumor has not breached the lateral wall of the right maxillary sinus (arrow).

Chordoma

Unenhanced axial CT is the method of choice for imaging the bone destruction caused by chordoma and for defining intratumoral calcifications and bone fragments. Chordoma generally shows moderate enhancement on post-contrast scans. CT is of limited value, however, for determining the extent of soft-tissue infiltration, especially in the region of the nasopharynx and parapharyngeal space.

On MRI, chordoma appears isointense or hypointense to muscle on T1-weighted images and hyperintense on T2-weighted images. It enhances markedly after the administration of Gd-DTPA. The extent of tumor infiltration is defined more accurately by MRI than by CT.

Chondroma and Chondrosarcoma

Chondroma. Conventional radiography and CT portray this tumor as a circumscribed, lobulated, predominantly extraskeletal mass. Ossifications or ring-like calcifications are also seen. Adjacent bone shows deformation and marginal sclerosis.

On MRI, this lesion shows intermediate signal intensity on T1-weighted images and high signal intensity on T2-weighted images. After contrast administration, the lesion shows intense homogeneous or nonhomogeneous enhancement.

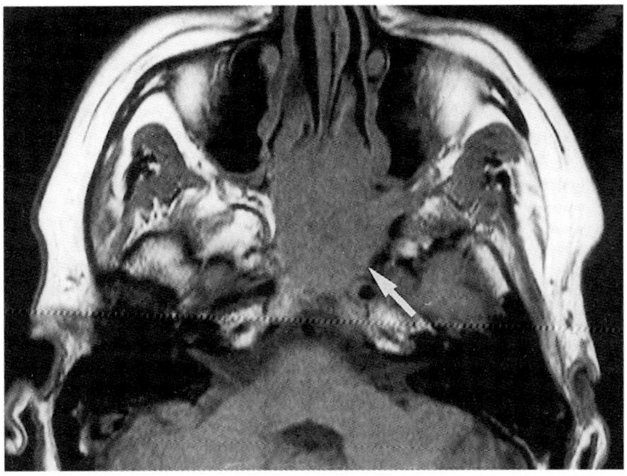

a

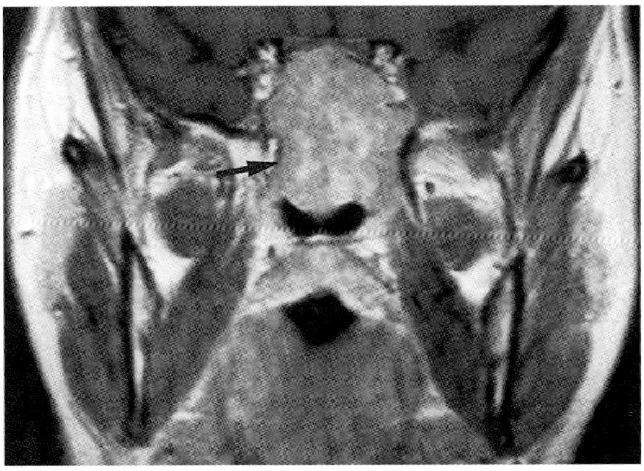

b

Figs. 6.**16 a, b** **Esthesioneuroblastoma with nasopharyngeal infiltration.**
(**a**) Unenhanced axial T1-weighted SE sequence (TR/TE = 700/15 ms) shows a uniformly isointense mass with smooth margins (arrow) in the region of the nasopharyngeal roof. The predominantly midline lesion shows anterior extension into the nasal cavity.
(**b**) Gd-enhanced coronal SE sequence (TR/TE = 700/15 ms) demonstrates moderate, nonhomogeneous enhancement of the mass (arrow), which does not show infiltrative margins. The mass completely fills the sphenoid sinus.

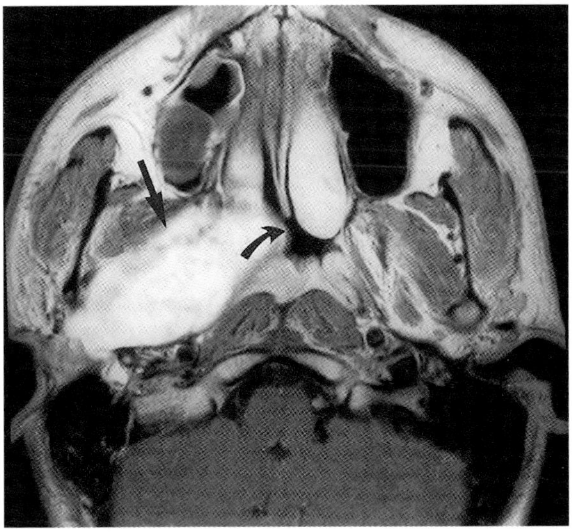

Fig. 6.**17** **Pleomorphic adenoma causing indentation of the nasopharynx.** Gd-enhanced axial T1-weighted SE sequence (TR/TE = 700/15 ms) demonstrates an extensive mass lesion of the parapharyngeal space (arrow) showing intense, homogeneous enhancement. Note the marked indentation of the nasopharynx (curved arrow) by this pleomorphic adenoma of the medial parotid lobe. The pressure defect refutes clinical suspicion of a primary lesion of the nasopharynx.

Table 6.**5** Signal characteristics of nasopharyngeal tumors

Tumor	T2-weighted SI	T1-weighted SI	Edema	Enhancement
Meningioma	↗	↙	+/-	↑↑
Carcinoma	↑	↓	++	↑ – ↑↑
Craniopharyngioma	↑↑	↑	+/-	↑
Chordoma	↑	↙	-	↑
Chondroma	↑↑	↓	+/-	↗
Chondrosarcoma	↑↑	↙	+	↑
Esthesioneuroblastoma (Fig. 6.**16 a**)	↗	↙	+/-	↑
Metastasis	↑	↓	+++	↑↑

↑ High SI or enhancement
↗ Isointense to hyperintense SI/moderate enhancement
↙ Hypointense to isointense SI
↓ Low SI/no enhancement
SI Signal intensity
\+ Moderate
++ Marked
+++ Intense
+/- Minimal
\- None

Chondrosarcoma. Unenhanced CT demonstrates chondrosarcoma as a slightly hyperdense mass with flocculent calcifications and nonspecific bone destruction. The tumor enhances only slightly on postcontrast scans, while MRI shows a slightly greater degree of enhancement. Even on unenhanced T2-weighted images, this relatively well-circumscribed tumor is conspicuous by its high signal intensity, which may be isointense to CSF and is a characteristic feature of this lesion. Chondrosarcoma appears isointense or hypointense on unenhanced T1-weighted images.

Inflammatory Lesions

Inflammatory lesions of the nasal cavity are the most common incidental finding on MR images of the skull. The nasal septum, turbinates, and all paranasal sinuses should be evaluated.

The following manifestations of acute or chronic inflammatory disease require differentiation:

- Mucosal hyperplasia.
- Polyp.
- Fluid (secretions).
- Retention cyst.
- Mucocele.

All acute inflammatory lesions and most chronic inflammatory changes display a high signal intensity on T2-weighted MR images. While mucosal hyperplasia appears as a diffusely hyperintense bulge of the sinus mucosa, polyps often product a mass effect. Mucosa and fluid secretions are indistinguishable on unenhanced T1-weighted images but can be differentiated on contrast-enhanced images. The secretions in a partially obstructed sinus always show slight, nonhomogeneous contrast enhancement, which provides a useful diagnostic criterion. A retention cyst of the maxillary sinus or sphenoid sinus shows extremely high signal intensity on T2-weighted images and is hypointense on T1-weighted images. Following the administration of Gd-DTPA, the cyst wall shows marked enhancement while the cystic fluid still appears hypointense. An abscess displays a typical pattern of intense rim enhancement, with T2-weighted images providing accurate delineation of accompanying edema.

Nonspecific osteomyelitis involving the nasopharynx or paranasal sinuses is usually a result of sinusitis or mastoiditis, so it most commonly affects the sphenoid bone or temporal bone. Conventional radiographs and CT scans demonstrate irregular foci of demineralization, patchy destructive changes, and isolated sequestra. Advanced cases present with increasing marginal sclerosis and reparative processes. Osteomyelitis of the calvaria tends to spread along sutures and blood vessels.

While conventional radiographs are important, they should be supplemented by CT or MRI to define foci of bony inflammation and evaluate infected soft tissues. The topographic relationships of the infected tissues should be closely analyzed to determine the origin of the inflammatory foci.

Iatrogenic Changes

Plain and contrast-enhanced MR images have a key role in the evaluation of posttherapeutic changes. T2-weighted images are particularly useful for differentiating residual posttherapeutic changes from a recurrent tumor, although it is difficult to distinguish these changes from a residual or recurrent tumor during the 2 to 6 week period after therapy.

After 8 weeks, a recurrent tumor shows high signal intensity on T2-weighted images and enhances after the administration of contrast medium. Scar tissue, on the other hand, has intermediate to low signal intensity on T2-weighted images and shows little or no contrast enhancement (Fig. 6.**18**).

CT and conventional radiography are of secondary importance in the diagnosis of recurrent soft-tissue tumors and are used only as adjuncts in patients with known or suspected osseous involvement. CT is superior to MRI, however, for detecting recurrent tumors that primarily involve bone and is more accurate in defining the extent of disease.

Conventional radiographs and CT also have substantial value in patients with suspected bone metastases, and both procedures can supplement radionuclide imaging in defining the precise location and topography of the lesions.

While CT portrays a recurrent soft-tissue tumor only as a nonspecific soft-tissue mass showing little or no enhancement, a bony metastasis or recurrent bone tumor appears as a progressive expansion or lytic area showing a variable degree of marginal sclerosis.

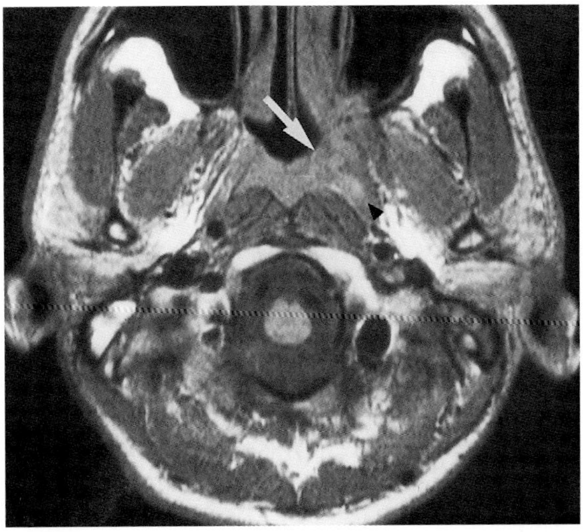

a

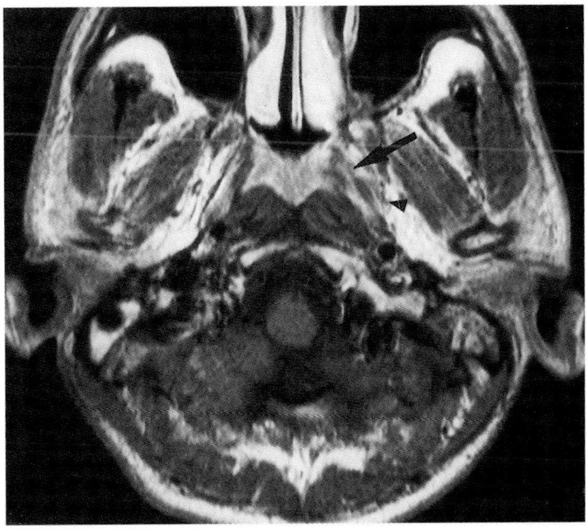

b

Figs. 6.**18 a, b** **Recurrent carcinoma of the lateral nasopharyngeal wall.**

(**a**) Unenhanced axial T1-weighted SE sequence (TR/TE = 700/15 ms) shows asymmetry and nonhomogeneities of the left lateral nasopharyngeal wall (arrow). The lesion is poorly demarcated from the parapharyngeal space (arrowhead).

(**b**) Gd-enhanced axial T1-weighted SE sequence (TR/TE = 700/15 ms) shows a nonhomogeneously enhancing tumor (arrow) of the lateral nasopharyngeal wall that has infiltrated adjacent parapharyngeal structures (arrowhead). There is no morphologic evidence that the tumor has crossed the midline.

Imaging Criteria and Their Differential Diagnosis

For lesions of the nasopharynx as well as the nasal cavity, *topography* is the key imaging criterion for making an accurate differential diagnosis (Fig. 6.**19**). There may also be other useful differentiating criteria such as structural changes, a change in signal intensity or density, and a destructive component, depending on the imaging modality used. The imaging criteria for the nasal cavity are closely tied to changes in the paranasal sinuses, thus Chapter 7 should also be consulted for differential diagnostic criteria. Whenever a morphologic change is found in the region of the nasopharynx, the basic determination to be made is whether the change is a primary incidental finding or requires further investigation as part of the diagnosis or staging of a clinically verified mass lesion.

Liquid Masses

A liquid mass is identified by its attenuation values on CT scans or its fluid-equivalent signal characteristics on MR images, i.e., low signal intensity in the T1-weighted SE sequence and high signal intensity in the T2-weighted SE sequence. The Thornwaldt cyst is the most common primary cystic mass that is detected incidentally in the nasopharyngeal region (Table 6.**6**), displaying smooth margins and moderate rim enhancement. Significant lymphoepithelial hyperplasia can lead to the formation of a lymphoepithelial cyst, whose frequent morphologic asymmetry serves to distinguish it from a primary medial or lateral cyst. The differential diagnosis should also include primary cystic masses such as dermoid cyst, cystic chordoma, or even necrotic liquefaction inside a malignancy.

Masses with Moderately High T2-Weighted Signal Intensity

The identification of a nasopharyngeal mass showing moderately increased signal intensity in the T2-weighted SE sequence is an important imaging criterion (Table 6.**7**). The two primary considerations in differential diagnosis are (1) the detection and differential diagnosis of lymphatic hyperplasia in the subacute or chronic stage and (2) the differentiation of a lymphoma or other primary or secondary nasopharyngeal mass. Lymphatic hyperplasia is recognized by the presence of markedly enhancing linear septa in post-contrast T1-weighted SE sequences, distinguishing it from the nonhomogeneous, finely stippled enhancement pattern observed in lymphomas.

Tumor Masses

This section reviews the general considerations that apply in the differential diagnosis of a nasopharyngeal tumor mass (Table 6.**8**). An etiologic distinction is drawn between primary masses such as cysts and primary or secondary benign or malignant tumor masses. It is also important to differentiate inflammatory processes, which may consist of abscessation or diffuse inflammatory involvement, and hematomas. These lesions may have a traumatic or iatrogenic (posttherapeutic, post biopsy) cause.

A unilateral or bilateral area of increased signal intensity in the mastoid air cells is an important sign of a nasopharyngeal mass and requires further inves-

Table 6.**6** Cystic masses of the nasopharynx

Finding	**Differential diagnostic criteria**
➤ Tornwaldt cyst (Fig. 6.**3**)	Symmetry, morphology, rim enhancement
➤ Lymphoepithelial cyst	Asymmetry, accompanied by lymphoepithelial hyperplasia
Benign tumor:	
➤ Dermoid cyst	Signal intensity, morphology, size
Malignant tumor, primary:	
➤ Squamous cell carcinoma with liquefaction (Fig. 6.**6 a**)	
➤ Metastases with liquefaction	Destruction, asymmetry, morphology
Inflammation:	
➤ Abscess	Broad enhancing rim, indistinct margins, perifocal edema
Trauma:	
➤ Submucous hematoma	Signal characteristics, intralesional hemorrhage
➤ Rare primary and secondary masses	

Table 6.7 Masses with moderately high T2-weighted signal intensity

Lesion	Differential diagnostic criteria
Lymphatic hyperplasia	Bilateral symmetry; intensely enhancing linear septations in post-contrast T1-weighted images; no destructive changes
Malignant non-Hodgkin or Hodgkin lymphoma	No enhancing septa; finely stippled enhancement pattern; no destructive changes
Lymphoepithelial carcinoma	Asymmetry, destructive changes, infiltration of skull base
Squamous cell carcinoma	Morphology, marked destructive changes

tigation. Topographic criteria are also important, since establishing the site of origin of a lesion allows for a more accurate differential diagnostic classification. Particularly with MRI, the signal characteristics of a lesion on T1- and T2-weighted images and its enhancement characteristics on post-contrast images can significantly advance the differential diagnosis of a tumor mass (Figs. 6.**17** and 6.**18**).

Bone Destruction

Lesions in proximity to the nasopharynx that are associated with bone destruction are described in Chapters 3 and 4, where the criteria for identifying these lesions are reviewed.

Abnormal Air Collections in the Nasopharynx

Rarely, localized air collections may be observed within primary or secondary lesions of the nasopharynx (Table 6.**9**). After iatrogenic changes following biopsy or other surgical or interventional procedures, the main diagnostic considerations are posttraumatic sequelae—especially those associated with complex basal skull fractures involving injury to the eustachian tube or other air-containing spaces—and superinfected inflammatory processes of the nasopharyngeal region.

Table 6.8 Tumor masses of the nasopharynx

Finding	Differential diagnostic criteria
Benign tumors:	
➤ Tornwaldt cyst	Homogeneity, morphology, symmetry
➤ Dermoid cyst	Morphology, topography
Malignant tumors:	
➤ Lymphoepithelial carcinoma	Morphology, destruction, signal characteristics
➤ Squamous cell carcinoma	Bone destruction
➤ Undifferentiated carcinoma	Bone destruction, infiltrative components
Inflammation:	
➤ Nasopharyngeal or parapharyngeal abscess	Broad enhancing rim, central liquefaction, air inclusions, displacement of key structures
➤ Phlegmonous inflammation	Structural change, morphology
➤ Lymphoepithelial cyst	
Trauma:	
➤ Hematoma	Signal or attenuation characteristics, accompanying bony injury
Vascular:	
➤ Internal or external carotid artery aneurysm	Signal characteristics, morphology, vascular structures
➤ Kissing carotid arteries with a retropharyngeal course (variation)	Course of vessels

Table 6.9 Air-containing structures in the nasopharyngeal region

Finding	Differential diagnostic criteria
Common:	
➤ Iatrogenic:	
–After biopsy or intervention	Morphology, air distribution
➤ Inflammatory complication:	
–Nasopharyngeal and parapharyngeal abscess	Morphology, topography, signal intensity or density
Rare:	
➤ Liquefaction of a primary or secondary tumor mass of the nasopharynx (squamous cell carcinoma, lymphoepithelial carcinoma)	Morphology, destruction, edema of surrounding structures
➤ Posttraumatic sequelae	Accompanying bone changes, key vascular structures

Summary and Diagnostic Strategy

The various MR sequences offer advantages over CT scans in differentiating tumors from inflammatory lesions of the nasopharynx and paranasal sinuses. T2-weighted SE sequences are essential for differentiating inflammatory tissue changes and fluid-containing structures. Images enhanced with Gd-DTPA can significantly improve the diagnosis of nasopharyngeal lesions, as normal mucosa enhances markedly after contrast administration, improving the delineation of the small nasopharyngeal muscles, the pharyngobasal fascia, and other anatomic details. While tumors and inflammatory tissue usually appear isointense on T1-weighted images, the tumor will generally show less enhancement than inflammatory lesions on post-contrast images. Cystic lesions show high signal intensities on T2-weighted images, and post-contrast images invariably show marked rim enhancement of the cyst with an absence of significant central enhancement.

The main advantage of Gd-DTPA is in evaluating the degree of vascularity of a mass, with some tumors showing an increase in signal intensity by a factor of 1.6–2.3. The greatest enhancement occurs in angiofibromas, glomus tumors, and highly vascularized angiomatous tumors. Necrotic tumor components usually occur at the center of the mass and show less enhancement than viable tumor. Despite the good soft-tissue discrimination of MRI, it can be difficult to appreciate superficial mucosal infiltration, because even healthy mucosa shows marked enhancement after the administration of Gd-DTPA. Subtraction images are helpful since tumor tissue generally shows less enhancement than normal mucosa.

The advantages of MRI make it superior to CT in the differential diagnostic analysis of nasopharyngeal lesions. A major reason for this is the paramagnetic contrast agent Gd-DTPA, which not only can discriminate among cysts, inflammatory lesions, and tumors but also contributes to the differential diagnosis of tumors based on differences in enhancement characteristics. Evaluation of the T1 and T2 times for various lesions is of limited value due to the very large range of variation, but it may provide helpful orientation.

In summary, the recommended diagnostic strategy for mass lesions of the nasopharynx and surrounding structures is to use unenhanced or Gd-enhanced MRI as a primary study and contrast-enhanced CT as a secondary study for the evaluation of fine bony details.

Three-dimensional MR imaging will bring important new advances in preoperative staging, while MRI combined with NMR (nuclear magnetic resonance) spectroscopy will open up new approaches to the assessment of therapeutic strategies (Tables 6.**10** and 6.**11**).

Table 6.**10** Comparison of MRI and CT in the evaluation of primary tumors of the nasopharynx and nasal cavity

Tumor	Noncontrast MRI	Gd-enhanced MRI	Comparison: MRI vs. CT	Enhancement factor
Carcinoma (Fig. 6.**4**)	2	3	+	~1.6
Lymphoepithelial carcinoma (Fig. 6.**7**)	2	3	+	~2.0
Juvenile angiofibroma (Fig. 6.**8**)	3	2	+	~2.3

Tumor visualization:
1 Acceptable
2 Good

Method:
+ MRI better than CT
0 MRI same as CT

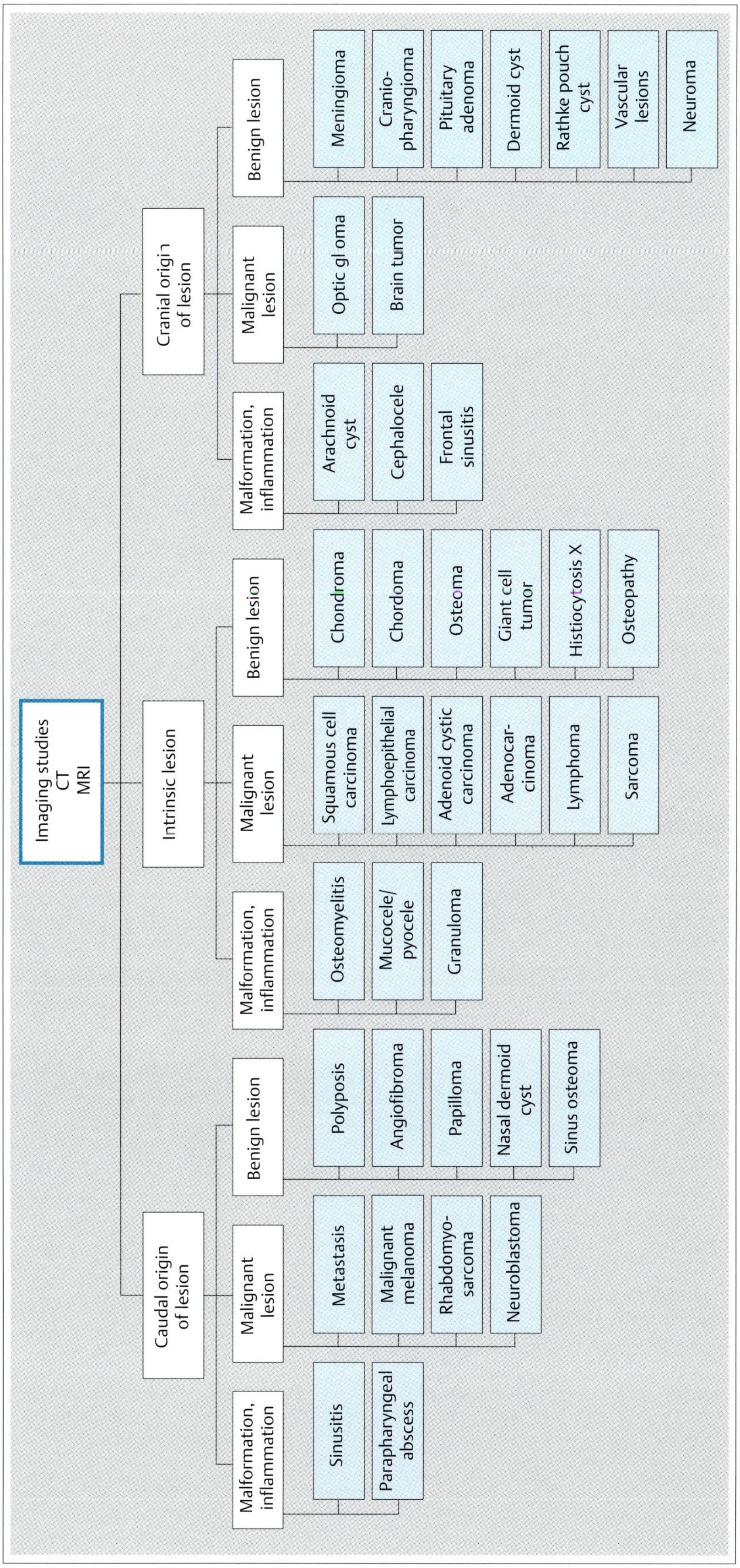

Fig. 6.19 **Differential diagnosis of nasopharyngeal lesions.**

Table 6.**11** Comparison of MRI and CT in the evaluation of secondary tumors of the nasopharynx and nasal cavity

Tumor	Noncontrast MRI	Gd-enhanced MRI	Comparison: MRI vs. CT
Intranasal tumor	2	2	0
Sphenoid/ethmoid meningioma	2	3	+
Esthesioneuroblastoma (Fig. 6.**16**)	2	3	+
Tonsillar carcinoma	2	3	+
Other tumors (e.g., lymphoma [Fig. 6.**11**], hemangioma)	2	3	+

Tumor visualization:
1 Acceptable
2 Good
3 Excellent, optimal

Method:
\+ MRI better than CT
0 MRI same as CT
\- MRI poorer than CT

References

1 Castelijns, J. A., M. W. van den Brekel: Magnetic Resonance Imaging evaluation of extracranial head and neck tumors. Magn Reson Q. 9 (1993) 113 - 128
2 Chapman, S., R. Nakielny: Aids to Radiological Differential Diagnosis, 3rd ed. 1995. Saunders, London 1995
3 Dähnert, W.: Radiology Review Manual, 3rd ed. Williams & Wilkins, Baltimore 1996
4 Dillon, W. P.: Magnetic Resonance Imaging of head and neck tumors. Cardiovasc Intervent Radiol. 8 (1986) 275 - 289
5 Dillon, W. P., C. M. Mills, B. Kjos, J. Degroot, M. Brant-Zawadski: Magnetic Resonance Imaging of the nasopharynx. Radiology 152 (1984) 731 - 738
6 Frey, K. W., K. Mees, T. J. Vogl: Bildgebende Verfahren in der HNO-Heilkunde. Enke, Stuttgart 1989
7 Harnsberger, H. R.: Handbook of Head and Neck Imaging, 2nd ed. Mosby Year Book, St. Louis 1995
8 Lanzieri, C. F., B. Bangert: Magnetic resonance imaging of the nasopharynx. Top Magn Reson Imaging 2 (1990) 39 - 47
9 Lufkin, R. B., W. N. Hanafee: MR reveals subtleties of head and neck pathology. Diagn. Imaging 8 (1986) 98 - 104
10 Lufkin, R. B., W. N. Hanafee: MRI of the head and neck. Magn. Reson Imaging 6 (1988) 69 - 88
11 Mafee, M. F., G. E. Valvassori et al.: High resolution and dynamic sequential computed tomography. Arch Otolaryngol. 109 (1983) 691 - 696
12 Mancuso, A. A., L. Bohmann, W. N. Hanafee, D. Maxwell: Computed Tomography of the Nasopharynx: normal and variants of normal. Radiology 137 (1980) 113 - 121
13 Mödder, U., M. Lenz: Klinische Radiologie: Gesichtsschädel, Felsenbein, Speicheldrüsen, Pharynx, Larynx, Halsweichteile. Diagnostik mit bildgebenden Verfahren. Springer, Berlin 1991
14 Naumann, H. H.: Differentialdiagnostik in der Hals-Nasen-Ohren-Heilkunde. Thieme, Stuttgart 1990
15 Som, P. M., R. T. Bergeron: Head and Neck Imaging, 2nd ed. Mosby Year Book, St. Louis 1991 (pp. 467 - 469, 875 - 924)
16 Valvassori, G. E., G. D. Potter, W. N. Hanafee, B. L. Carter, R. A. Buckingham: Radiology of the Ear, Nose and Throat. Thieme, Stuttgart 1982
17 Valvassori, G. E., R. A. Buckingham, B. L. Carter, W. N. Hanafee, M. F. Mafee: Head and Neck Imaging. Thieme, Stuttgart 1988
18 Vogl, T. J.: MRI of the Head and Neck. Springer, Berlin 1991
19 Vogl, T. J., S. Dresel: Advances in radiologic diagnosis of nasopharyngeal tumors. Curr Opin Radiol. 2 (1990) 93 - 99
20 Vogl, T. J., S. Dresel: MR Imaging of the nasopharynx and the face: new developments. Curr Opin Radiol. 3 (1991) 61 - 65
21 Vogl, T. J., S. Dresel: Diagnostic procedures in nasopharyngeal illness. Curr Opin Radiol. 4 (1992) 127 - 135
22 Vogl, T. J., R. Felix: Head and neck tumors: MR-guided laser-induced thermotherapy (LITT). In Lufkin, R., R. Black: Interventional MRI, Med Publisher, Los Angeles 1994 (pp. 58 - 60)
23 Vogl, T. J., J. O. Balzer: Base of skull, nasopharynx, and parapharyngeal space. In Yousem, D. M.: Head and Neck imaging. Neuroimaging Clin North Am. 6 (1996) 357 - 378
24 Vogl, T. J., S. Dresel, L. T. Bilaniuk, G. Grevers, K. Kang, J. Lissner: Tumors of the nasopharynx und adjacent areas: MR Imaging with Gd-DTPA. AJNR 11 (1990)

7 Paranasal Sinuses and Adjacent Facial Skeleton

With the advent of modern therapeutic procedures such as functional sinus surgery (FSS), sectional imaging modalities have assumed major importance in diagnosis as well as treatment planning, especially in patients with chronic inflammatory diseases such as maxillary, ethmoid and frontal sinusitis. Today it is common practice to precede planned interventions with a computed tomography (CT) examination, which affords maximum spatial resolution for defining key bony structures and aerated spaces. In problem cases such as chronic inflammation or complete paranasal sinus obstruction, magnetic resonance imaging (MRI) makes an excellent adjunct for differentiating inflammatory and neoplastic processes.

In the evaluation of sinonasal pathology, it is important to note that the development of the paranasal sinuses and nasal cavity is not completed until puberty. A precise knowledge of the various developmental stages of the paranasal sinuses will help to avoid errors of interpretation, especially on conventional radiographs. In infants younger than 1 year of age, it is normal for X-ray films to show clouding or incomplete development of the paranasal sinuses. Thus, clinical significance cannot be attributed to sinus opacification in this age group, and radiologic evaluation of the paranasal sinuses for inflammatory changes should be avoided. In children older than 3 years, paranasal sinus opacification or air–fluid levels are considered a reliable indicator of inflammatory sinus disease. Between 1 and 3 years of age, radiologic studies should be interpreted with caution due to the limitations stated above.

Normal Anatomy

The paranasal sinuses are lined with a thin ciliated epithelium. The mucociliary flow is directed toward the ostia to cleanse the sinus cavities, i.e., upward in the maxillary sinus and downward in the frontal sinus.

The interior of the nose is divided by the nasal septum into a right and left nasal cavity. The common anterior opening of the bony nasal cavities, the piriform aperture, is bounded by both maxillae and the two nasal bones. The paired posterior orifices, or choanae, open into the nasopharynx. The narrow roof of the bony nasal cavity is formed by the cribriform plate of the ethmoid bone. It merges anteriorly with the downsloping nasal part of the frontal bone and the nasal bone, and posteriorly with a short posterior wall formed by the almost vertical anterior surface of the body of the sphenoid bone. The medial wall (nasal septum) consists of a bony portion (perpendicular plate of ethmoid bone, vomer) and a cartilaginous portion (cartilaginous septum). The floor of the nasal cavity is also the roof of the mouth (palate), formed anteriorly by the palatine process of the maxilla and posteriorly by the horizontal plate of the palatine bone. Anteriorly, next to the septum, the nasal floor is traversed by the incisive canal.

The ostia are the excretory ducts that connect the paranasal sinuses with the nasal cavity. All the paranasal sinuses except the maxillary sinus border directly on the cranial cavity, and their proximity to the meninges poses the inherent risk of an ascending inflammatory process.

Maxillary Sinus

The maxillary sinus is shaped like a four-sided pyramid, the base being the medial sinus wall. The ostium, located in an unfavorably high position, opens into the ethmoid infundibulum. The sinus drains into the nose through the infundibulum and the semilunar hiatus of the middle meatus.

Ethmoid Sinus

The ethmoid sinus consists of eight to ten air cells bordered anterosuperiorly by the frontal sinus, superiorly by the skull base, laterally by the orbit, medially by the upper portions of the lateral nasal wall, posteriorly by the sphenoid sinus, and inferolaterally by the maxillary sinus. The anterior ethmoid cells drain through the ethmoid infundibulum into the middle meatus, and the posterior ethmoid cells drain into the superior meatus.

Frontal Sinus

The frontal sinus develops between the laminae interna and externa of the frontal bone. The right and left sinuses, separated by the interfrontal septum, are often of different sizes and may contain numerous recesses and intrasinus septa. Aplasia of the frontal sinuses is occasionally seen. The floor of the sinus borders on the orbit, and its posterior wall forms part of the anterior skull base.

Sphenoid Sinus

The sphenoid sinus is located in the right and left portions of the body of the sphenoid bone, a septum dividing it into two cavities that are usually of unequal size. The floor of the sphenoid sinus is the roof of the nasopharynx, the posterior wall is the very thick clivus, and the roof borders on the sella turcica and the anterior and middle cranial fossae. The lateral wall relates closely to the internal carotid artery, optic canal, and cavernous sinus.

The section on the facial skeleton deals with the forehead, upper lid, cheek, lower lid, and maxilla. Diseases of the orbit, parotid gland, and temporomandibular joint are discussed in Chapters 8, 11, and 12.

Clinical Signs and Symptoms

Observable morphologic changes, injuries, and swellings can contribute significantly to the diagnostic evaluation of paranasal sinus diseases.

The clinical evaluation of sinonasal disease relies mainly on inspection, palpation, and percussion, which may disclose any of the following *cardinal symptoms:*

Nasal-airway obstruction:
- Acute or chronic rhinitis
- Rhinopathy
- Sinusitis
- Congenital or acquired septal deviation
- Fracture of nasal pyramid
- Perforated septum
- Nasal polyposis
- Foreign bodies
- Adenoids
- Tumors
- Meningoencephalocele or other anomalies
- Choanal atresia
- Specific drugs

Rhinorrhea may signify:
- Chronic rhinitis
- Allergic rhinopathy
- Cerebrospinal-fluid (CSF) leak from a frontobasal fracture

Epistaxis:
- Infectious diseases
- Hypertension
- Coagulation disorders
- Malignant diseases

Dry nose:
- Viral rhinitis
- Previous surgery
- Drugs
- Previous radiotherapy

Olfactory dysfunction:
- Mechanical obstruction
- Damage to olfactory epithelium
- Trauma
- Infection
- Vascular
- Iatrogenic
- Psychological
- Congenital
- Endocrine

Headache:
- Acute maxillary sinusitis
- Ethmoid, frontal or sphenoid sinusitis

The diagnosis of facial pathology starts with the clinical examination (Fig. 7.**1 a**). Changes in shape or color, cutaneous changes, facial paralysis, craniofacial pain, facial malformations, and the overall facial appearance can yield important diagnostic clues.

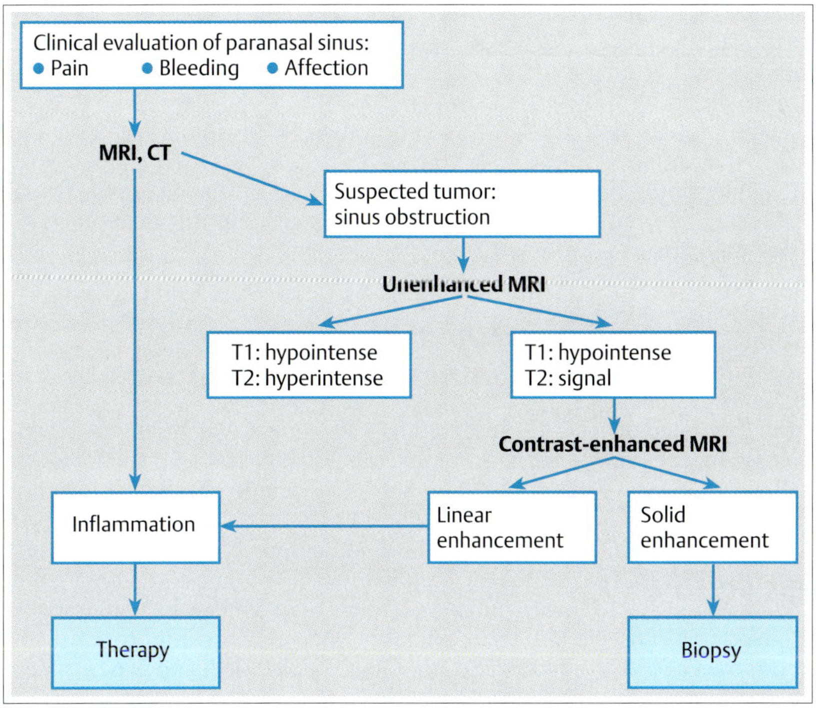

Fig. 7.**1 a** **Flowchart for the evaluation of paranasal sinus disease.**

Imaging Evaluation and Differential Diagnosis

The following imaging modalities have varying applications in the diagnosis of paranasal sinus diseases:

Ultrasound

Ultrasonography is best for evaluating diseases of the maxillary sinus and has somewhat less value in examinations of the frontal sinus and anterior ethmoid bone. A 3.5- to 5-MHz transducer is generally used for examinations of the paranasal sinuses. The posterior ethmoid bone and sphenoid sinus cannot be evaluated. Ultrasound can demonstrate mucosal swelling, intrasinus secretions, cysts, celes, and tumors of the paranasal sinuses. It is used mainly for evaluating acute and chronic sinus diseases, especially in children and pregnant patients, and for monitoring therapeutic response. The disadvantage of ultrasound is that it provides less detailed findings than conventional radiography and CT.

Conventional Radiography

Standard paranasal sinus films are obtained in the occipitofrontal and occipitomental projections. The occipitofrontal view demonstrates the frontal sinus and ethmoid cells, while the occipitomental view demonstrates the maxilla and maxillary sinus. Conventional radiographs are mainly indicated in patients with inflammatory, cystic, neoplastic, or traumatic lesions of the facial skeleton, nose, and paranasal sinuses. As a rule, X-ray films provide little detailed information because of their relatively low sensitivity and specificity. Their main role is to exclude frank paranasal sinus disease (including sinobronchial syndrome) and to screen for infectious foci in clinically asymptomatic patients.

Computed Tomography (CT)

When diagnostic problems arise, CT is the procedure of first choice for evaluating the nose and paranasal sinuses. With its excellent bone–soft tissue discrimination, CT is generally superior to MRI for paranasal sinus imaging. It is used mainly for the evaluation of acute and chronic inflammatory processes (Fig. 7.**3**), the determination of tumor extent and infiltration, the evaluation of frontobasal fractures, and the planning of surgical procedures on the nose and paranasal sinuses. Both axial and coronal scans are obtained. If dental artifacts obscure image details, axial spiral CT with secondary reconstruction should be performed.

The slice thickness depends on the nature of the clinical problem. While 4- or 5-mm slices are adequate for primary studies, a 2-mm slice thickness is recommended prior to functional endoscopic surgical procedures. Spiral CT scanning, which entails a slight reduction in bony contrast, has become the preferred technique. In any case the scanning angle should be adjusted to place troublesome metallic implants outside the volume of interest. Contrast medium generally adds little to the assessment of sinonasal infiltration by squamous cell carcinoma due to the similar attenuation values of tumor, inflammatory lesions, and normal soft tissues. Contrast medium should be used, however, to define the extent of intracranial infiltration, to distinguish between solid and necrotic tumor, and to differentiate tumor components from normal orbital tissues (Figs. 7.**22 c, d**).

Digital Subtraction Angiography (DSA)

DSA is indicated in patients with "intractable" nosebleed or a suspected hypervascular tumor such as juvenile nasopharyngeal fibroma. It also affords an opportunity for interventional therapeutic procedures (Figs. 7.**24 c, d**).

Magnetic Resonance Imaging (MRI)

MRI provides excellent discrimination of tumor tissue from surrounding soft tissues, inflammatory changes, and retained fluids in the paranasal sinuses. This and the capacity for multiplanar imaging help make MRI superior to CT for diagnosing tumor masses of the nasal cavity and paranasal sinuses. The recommended protocol consists of unenhanced T1- and T2-weighted spin-echo (SE) sequences and contrast-enhanced T1-weighted sequences. CT is preferred only for evaluating chronic sinusitis in which bony changes are of primary interest. MRI provides a more confident benign–malignant differentiation of sinonasal lesions based on differences in signal characteristics. The use of a paramagnetic contrast agent can further improve the diagnostic accuracy of MRI.

Imaging Findings

Table 7.**1** lists the various differential diagnoses that should be considered in patients with paranasal sinus disease. The various diseases that may involve the paranasal sinuses are listed according to frequency in Table 7.**2**.

Congenital Variations and Malformations

The most common congenital variations and malformations are *aplasias*, *hypoplasias*, and the *abnormal enlargement of individual paranasal sinuses* (Table 7.**3**). In most cases the diagnosis can be made from conventional radiographs. *Pneumosinus dilatans* refers to the abnormal dilatation of a frontal sinus with bulging of the anterior sinus wall. Rarely, maxillary sinus dilatation may also occur. In contrast to a mucocele, the sinus is air-filled and has a patent ostium. Conventional radiographs show exceptionally sharp delineation of the sinus boundaries.

Malformations of the facial skeleton can be extremely diverse, ranging from medial and lateral cleft anomalies and isolated nasal dysplasias to the most severe types of anomaly (e.g., craniomandibulofacial dysostoses, craniosynostoses, otomandibular and otopalatinodigital anomalies, mandibular arch syndromes, etc.).

Congenital nasal glioma is a rare anomaly representing an extracranial residua of glial tissue and not a true neoplasm. Only 15% of these lesions have a fibrous connection to the subarachnoid space. The radiologic findings are nonspecific. Images usually show a soft-tissue mass of benign appearance in the nasal septum without associated bone destruction.

Nasal dermoid tumors have a pleomorphic imaging appearance and usually display the radiographic density or signal characteristics of fat.

In diagnosing *anterior cephaloceles* (Fig. 7.**1 b**) in the paranasal sinuses, it is important to distinguish between a meningocele, which denotes the herniation of meninges, and an encephalocele, which denotes the herniation of meninges and brain substance through a cranial defect. Another distinction may be drawn between externally visible cephaloceles and those that cannot be seen without the aid of CT or MRI. The great majority of cephaloceles (70%) are occipital. Only about 15% of all cephaloceles involve the anterior skull base and ethmoid sinus. In the diagnosis of meningoceles and encephaloceles, axial or coronal CT scans can define the bony defect through which the cephalocele passes. With MRI, sagittal and coronal images are best for documenting the soft-

Table 7.1 Differential diagnosis of paranasal sinus diseases

Disease group	Differential diagnoses	Imaging modalities*
Congenital malformations	➤ Choanal atresia ➤ Choanal stenosis ➤ Dermoid cyst ➤ Meningocele, meningoencephalocele (Fig. 7.**1 b**) ➤ Cleft palate, alveolus ➤ Kartagener syndrome	➤ Ultrasound ➤ CT ➤ MRI ➤ Conventional radiographs
Malignant tumors	➤ Squamous cell carcinoma (Fig. 7.**22**) ➤ Adenoid cystic carcinoma (Fig. 7.**25**) ➤ Adenocarcinoma ➤ Osteosarcoma (Fig. 7.**9**) ➤ Malignant lymphoma ➤ Chondrosarcoma (Fig. 7.**20**) ➤ Basal cell carcinoma (secondary) ➤ Eosinophilic granuloma and other forms of histiocytosis X ➤ Malignant melanoma ➤ Metastases (Fig. 7.**2 a**)	➤ MRI ➤ CT
Benign tumors	➤ Osteoma ➤ Papilloma (Fig. 7.**28**) ➤ Fibroma ➤ Chondroma ➤ Myxoma ➤ Lipoma ➤ Hemangioma ➤ Lymphangioma ➤ Teratoma ➤ Adenoma ➤ Cystadenolymphoma (Warthin tumor) ➤ Inverted papilloma (Fig. 7.**16**) ➤ Plasma cell granuloma (pseudotumor) ➤ Bone cyst (pseudotumor)	➤ MRI ➤ CT ➤ Conventional radiographs ➤ Ultrasound
Inflammatory diseases	➤ Acute sinusitis ➤ Chronic sinusitis (Fig. 7.**15**) ➤ Mucocele (Figs. 7.**13**, 7.**23**) ➤ Pyocele ➤ Specific inflammation (syphilis, tuberculosis, sarcoidosis)	➤ Ultrasound ➤ Conventional radiographs ➤ CT ➤ MRI
Degenerative changes	Extremely rare	
Trauma	➤ Lateral midfacial fractures ➤ Frontobasal fractures	➤ Conventional radiographs ➤ CT
Iatrogenic changes		➤ CT ➤ Conventional radiographs ➤ MRI

* Listed in order of diagnostic importance

Table 7.2 Frequency of sinonasal diseases

Common	Rare
➤ Carcinoma (squamous cell carcinoma [Fig. 7.**22**], adenoid cystic carcinoma, adenocarcinoma) ➤ Encapsulated exudate, pus (Fig. 7.**3**) or blood ➤ Extrinsic neoplasm infiltrating the paranasal sinuses (e.g., pituitary, orbit, oropharynx, nasopharynx, chordoma, juvenile angiofibroma, lymphoepithelioma, Burkitt tumor) ➤ Fracture with hematoma (e.g., blowout fracture [Figs. 7.**4**, 7.**5**]) ➤ Impacted tooth (maxillary sinus) ➤ Mucocele (Fig. 7.**13 a**) (especially of frontal or ethmoid sinus) ➤ Mucosal edema or inflammation (allergic sinusitis, infection) ➤ Retention cyst ➤ Osteoma (especially of frontal or ethmoid sinus) ➤ Polyp or pseudopolyp (Fig. 7.**14 a**)	➤ Antrochoanal polyp (maxillary sinus) ➤ Barotrauma ➤ Benign neoplasm (osteochondroma, hemangioma, hemangiopericytoma, dermoid, lipoma, ossifying fibroma, giant cell tumor, aneurysmatic bone cyst) ➤ Encephalocele (Fig. 7.**1 b**) ➤ Epithelial papilloma (squamous cell papilloma, inverted papilloma [Fig. 7.**16 a**]) ➤ Granulomatous disease (tuberculosis, syphilis, mycosis, sarcoidosis, rhinosclerosis, giant cell granuloma) ➤ Histiocytosis X ➤ Metastasis (especially from kidneys [Fig. 7.**2 a**]) ➤ Myeloma, plasmacytoma (extramedullary) ➤ Neurogenic tumor, schwannoma, neurofibroma, neurocele, meningioma) ➤ Odontogenic cyst or tumor ➤ Polypoid rhinosinusitis ➤ Wegener granulomatosis ➤ Previous paranasal sinus surgery (Caldwell–Luc procedure)

Table 7.3 Common variations and malformations

	Common	Rare
Hypoplasia or aplasia of paranasal sinuses (usually the frontal sinus)	➤ Congenital aplasia or hypoplasia ➤ Cretinism, hypothyroidism ➤ Kartagener syndrome ➤ Trisomy 21 (Down syndrome)	➤ Cleidocranial dysplasia ➤ Cockayne syndrome ➤ Craniodiaphyseal dysplasia ➤ Frontometaphyseal dysplasia ➤ Hyperphosphatasia ➤ Hypopituitarism ➤ Binder syndrome ➤ Median cleft syndrome ➤ Melnick-Needles syndrome ➤ Prader–Willi syndrome ➤ Schwarz–Lelek syndrome ➤ Treacher–Collins syndrome
Conditions marked by excessive bone growth	➤ Fibrous dysplasia (Fig. 7.**21**) ➤ Paget disease ➤ Hemolytic anemia	

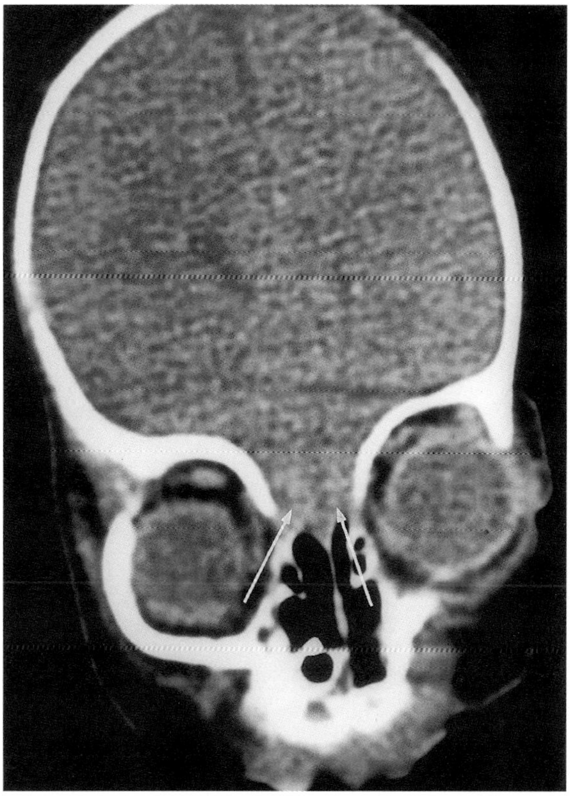

Fig. 7.**1 b** **Anterior encephalocele.** Coronal CT scan with a soft-tissue window shows the defect in the anterior skull base (arrows) through which meninges and brain (encephalocele) have herniated into the ethmoid sinus.

tissue portion of the cephalocele and differentiating between a meningocele and an encephalocele.

Tumors

Benign Tumors

Benign tumors are an uncommon finding in the paranasal sinuses (Tables 7.**4**, 7.**5**).

Osteoma

Occurring mainly in the frontal and ethmoid sinuses, osteomas consist of very dense compact bone or lamellar bone with intertrabecular fibrotic tissue. Fibrotic osteoma appears less dense on conventional radiographs and may be mistaken for a cyst. While usually asymptomatic, osteomas may obstruct the sinus ostium leading to secondary infection or may extend into an adjacent region such as the orbit. The optimum imaging procedure for detection, localization, and differentiation from other masses is spiral CT.

Papilloma (Fig. 7.**16 a**)

Papillomas arising from the nasal or sinus mucosa may be of the *fungiform* (50%), *inverted* (47%) (Fig. 7.**16 a**) or *cylindrical-cell* type (3%). Fungiform papillomas arise from the nasal septum, have a verrucous appearance, and are not considered premalignant.

Inverted papillomas (Figs. 7.**16 a, b**) are usually unilateral, arise on the middle turbinate, and spread into the ethmoid and maxillary sinuses. Though histologically benign, inverted papillomas may cause bone destruction (Fig. 7.**16 c**) and tend to recur after incomplete removal. Approximately 15% of inverted papillomas are associated with squamous cell carcinoma. Inverted papillomas display a higher signal intensity than malignant tumors when imaged on T2-weighted MR sequences. On post-contrast images they show a laminar pattern of enhancement caused by nodular protrusions and depressions in the mass.

Adenoma

Adenomas may arise in any epithelial tissue that contains glandular elements. Those occurring in the nose, paranasal sinuses, or nasopharynx may have the appearance of a simple polyp. They are locally invasive, however, and tend to recur after incomplete resection. Pleomorphic adenomas derived from the minor salivary glands may arise from the palate or from ectopic salivary gland rests. Malignant mixed tumors are far more common in the minor salivary glands than in the major salivary glands. Adenomas are indistinguishable from polyps (Fig. 7.**14**) in sectional imaging studies and conventional radiographs.

Neurogenic Tumors

Tumors with a neurogenic origin occur very rarely in the nose and paranasal sinuses. Peripheral nerve-sheath tumors may be classified as *schwannomas*, *neurofibromas*, or *neurogenic sarcomas*.

The typical CT appearance of schwannoma is that of a smoothly marginated, homogeneous mass that shows moderate enhancement after the intravenous administration of contrast medium.

On MRI, these tumors appear hypointense to isointense on T1-weighted images and hyperintense on T2-weighted images. They show moderate enhancement following the injection of gadolinium (Gd)-DTPA. Most schwannomas show a homogeneous internal structure, but cystic components may be present depending on the particular tumor histology.

Schwannomas typically cause displacement and remodeling of bony structures. Signs of aggressive bone destruction are suggestive of malignant transformation.

Table 7.4 Benign and malignant tumors of the paranasal sinuses

	Common	Rare
Benign tumors and tumor-like lesions	➤ Polyp (Fig. 7.**14a**) (inflammatory), polypoid rhinosinusitis ➤ Juvenile angiofibroma (Fig. 7.**24**) ➤ (Lymphatic tissue, adenoids) ➤ Mucocele (Fig. 7.**13a**) ➤ Retention cyst ➤ Osteoma	➤ Adenoma ➤ Ameloblastoma ➤ Amyloidosis ➤ Antrochoanal polyp ➤ Branchiogenic cyst ➤ Chondroma ➤ Dermoid, teratoma ➤ Encephalocele (Fig. 7.**1b**) ➤ Inverted papilloma (Fig. 7.**16a**) ➤ Fibroma ➤ Giant cell tumor ➤ Granuloma (tuberculosis, sarcoidosis) ➤ Hamartoma ➤ Hemangioma ➤ Histiocytosis X ➤ Lipoma ➤ Lymphangioma ➤ Nasoalveolar cyst ➤ Neurogenic tumor (neuroma of cranial nerves IX, X, XI ➤ Odontoma ➤ Rhinolith, foreign body
Malignant tumors and tumor-like lesions	➤ Carcinoma (squamous cell carcinoma [Fig. 7.**22**], lymphoepithelial carcinoma [Fig. 7.**26**]) ➤ Lymphoma ➤ Metastsis (Fig. 7.**2a**)	➤ Chordoma ➤ Esthesionneuroblastoma (Fig. 7.**27**) ➤ Hermangiopericytoma ➤ Malignant histiocytoma ➤ Melanoma ➤ Extramedullary plasmacytoma ➤ Salivary gland tumor (carcinoma, mixed tumors) ➤ Sarcoma (Fig. 7.**20**) (neurosarcoma, rhabdomyosarcoma, osteogenic sarcoma [Fig. 7.**9**], spindle cell sarcoma, fibrosarcoma [Fig. 7.**18a**]) ➤ Wegener granulomatosis

Angiofibroma (Fig. 7.**24**)

Angiofibromas are benign, highly vascularized, unencapsulated neoplasms that occur exclusively in male adolescents and young adults and show a 20–36% incidence of intracranial involvement. These tumors are clinically benign but locally aggressive. Most originate in the area of the pterygopalatine fossa in the nasopharynx. The tumor may then extend into the maxillary sinus, nasal cavity, sphenoid sinus, ethmoid sinus, or infratemporal fossa, into the orbit through the inferior orbital fissure, or into the cranial cavity through the foramen rotundum, pterygoid canal, or superior orbital fissure. The diagnosis is established by the clinical data (age, sex, symptoms) and by CT, MRI, or angiography. Angiofibromas appear very hyperdense on early contrast-enhanced CT scans. They appear hypointense to isointense on noncontrast T1-weighted MR images (Fig. 7.**24b**) and proton-density images, and isointense to hyperintense on T2-weighted images. It is common to see linear areas of signal void (flow voids) caused by rapid flow within tumor vessels. Intense enhancement is consistently seen after the intravenous injection of paramagnetic contrast medium.

Hemangioma (Fig. 9.**10**)

This lesion should be considered whenever coarse vascular structures are detected within a mass. The histologic types—capillary and cavernous hemangiomas—may occur in isolation or as part of a syndrome (Osler–Weber–Rendu syndrome). Hemangiomas of the cartilaginous septum are highly aggressive and tend to recur after incomplete resection.

Giant Cell Tumors

Giant cell tumors of the paranasal sinuses show a locally expansive, destructive pattern of growth.

Table 7.5 Benign and malignant tumors of the facial region

Benign	Malignant
Benign epithelial tumors: ➤ Sebaceous adenoma ➤ Keratocanthoma ➤ Melanocanthoma ➤ Nevi (various types) ➤ Papilloma ➤ Verruca vulgaris ➤ Xanthelasma (Fig. 7.**29**)	**Malignant epithelial tumors:** ➤ Basal cell carcinoma ➤ Squamous cell carcinoma (spindle cell carcinoma) ➤ Secondary skin cancers (metastatic carcinomas) ➤ Malignant melanoma
Benign mesenchymal tumors: ➤ Angioma (hemangioma, less commonly lymphangioma) ➤ Fibroma ➤ Granular cell tumor ➤ Keloid ➤ Lipoma ➤ Neurofibroma	**Malignant mesenchymal tumors:** ➤ Malignant lymphoma of skin ➤ Cutaneous manifestations of leukemia ➤ Malignant histiocytosis of skin ➤ Kaposi sarcoma (with or without HIV infection) **Neoplasms secondarily involving the face:** ➤ Nose and paranasal sinuses ➤ Oral cavity ➤ Maxilla, mandible, and teeth ➤ Parotid gland ➤ Ear

Other Tumors

Myxomas and *meningiomas* are very rare tumors of the nasal cavity and paranasal sinuses.

Fibrous dysplasia (Fig. 7.**21**) of the facial skeleton may involve a single or multiple bones and can cause marked expansion of the affected bony structures. While conventional radiographs and CT scans can demonstrate the morphologic criteria of fibrous dysplasia (Fig. 7.**21**), it is also important to note its characteristic MR features, since fibrous dysplasia is frequently misinterpreted as an aggressive paranasal sinus tumor or intracranial tumor. The lesions of fibrous dysplasia appear hypointense on T2-weighted images (Fig. 7.**21 a**), isointense to brain on T1-weighted images, and show nonhomogeneous enhancement after contrast administration (Fig. 7.**21 b**).

Ossifying fibromas may contain coarse granular calcifications. *Chordomas* and *eosinophilic granulomas* may occur in rare cases.

Additionally, a variety of *odontogenic cysts* and *tumors* may arise from the maxilla (Fig. 7.**12**) and mandible. *Radicular cysts* (30 times more common than follicular cysts) arise from an inflamed root granuloma, while *follicular cysts* develop from an anomalous tooth bud and contain dental elements. Multiple odontogenic cysts, especially the *keratocyst* (Figs. 7.**10**, 9.**11 a**), can occur in the setting of various syndromes and may undergo malignant transformation.

Malignant Tumors

Most malignant neoplasms of the nose and paranasal sinuses are epithelial tumors. These lesions can be further subdivided into tumors with an epithelial origin and tumors arising from salivary glands. The main histologic types of malignant epithelial tumors are *squamous cell carcinoma* (Fig. 7.**22**), *adenocarcinoma*, and *anaplastic carcinoma*. Malignant tumors arising from salivary glands consist of *adenoid cystic carcinoma* (Fig. 7.**25**), *acinar cell carcinoma*, and *mucoepidermoid carcinoma*.

Less common are malignant tumors of mesenchymal origin such as *osteosarcoma*, *malignant lymphoma*, and *chondrosarcoma*.

Squamous Cell Carcinoma (Fig. 7.22)

These tumors are approximately twice as common in males as females, with a peak incidence between 50 and 70 years of age. Cases present clinically with unilateral nasal obstruction or a purulent nasal discharge. Squamous cell carcinoma of the sphenoid sinus often leads to nerve deficits with frequent involvement of the abducent nerve. Carcinoma of the maxillary sinus tends to infiltrate the orbit, ethmoid sinus, pterygopalatine fossa, or infratemporal fossa. Squamous cell carcinoma of the ethmoid sinus is rare, and most ethmoid sinus carcinomas are of the adenoid cystic type. Infiltration of the orbit or pterygoid fossa or metastasis to cervical lymph nodes implies a poor prognosis.

Tumors of the minor salivary glands account for 4–10% of malignant neoplasms. They may occur in

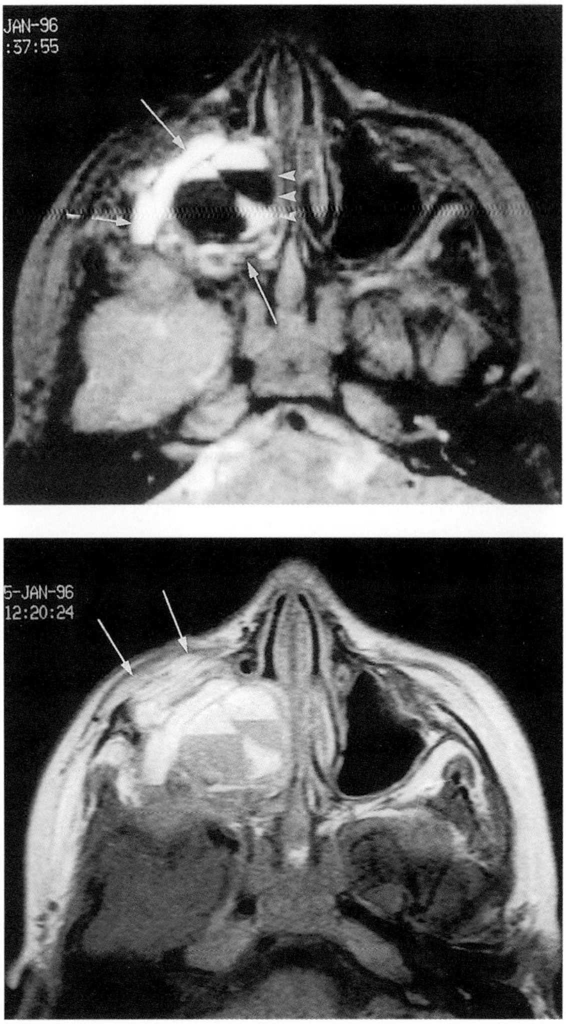

a

b

Fig. 7.**2 a, b** **Metastatic neuroblastoma (from renal tumor) in the right maxillary sinus.**
(**a**) Axial T2-weighted sequence (TR/TE = 3000/90 ms) shows a loculated mass of mixed high and low signal intensity in the right maxillary sinus (arrows). The posterior sinus wall is ill defined, and the right nasal turbinates also show destructive changes (arrowheads).
(**b**) Axial T1-weighted sequence (TR/TE = 700/15 ms) after contrast administration shows zones of marked enhancement along with central, loculated areas of intermediate signal intensity. Perifocal edema is evident in the overlying facial soft tissues (arrows).

the nasal cavity and any of the paranasal sinuses, but most tumors arise from the minor salivary glands of the palate. The cancers may be adenoid cystic carcinoma (Fig. 7.**25**), mucoepidermoid carcinoma, acinar cell carcinoma, or mixed neoplasms.

Esthesioneuroblastoma (Fig. 7.**27**)

Esthesioneuroblastomas (olfactory nerve neuroblastomas) are rare malignant nasal tumors that are most prevalent between 30 and 50 years of age and show an equal sex distribution. Most arise from the olfactory mucosa in the upper third of the nasal vault and subsequently infiltrate the ethmoid cells, orbit, and anterior cranial fossa (Fig. 7.**27**). With invasion of the frontal skull base, brain abscesses may form. Because these tumors are highly vascularized, they show intense enhancement on post-contrast CT scans. Intratumoral calcifications are occasionally seen. Esthesioneuroblastoma is predominantly isointense on noncontrast T1- and T2-weighted MR images. It enhances intensely on post-contrast images and thus can be difficult to distinguish from the brightly enhancing mucosa. Although the extent of bone destruction is often difficult to appreciate on MRI, this modality makes a useful primary study because sagittal and coronal images in particular can accurately define the extent of spread into the anterior cranial fossa.

Hemangiopericytoma

Hemangiopericytomas of the paranasal sinuses are rare, their most common symptoms being *nasal obstruction* and *epistaxis*. Treatment consists of wide local excision.

CT demonstrates the lesion as a moderately to intensely enhancing mass with small central calcifications. The tumor may attain considerable size and cause erosion of bone. It is hypointense to isointense on T1-weighted MR images, isointense to hyperintense on T2-weighted images, and shows moderate to intense enhancement after the administration of Gd-DTPA.

Hemangiopericytoma may be a primary sinus tumor or may invade the sinuses secondarily from bordering spaces or by metastasis (Fig. 7.**2**).

Inflammatory Lesions (Fig. 7.**15**)

The most common inflammatory disease of the paranasal sinuses is *acute* or *chronic sinusitis*. The diagnosis of sinusitis is not necessarily based on imaging studies alone, since a history of previous infections, prior surgery, or antecedent trauma may suggest the correct diagnosis. *Thickening of the mucosa* is the most common imaging finding and is suggestive of chronic sinonasal disease. Inflammatory sinus changes are noted in 20–40% of patients who undergo MRI examination of the head and neck region. *Viral infection* is the leading cause of acute sinusitis. Another frequent cause of sinusitis is *bacterial infection* with *Streptococcus pneumoniae* or *Haemophilus influenzae.* An isolated inflammatory reaction in the maxillary sinus usually signifies an infection arising from the teeth or periodontal tissues. Sinusitis may take a severe course in diabetic and immunosuppressed patients and may be complicated by *fungal infection* (e.g., aspergillosis) resulting in *extensive tissue destruction* and *osteomyelitis* (Fig. 7.**3**).

Standard occipitomental and occipitofrontal radiographic projections are still used in the workup of acute sinusitis, for which the presence of air-fluid levels is considered pathognomonic. Chronic sinusitis is usually evaluated by coronal CT, and MRI is added if complete sinus opacification is found.

The complications of sinusitis may consist of local mucosal complications such as polyps (Fig. 7.**14**), retention cyst, mucocele (Fig. 7.**23**), osteomyelitis (Fig. 7.**3**), or regional intracranial complications such as orbital cellulitis, orbital abscess, optic neuritis, meningitis, subdural empyema, brain abscess, and cavernous sinus thrombosis.

Traumatic Lesions (Figs. 7.**4**–7.**8**)

Isolated injuries of the nose (Fig. 7.**6**) or paranasal sinuses (Fig. 7.**5**), like injuries of the midface (Fig. 7.**8**) and anterior skull base, are usually accompanied by unilateral or bilateral nasal airway obstruction caused by mucosal swelling or displaced fragments. Injuries of the nose and paranasal sinuses may lead to hematomas and septal abscesses, with most hematomas occurring on the anterior part of the nasal septum.

Posttraumatic changes in facial shape or symmetry usually pose no difficulties in terms of differential diagnosis, since the patient will usually be aware of the change and clinical examination will disclose soft-tissue scars, displaced or nondisplaced fracture lines, indentations, deviations, or deformities of the bony and cartilaginous facial skeleton. Conventional radiographs and CT scans are excellent for documenting complex bony injuries.

The differential diagnosis of facial injuries can be difficult in certain cases of acute blunt-force trauma and is often difficult in children with facial trauma.

The following *fracture types* may be encountered in the facial region:

Frontal skull fracture. This is a depressed fracture involving the frontal bone and frontal sinus with lateral and/or posterior displacement of the fragments.

Differentiation is required from a frontobasal fracture involving injury to the dura and brain, and concomitant injuries of the ethmoid and sphenoid sinuses, the orbit and its contents (Figs. 7.**4**, 7.**5**), and cranial nerves I to VI should be excluded.

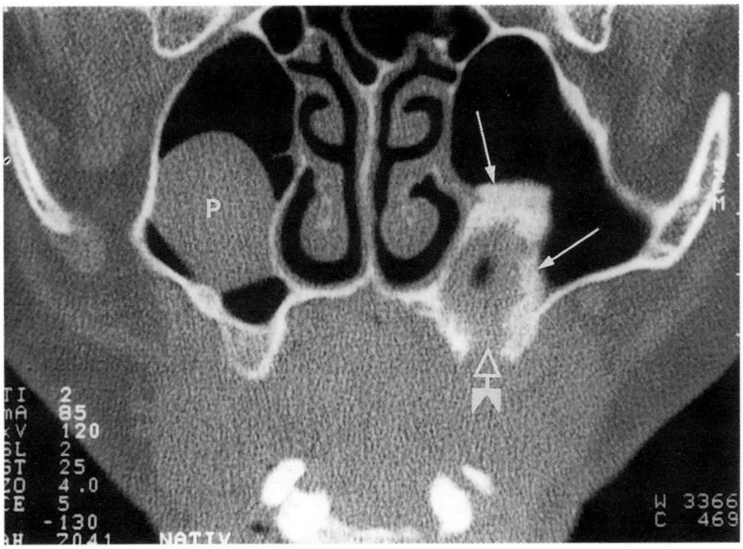

Fig. 7.**3** **Osteomyelitis with a fistulous tract.** Coronal CT scan with a bone window shows destruction of the maxillary cortex (arrows) with rarefaction and indistinctness of cortical structures in the maxillary sinus floor. The osteomyelitis is secondary to a fistulous tract (open tailed arrow) that developed in the maxilla after a previous tooth extraction. As an incidental finding, the image documents a polyp in the right maxillary sinus, which shows no evidence of bone destruction in the medial or lateral sinus wall or in the maxilla.
P Polyp in the maxillary sinus.

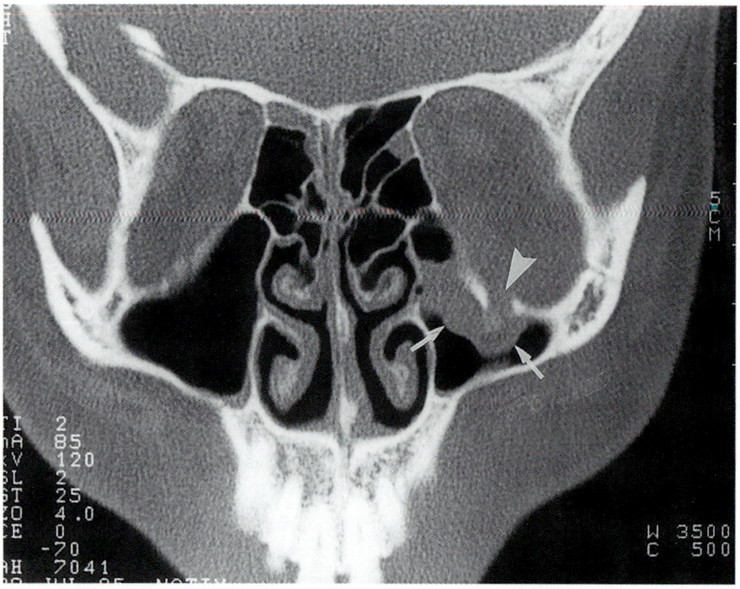

Fig. 7.4 **Orbital blowout fracture.** Coronal CT scan with a bone window shows a bony discontinuity in the floor of the orbit (arrowhead) with herniation of orbital fat (arrows) into the left maxillary sinus.

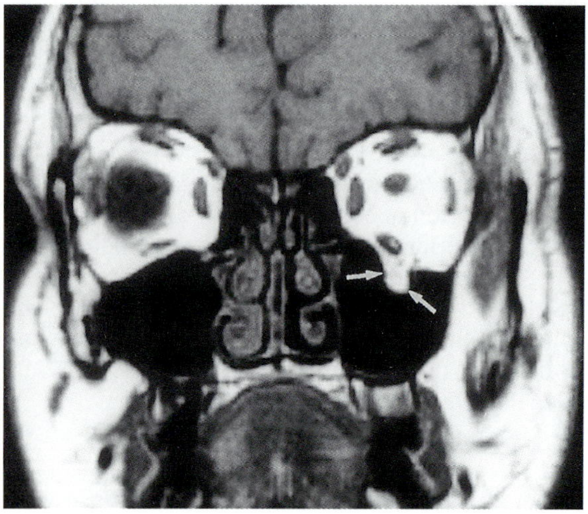

Fig. 7.5 **Orbital blowout fracture.** Coronal T1-weighted sequence (TR/TE = 700/15 ms) shows orbital fat (arrows) herniating into the left maxillary sinus. The bone defect is not demonstrated by MRI, so the diagnosis of the blowout fracture must be based on secondary fracture signs.

Midfacial fractures. These fractures may be medial or lateral, isolated or combined, and may involve the maxilla and sinuses, orbit, nasal bone, and/or the zygoma (Fig. 7.**8**):

- *Nasal fractures:* A fracture of the nasal bone (Fig. 7.**6**) may be associated with simple lateral displacement of the bony and often the cartilaginous nasal pyramid and with septal dislocation. Depressed fractures and fracture-separations also may occur and may be marked clinically by a flattened, indriven nose.

- *Maxillary fractures:* Most of these injuries are horizontal (Guérin-type) fractures.

- *Medial midfacial fractures,* known also as *Le Fort fractures,* are classified as follows:
  - Le Fort I: deep maxillary Guérin fracture with detachment of the upper alveolar process and malocclusion (Fig. 7.**7**).
  - Le Fort II: pyramidal fracture with separation of the body of the maxilla and involvement of the nasal bone, the frontal processes of the maxilla, the orbital floor, and the zygomatic-maxillary junction.
  - Le Fort III: separation of the facial skeleton from the skull base. The fracture line follows the nasofrontal, maxillofrontal and zygomaticofrontal sutures and frequently involves all paranasal sinuses, the anterior skull base, the orbit, and the zygomata (Fig. 7.**8**).

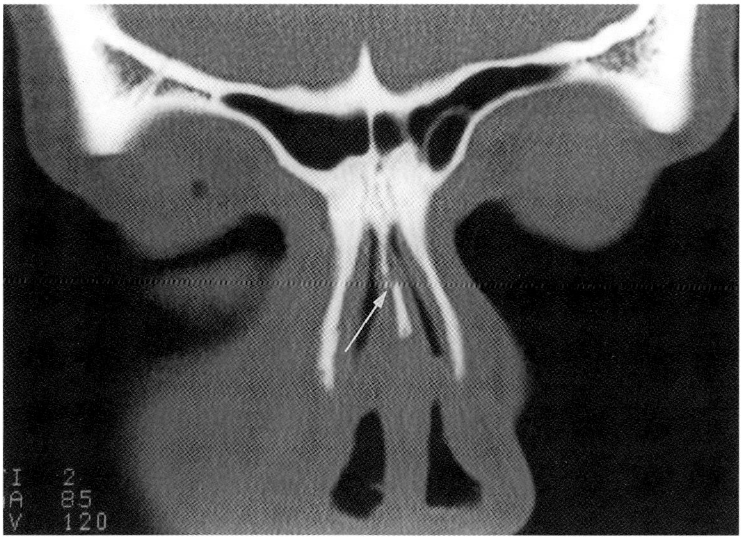

Fig. 7.**6** **Nasal fracture.** Coronal CT scan with a bone window demonstrates a fracture of the nasal bone (arrow) in which the distal fragment is displaced toward the left side.

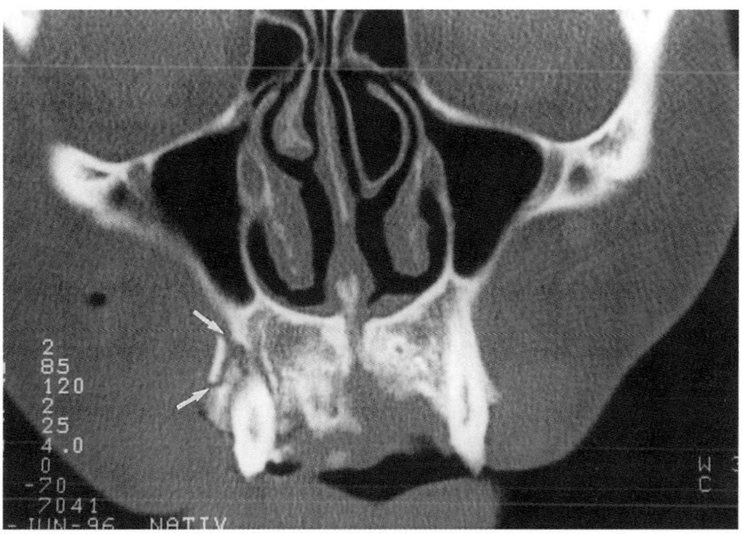

Fig. 7.**7** **Le Fort I fracture.** Coronal CT scan with a bone window shows a Le Fort I fracture of the right dental ridge (arrows) with a detached bone fragment caused by frontal trauma.

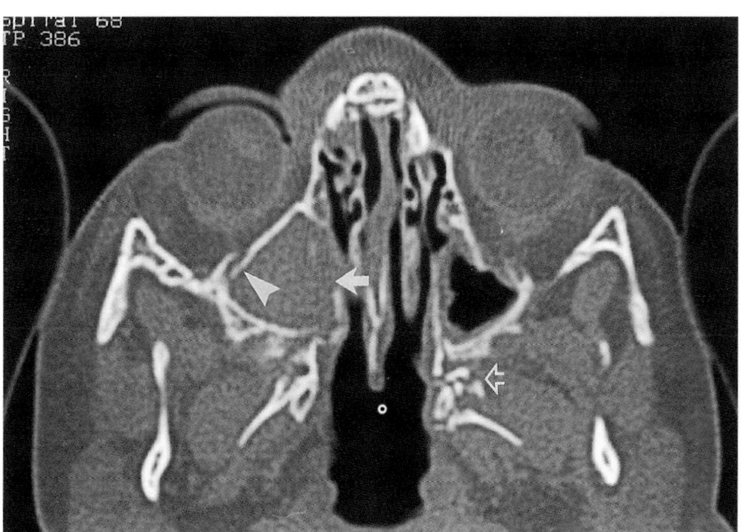

Fig. 7.**8** **Complex facial fracture (Le Fort III) in a multiply injured patient.** Axial CT scan with a bone window demonstrates a complex midfacial fracture involving the medial wall of the right orbit (arrowhead) and medial maxillary sinus wall (arrow) with an associated hematoma. A complex comminuted fracture of the sphenoid bone is visible on the left side (open arrow).

- *Lateral midfacial fractures* may consist of a zygomatic fracture ("tripod" fracture) with displacement of the zygoma; an isolated zygomatic arch fracture, often associated with depression of the bone fragments; and an isolated blowout fracture of the orbital floor (Figs. 7.**4** and 7.**5**).

Iatrogenic Changes

Surgery of the nose and paranasal sinuses can leave a variety of tissue defects including the absence of turbinates, the absence of a maxillary sinus wall, or extensive defects after tumor resections. In cases where reconstruction has been performed after a tumor resection, imaging procedures have a key role in distinguishing postoperative and posttherapeutic changes from residual or recurrent tumor. Even today, this can be a very challenging task. MRI is strongly recommended as a follow-up procedure owing to its excellent capacity for tissue discrimination.

Imaging Criteria and Their Differential Diagnosis

The diagnoses that are of key importance in the differential diagnosis of sinonasal pathology are reviewed below according to their morphologic appearance in imaging procedures.

Deformity or Asymmetry of the Paranasal Sinuses (Tables 7.**6** and 7.**7**)

Noncontrast CT, especially using spiral technique, is the procedure of choice for confirming deformity or asymmetry of one or more paranasal sinuses, as it provides optimum contrast between air-containing structures and bone. Common variations include deformity of the nasal septum and partial hypoplasia or hyperplasia of the paranasal sinuses leading to the deformation of surrounding structures. A variety of benign and malignant tumor masses can also cause asymmetry or deformity of the paranasal sinuses (Fig. 7.**9**).

The detection of an air-containing mass is usually accomplished with conventional radiography or CT. The most common findings fall under the heading of variations. Pneumatocele and ethmoid bulla in particular should be considered in the differential diagnosis.

Traumatic lesions of the paranasal sinuses (Fig. 7.**8**) with air inclusions are frequently associated with a perforation of the lamina papyracea.

Table 7.**6** Deformity, asymmetry, or opacification of the nasal cavity and paranasal sinuses

Common	**Rare**
➤ Congenital deformity of the nasal septum ➤ Fracture of the nasal roof or septum (Fig. 7.**6**) ➤ Mucosal swelling (inflammatory, allergic, traumatic) ➤ Polyp or pseudopolyp (Fig. 7.**14 b**) (including allergic polyposis, polypoid rhinosinusitis, cystic fibrosis) ➤ Rhinolith, foreign body ➤ Turbinate pathology (enlargement, congenital aplasia)	➤ Antrochoanal polyp ➤ Benign tumor (e.g., fibroma, neurofibroma, osteoma) ➤ Nasal carcinoma ➤ Choanal atresia or stenosis ➤ Dermoid cyst ➤ Encephalomeningocele (Fig. 7.**1 b**) ➤ Esthesioneuroblastoma (Fig. 7.**27**) ➤ Hypoplasia of nasal bones in various congenital syndromes ➤ Inverted papilloma (Fig. 7.**16 a**) ➤ Lymphoma ➤ Mucocele (Fig. 7.**13 a**) ➤ Rhinoscleroma ➤ Wegener granulomatosis

Table 7.7 Deformity and asymmetry of the aerated paranasal sinuses

Findings	Differential diagnostic criteria
Common:	
➤ Variation:	
—Congenital deformity of the nasal septum	Topography, morphology
—Bony hypoplasia of nose or paranasal sinuses	Topography, bony structures
—Congenital aplasia of nasal turbinates	Topography
➤ Tumor:	
—Adenoma	Density, signal intensity
➤ Inflammation:	Density, morphology
—Polyp or pseudopolyp (Fig. 7.**14 a**): allergic polyposis, polypoid rhinosinusitis, cystic fibrosis, mucosal swelling, mucocele (Fig. 7.**13 a**)	
Rare:	
➤ Malformations:	
—Choanal atresia or stenosis	
—Encephalomeningocele (Fig. 7.**1 b**)	
➤ Tumor:	
—Antrochoanal polyp	
—Benign (fibroma, neurofibroma, osteoma)	Density, signal intensity
—Esthesioneuroblastoma (Fig. 7.**27**)	Bone destruction
—Inverted papilloma (Fig. 7.**16 a**)	Signal intensity, morphology
—Lymphoma	Morphology
➤ Inflammation:	
—Wegener granulomatosis	Morphology

Liquid Sinus Masses on CT

Fluid in the paranasal sinuses, with or without an associated mass effect, is a common finding in CT and MRI. The role of noncontrast CT is to determine the primary density of a lesion. On MRI, a liquid lesion or mass in the paranasal sinuses typically shows increased signal intensity on T2-weighted images, low signal intensity on T1-weighted images, and frequent rim enhancement on post-contrast images (Fig. 7.**15 a**). The most common lesion is a cystic mass (Figs. 7.**10** – 7.**12**). The principal differential diagnoses for liquid sinus masses are listed in Table 7.**8**.

Sinus Tumor Masses on CT or MRI

(Table 7.**9**)

A major problem in the diagnosis of sinonasal tumor masses is that the lesion is frequently obscured by chronic sinusitis (Fig. 7.**15 a**) or an allergic reaction. Although modern CT techniques can distinguish tumor masses from accompanying inflammatory changes, this differentiation can still be difficult in some cases. MRI is superior to CT for delineating tumor masses in these cases, as it can discriminate more effectively between inflammatory changes and neoplastic tissue. This is best accomplished with T2-weighted sequences (Figs. 7.**9**, 7.**22 a**); here inflammatory changes show a very high signal intensity that contrasts with the intermediate signal intensity of tumor masses, which tend to be very cellular in the sinus region. In terms of differential diagnosis, it is important to note that a number of benign and gland-like tumors such as polyps (Fig. 7.**14 a**), papillomas (Fig. 7.**28**), inverted papillomas (Fig. 7.**16 a**), minor salivary gland tumors, and schwannomas have a high water content and may display a very high signal intensity on T2-weighted images. Conventional radiographs are still a useful screening tool for various sinonasal lesions and can direct the selection of further studies such as CT or MRI. For example, chronic sinusitis (Fig. 7.**15**) is consistently associated

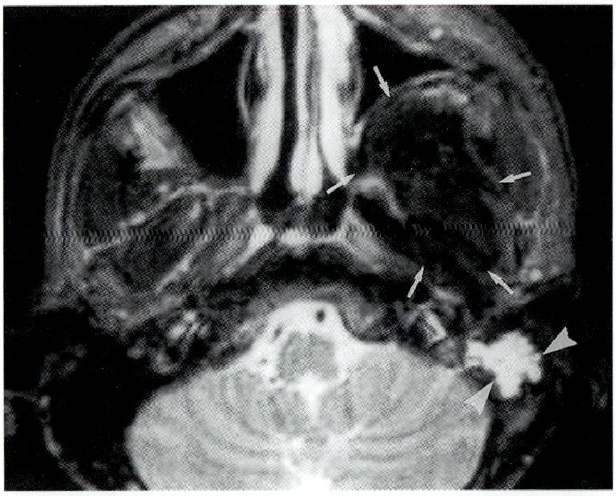

a

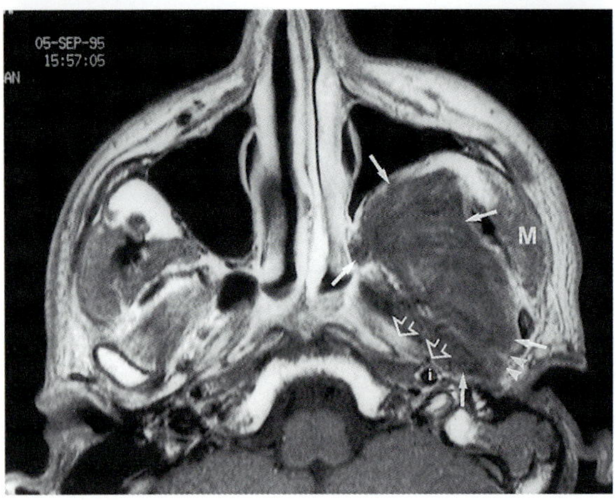

b

Figs. 7.**9 a, b** **Osteogenic sarcoma.**
(**a**) Axial T2-weighted sequence (TR/TE = 3000/90 ms) shows a mass with indistinct margins (arrows) indenting the posterior wall of the left sphenoid sinus. The mass appears markedly hypointense in the T2-weighted sequence. The tumor has compressed and effaced much of the fat in the parapharyngeal space and obstructed the eustachian tube, causing fluid retention in the left mastoid cells (arrowheads). The neurovascular sheath is displaced medially and posteriorly.
(**b**) Contrast-enhanced axial T1-weighted image (TR/TE = 700/15 ms) again documents the tumor mass (arrows), its impression on the posterior wall of the maxillary sinus, and the concomitant involvement and edematous reaction of the left masseter muscle. The mass extends posteriorly to the medial pole of the parotid gland (arrowheads), displacing the internal carotid artery and parapharyngeal fat (open arrows) medially and posteriorly. The mass shows minimal contrast enhancement.
M Masseter muscle
i Internal carotid artery

Table 7.**8** Liquid sinus masses on CT or MRI

Findings	**Differential diagnostic criteria**
Variation:	
➤ Meningoencephalocele (Fig. 7.**1 b**)	Topography, morphology
Tumor:	
➤ Cyst: odontogenic, keratocyst (Fig. 7.**10**), dermoid cyst	Density, signal intensity, morphology
➤ Necrotic malignant tumors (Fig. 7.**22**)	Signal intensity, density, morphology
Inflammation:	Density, morphology
➤ Acute sinusitis	
➤ Mucocele (Fig. 7.**13 a**)	Density, expansion
Trauma:	
➤ Acute paranasal sinus trauma (Figs. 7.**4**, 7.**5**)	
➤ Fracture of sinus wall (Fig. 7.**8**)	Topography, morphology
Iatrogenic:	
➤ Previous tooth extraction	
➤ Previous sinus surgery	

a

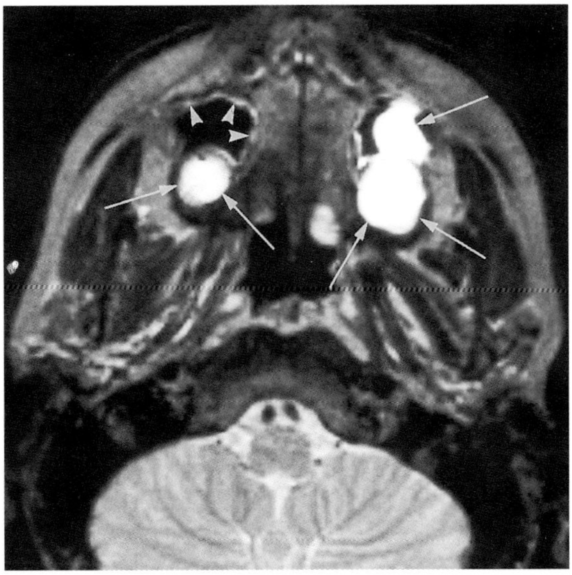

b

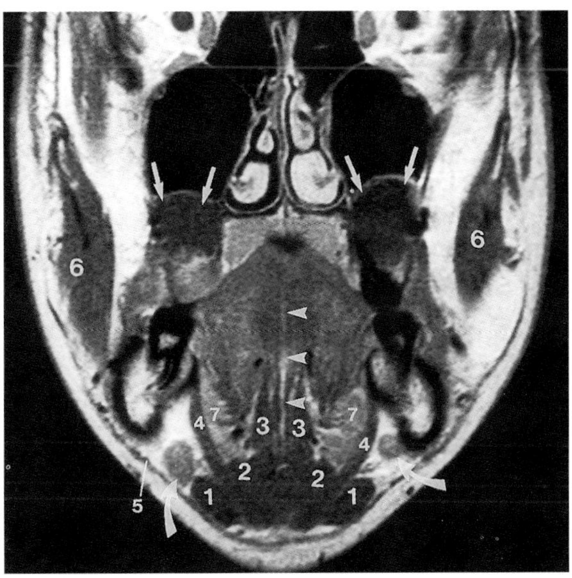

Figs. 7.**10 a, b** **Bilateral keratocysts in the maxilla.**
(**a**) Axial T2-weighted MR image (TR/TE = 3000/90 ms) shows well-circumscribed masses of very high signal intensity in the lower portions of the maxillary sinus on both sides (arrows). The image also shows a subtle inflammatory reaction of the mucosae (arrowheads) in the still-aerated portions of the maxillary sinuses.
(**b**) Contrast-enhanced T1-weighted MR image in the coronal plane shows rim enhancement of the cystic masses in the lower portions of the maxillary sinuses (arrows). The coronal image clearly documents the relation of the keratocysts to the maxilla. Additionally, there is reactive enlargement of the submandibular lymph nodes on each side (curved arrows). Note also the excellent documentation of normal oral floor anatomy on the coronal plane.
1 Digastric muscle
2 Geniohyoid muscle
3 Genioglossus muscle
4 Mylohyoid muscle
5 Platysma
6 Masseter muscle
7 Sublingual gland
Arrowheads: lingual septum

with marked thickening of the mucosa and occasionally with prominent sclerosis of the bony sinus walls. As polyps of the nasal cavity and paranasal sinuses (Fig. 7.**14**), mucoceles (Figs. 7.**13** and 7.**23**), and other benign masses slowly enlarge, they can displace surrounding structures and also cause atrophy or erosion of adjacent bone. These changes are consistently demonstrable on CT scans in patients with large polyps and mucoceles (Fig. 7.**13 b**).

Epithelial tumors of the nose and paranasal sinuses usually present with symptoms similar to those of chronic sinusitis. Thus, persistent unilateral symptoms warrant further investigation by a radiologic workup consisting of CT, MRI, or both. MRI can accurately demarcate the tumor from surrounding soft tissues and can discriminate among tumor, inflammatory changes, and retained fluids, while CT can accurately define bony structural details and sites of osseous involvement (Figs. 7.**16 c**, 7.**20**, 7.**22 c, d**).

Images on the coronal or sagittal plane have become an important adjunct for detecting possible infiltration of the skull base (Fig. 7.**27 b**).

DSA is rarely necessary today for the differential diagnosis of sinonasal pathology, which is adequately accomplished by CT or MRI. It is still used, however, in interventional procedures for mass lesions (Fig. 7.**24**) as part of an interdisciplinary therapeutic approach.

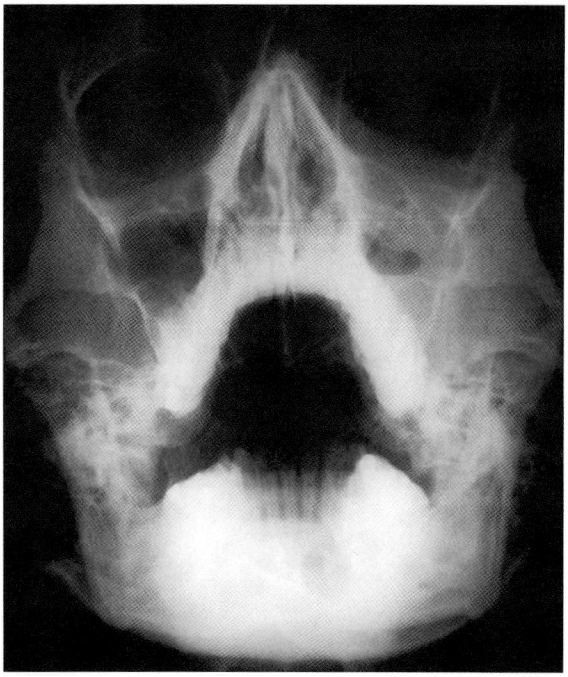

a

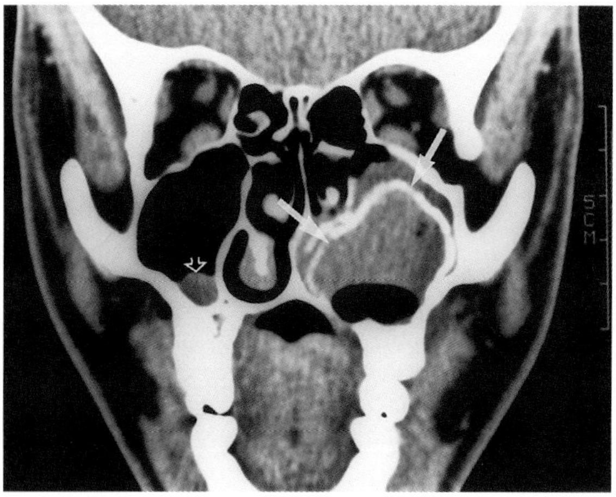

b

Figs. 7.**11 a, b** **Granulation cyst of the left maxillary sinus.**
(**a**) Conventional sinus radiograph demonstrates opacity of the left maxillary sinus.
(**b**) Coronal CT scan with a soft-tissue window shows a cystic mass arising from the maxilla and extending into the left maxillary sinus (arrows). The right maxillary sinus mucosa shows inflammatory thickening (open arrow).

Radiographically Dense Sinus Lesions

(Table 7.**10**)

In clinical and radiologic evaluations of the paranasal sinuses, a radiographically dense sinus lesion detected on plain films or CT scans provides an important basis for differential diagnostic considerations. The most common isolated mass lesion found within or bordering on the paranasal sinuses is a primary sinus osteoma. The differential diagnosis should also include iatrogenic changes and foreign bodies. Diffuse wall changes may signify processes such as chronic sinusitis (Fig. 7.**15**), chronic osteomyelitis (Fig. 7.**3**), or primary osseous diseases of the bony walls or cartilaginous structures of the paranasal sinuses. If complex and extensive sinus changes are found, the bony structures should always be evaluated for signs of malignant infiltration by processes such as plasma cell leukemia (Fig. 7.**17**). Malignant infiltration should be suspected whenever low signal intensity on noncontrast T1-weighted MR images gives way to marked enhancement on post-contrast images. Even severe chronic sinusitis generally is not associated with extensive cancellous bone hypointensity on T1-weighted sequences.

Most of the differential diagnostic criteria presented in the sections on the middle skull base apply to the lesions described above.

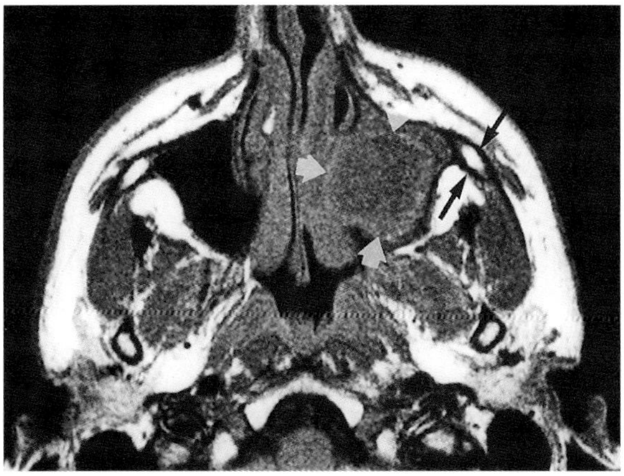

a

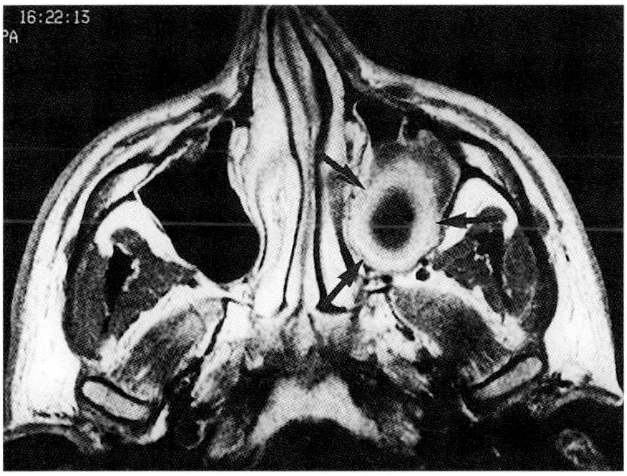

b

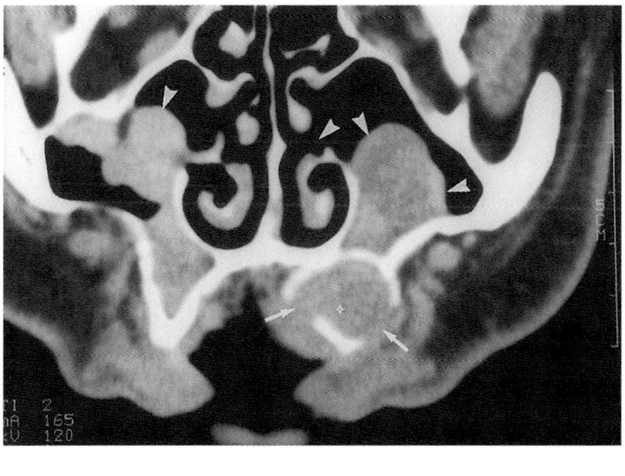

c

Figs. 7.**12 a – c** **Globulomaxillary cyst in the left maxillary sinus.**

(**a**) Unenhanced T1-weighted image (TR/TE = 700/15 ms) shows a mass with smooth, slightly hyperintense margins (thick arrows) causing slight compression of the nasal turbinates. Bone destruction is not appreciated on the MR image. (Thin arrows = zygoma).

(**b**) After the administration of 0.1 mmol/kg bw Gd-DTPA, the mass displays a nonenhancing center and an intensely enhancing rim (arrows). The medial aspect of the mass is clearly demarcated from the turbinate on the post-contrast image.

(**c**) Coronal CT scan with a soft-tissue window shows that the cyst (arrow) has expanded the bony structures of the maxilla and contains protein-rich material. The scan also shows polypoid and postoperative changes in the right and left maxillary sinuses (arrowheads).

Table 7.**9** Benign and malignant tumors and tumor-like lesions of the nasal cavity and paranasal sinuses

Benign	Malignant
➤ Polyp (inflammatory), polypoid rhinosinusitis (Fig. 7.**14 a**) ➤ Juvenile angiofibroma (Fig. 7.**24**) ➤ (Lymphatic tissue, adenoids) ➤ Mucocele (Fig. 7.**13 a**) ➤ Retention cyst ➤ Osteoma	➤ Adenoma ➤ Ameloblastoma ➤ Amyloidosis ➤ Antrochoanal polyp ➤ Arteriovenous fistula ➤ Branchiogenic cyst ➤ Chondroma ➤ Dermoid, teratoma ➤ Encephalocele (Fig. 7.**1 b**) ➤ Inverted papilloma (Fig. 7.**16 a**) ➤ Fibroma ➤ Giant cell tumor ➤ Granuloma (tuberculosis, sarcoidosis) ➤ Hamartoma ➤ Hemangioma ➤ Histiocytosis X (Fig. 10.**9**) ➤ Lipoma ➤ Lymphangioma ➤ Nasoalveolar cyst ➤ Neurogenic tumor (neuroma of cranial nerves IX, X, XI) ➤ Odontoma ➤ Rhinolith, foreign body
➤ Carcinoma (squamous cell carcinoma [Fig. 7.**22**], lymphoepithelial carcinoma [Fig. 7.**26**]) ➤ Lymphoma ➤ Metastasis (Fig. 7.**2 a**)	➤ Chordoma ➤ Esthesioneuroblastoma (Fig. 7.**27**) ➤ Hemangiopericytoma ➤ Malignant histiocytoma ➤ Melanoma ➤ Extramedullary plasmacytoma ➤ Salivary gland tumor (carcinoma, mixed tumors) ➤ Sarcoma (neurosarcoma, rhabdomyosarcoma, osteogenic sarcoma [Fig. 7.**9**], spindle cell sarcoma, fibrosarcoma [Fig. 7.**18 a**]) ➤ Wegener granulomatosis

Table 7.**10** Radiographically dense lesions of the paranasal sinuses

Findings	Differential diagnostic criteria
Variation:	
➤ Dysplastic sinus with increased wall density	Morphology, topography
Tumor:	
➤ Benign: osteoma, chondroma, ossifying fibroma	Density, signal intensity, morphology
➤ Malignant: osteosarcoma (Fig. 7.**9**)	Bone destruction, nonhomogeneity, metastasis
Inflammation:	
➤ Chronic osteomyelitis (Fig. 7.**3**)	Nonhomogeneous structure
Traumatic:	
➤ Chronic trauma sequelae	Displacement
Iatrogenic:	
➤ Synthetic materials	Morphology, trauma, foreign body introduced at operation

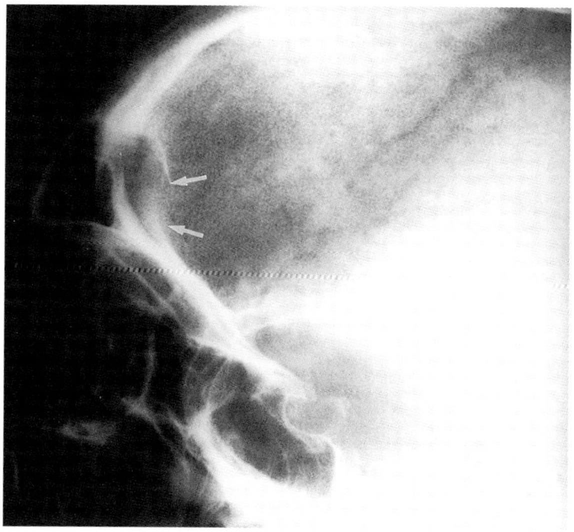

a

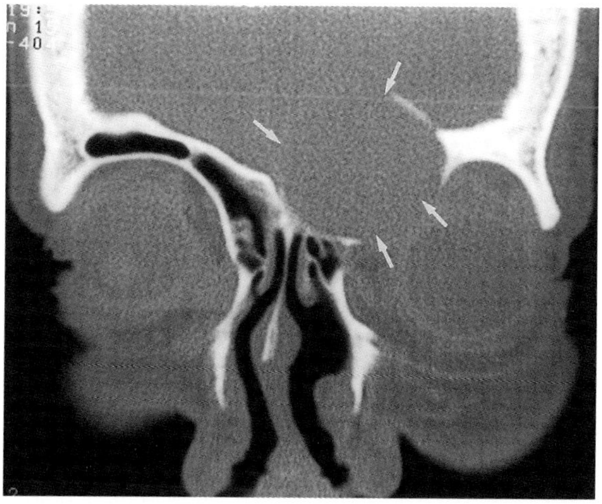

b

Figs. 7.**13 a, b** **Mucocele in the left frontal sinus.**
(**a**) Lateral skull radiograph shows thinning of the posterior bony wall of the frontal sinus (arrows), suggesting that the sinus has been expanded by a space-occupying lesion.
(**b**) Coronal CT scan with a bone window shows a rounded mass in the left frontal sinus that has thinned the sinus walls superiorly and inferiorly (arrows). The CT findings do not suggest a malignant mass but are consistent with a mucocele. This was confirmed at operation.

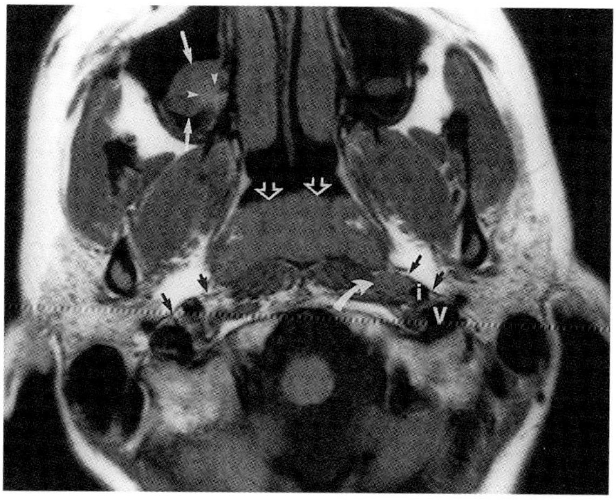

a

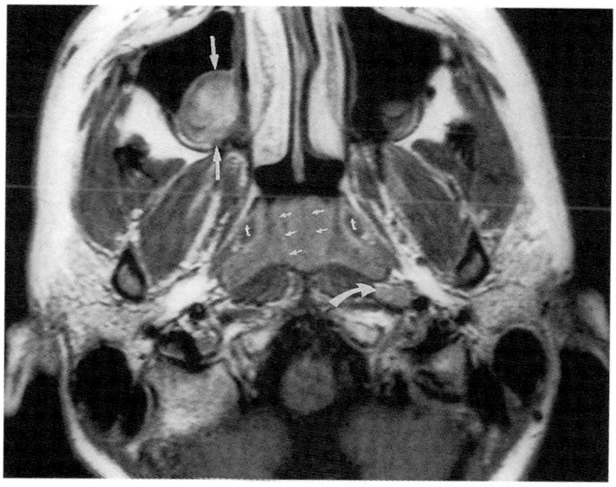

b

Figs. 7.**14 a, b** **Polyp of the left maxillary sinus.**
(**a**) Unenhanced T1-weighted image (TR/TE = 700/15 ms) shows an approximately 2-cm polyp in the left maxillary sinus (white arrows). A small hemorrhagic area at the center of the mass shows increased signal intensity (arrowheads). Lymphatic hyperplasia is visible in the nasopharynx (open arrows), and an islet of adenoid tissue appears in the post-styloid compartment (curved arrow).

i	Internal carotid artery
V	Internal jugular vein
Black arrows	Stylopharyngeal diaphragm

(**b**) Contrast-enhanced T1-weighted image after the administration of 0.1 mmol/kg bw Gd-DTPA (TR/TE = 700/15 ms) in a 12-year-old girl shows an approximately 2-cm polyp (arrows) in the left maxillary sinus. The polyp has smooth, well-defined margins with no signs of infiltration or bone destruction. The image also shows lymphatic hyperplasia in the nasopharynx with highly vascularized septa (see also Ch. 6) and heterotopic adenoid tissue (curved arrow) on the left side.
t Torus tubarius

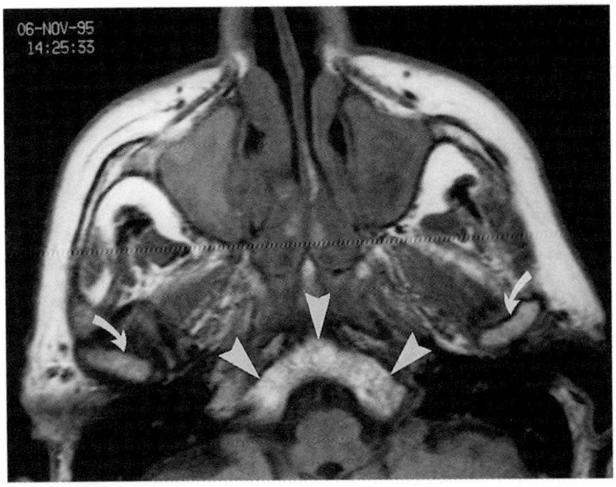

a

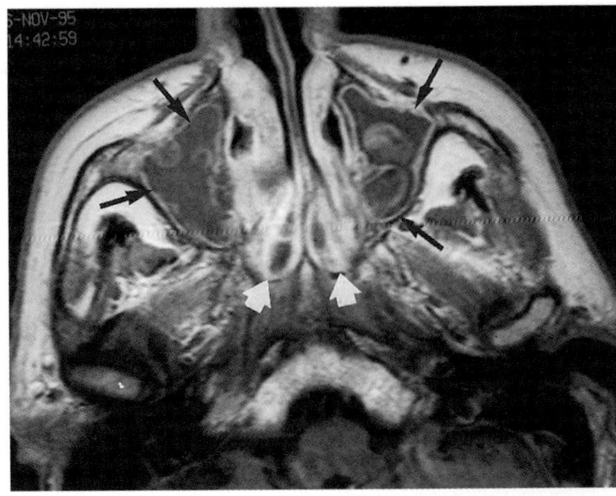

b

Figs. 7.**15 a, b** **Chronic bilateral maxillary sinusitis.**
(**a**) Contrast-enhanced axial T1-weighted image (TR/TE = 700/15 ms) shows marked, bilateral soft-tissue proliferation in the maxillary sinuses and nasal cavity. Compared with Fig. 7.**17 a**, there is no reduction of signal intensity in the mandibular condyles (curved arrows) or clivus (arrowheads).

(**b**) Contrast-enhanced axial T1-weighted image (TR/TE = 700/15 ms) shows markedly swollen, intensely enhancing mucosa (black and white arrows) in both maxillary sinuses and the nasal cavity with retained fluid. MRI shows no evidence of bone destruction or a tumor mass.

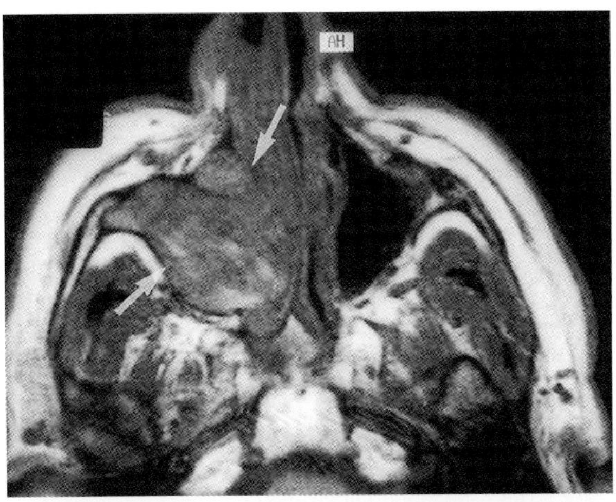

a

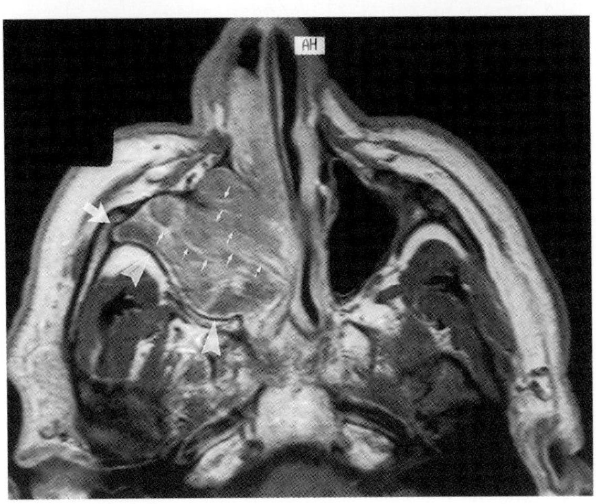

b

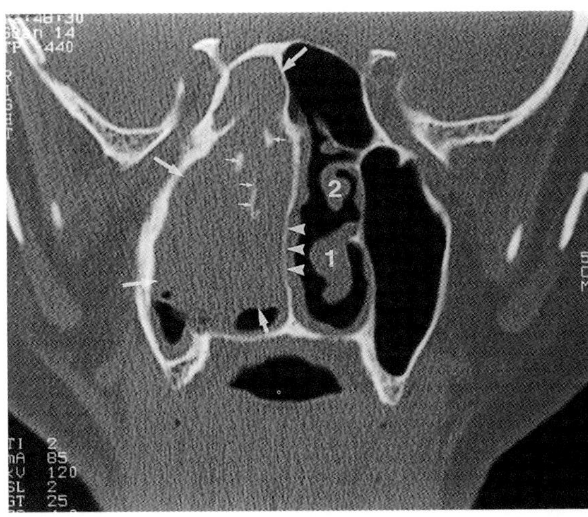

c

Figs. 7.**16**

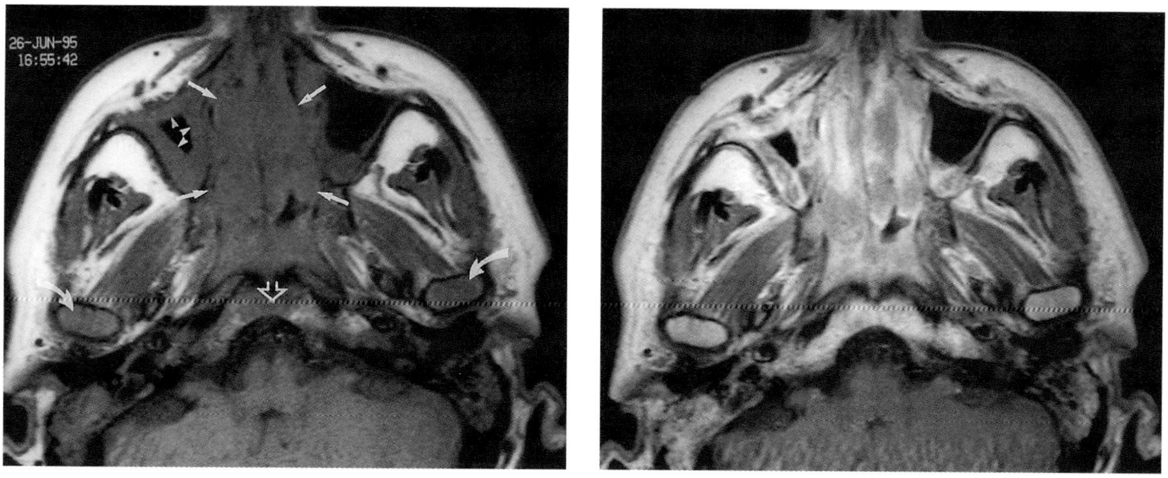

a b

Figs. 7.**17 a, b** **Infiltration by plasma cell leukemia.**
(**a**) Axial T1-weighted image (TR/TE = 700/15 ms) shows prominent soft-tissue masses in the nasal cavity (arrows) and nasopharynx. Note also the marked mucosal swelling in the right maxillary sinus (arrowheads) and milder swelling in the left sinus. Additionally, the signal intensity of the cancellous bone in the mandibular condyles (curved arrows) and clivus (open arrow) is markedly decreased relative to the normal population.
(**b**) Contrast-enhanced T1-weighted image (TR/TE = 700/15 ms) shows marked enhancement in the nasal cavity, maxillary sinus, nasopharynx, and also in the mandibular condyles and clivus. Histologic examination identified plasma cell leukemic infiltration of the nasal cavity, nasopharynx, and the cancellous bone of the temporomandibular joint and clivus. The mucosal enhancement in the right maxillary sinus is interpreted as an inflammatory response.

◁ Fig. 7.**16 a–c** **Inverted papilloma of the right maxillary and ethmoid sinus.**
(**a**) Unenhanced T1-weighted image (TR/TE = 700/15 ms) shows a nonhomogeneous mass (arrows) that is predominantly isointense to muscle tissue.
(**b**) After the administration of 0.1 mmol/kg bw Gd-DTPA, the mass shows a laminar pattern of contrast enhancement (small arrows). The papilloma completely fills the right maxillary sinus and has expanded the sinus wall posteriorly without bone destruction (arrowheads). There is obvious remodeling of the zygomatic bone (arrow). Contrast administration has produced a laminar pattern of alternating high and low signal intensity within the tumor.
(**c**) Coronal CT scan with a bone window shows an inverted papilloma (arrows) in the right maxillary and ethmoid sinuses (compare with the mass in Fig. 7.**23**). CT documents the deformation of the bony sinus structures by the tumor, particularly the medial bone thinning (arrowheads). The scan also shows central flecks of calcification (small arrows) that appear as hypointense areas on MRI.
1 Inferior turbinate
2 Middle turbinate

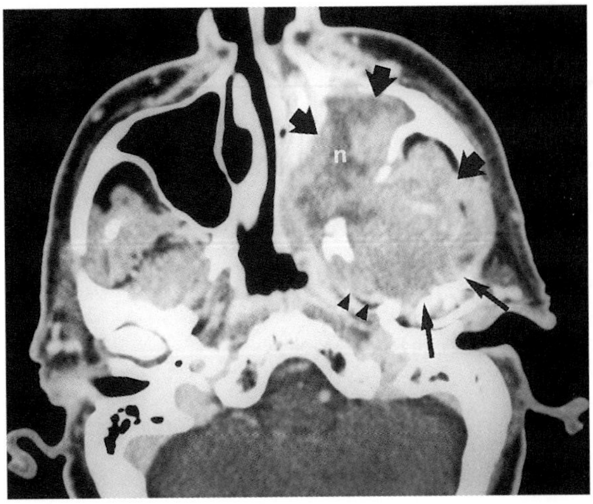

a

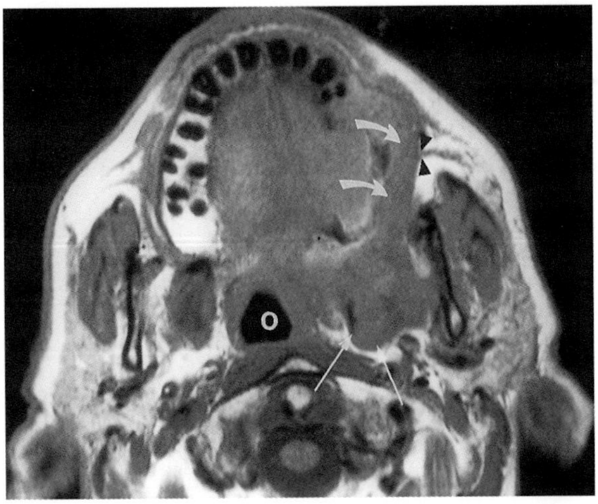

b

Figs. 7.**18 a, b** **Left-sided fibrosarcoma.**
(**a**) Axial CT scan with a soft-tissue window shows an extensive fibrosarcoma (thick black arrows) in the left maxillary sinus that has destroyed the posterior sinus wall (arrow heads) and invaded the masticator space. The mass extends posteriorly as far as the mandibular condyle (this black arrows) and has compressed the fat plane in the parapharyngeal space (arrowheads). The intrasinus portion of the mass contains a central area of necrotic liquefaction (n).

(**b**) Unenhanced axial T1-weighted image (TR/TE = 700/15 ms) shows the fibrosarcoma invading the masticator space (infiltrating the medial pterygoid muscle) and extending into the buccal space (curved arrows). The tumor has also infiltrated the maxilla and buccal muscle on the left side and the distal portion of the parotid duct (arrowheads). The mass extends posteriorly into the prestyloid compartment of the parapharyngeal space, causing displacement of the parapharyngeal fat (this arrows). Displacement of the naso-oropharyngeal air column (O) is also seen.

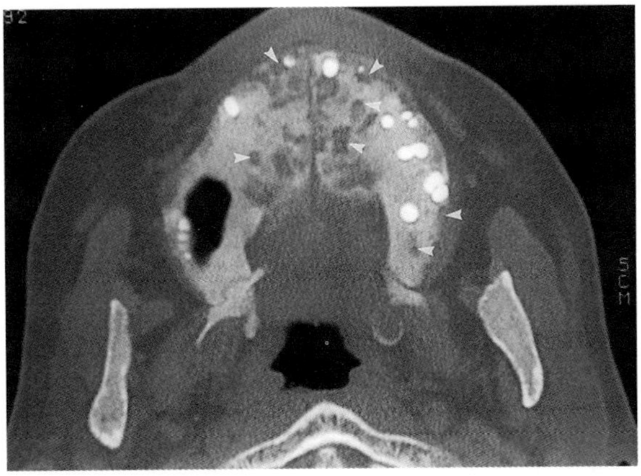

Fig. 7.**19** **Secondary hyperparathyroidism in diabetes mellitus.** Axial CT scan with a bone window demonstrates multiple osteolytic foci (arrowheads) in the hard palate and maxilla representing "brown tumors" due to hyperparathyroidism.

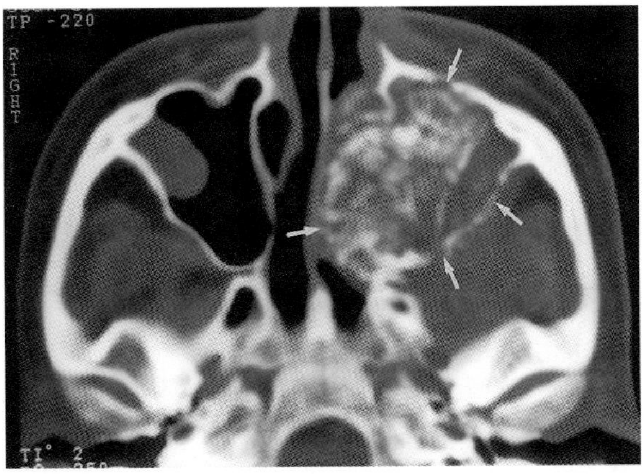

Fig. 7.**20** **Chondrosarcoma of the left maxillary sinus.** Axial CT scan with a soft-tissue window shows destruction of the bony walls of the left maxillary sinus (arrows) similar to that caused by squamous-cell carcinoma. Arising from the maxilla, the chondrosarcoma differs from squamous cell carcinoma (compare with Figs. 7.**22 c, d**) in the presence of prominent central calcifications.

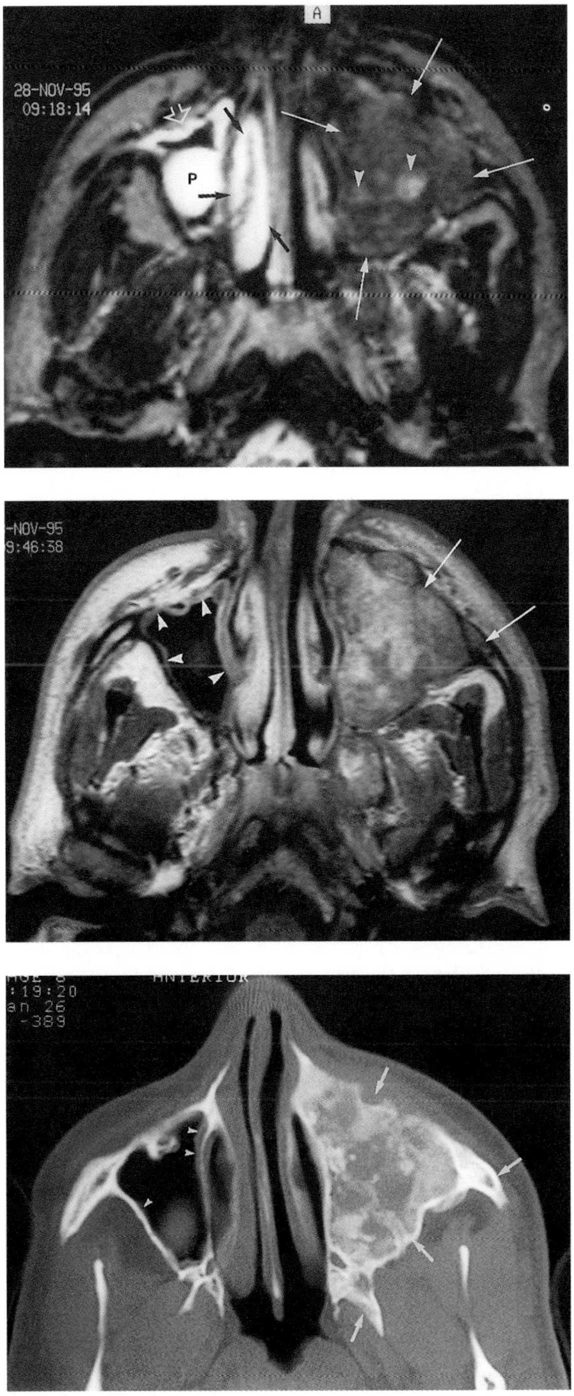

a

b

c

Figs. 7.**21 a–c** **Fibrous dysplasia of the left maxillary sinus.**
(**a**) Unenhanced T2-weighted image (TR/TE = 2500/90 ms) shows a hypointense lesion (arrows) in the left maxillary sinus. The mass contains small patchy areas (arrowheads) of slightly greater signal intensity. A polyp (P) is visible in the right maxillary sinus. The image also documents inflammatory changes in the right maxillary sinus with prominent mucosal thickening (open arrow) and in the right nasal cavity (black arrows).
(**b**) T1-weighted image (TR/TE = 700/15 ms) after the administration of 0.1 mmol/kg bw Gd-DTPA shows nonhomogeneous enhancement of the lesion. The inflamed mucosae of the right maxillary sinus (arrowheads) show marked enhancement. Note also the involvement of adjacent bony structures such as the lateral maxillary sinus wall and zygoma (arrows).
(**c**) Axial CT scan with a bone window documents the characteristic changes, showing patchy increased density and irregularity of the bone structure and scaly calcifications. Note the expansion of the affected bones (maxillary sinus walls, lateral and medial plates of left pterygoid process, zygoma). Arrowheads = inflamed mucosa of right maxillary sinus

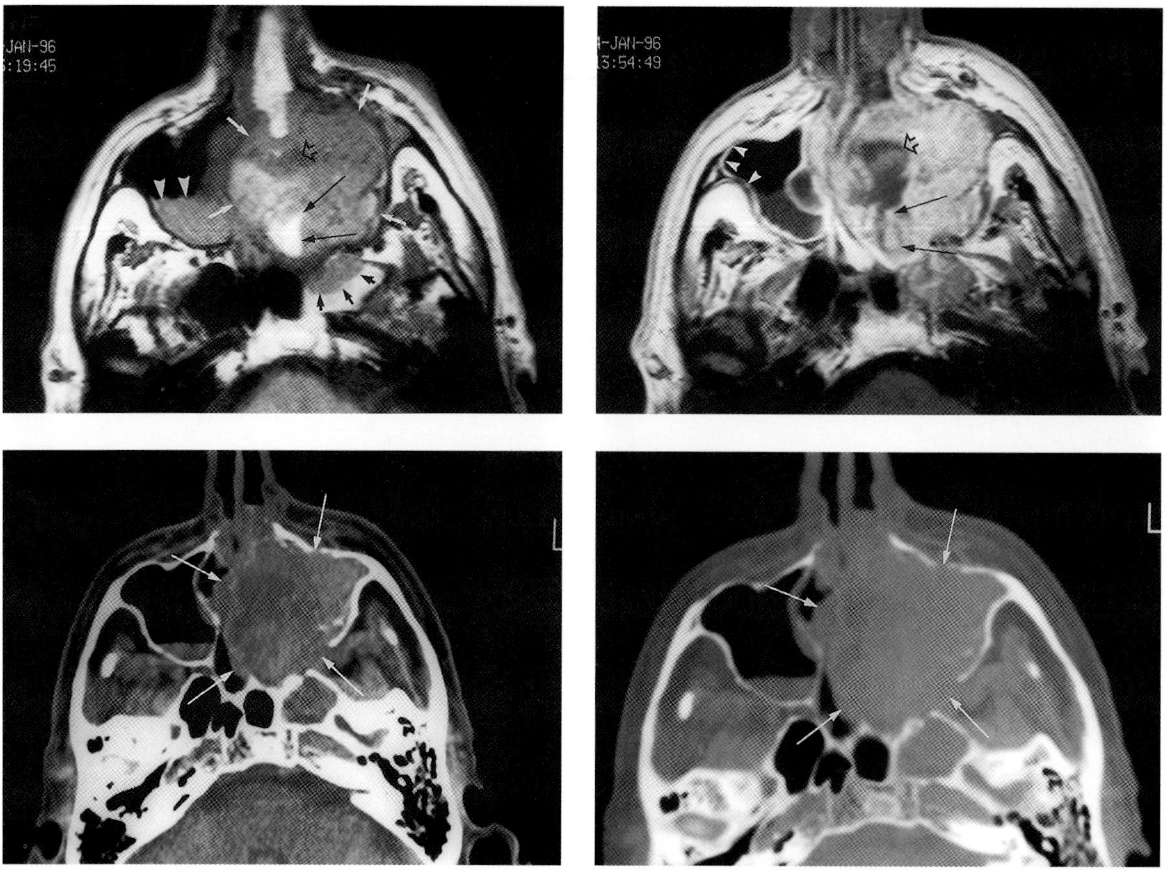

a b c d

Figs. 7.**22 a – d** **Squamous cell carcinoma of the left maxillary sinus.**
(**a**) Unenhanced T1-weighted image (TR/TE = 700/15 ms) shows a mass (white arrows) containing hypointense necrotic areas (open black arrow) and hyperintense hemorrhagic areas (thin black arrows). The tumor has penetrated the bony walls of the maxillary sinus and invaded the left sphenoid sinus (small black arrows). Inflammatory changes are evident in the right maxillary sinus (white arrowheads).
(**b**) T1-weighted image after the administration of 0.1 mmol/kg bw Gd-DTPA (TR/TE = 700/15 ms) shows marked nonhomogeneous enhancement of the mass. The initially hypointense necrotic areas (open arrow) still appear hypointense after contrast administration and are more clearly delineated. The initially hyperintense hemorrhagic areas (black arrows) remain hyperintense on the contrast-enhanced image. An ordered internal structure cannot be discerned. The medial bony wall of the maxillary sinus is undefined. The thickened, inflamed mucosa (arrowheads) of the right maxillary sinus shows marked enhancement.
(**c**) Axial CT scan with a soft-tissue window defines the sites of bone destruction by the squamous cell carcinoma in the anterior, medial, and posterior walls of the maxillary sinus (arrows). There is no sign of intratumoral calcifications.
(**d**) Axial CT scan with a bone window again defines the lytic portions of the anterior, medial, and posterior sinus walls (arrows). There is no sign of intratumoral calcifications.

Sinus Lesions with High T2-Weighted Signal Intensity

The presence of soft-tissue lesions or pathologic processes with prolonged T2 relaxation times on MR images can significantly advance the differential diagnosis. The most likely entities are chronic inflammatory changes and hematomas.

High T2-weighted signal intensity is characteristic of mucoceles that are not yet inspissated. These lesions also show high T1-weighted signal intensity due to their high protein content (Fig. 7.**23**). As the contents of the mucocele become inspissated, the lesion generally shows a definite change in signal intensity, appearing markedly hypointense on both T1- and T2-weighted MR images.

The antrochoanal polyp is a benign sinus tumor that also appears hyperintense on T2-weighted images. The radiologic presentation of an antrochoanal polyp is usually characteristic. Conventional X-ray films show unilateral opacification of a paranasal sinus or nasal cavity. CT demonstrates a lesion of mucus attenuation usually appearing in the maxillary sinus, ipsilateral nasal cavity, and nasopharynx. This mass usually appears hypointense on T1-weighted images.

The most common differential diagnoses are a cyst, polyp (Fig. 7.**14**), or papilloma (Fig. 7.**28**).

Sinus Lesions with Low T2-Weighted Signal Intensity

Lesions with low signal intensity on T2-weighted MR images may belong to one of several groups:

- Variations: celes.
- Tumors: osteoma, fibrous dysplasia (Fig. 7.**21**).
- Fungal sinusitis: aspergilloma.

Conventional radiographs and CT scans of fungal sinusitis (aspergillosis) usually show involvement of multiple paranasal sinuses with nodular mucoperiosteal thickening. Calcifications are occasionally seen. The lesions may grow invasively and cause focal bone destruction, simulating an aggressive malignant process. Aspergillus infections may incite a vasculitis, eventually leading to thrombosis or hemorrhagic infarction of adjacent brain areas. Aspergillomas tend to show very low signal intensity in both T1- and T2-weighted sequences, and this is considered a characteristic imaging feature of fungal sinusitis. Other noninfectious forms of sinusitis may occur in association with Wegener granulomatosis. Imaging studies in these cases show marked mucosal thickening with soft-tissue nodules throughout the paranasal sinuses and nasal cavity. Usually the maxillary sinus is affected, and bone destruction is common.

Osteomas are clinically asymptomatic in most patients, appearing on conventional radiographs and CT scans as a well-circumscribed mass of osseous density. They most commonly occur in the frontal or ethmoid sinus and can range from a few millimeters to several centimeters in size. Complications are very rare with osteomas and usually result from obstruction of the nasofrontal duct. This can lead to the development of a mucocele-like structure, or pneumocephalus may result from erosion of the posterior wall of the frontal sinus.

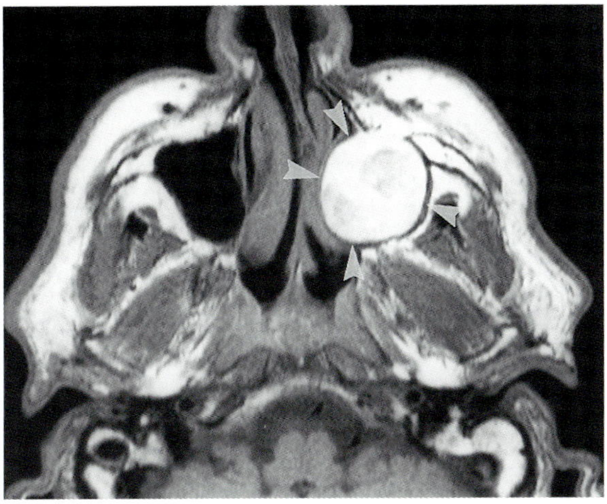

Fig. 7.**23** **Mucocele in the left maxillary sinus.** Unenhanced axial T1-weighted image demonstrates a smooth-bordered mass of very high signal intensity in the left maxillary sinus that almost completely fills the sinus and causes expansion of its posterior, lateral, and medial walls. The spherical mass is surrounded by a thick wall (arrowheads).

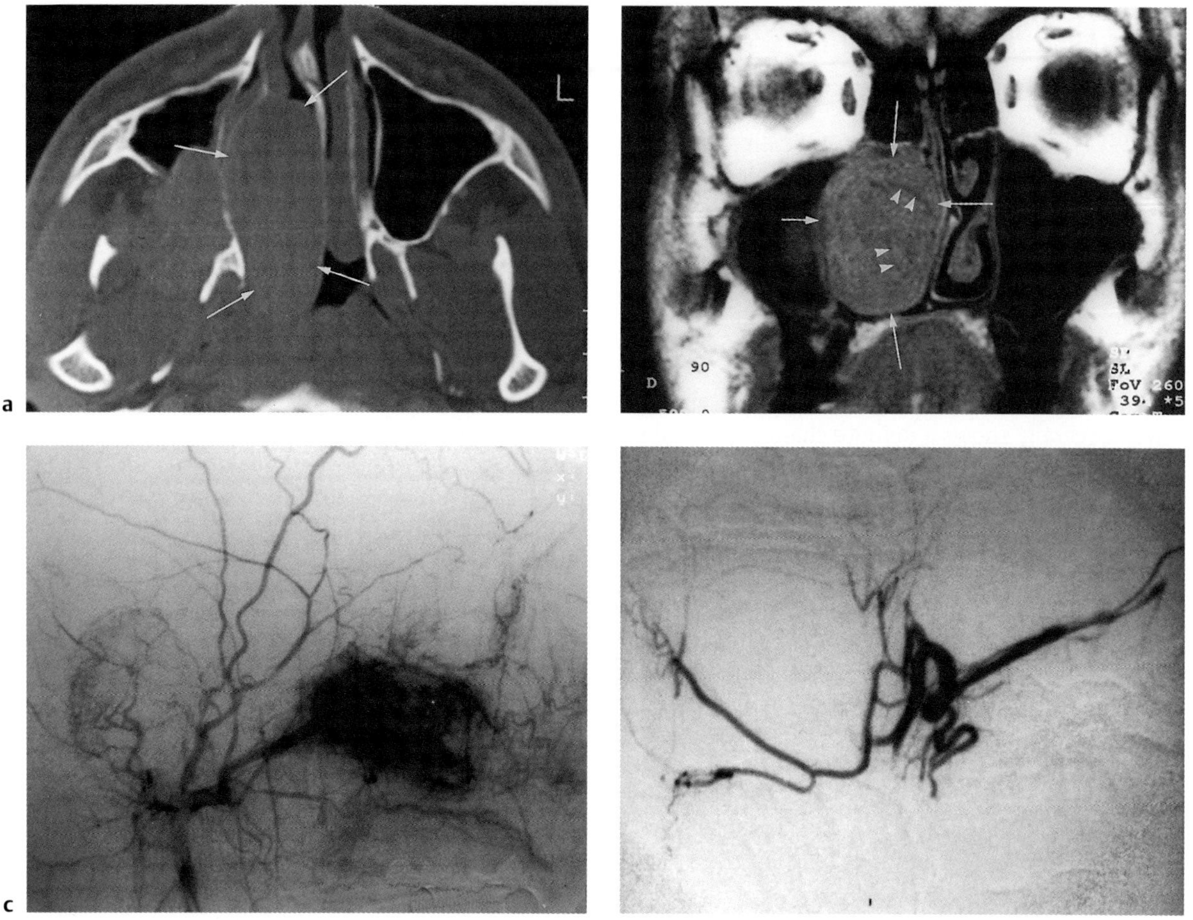

Figs. 7.**24a–d** **Angiofibroma.**
(**a**) Axial CT scan with a bone window demonstrates the mass (arrows) in the right nasal cavity displacing the lateral and medial nasal walls.
(**b**) Unenhanced T1-weighted image (TR/TE = 500/15 ms) shows the smooth-bordered mass (arrows) in the right nasal cavity. Vascular structures appear as linear signal voids (arrowheads) within the mass.
(**c**) Pre-embolization DSA defines the very rich vascular supply of the angiofibroma.
(**d**) Postembolization DSA confirms complete preoperative occlusion of the tumor-feeding vessels.

Fibrous dysplasia (Fig. 7.**21**) is a relatively common benign skeletal lesion that predominantly affects adolescents and young adults (75% of patients are under 30 years of age). Fibrous dysplasia may be clinically asymptomatic or may cause painful swelling. CT demonstrates marked thickening and sclerosis of the affected bone, which tends to show uniform density but may contain cystic regions, especially in the early, active phase of the disease. MRI demonstrates areas of marked bone expansion that appear hypointense in both T1- and T2-weighted sequences. Active cystic elements in affected bone show a mixed hypointense and hyperintense pattern in both sequences.

Circumscribed Facial Swelling

Circumscribed swelling in the facial region can be classified according to the clinical site of involvement, as in Table 7.**11**.

Bone Destruction

CT is still the best modality for making an accurate assessment of bone destruction. Intracranial infiltration by paranasal sinus tumors can be quite extensive and inaccessible to endoscopic diagnosis. The most critical sites in this regard are the bony orbital wall, the cribriform plate, the fovea ethmoidalis, the posterior wall of the ethmoid sinus, the pterygopalatine fossa, the walls of the sphenoid sinus, and the posterior wall of the frontal sinus. The presence of bone erosion in these areas should always be interpreted as signifying tumor infiltration outside the nasal cavity and paranasal sinuses (Fig. 7.**18**).

Bone destruction can also be caused by primary osseous lesions such as fibrous dysplasia (Fig. 7.**21**) and osteomyelitis (Fig. 7.**3**). Depending on the patient's history, multiple osteolytic foci should raise the possibility of multifocal metastatic invasion or an endocrine disorder such as diabetes mellitus with secondary hyperparathyroidism in patients with chronic renal disease (Fig. 7.**19**).

Table 7.**11** Circumscribed facial swelling

Involving the forehead and upper eyelid:

- Frontal sinusitis (including spread to external tissues)
- Osteomyelitis of flat cranial bones
- Mucocele and pyocele (Fig. 7.**13 a**)
- Pnemosinus dilatans
- Trauma and its sequelae (Fig. 7.**8**)
- Neurofibromatosis (Recklinghausen type) of the face
- Pierre-Marie syndrome
- Paget disease of bone
- Encephalocele (meningoencephalocele) (Fig. 7.**1 b**)
- Glioma

Involving the maxilla, cheek, and lower eyelid:

- Ethmoid and/or maxillary sinusitis (Fig. 7.**15 a**)
- Zygomaticitis
- Maxillary osteomyelitis (Fig. 7.**3**)
- Mucocele and/or pyocele of the maxillary sinus
- Fibrous dysplasia (Fig. 7.**21 a**)
- Ossifying fibroma
- Odontogenic cysts
- Xanthomas (Fig. 7.**29**)
- Benign and malignant tumors

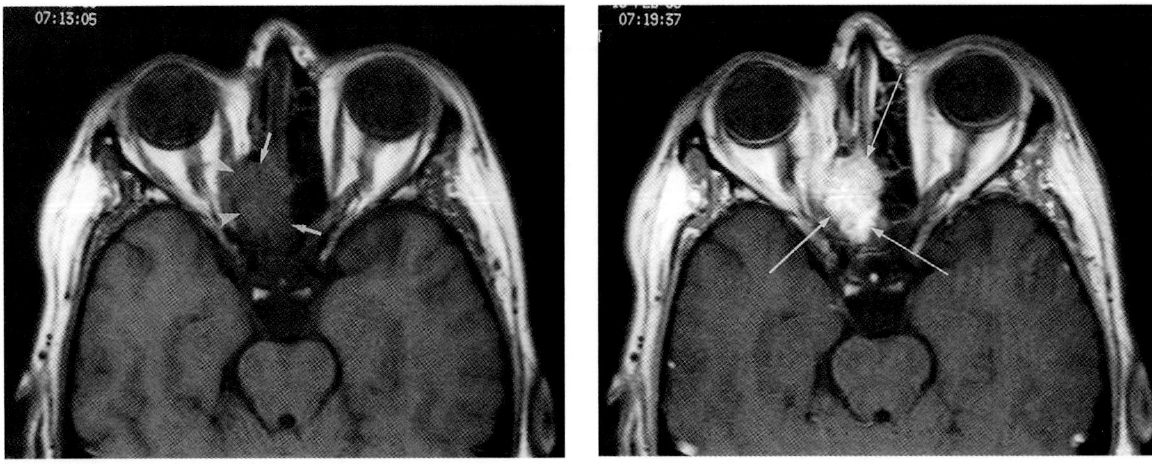

a b

Figs. 7.25 a, b **Adenoid cystic carcinoma.**
(**a**) Unenhanced axial T1-weighted image (TR/TE = 700/15 ms) documents an adenoid cystic carcinoma (arrows) in the right ethmoid sinus with erosion of the medial orbital wall (arrowheads).

(**b**) Contrast-enhanced axial T1-weighted image (TR/TE = 700/15 ms) shows intense enhancement of the adenoid cystic carcinoma (arrows) in the right ethmoid sinus. The mass contains no discernible linear hypointense structures.

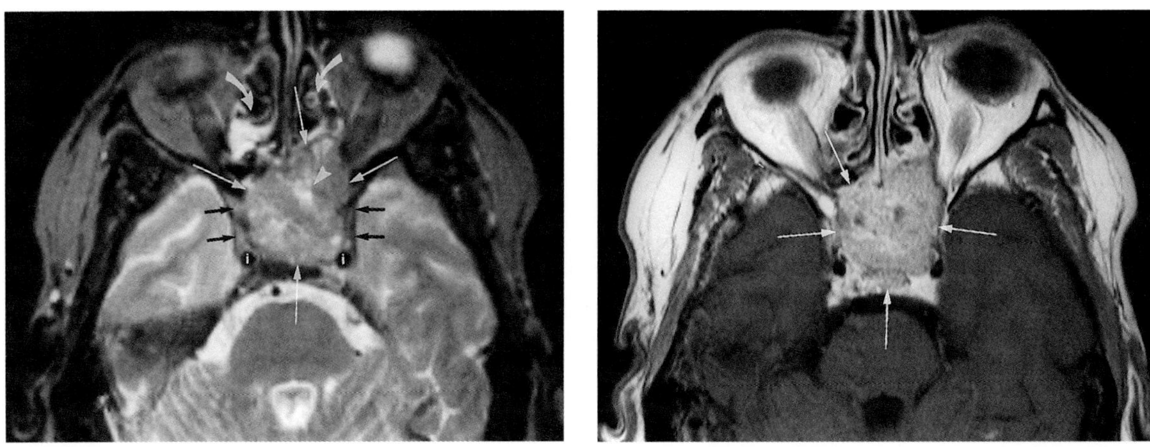

a b

Figs. 7.26 a, b **Lymphoepithelial carcinoma.**
(**a**) Unenhanced T2-weighted image (TR/TE = 2500/90 ms) depicts the mass (arrows) and its relation to the cavernous sinus. The tumor shows a nonhomogeneous internal structure with small necrotic areas (arrowhead) of increased signal intensity. Inflammatory changes are visible in the ethmoid sinus on both sides (curved arrows).
i Internal carotid artery

(**b**) T1-weighted image after the administration of 0.1 mmol/kg bw Gd-DTPA (TR/TE = 700/15 ms) shows marked enhancement of the mass (arrows). The small necrotic areas appear hypointense.

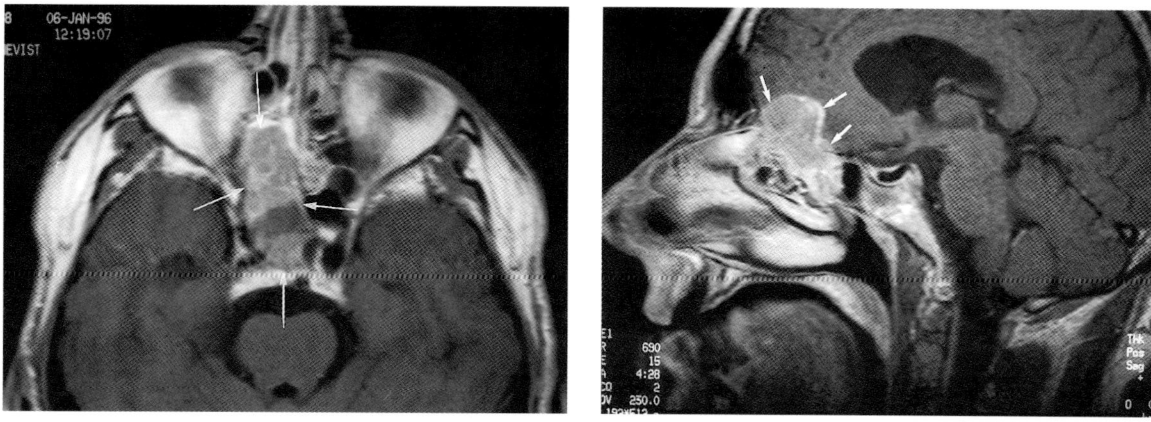

a b

Figs. 7.**27 a, b** **Recurrence of esthesioneuroblastoma.**
(**a**) Contrast-enhanced axial T1-weighted image (TR/TE = 700/15 ms) shows a nonhomogeneous enhancing mass (arrows) in the region of the right ethmoid sinus.

(**b**) Contrast-enhanced sagittal T1-weighted image documents infiltration of the anterior skull base by the esthesioneuroblastoma (arrows).

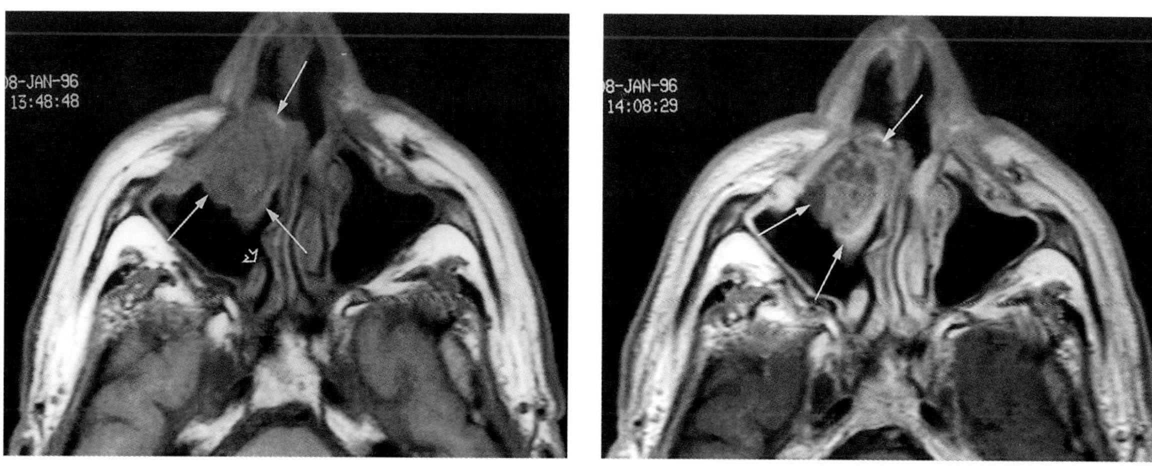

a b

Figs. 7.**28 a, b** **Papilloma of the right maxillary sinus.**
(**a**) Unenhanced T1-weighted image (TR/TE = 700/15 ms) demonstrates a recurrent papilloma (arrows) in the right maxillary sinus. A postoperative turbinectomy remnant is visible in the nasal cavity (open arrow). The mucosa in both maxillary sinuses appears thickened due to an accompanying inflammatory reaction.

(**b**) T1-weighted image after the administration of 0.1 mmol/kg bw Gd-DTPA (TR/TE = 700/15 ms) shows nonhomogeneous enhancement of the papilloma (arrows) with a laminar pattern of hyperintense and hypointense zones. This enhancement pattern is very similar to that seen in inverted papillomas.

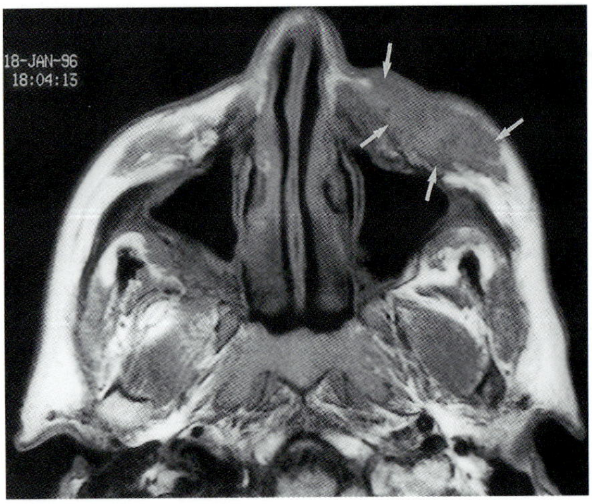

Fig. 7.**29** **Fibroxanthoma.** Unenhanced axial T1-weighted image (TR/TE = 700/15 ms) demonstrates a subcutaneous mass that is isointense to muscle tissue (arrows). The mass showed marked homogeneous enhancement after the administration of contrast medium.

Summary and Diagnostic Strategy

There are situations in which CT or MRI should supplement the clinical examination in differential diagnostic evaluations of the paranasal sinuses. In patients with chronic sinusitis, CT should be used preoperatively to evaluate the status of bony sinus structures. In patients with a questionable tumor mass, a special MR imaging protocol should be performed as part of the primary workup. The CT evaluation of a tumor mass is best accomplished with coronal scans using a 2-mm slice thickness. The MR examination should start with axial T2- and T1-weighted sequences, followed by Gd-enhanced T1-weighted sequences in the axial and coronal planes. Coronal T1-weighted fat-suppression sequences may then be added to check for possible orbital involvement. Key morphologic criteria for the radiologic differentiation of benign and malignant masses are the location of the mass and the presence or absence of bone destruction. If images show simple mucosal swelling without bone destruction and without suspicious calcification patterns within the mass, the lesion may be considered to be a benign inflammatory reaction and treated accordingly. A solid enhancing lesion, especially when extensive, should be biopsied so that a preoperative histologic diagnosis can be established and adequate preoperative chemotherapy can be provided to reduce the extent of the resection and improve the postoperative prognosis.

References

1 Alvarez, I., C. Suarez, J. P. Rodrigo, F. Nunez, M. J. Caminero: Prognostic factors in paranasal sinus cancer. Am J Otolaryngol. 16 (1995) 109 - 114
2 Ataman, M., K. Ayas, B. Gursel: Giant osteoma of the frontal sinus. Rhinology 31 (1993) 185 - 187
3 Cannon, C. R., B. McCay, J. R. Haltom: Paranasal sinus development in children and its relationship to sinusitis. J Miss State Med Assoc. 36 (1995) 40 - 43
4 Ferguson, B. J.: Fibrous dysplasia of the paranasal sinuses. Am J Otolaryngol. 15 (1994) 227 - 230
5 Hasso, A. N., D. Lambert: Magnetic Resonance Imaging of the paranasal sinuses and nasal cavities. Top Magn Reson Imaging 6 (1994) 209 - 223
6 Hesselink, J. R., P. F. J. New, K. R. Davis et al.: Computed Tomography of the paranasal sinuses and face II: pathological anatomy. J Comput Assist Tomogr. 2 (1978) 568 - 576
7 Kingdom, T. T., M. J. Kaplan: Mucosal melanoma of the nasal cavity and paranasal sinuses. Head Neck Surg. 17 (1995) 184 - 189
8 Naguib, M. T., J. M. Byers. L. N. Slater: Paranasal sinus infection due to atypical mycobacteria in two patients with AIDS. Clin Infect Dis. 19 (1994) 789 - 791
9 Saeed, S. R., G. B. Brookes: Aspergillosis of the paranasal sinuses. Rhinology 33 (1995) 46 - 51
10 Sercarz, J. A., R. J. Mark, L. Tran, I. Storper, T. C. Calcaterra: Sarcomas of the nasal cavity and paranasal sinuses. Ann Otol. 103 (1994) 699 - 704
11 Shapiro, M. D., P. M. Som: MRI of the paranasal sinuses and nasal cavity. Radiol Clin North Am 27 (1989) 447 - 475
12 Weissman, J. L., H. D. Curtin, D. E. Eibling: Double mucocele of the paranasal sinuses. AJNR 15 (1994) 1263 - 1264
13 Woodruff, W. W., D. P. Vrabec: Inverted papilloma of the nasal vault and paranasal sinuses: spectrum of CT findings. AJR 162 (1994) 419 - 423
14 Yousem, D. M.: Imaging of sinonasal inflammatory disease. Radiology 188 (1993) 303 - 314

8 The Orbit

Before the advent of modern sectional imaging techniques, only limited means were available for examining the orbit and its contents, the orbital nerve, and the optic chiasm. In particular, modern sectional imaging has greatly facilitated the accurate differentiation of neurovascular structures and the intraorbital muscles.

While conventional radiographs are useful for demonstrating bony structures and traumatic orbital lesions, often they cannot detect a neoplastic or inflammatory lesion or accurately define its extension into adjacent soft tissues.

Ultrasonography of the orbital region is a noninvasive modality that can detect lesions of the globe and its anterior segment, but it cannot adequately visualize the posterior part of the orbit or osseous structures.

Conventional angiography and venography of the orbital region still have a role in the diagnosis of arteriovenous malformations and arteriovenous fistulas. Even these lesions, though, are increasingly being evaluated with specialized techniques of computed tomography (CT) and magnetic resonance imaging (MRI).

The use of CT in orbital investigations is based on the increasing, widespread availability of this modality and on improvements in data acquisition and image postprocessing, including thin-slice scanning and multiplanar reconstructions. Even modern CT scanners, however, are susceptible to partial-volume artifacts and may deliver a significant radiation dose to the lens.

Meanwhile, advances in MR technology have influenced the use of this modality in diseases of the orbit, and today MRI has become the method of choice for the diagnosis or orbital lesions. The introduction of fast, high-resolution multiplanar sequences and the development of high-definition orbital surface coils have expanded the indications for MRI while greatly increasing its sensitivity and specificity.

Normal Anatomy

In this section we shall briefly review the essential anatomic features of the orbit before proceeding to individual symptoms and lesions of the orbital region and establishing criteria for differential diagnosis.

Globe

The globe, consisting of the *lens*, *vitreous body*, *retina*, *uvea*, and *sclera*, can be imaged by high-resolution CT and MRI, but only high-resolution axial and sagittal MR images acquired with a special surface coil can accurately differentiate the various components of the eye. The lens, composed of approximately two-thirds water and one-third protein, shows an intermediate signal intensity on T1-weighted MR images and is surrounded by the hypointense ocular chambers and vitreous body. These signal intensities are reversed on T2-weighted images, the ocular chambers and vitreous body displaying high signal intensity because of their high water content (98.5%).

The sclera appears hypointense in all MR sequences, but lesions of the sclera are best appreciated on T2-weighted images. The choroid and retina show a high T1-weighted signal intensity and an intermediate T2-weighted signal intensity.

Orbital Nerves

The *ophthalmic nerve* (cranial nerve VI) and its branches (the lacrimal, frontal, and nasociliary nerves) run from the trigeminal ganglion through the superior orbital fissure into the orbit.

The frontal branch of the ophthalmic nerve can be identified as a hyperintense structure on coronal T1-weighted images. The oculomotor nerve (cranial nerve III), which also traverses the superior orbital fissure, innervates all the extraocular muscles but the superior oblique and lateral rectus, so it is chiefly responsible for ocular movements.

The *trochlear nerve* (cranial nerve IV) also passes through the superior orbital fissure, supplying motor innervation to the superior oblique muscle.

The *abducens nerve* (cranial nerve VI) supplies only the lateral rectus muscle and accompanies the superior ophthalmic vein through the superior orbital fissure.

The *optic nerve* (cranial nerve II), an extension of the cerebral white matter, is enclosed in three meningeal sheaths and, at the back of the globe, by the sclera. The nerve runs backward and medially in a sinuous course to the orbital apex and accompanies the ophthalmic artery through the optic foramen to the middle skull base, where it joins the optic chiasm. MRI is superior to CT for defining the intracanalicular and prechiasmatic segments of the optic nerve.

The signal intensity of the optic nerve is similar to that of the normal cerebral white matter in T1- and T2-weighted sequences. The sharp hypointense bands often seen accompanying the optic nerve are chemical-shift artifacts.

The optic chiasm is usually delineated best in sagittal or coronal T1-weighted sequences. Like the nerve, it displays a high signal intensity equivalent to that of normal cerebral white matter.

Lesions at the level of the optic chiasm present clinically with bitemporal hemianopsia or heteronymous visual field defects. Postchiasmatic nerve lesions typically cause homonymous hemianopsia due to the decussation of the fibers in the chiasm.

Orbital Vessels

The *superior ophthalmic vein* is the largest and most easily visualized of the orbital vessels. It takes a tortuous course from the trochlea to the orbital apex, passes through the superior orbital fissure, and drains into the cavernous sinus through supraorbital veins.

The ophthalmic artery arises from the internal carotid artery and courses with the optic nerve through the optic canal. The nerve usually appears cranial to the vessel on imaging studies.

Muscles and Orbital Fat

Eye movements are coordinated by six extraocular skeletal muscles. The *superior, inferior, lateral* and *medial rectus muscles* originate from an annular ligament called the common tendinous ring (anulus of Zinn). The *inferior oblique* is the only extraocular muscle that arises not from the orbital apex but from the orbital floor near the nasolacrimal duct. The largest of the six extraocular muscles, the *superior oblique*, is supplied by the trochlear nerve; the *lateral rectus* is supplied by the abducens nerve, and the remaining four muscles by the oculomotor nerve. All the extraocular muscles are clearly depicted on T1-weighted MR images owing to their low signal intensity relative to the surrounding fat. Coronal and parasagittal images can further differentiate the superior rectus and levator palpebrae muscles.

Lacrimal Gland

Depending on the amount of fat between the individual lobules, the lacrimal gland appears on MRI as a nonhomogeneous structure of moderate signal intensity in T1- and T2-weighted spin-echo (SE) sequences. Axial images best demonstrate the gland, which lies in the lacrimal fossa superolateral to the anterior orbit

Bony Boundaries of the Orbit

The roof of the orbit is formed by the *frontal bone* and the *lesser sphenoid wing*. The lateral orbital wall is formed by the *zygoma* and the *greater sphenoid wing*. The floor is comprised of the *maxilla* and the *orbital process* of the *palatine bone*, and the medial wall is formed chiefly by portions of the *ethmoid bone* and *lacrimal bone*. Radiologically important communications between the orbit and cranial cavity include the *superior orbital fissure*, the *optic canal*, and the *inferior orbital fissure*, which is connected by an anterior sulcus with the *infraorbital foramen*. The orbit contains the *globe, retrobulbar fat, extraocular muscles, lacrimal gland*, and *optic nerve* with accompanying orbital nerves and vessels. The principal fibers of the optic nerve pass from the back of the globe through the optic canal to the optic chiasm, where the nerve fibers from the nasal half of each retina cross the median plane and enter the optic tract of the opposite side.

Clinical Signs and Symptoms

The orbit is an anatomic crossroads for several medical specialties, so interdisciplinary teamwork is needed in the diagnosis and treatment of orbital disease. The evaluation of an orbital lesion requires an accurate clinical examination of the affected eye, and ultrasound must often be used as the primary imaging modality. Conventional radiographs and modern sectional imaging procedures are generally reserved for cases with a suspected primary or secondary mass lesion of the orbit.

The main clinical symptoms of a soft-tissue mass, trauma, or inflammatory disease of the orbital region are as follows:

- Displacement of the globe: protrusion, exophthalmos, enophthalmos.
- Changes in the globe: congestion of orbital veins, globe compression, optic nerve compression.
- Limitation of eye movements in one or all directions.
- Pupillary lesion: absence of light reaction (absolute or amaurotic).
- Vitreous changes: leukokoria (Table 8.**1**).

Table 8.1 Differential diagnosis of leukokoria

Lesion	Morphology
Retinoblastoma	Contrast enhancement, often bilateral, calcifications, low signal intensity in T1- and T2-weighted sequences
Coats disease	No contrast enhancement, unilateral, intermediate T1-weighted signal intensity, high T2-weighted signal intensity, complete retinal detachment
Older subretinal hemorrhage	Signal depends on age of collection; high T1- and T2-weighted signal intensity
Retinopathy of prematurity (retrolental fibroplasia)	Ophthalmoscopic features
Endophthalmitis	Laboratory findings (ELISA*), unilateral microphthalmia, occasional contrast enhancement

* Enzyme-linked immunosorbent assay

- Changes in the optic fundus: retinal detachment, papilledema.

Imaging Evaluation and Differential Diagnosis

Conventional Radiography

Skull radiographs in the anteroposterior (AP) and lateral projections can delineate the bony boundaries of the orbit. The occipitomeatal projection of the paranasal sinuses is often more rewarding, particularly for evaluating the orbital floor. The technical parameters are like those described for conventional X-ray films in Chapters 3 and 4. The following special views may be indicated in selected cases:

Oblique Rhese Projection

This projection is used to evaluate the posterior part of the orbit and optic canal. Bilateral films are taken to allow for right–left comparison. The patient is positioned prone with the head turned 50° toward the examined side and resting on the nose and zygoma.

Dacryocystography

In this study a water-soluble contrast medium is instilled into the lacrimal apparatus to reveal sites of stenosis, occlusion, or ectasia in the lacrimal sac and duct. It also yields information on the condition of the lacrimal sac. Usually the study is performed during the inflow phase using a subtraction technique, much as in digital subtraction angiography (DSA), and is often followed by intraluminal balloon dilatation of the lacrimal duct (dacryocystoplasty) for treatment of epiphoria.

Computed Tomography (CT)

CT scans can clearly demonstrate the bony orbital structures, the extraocular muscles, the globe, and the retrobulbar fat, provided the slice thickness does not exceed 2 mm. CT is also excellent for detecting and locating intraorbital foreign bodies. CT accurately portrays all structures of the orbit and is particularly useful after trauma. Besides axial scans for evaluating the lamina papyracea, scans in the coronal plane are often performed to evaluate the orbital floor. Even a complete CT examination of the orbit delivers a radiation dose (3.2 cGy) to the lens that is far below the cataractogenic threshold (150 cGy).

Magnetic Resonance Imaging (MRI)

When MRI is performed with a special eye coil and thin slices (less than 3 mm), the orbit can be evaluated in all three planes with no radiation exposure. The high soft-tissue contrast in T1- and T2-weighted sequences makes MRI excellent for diagnosing intrabulbar and extrabulbar inflammations and tumors, evaluating the optic nerve and extraocular muscles, and defining the intracranial optic chiasm. A combination of fat suppression and contrast enhancement is optimum for evaluating the fatty retrobulbar space.

The MR examination may be performed with a head coil or a special surface coil placed over one or both eyes, depending on the nature of the inquiry. The "penetration depth" of this study correlates directly with coil diameter. While the various types of surface coil provide a better signal-to-noise ratio and higher resolution, they are more susceptible than head coils to motion artifacts. The head coil is also better for evaluating deeply placed anatomic structures in both eyes and the optic chiasm.

The effect of motion artifacts can be minimized by keeping the imaging time as short as possible, for example by using short TR times of 500–700 ms and one or two acquisitions with a 256 x 256 or 512 x 256 matrix. Spatial resolution can be increased by using a slice thickness of 3 – 5 mm and a 150- to 190-mm field of view. T2-weighted images are usually obtained with a long TR of approximately 2000 ms and a long TE of 90/22 ms using double-echo technique. Alternatively, a T2-weighted turbo spin-echo (TSE) sequence may be performed when a head coil is used.

With axial MR imaging, both eyes can be directly compared on the same image and correlated with CT findings. Axial images may have to be supplemented by coronal, sagittal, or parasagittal scans so that the extent of a lesion can be more accurately assessed.

The use of gradient-echo sequences with TR/TE = 300 to 500/15 ms and a variable flip angle may yield additional information in evaluations of various vascular abnormalities such as capillary hemangiomas and orbital varices. This technique can also demonstrate the T2 effect of calcifications and aid in the diagnosis of retinoblastoma.

Ultrasound

Intrabulbar lesions, especially neoplasms, can be diagnosed by standard ultrasound techniques like those used in ophthalmology. Usually a standard A-scan is obtained in conjunction with a contact B-scan, and Doppler techniques may be used for flow investigations.

Diagnostic Angiography and Interventional Procedures

Arteriographic or venographic imaging of the orbital vessels is rarely indicated but may be used to define angiomatous lesions or venous varices. Selective subtraction angiography of the external carotid artery is usually sufficient, but the internal carotid artery may also be visualized in suspected cases of carotid-cavernous fistula. If a fistula is confirmed, it can be obliterated in the same sitting by transcatheter embolization (coils, balloons). Some cases may require fluorescein angiography to investigate the flow dynamics of the fundic vessels and the perfusion of structures that the vessels supply.

Imaging Findings

The following sections deal with the morphologic imaging features of the principal types of orbital lesion, regardless of their site of origin.

Congenital Variations, Malformations, and Congenital Lesions

The orbital region is subject to *congenital hypoplasia* or *aplasia* and primary congenital lesions such as *Coats disease* and *retinoblastoma* as well as manifestations of other hereditary disorders. Among the most important hereditary diseases that show primary involvement of the facial skeleton and orbit are *hemangioblastoma* and *lymphangioma*.

The phakomatoses also present with orbital manifestations. *Neurofibromatosis* and *Hippe–Lindau syndrome* in particular are associated with optic nerve gliomas, orbital neurofibromas, and hemangioblastomas.

Dermoids (Fig. 8.**1**)

In cases where imaging documents a dermoid near the frontozygomatic suture, it cannot always be determined whether a mass in the lacrimal fossa has arisen from the lacrimal gland or from a subperiosteal or extraconal origin. Dermoids are also known to occur in the eyelids.

Most dermoid tumors have a fatty consistency that produces negative attenuation values on CT scans and is predominantly hyperintense on T1-weighted MR images. Occasionally, especially after rupture, the lesion appears as a soft-tissue mass showing higher CT density and low T1-weighted signal intensity.

Coats Disease

A typical ocular manifestation of fully established Coats disease is *leukokoria*. In some advanced cases, imaging should be performed to exclude a *retinoblastoma*. The incidence is biphasic, showing a peak at approximately 10 years of age and between 40 and 60 years of age; males are more commonly affected. The pathophysiology of the syndrome is based on a loss of pericytes and endothelial cells in the retinal vessels, with leakage of a cholesterol-rich exudate leading to retinal detachment.

Generally the disease is in an advanced stage at the time of radiologic diagnosis. Both CT and MRI can demonstrate the exudative retinal detachment.

CT shows a hyperdense, often nonhomogeneous mass completely filling the subretinal space. On MRI, the subretinal space appears hyperintense in

T1- and T2-weighted sequences. Both modalities can document the V-shaped retinal detachment and lack of contrast enhancement that are characteristic of Coats disease. In cases with long-standing retinal detachment, CT and MRI typically show unilateral heterogeneous changes due to the presence of hemorrhagic elements and cholesterol in the subretinal fluid.

The main lesion to be considered in the differential diagnosis is retinoblastoma, which is distinguished from Coats disease by the presence of calcifications on CT and by its predominantly low signal intensity on T2-weighted MR images. The most important differentiating criterion, however, is the absence of contrast enhancement in Coats disease.

Optic Nerve Glioma

Optic nerve glioma may be *unilateral* or *bilateral*. The bilateral form is relatively common in patients with *neurofibromatosis type I* (Recklinghausen disease), and up to 50% of patients with optic nerve glioma have neurofibromatosis type I. The clinical approach depends on the location and extent of the tumor, and purely intraorbital lesions should be differentiated from tumors showing intracanalicular or intracranial extension or tumors that involve the optic chiasm.

Optic nerve glioma is manifested earlier in patients with neurofibromatosis than in patients with the sporadic form, and clinical symptoms may appear during the first 10 years of life. The clinical course may span several decades.

Histologically, optic nerve glioma is composed chiefly of astrocytes and less commonly of oligodendrocytes. The pattern of tumor growth appears to be determined by the presence or absence of an association with neurofibromatosis.

In patients who have neurofibromatosis, the tumor tends to show a circumferential, perineural pattern of spread, growing predominantly in the subarachnoid space and leaving the optic nerve largely intact. In patients who do not have neurofibromatosis, the tumor tends to show a diffuse, infiltrative type of growth that causes optic nerve expansion. MRI can differentiate these two forms in individual cases.

If intracranial extension has occurred, the Rhese film will demonstrate enlargement of the optic canal. Expansion of the optic foramen is more common with optic nerve glioma than with optic-nerve-sheath meningioma, although dysplasia of the sphenoid wing in neurofibromatosis patients can simulate an expanded foramen. The lateral skull film or special views can show erosion of the anterior clinoid process or prechiasmatic sulcus.

On CT scans, optic nerve glioma appears as a homogeneous expansion of the optic nerve to more than 5 mm in diameter. The optic nerve segment surrounded by tumor is not demarcated as a separate structure. A significant percentage of optic nerve gliomas shows contrast enhancement, but generally this will not differentiate tumor from nerve. Contrast administration is useful for defining necrotic areas and cystic components.

MRI of the intraorbital form demonstrates a homogeneous fusiform, eccentric, or tubular expansion of the optic nerve. The tumor is isointense to the normal optic nerve or cerebral white matter on T1-weighted images and is usually hyperintense on T2-weighted images. It shows marked contrast enhancement and, unlike optic sheath meningioma, is not demarcated from the optic nerve by the relatively low signal intensity of the nerve.

MRI is usually better than CT for diagnosing intracanalicular extension, since MRI visualization of the optic canal is not hampered by beam-hardening artifacts. With a tumor that shows minimal contrast enhancement, however, the intracanalicular component is difficult to appreciate even with MRI. It may be helpful in these cases to correlate MR findings with a conventional Rhese radiograph.

Chiasmal involvement is manifested by expansion of the chiasm, which is easily recognized in unilateral cases by a right–left comparison. Contrast enhancement, if present, is helpful in cases of bilateral involvement.

Neurofibroma

The form of neurofibroma that occurs outside Recklinghausen disease is typically located in the extraconal compartment. The tumor is encapsulated, so its borders are smooth (Fig. 8.**3**). The lesions are usually multiple and have a tendency to invade the cranial cavity through the superior orbital fissure (Fig. 8.**4**).

Conventional radiographs show an increase in the volume of the affected orbit.

On CT scans, neurofibromas are approximately isodense to brain tissue and are well demarcated by their smooth borders.

An inflammatory pseudotumor is mainly distinguished from neurofibroma by its intraconal site of occurrence.

The specific morphologic criteria for neurofibroma and its appearance on CT and MRI were covered in Chapter 4.

Hemangioblastoma

Hemangioblastoma is an uncommon central nervous system (CNS) tumor that predominantly involves the posterior cranial fossa. The *multifocal* form in particular has an association with *Hippel–Lindau syndrome* of the phakomatosis group. Ocular involvement in Hippel–Lindau disease consists of retinal angiomas, which coexist with hemangioblastomas in other or-

Figs. 8.**1 a–d** **Dermoid of the right eye.**
(**a**) Unenhanced axial T2-weighted SE sequence (TR/TE = 3000/90 ms) shows a predominantly hypointense mass with scalloped borders (arrow) displacing the globe on the right side.
(**b**) Unenhanced axial T1-weighted SE sequence (TR/TE = 700/15 ms) shows a well-circumscribed, uniformly hyperintense mass (arrow) displacing the medial rectus muscle (arrowheads).
(**c**) Gd-enhanced sagittal SE sequence (TR/TE = 700/15 ms) shows downward displacement of the globe (arrow) and optic nerve (curved arrow) by the moderately enhancing tumor with no signs of invasion.
(**d**) Gd-enhanced coronal SE sequence (TR/TE = 700/15 ms) through the posterior part of the orbits shows retrobulbar displacement and deformation of the superior rectus muscle (arrow). There is no sign of muscle invasion by the tumor.

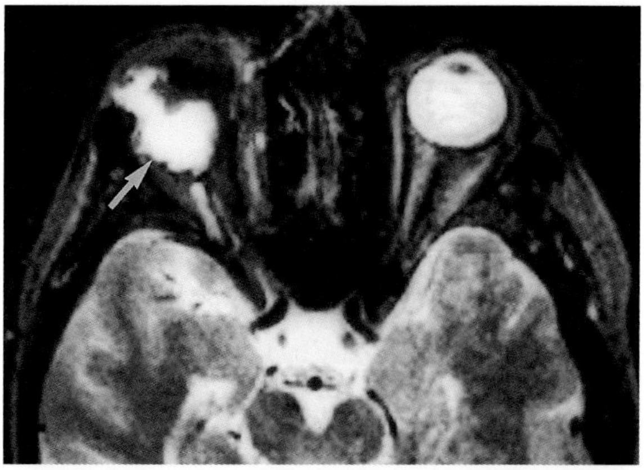
a

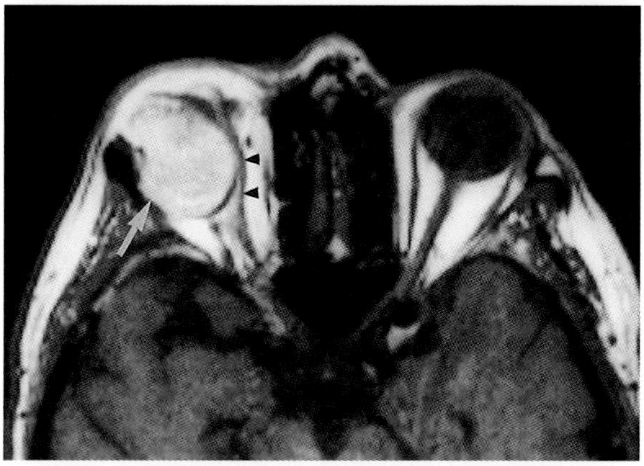
b

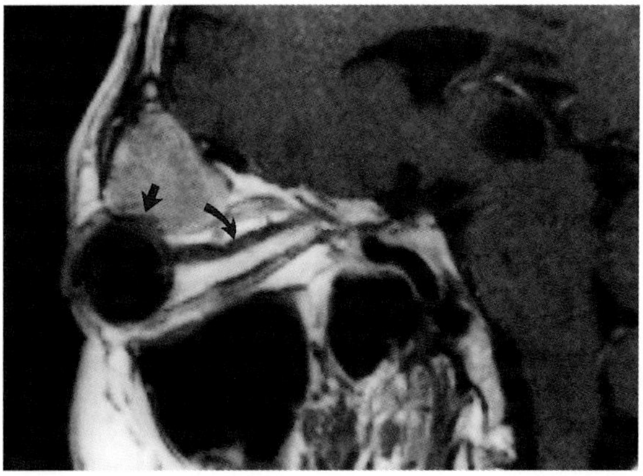
c

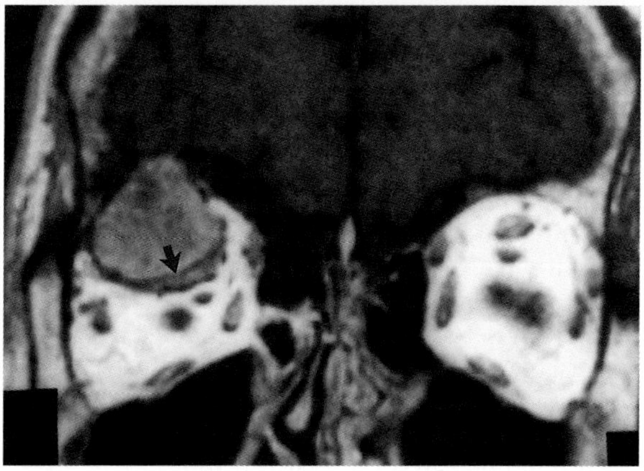
d

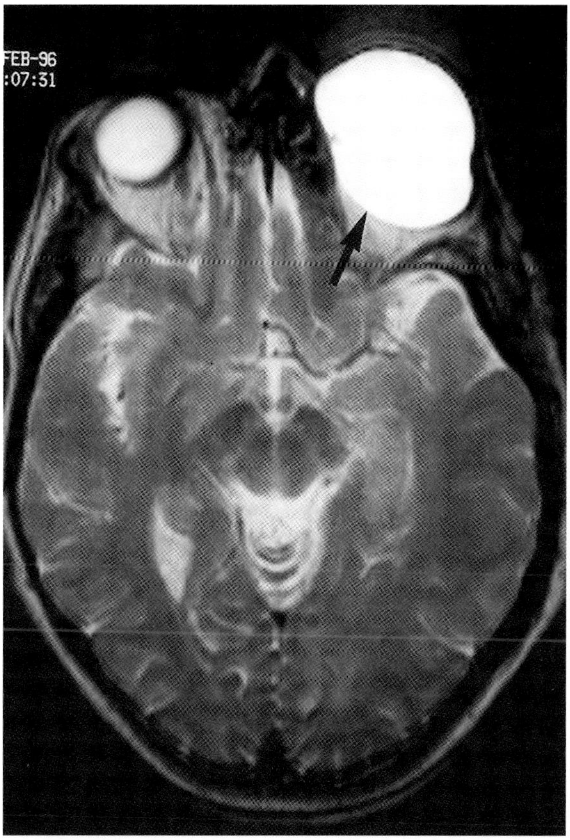

a

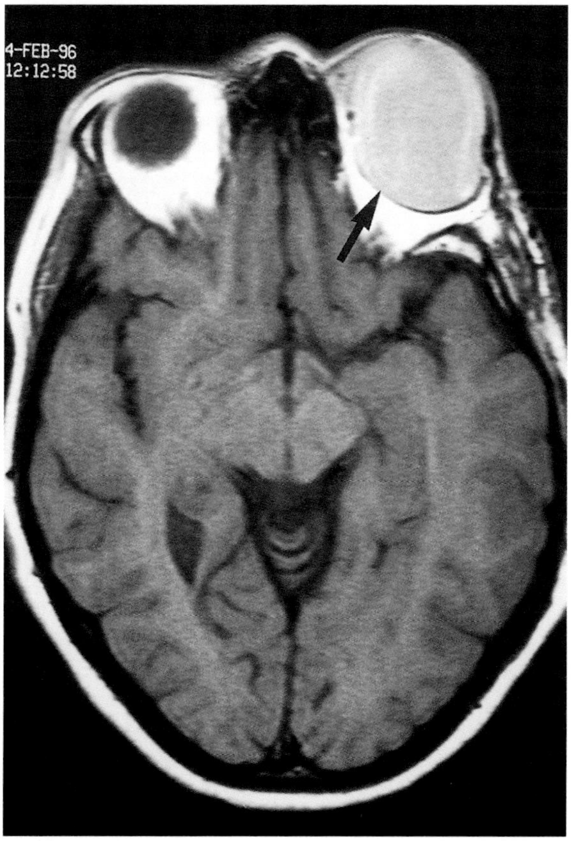

b

Figs. 8.**2 a, b** **Ocular prosthesis.**
(**a**) Unenhanced axial T2-weighted SE sequence (TR/TE = 3000/90 ms) shows a homogeneous mass of very high signal intensity (arrow) occupying the left orbit. Besides an inflammatory or neoplastic fluid collection, the differential diagnosis should include an ocular prosthesis.
(**b**) Unenhanced axial T1-weighted SE sequence (TR/TE = 700/15 ms) also depicts the silicone prosthesis as a hyperintense mass (arrow).

gans. Isolated cases of optic nerve hemangioblastoma have also been documented.

Approximately 30% of hemangioblastomas are *solid, cystic,* or purely cystic lesions with mural nodules. Calcifications are unusual.

On CT, the cystic form appears as a well-circumscribed mass of central fluid attenuation, while the solid form is isodense to cerebral white matter. Following contrast administration, lesions with *mural nodules* show homogeneous enhancement of the nodules while the solid form shows intense, homogeneous enhancement.

MRI is superior to CT for demonstrating the full spectrum of tumor morphology. Thus, T1- and T2-weighted images can define hemorrhagic areas, cysts, and angiomatous vessels within the hemangioblastoma and can identify the feeding and draining vessels.

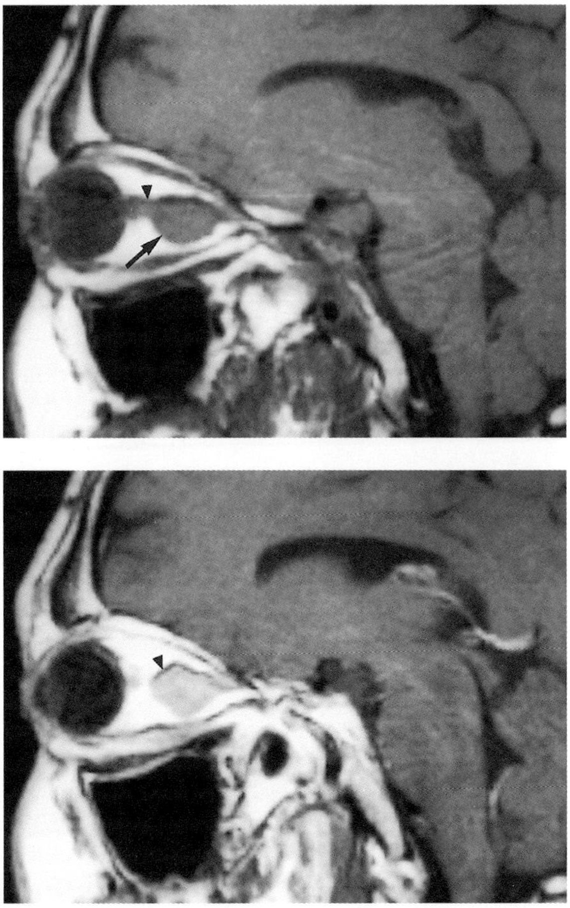

Figs. 8.**3 a, b** **Neurofibroma of the optic nerve.**
(**a**) Unenhanced sagittal T1-weighted SE sequence (TR/TE = 700/15 ms) shows a well-circumscribed, uniformly isointense mass (arrow) that arises from the optic nerve (arrowhead) from which it is not demarcated.
(**b**) Gd-enhanced sagittal SE sequence (TR/TE = 700/15 ms) shows intense, uniform enhancement of the neuroma. The dark band at the top of the lesion is a chemical-shift artifact (arrowhead).

Tumors

Tumors of the optic nerve and its sheath can be classified by their location as *bulbar, intraconal,* or *extraconal. Malignant intrabulbar tumors* include retinal melanoma, retinoblastoma, and other epithelial and mesenchymal neoplasms. *Benign intrabulbar tumors* are rare except for hemangioma. *Primary intraorbital tumors* include optic-nerve-sheath meningioma and pilocytic astrocytoma. Tumors that invade the orbit *secondarily* include paranasal sinuses tumors, meningioma (Fig. 8.**9**), and esthesioneuroblastoma. The globe and orbit are also subject to involvement by *metastases*, and any of the foregoing primary tumors may involve the extraorbital optic nerve as far as the optic chiasm. In most cases a histologic diagnosis cannot be made from radiologic findings alone, but CT and MRI are still essential for demonstrating morphology, extent, and associated changes.

Melanoma

Uveal melanoma is the most common primary ocular neoplasm in adults, with a peak incidence between 50 and 70 years of age. Melanomas may occur in all three components of the uvea: the choroid, ciliary body, and iris. The choroid is most commonly affected, followed by the ciliary body.

Melanoma is frequently associated with retinal detachment and is difficult to diagnose by CT. MRI, however, can accurately diagnose this tumor by its signal intensity on T1- and T2-weighted images and its enhancement after the administration of gadolinium (Gd)-DTPA (Fig. 8.**5**). The signal intensity of the lesion depends on its melanin content. The rule of thumb is that the higher the melanin content of a lesion, the lower its MRI signal intensity. Melanoma is predominantly hypointense on T2-weighted images and is moderately intense to hyperintense on T1-weighted images.

The differential diagnosis includes angiomas of the choroid and retina (e.g., in the setting of Hippel–Lindau syndrome), hamartomas, medulloepithelioma, hemangioma, and metastases.

The emphasis in modern sectional imaging, besides differentiating melanoma from other lesions, is on accurately determining the size of the tumor and the extent of tumor invasion.

On noncontrast CT scans, melanoma is hyperdense to the vitreous, usually has a broad base, and presents a biconvex elliptical, round, or discoid shape, generally with well-defined margins. On postcontrast CT, melanoma shows rapid enhancement followed by a gradual fading of intensity. Its attenuation

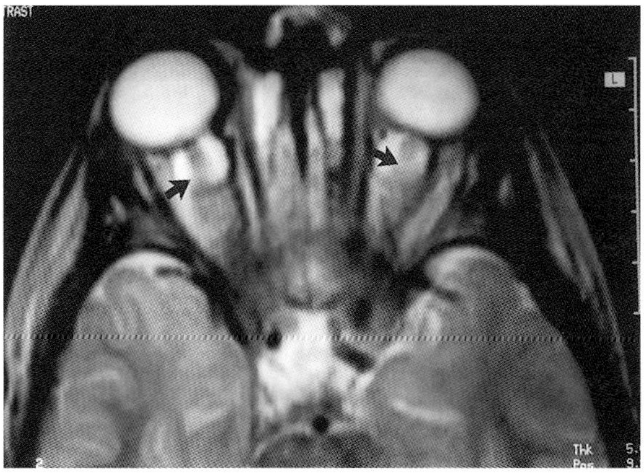

a

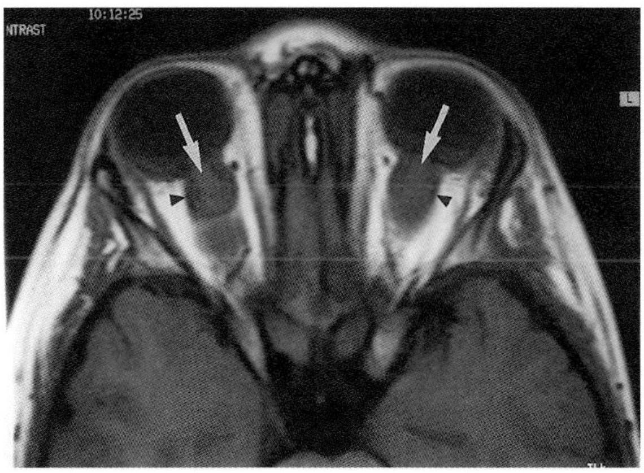

b

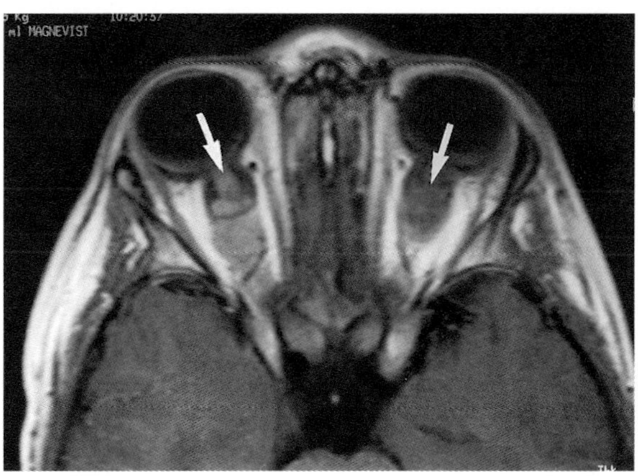

c

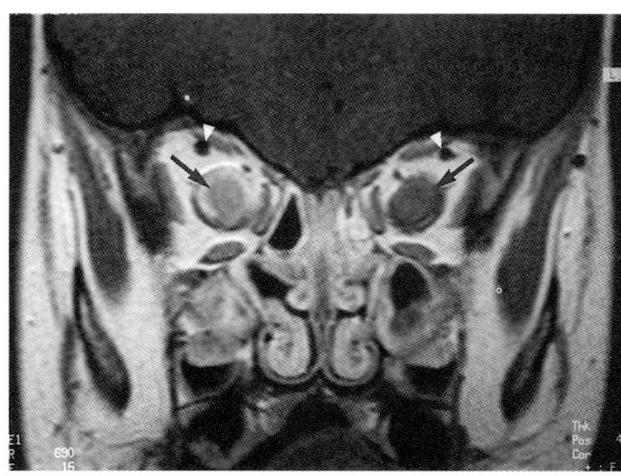

d

Figs. 8.**4 a–d** **Bilateral optic neuroma.**
(**a**) Unenhanced axial T2-weighted SE sequence (TR/TE = 3000/90 ms) shows nonhomogeneously isointense expansion of both optic nerves (arrows) with adjacent expansion of the subarachnoid space.
(**b**) Unenhanced axial T1-weighted SE sequence (TR/TE = 700/15 ms) shows isointense expansion of the optic nerves (arrows) with hypointense expansion of the subarachnoid space (arrowheads).
(**c**) Gd-enhanced axial SE sequence (TR/TE = 700/15 ms) documents moderate to intense enhancement of the optic nerves (arrows). The overall impression is that of a well-circumscribed lesion with noninfiltrating margins confined to the optic nerve.
(**d**) Gd-enhanced coronal SE sequence (TR/TE = 700/15 ms) documents the expansion of the optic nerves on the coronal plane (arrows) and their variable enhancement. A large ophthalmic vein is present on each side (arrowheads) as an incidental finding.

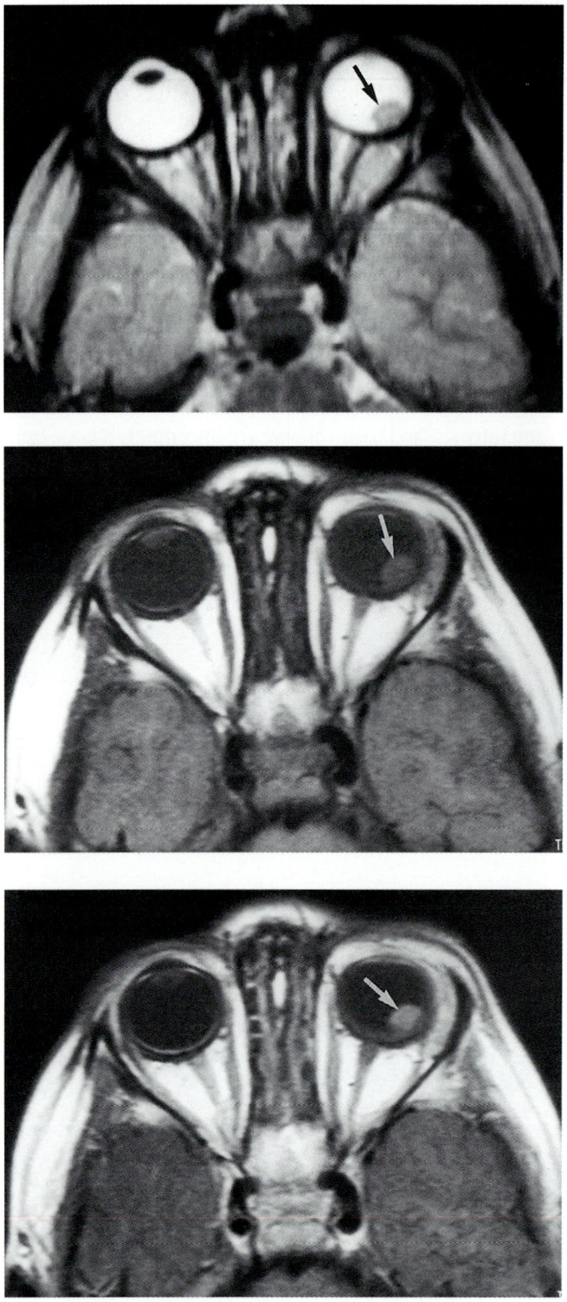

a

b

c

Figs. 8.**5 a – c** **Choroidal melanoma of the left eye.**
(**a**) Unenhanced axial T2-weighted SE sequence (TR/TE = 3000/90 ms) shows a well-circumscribed choroidal mass that is hypointense to the vitreous (arrow).
(**b**) In the unenhanced axial T1-weighted SE sequence (TR/TE = 700/15 ms), the choroidal melanoma of the left eye (arrow) appears isointense to brain tissue and hyperintense to the vitreous.
(**c**) Gd-enhanced axial SE sequence (TR/TE = 700/15 ms) shows marked, homogeneous enhancement of the tumor (arrow).

is approximately 50 HU on plain scans and rises to 65 – 100 HU after intravenous contrast administration.

On MRI, pigmented melanoma appears hyperintense to the globe on T1-weighted images and hypointense on T2-weighted images. Amelanotic melanoma and very small lesions (< 2 mm) are difficult to diagnose, especially in the iris. It can also be difficult in some cases to differentiate the tumor itself from hemorrhagic areas.

Small lesions can sometimes be defined on MRI by using a special high-resolution orbital coil. Postcontrast images can differentiate amelanotic melanoma from hemorrhagic areas, which do not enhance after contrast administration.

Differentiation is required from retinoblastoma, subacute choroidal hemorrhage, and senile macular degeneration.

The extent of scleral infiltration, which occurs even with very small melanomas, is an important prognostic indicator. The signs of scleral invasion are subtle and variable and consist of increased signal intensity and either an increase or decrease in scleral thickness.

Osteoma

Osteomas of the orbital region are slow-growing tumors that are most common in middle-aged adults, predominantly affect women, and tend to occur near the optic disk. Involvement is bilateral in approximately 25 % of cases.

CT portrays osteoma as a crescent-shaped choroidal lesion of calcific density whose size is depicted more accurately by CT than by ultrasound. Soft-tissue invasion does not occur.

The differential diagnosis should include drusen, calcification due to toxoplasmosis, and calcified hemangioma of the choroid. With retinoblastoma, the typical age of occurrence and presence of soft-tissue components will generally distinguish that tumor from osteoma.

Retinoblastoma

Retinoblastoma is the most common intraocular tumor of childhood and accounts for some 80 % of malignant eye tumors in children under 15 years of age. Approximately 50 % of the tumors are *hereditary* and 50 % are *spontaneous*. Only the hereditary form is bilateral and may coexist with a tumor of the pineal body. Histologically, the following *growth patterns* may be observed:

- *Endophytic* (toward the vitreous).
- *Exophytic* (toward the subretinal space, leading to retinal detachment).
- *Plaquelike* within the retina.

A 5-year-survival rate of up to 90% can be achieved at present, depending on the time of diagnosis. Retinoblastoma may spread by the hematogenous route or along the optic nerve in the subarachnoid space, leading to leptomeningeal involvement. The diagnosis may be suggested clinically by leukokoria or strabismus.

The detection of calcifications is the most important aid to differential diagnosis. Calcifications are present histologically in 95% of retinoblastomas, and high-resolution CT can detect these in more than 80% of patients. They are consistently present in tumors that have attained a certain size. In patients age 2 years or under, the presence of calcifications on CT scans combined with leukokoria is virtually pathognomonic for retinoblastoma. Advanced tumor stages are characterized histologically by involvement of the choroid, sclera, or optic nerve through the scleral lamina cribrosa, but this cannot be documented by sectional imaging studies. Only extensive involvement of the retrobulbar space, including the optic nerve, and intracranial extension can be appreciated on sectional images.

Conventional radiographs can show only extensive calcifications that have developed in larger tumors.

CT usually displays retinoblastoma as an intrabulbar mass that is hyperdense to the vitreous. Often it is posterior to the equator of the globe, but large tumors will extend past the equator. Larger tumors tend to have multiple large calcifications, while small tumors often contain only one calcification with a homogeneous appearance. The tumor shows only slight enhancement on post-contrast scans. Attention should be given to possible infiltration of the optic nerve or retrobulbar space, involvement of the contralateral eye, and pineal body masses.

The role of MRI is still unclear. Given the critical importance of calcifications in the initial workup and the relative insensitivity of MRI to calcific structures, CT is the modality of choice in the diagnosis of retinoblastoma. T1-weighted MR images show the tumor as a hypointense mass that is virtually indistinguishable from the vitreous, but its signal intensity on T2-weighted images is markedly lower than that of the vitreous. An accompanying exudative or hemorrhagic retinal detachment and other associated changes are better visualized with MRI than CT.

Optic-Nerve-Sheath Meningioma

Optic nerve-sheath meningioma can usually be distinguished from sphenoid wing meningioma (Fig. 8.**9**) by its location or origin, but the differentiation of very advanced forms is sometimes difficult.

Optic nerve-sheath meningioma is a rare tumor that predominantly affects middle-aged women. It occasionally occurs in children and adolescents with neurofibromatosis type II.

The tumor arises from cells of the arachnoid layer of the optic nerve sheath and spreads within the subarachnoid space of the optic nerve. It appears on CT and MRI as a tubular (Fig. 8.**6**) or fusiform expansion of the optic nerve. In later stages the tumor may become excrescent and penetrate the dura. Early cases present clinically with progressive visual loss, papilledema or optic atrophy, and occasional shunt vessels on the surface of the optic disk. Exophthalmos is less commonly observed and is less pronounced than in patients with optic nerve glioma.

Optic nerve-sheath meningioma may occasionally cause enlargement of the optic canal accompanied by thinning or destruction of the cortical bone, which does not occur with optic nerve glioma. These osseous changes may be documented at the margin of the optic canal or may involve the anterior clinoid processes.

Another less conspicuous osseous change is hyperostosis similar to that occurring with intracranial meningiomas. Conventional tomography can detect these bony changes and can also demonstrate intratumoral calcifications, which are pronounced in some cases.

Criteria for the CT diagnosis of optic-nerve-sheath meningioma are an optic nerve mass of increased density on unenhanced scans, frequent pronounced intratumoral calcification, concomitant hyperostosis of the ipsilateral anterior clinoid process, and intense enhancement after intravenous contrast administration.

The main disease to be considered in the differential diagnosis is perineuritis. Optic nerve-sheath meningioma is readily distinguished from optic nerve glioma by its "tram track" appearance on axial images, although this sign is by no means pathognomonic for meningioma and may occur with perineuritis and pseudotumors. The "tram track" sign on CT and MR images is caused by the greater attenuation, signal intensity, and contrast enhancement of the tumor in relation to the optic nerve.

The MRI signal characteristics of optic nerve-sheath meningioma are almost identical to those of intracranial meningiomas (see Ch. 3).

A small optic nerve-sheath meningioma (Fig. 8.**6**) is difficult to diagnose with CT or MRI. The differential diagnosis should include perineuritic changes associated with an orbital pseudotumor, in which case the obvious clinical manifestations of pseudotumor, including pain and exophthalmos, and its multifocality will suggest the correct diagnosis.

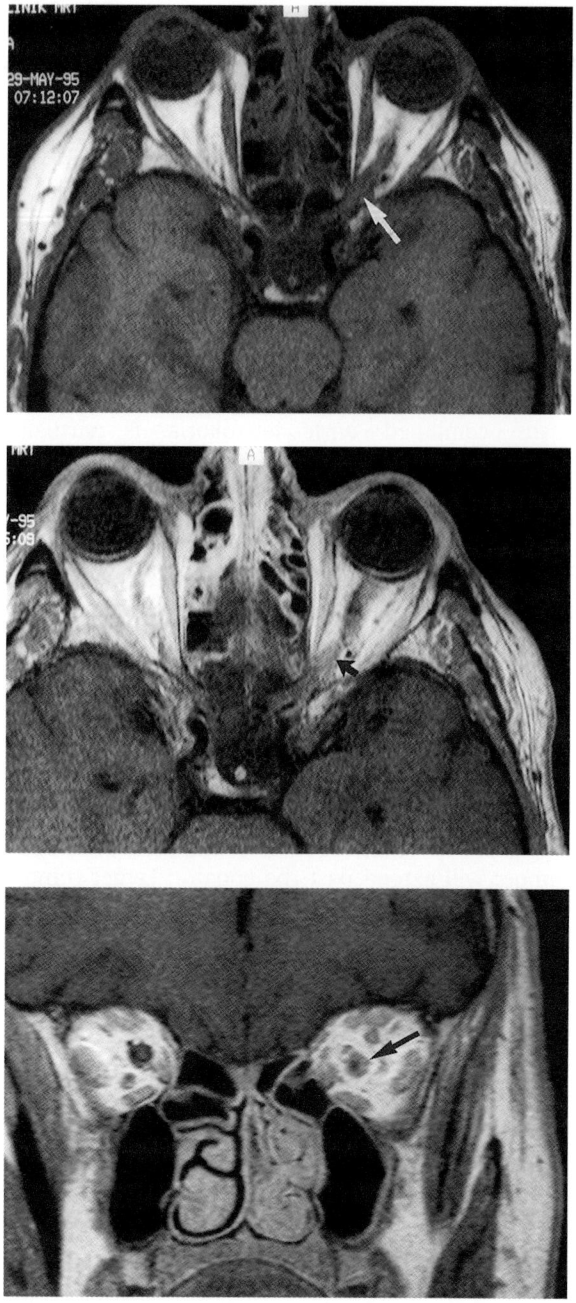

Figs. 8.**6 a – c** **Meningioma of the left optic nerve sheath.** (**a**) Unenhanced axial T1-weighted SE sequence (TR/TE = 700/15 ms) shows slight, homogeneous expansion of the left optic nerve (arrow) extending to the chiasm.
(**b**) Gd-enhanced axial SE sequence (TR/TE = 700/15 ms) shows homogeneous enhancement of the optic nerve lesion (arrow) with no evidence of infiltrative growth.
(**c**) Gd-enhanced coronal SE sequence (TR/TE = 700/15 ms) clearly shows the uniformly enhancing sheath tumor (arrow) surrounding the central, nonenhancing optic nerve.

Metastases

Lung and breast carcinomas are the most common primary tumors that metastasize to the eye and orbit, but virtually any tumor may metastasize to this region.

The principal sites of metastatic involvement are the bony orbit, the choroid, and the retrobulbar space. Smaller lesions are often asymptomatic, and postmortem findings show that ocular metastases are more common than clinical experience would suggest.

Isolated involvement of the intraconal compartment is unusual, and the infiltrative lesions tend to involve multiple sites that may include the choroid, optic nerve, bony orbit, and extraconal compartment.

Orbital metastases appear on plain CT scans as multiple ill-defined lesions that are hyperdense to orbital fat and, in some cases, to the extraocular muscles. They show marked enhancement, sometimes nonhomogeneous, after contrast administration.

Metastases are isointense to muscle on T1-weighted MR images and hyperintense on T2-weighted images. The high T2-weighted signal intensity is characteristic and serves to distinguish metastases from morphologically similar lesions such as inflammatory pseudotumor.

Hemangiopericytoma

Hemangiopericytoma should be considered in the differential diagnosis of rounded, well-circumscribed intraconal masses. The tumor is manifested clinically by a slowly progressive exophthalmos. Histologic examination reveals bundles of smooth muscle cells that presumably arise from the vessel walls. Vascular components may be present in varying degrees. The tumor has the same CT and MRI appearance as cavernous hemangioma. Its enhancement characteristics are not precisely known, but enhancement would be expected in tumors that have a marked vascular component. Extraconal occurrence is uncommon.

Lymphoma

Lymphoma of the eye and orbit is an extranodal form of the disease that most commonly involves the subconjunctival space, lacrimal gland, eyelid, and orbit. A distinction is drawn between *benign reactive lymphatic hyperplasia* and *malignant lymphoma*. Lymphoma cannot always be clearly differentiated from an *inflammatory pseudotumor*.

In contrast to lymphomas of the nasopharynx, imaging procedures are unable to distinguish between benign and malignant orbital lymphomas.

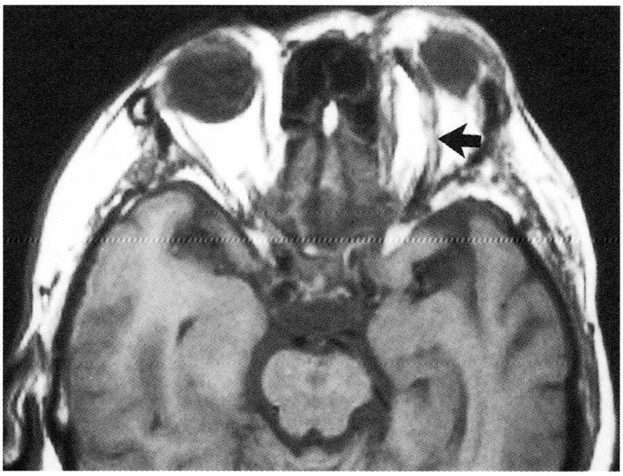

a

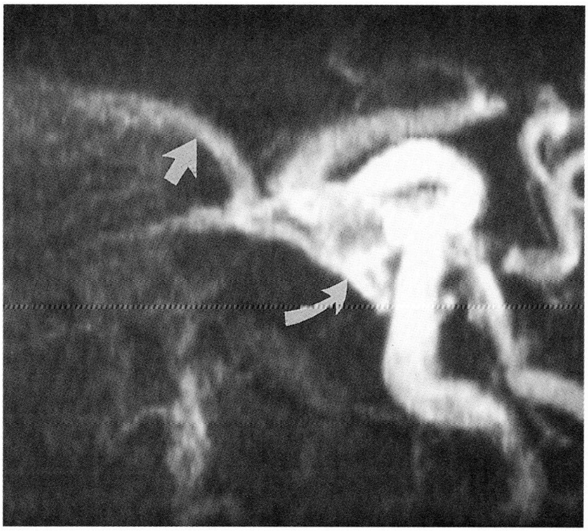

c

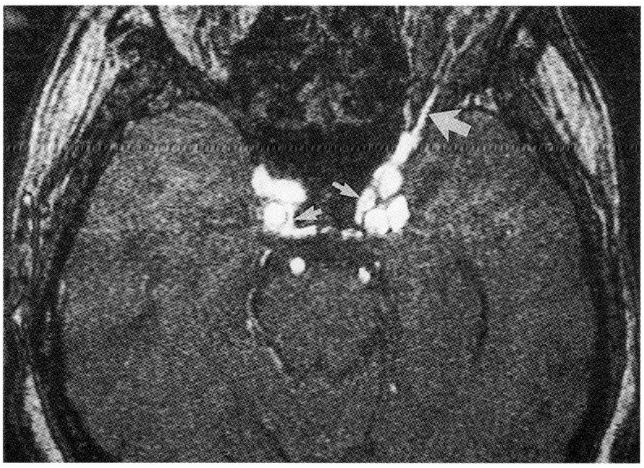

b

Figs. 8.**7 a–c** **Left-sided carotid-cavernous fistula.**
(**a**) Unenhanced axial T1-weighted SE sequence (TR/TE = 700/15 ms) shows a dilated left ophthalmic vein (arrow), considered pathognomonic for this arteriovenous fistula.
(**b**) Unenhanced axial TONE MRA (TR/TE = 43/8 ms, flip angle $\alpha = 15°$). The original MRA data set shows an arterial perfusion pattern in both the left ophthalmic vein (arrow) and the cavernous sinus (small arrows).
(**c**) Sagittal reconstruction of the unenhanced axial TONE MRA (TR/TE = 43/8 ms, flip angle $\alpha = 15°$) shows normal circle of Willis vessels, the left ophthalmic vein (arrow), and arterial blood flow in the cavernous sinus (curved arrow).

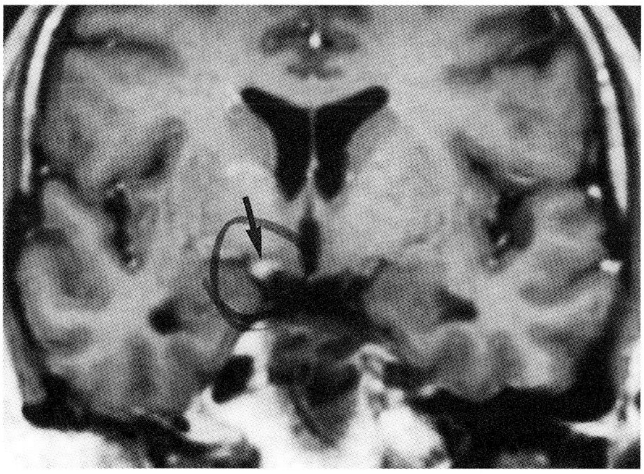

Fig. 8.**8** **Optic neuritis.** Gd-enhanced coronal T1-weighted SE sequence (TR/TE = 700/15 ms) shows circumscribed enhancement (arrow) of the right optic nerve with no signs of surrounding infiltration or significant volume increase, consistent with optic neuritis. The left optic nerve appears normal.

The clinical onset is usually insidious and is marked by a slowly progressive *exophthalmos*. Pain similar to that experienced with an acute inflammatory pseudotumor is unusual. Most lymphomas are comparable to acute inflammatory pseudotumor in their favorable response to cortisone therapy.

Some lymphomas, especially the highly malignant forms, are associated with *bone destruction* that is visible on conventional radiographs. The great majority of lymphomas do not cause bone destruction, however, and do not erode or expand the bony orbit.

Orbital lymphomas frequently occur in the cranial portions of the orbit. They are manifested clinically by displacement of the globe forward (exophthalmos) and downward. On axial CT scans, smaller lymphomas may be mistaken for an enlargement of the superior rectus or levator palpebrae superioris muscle, or may be missed entirely. They are better visualized on coronal scans, which can differentiate the tumor from the extraocular muscles and orbital roof.

Differentiation from other tumors is aided by the frequent discrepancy between the large size of the mass and the minimal displacement of orbital structures. The lymphoma has a smooth interface with the orbital roof, extraocular muscles, or globe and follows the contours of contiguous structures. Its interface with the retrobulbar fat is more irregular and shows small linear extensions. Post-contrast CT scans usually show a moderate degree of enhancement.

On MRI, orbital lymphomas are clearly delineated on coronal and parasagittal images. They are approximately isointense to the extraocular muscles in T1- and T2-weighted sequences. They enhance more intensely than on CT scans, and their morphologic features are the same as on CT.

Lymphomatous involvement of the optic nerve is an intracranial process that does not cause displacement of adjacent structures. The lesions are hyperdense to orbital fat on CT scans, hypointense on T1-weighted MR images, and hyperintense on T2-weighted images. Marked enhancement may be seen after contrast administration. Differentiation is mainly required from inflammatory pseudotumor and sarcoidosis.

Schwannoma (Fig. 8.**4**)

Orbital schwannomas arise from the Schwann cells of cranial nerves III through VII but not from the optic nerve. Orbital schwannomas are slow-growing *benign tumors of adults*. Pathologically, they are encapsulated tumors of a relatively soft consistency that have varicose vessels on their surface.

Conventional radiographs generally do not show changes in the bony orbit.

CT shows a sharply circumscribed, markedly enhancing mass that is hyperdense to the retrobulbar fat. Even large schwannomas may cause very little deformation or displacement of surrounding orbital structures.

On MRI, schwannomas have a low T1-weighted signal intensity and a very high T2-weighted signal intensity. Both CT and MRI show marked enhancement after intravenous contrast administration.

Cavernous Hemangioma (Fig. 8.**11**)

Cavernous hemangioma is the most common orbital tumor. It occurs chiefly in middle-aged adults and predominantly affects females. *Visual loss* and *proptosis* are almost always present to a degree, but the clinical presentation is rarely dramatic. Radiologic studies can define the precise relation of the tumor to neighboring structures and can usually establish a diagnosis based on typical imaging features.

A large percentage of cavernous hemangiomas are intraconal, and many are located directly behind the globe. Intraconal lesions at the orbital apex and extraconal lesions are much less common.

CT shows cavernous hemangioma as a rounded, sharply circumscribed, dense mass that spares the orbital apex and shows homogeneous contrast enhancement (Fig. 8.**10**). Large lesions may deform and erode the bony orbit, but bone destruction does not occur.

MRI better delineates the relation of the tumor to the optic nerve and extraocular muscles. Cavernous hemangioma of the orbit is isointense to muscle on plain T1-weighted images and hyperintense on T2-weighted images. It shows nonhomogeneous enhancement after the administration of Gd-DTPA (Fig. 8.**11**).

Capillary Hemangioma

Capillary hemangioma occurs during the 1st year of life. Usually it is first noticed as a *small lesion of the eyelids* in the newborn and enlarges during subsequent months. *Superficial* capillary hemangiomas, which often involve the upper medial portion of the face, are distinguished from *deep forms*. The latter may involve the extraocular muscles and other orbital structures.

CT demonstrates capillary hemangioma as a nonhomogeneous retrobulbar mass. Consistent with its vascular origin, the tumor may enhance intensely after intravenous contrast administration.

On MRI, capillary hemangioma appears as a nonhomogeneous mass in T1- and T2-weighted sequences. The tumor is poorly demarcated from its surroundings and readily transgresses the boundaries between orbital compartments. Perfused vascular segments appear as signal voids in selected sequences. Normal vascular structures of the orbit may be dilated.

Capillary hemangioma is isointense or slightly hyperintense to the extraocular muscles on T1-weighted images. Its T2-weighted signal intensity is very high.

Rhabdomyosarcoma (Fig. 6.**13**)

The *skeletal* and *orbital* forms of rhabdomyosarcoma correlate with patient age: skeletal rhabdomyosarcoma is a tumor of adults, while the orbital forms mainly affect children, usually males. Few if any cases are seen after 18 years of age.

Rhabdomyosarcoma is manifested clinically by a rapidly progressive exophthalmos. Epistaxis occurs in a small percentage of patients. This symptom, caused by invasion of the nasal cavity, distinguishes rhabdomyosarcoma from other orbital tumors.

The histologic types of rhabdomyosarcoma are *embryonic*, *alveolar*, and *pleomorphic*.

Conventional radiographs may occasionally show enlargement of the bony orbit or bone destruction.

The differential diagnosis includes most tumors that are encountered in this age group.

Lymphangioma

Lymphangioma is distinguished from hemangioma by its clinical presentation and histologic features. Unlike cavernous hemangioma, lymphangioma is not encapsulated. Histologically, it is composed of endothelium-lined lacunae whose lumina are filled with serous fluid or blood of variable age.

Lymphangioma is a *pediatric tumor*, with most cases presenting before 15 years of age. Many tumors become symptomatic because of their bleeding tendency. MRI will consistently show hematoma of varying duration within the tumor. Larger hematomas may cause obvious proptosis. It is typical for lymphangiomas to transgress the boundaries between orbital compartments (orbital septum and muscle cone).

Lymphangioma appears on CT as a lobular soft-tissue mass of variable density. Post-contrast scans show moderate enhancement of the rim and septa. The bony orbit is often expanded, and calcifications are occasionally seen. Lymphangiomas are rarely infiltrative.

On MRI, lymphangioma displays the same nonhomogeneous morphologic criteria. Its signal intensity depends on the age of the intratumoral hemorrhage and may be very high, even on T1-weighted images. T2-weighted images should be obtained in these cases to differentiate the tumor from dermoids and other extraconal lesions.

Inflammatory Lesions (Fig. 8.**8**)

Primary inflammatory lesions such as dacryoadenitis and myositis of the extraocular muscles are distinguished clinically from *secondary inflammatory disease* that has spread to the orbital region, where it may incite an orbital cellulitis or intraorbital abscess. These secondary inflammatory lesions most commonly result from trauma or acute sinusitis. Another inflammatory manifestation of major clinical significance is *retrobulbar optic neuritis.*

Mild ocular inflammatory disease is manifested initially by pain, increased lacrimation, visual deterioration, and possible unilateral exophthalmos. Myositis of the extraocular muscles often causes restriction of ocular movements. Optic neuritis is most common in the setting of multiple sclerosis and is manifested by visual deterioration of abrupt onset with no discernible changes in the optic fundus. Advanced bacterial inflammations can lead to severe complications such as loss of vision, venous sinus thrombosis, meningitis, and intracranial abscess formation.

Conventional radiographs are useful for excluding bony changes. Axial and coronal CT scans are best for evaluating the bony orbital boundaries and lamina papyracea.

MRI reveals intraorbital abscesses and inflammatory infiltrates as areas of altered signal intensity in the retro-orbital fat. The fat itself shows high signal intensity on T1-weighted images. Inflammatory structures appear hypointense on T1-weighted images and hyperintense on T2-weighted images, especially in the fat suppression sequence. The changes associated with retrobulbar optic neuritis are best demonstrated by fat-suppressed MR sequences. Venous magnetic resonance angiography (MRA) yields additional information on blood flow in the ophthalmic vein.

Orbital Infections

Orbital infections are manifested by clinical signs of inflammation, but imaging studies cannot always demonstrate a correlative mass lesion. Less severe conditions that require differentiation from true orbital inflammations involving the retrobulbar space are *subperiosteal abscesses* and *infections* localized to the *preseptal area*. The dominant clinical feature of preseptal inflammations is an inflammatory reaction of the eye and eyelid, whereas postseptal inflammations lead to optic-nerve involvement and to impaired ocular motility if a localized mass develops.

Inflammatory lesions of the paranasal sinuses are the most common source of orbital inflammatory disease. The ethmoid cells are a frequent source of orbital involvement due to spread through the very thin lamina papyracea. Spread through valveless veins has also been postulated.

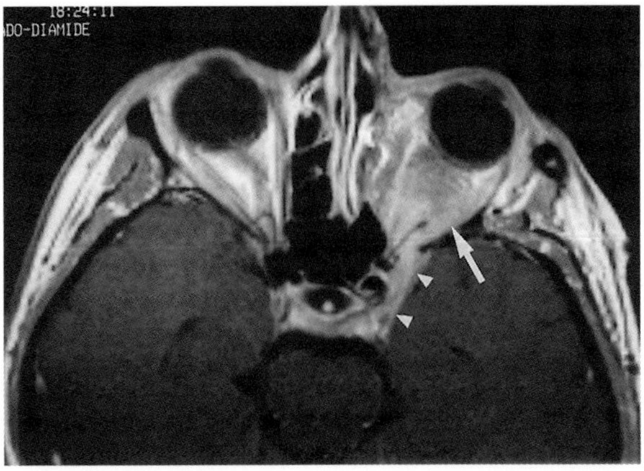

Fig. 8.**9** **Sphenoid wing meningioma infiltrating the orbit.** Gd-enhanced axial T1-weighted SE sequence (TR/TE = 700/15 ms) demonstrates a conspicuous tumor mass (arrow) of the left orbit showing predominantly homogeneous enhancement. Tumor components are also visible in the cavernous sinus area (arrowheads). Findings are consistent with a sphenoid wing meningioma that has invaded the left orbit.

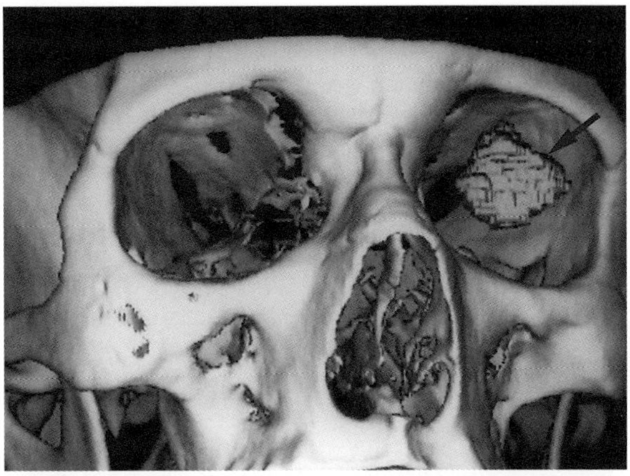

a

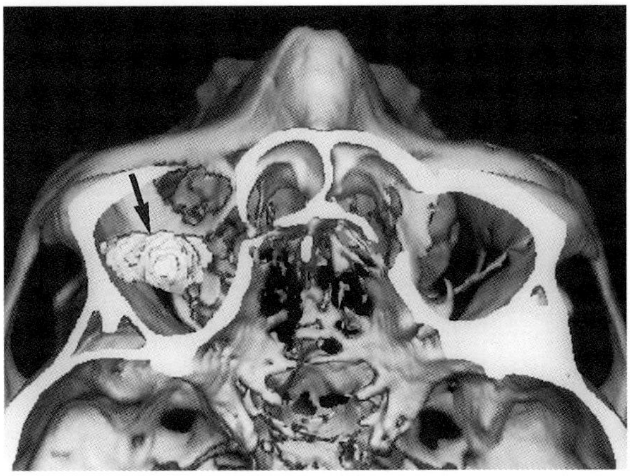

b

Figs. 8.**10 a, b** **Cavernous hemangioma of the left eye.**
(**a**) 3-D shaded surface reconstruction of post-contrast axial CT scans (100 mL Ultravist 370) shows a well-circumscribed, intensely enhancing cavernous hemangioma (arrow) of the left eye.
(**b**) 3-D shaded surface reconstruction of post-contrast axial CT scans (100 mL Ultravist 370) in the superior view demonstrates the relation of the cavernous hemangioma (arrow) to the bony orbital boundaries.

Mucoceles

Mucoceles are *retention cysts* of the paranasal sinuses caused by the obstruction of a sinus ostium due to inflammation or, less commonly, by neoplastic disease. The obstruction leads to the retention of secretions in the affected sinus, which becomes distended and impinges on neighboring structures.

Most mucoceles are round or oval and have smooth margins. The sinuses often show associated changes such as mucosal swelling and fluid levels.

Conventional radiographs show opacification of the paranasal sinuses. The mucocele itself may be identifiable as an expanded sinus cell. Mucoceles of long standing lead to thinning of adjacent bony structures.

CT reveals paranasal sinus opacity, usually of intermediate density, and may show distension and erosion of bony structures. In some cases this erosion

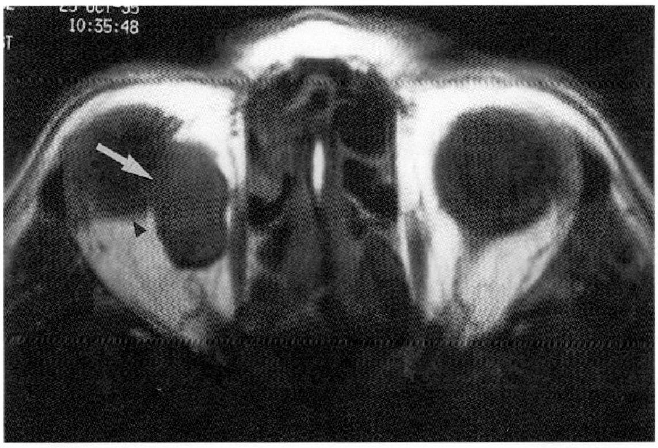

a

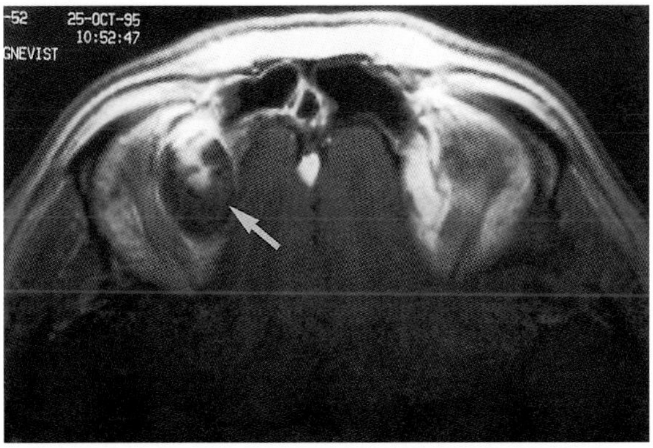

b

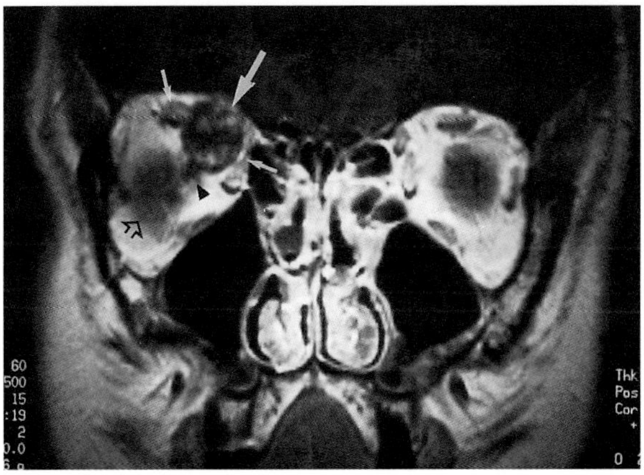

c

Figs. 8.**11 a–c** **Cavernous hemangioma of the right eye.** (**a**) Unenhanced axial T1-weighted SE sequence (TR/TE = 700/15 ms) with a high-resolution orbital coil shows the cavernous hemangioma (arrow) as a well-circumscribed mass, isointense to muscle, that is indenting and laterally displacing the globe (arrowhead).
(**b**) Gd-enhanced axial SE sequence (TR/TE = 700/15 ms) shows intense, nonhomogeneous enhancement spreading from the periphery of the lesion toward its center (arrow).
(**c**) Gd-enhanced coronal image (TR/TE = 700/15 ms) accurately defines the relation of the cavernous hemangioma (large arrow) to the extraocular muscles (small arrows), optic nerve (arrowhead), and globe (open arrow).

may cause mucocele to simulate an extraconal mass that has spread secondarily to the paranasal sinuses.

On MRI, mucoceles are usually isointense or hypointense on T1-weighted images, hyperintense on T2-weighted images, and show a narrow enhancing rim on post-contrast images. This typical pattern is seen in mucoceles with serous contents. Hemorrhage within the mucocele causes high signal intensity even on T1-weighted images, while inspissation of the liquid contents produces low signal intensity on T1- and T2-weighted images.

Subperiosteal Abscess

The most common sources of inflammatory orbital lesions are *sinusitis* and foreign bodies. CT is the initial imaging procedure for the assessment of acute cases.

Special importance is placed on the early diagnosis of an abscess, since the formation of an abscess is the signal to discontinue antibiotic therapy and proceed with surgical evacuation.

Some patients have a known history of dental extractions or craniofacial trauma. *Infections due to foreign bodies* naturally depend on the route of access and the definitive location of the foreign body (Fig. 8.**13**).

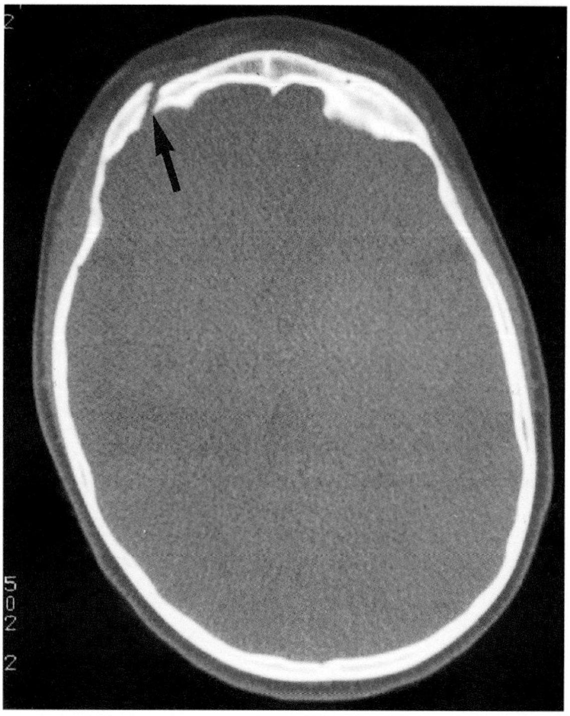

a

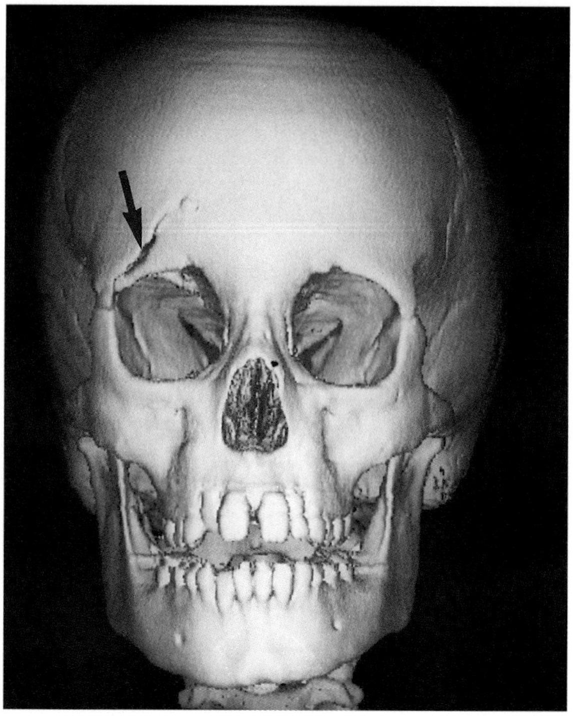

b

Figs. 8.**12 a, b** **Fracture of the right orbital roof.**
(**a**) Axial unenhanced cranial CT scan with a bone window shows a gaping fracture line (arrow) through the anterior calvaria on the right side. Image at this level shows no sign of free intracranial air that would indicate open craniocerebral trauma.

(**b**) 3-D shaded surface reconstruction of unenhanced axial CT scans defines the extent of the fracture line in the anterior skull base, showing extension of the fracture into the right orbital roof (arrow). Note the marked dehiscence of the fracture site.

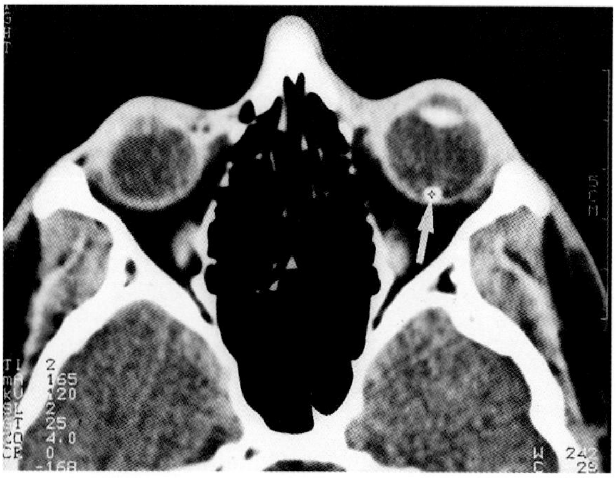

Fig. 8.**13** **Intraorbital foreign body.** Axial cranial CT scan with a bone window after contrast administration (100 mL Ultravist 370) shows a mass of metallic density (arrow) near the optic disk of the left eye.

Conventional radiographs show paranasal sinus opacities and in severe cases may show erosion of the bony orbital wall and soft-tissue densities projected over the orbit.

On CT, a subperiosteal abscess originating from the ethmoid cells appears as a soft-tissue mass along the medial orbital wall. The medial rectus muscle is frequently enlarged, and large abscesses may affect other extraocular muscles as well. After contrast administration the mass shows faint enhancement, sometimes with a nonenhancing center, and is poorly demarcated from surrounding structures. As a result, cellulitic inflammations and abscesses are not always distinguishable on CT scans.

Intracranial spread of the inflammatory process represents a life-threatening complication of orbital infections. Sites of bone destruction are not necessarily detectable in early stages.

Tolosa-Hunt Syndrome

Tolosa–Hunt Syndrome is a *painful ophthalmoplegia* caused by nonspecific granulomatous tissue in the cavernous sinus, orbital apex, or superior orbital fissure. It bears some similarity to an inflammatory pseudotumor.

Digital subtraction angiography (DSA) and possibly MRA can document occlusions of the ophthalmic vein before its entry into the cavernous sinus and changes in the wall of the internal carotid artery. CT and MRI can demonstrate granulomatous tissue in the cavernous sinus. The parasellar tissue is well defined on coronal MR images and shows predominantly homogeneous contrast enhancement.

Endocrine Orbitopathy

Endocrine orbitopathy is today considered a separate disease entity, although it most commonly results from thyroid dysfunction states with elevated levels of TSH (thyroid stimulating hormone). Often the clinical picture is dominated by *pronounced exophthalmos* and classic *ocular signs of thyroid dysfunction* (i.e., Möbius, Graefe, Stellwag, Dalrymple). The morphologic basis of endocrine orbitopathy involves the deposition of mucopolysaccharides in the retrobulbar space.

Ultrasonography is the initial diagnostic study. Further information is provided by CT and MRI, which can accurately evaluate the retrobulbar space, orbital apex, and adjacent areas of the skull base and brain.

For reasons still unclear, endocrine orbitopathy usually occurs in association with Graves disease. Thus, diagnostic imaging should be performed in a patient with known Graves disease who develops unilateral exophthalmos that does not show a close temporal correlation with hyperthyroidism. MRI is superior to CT for demonstrating specific ocular muscle changes.

Endocrine orbitopathy typically leads to bilateral, almost symmetric enlargement of extraocular muscles. In a patient with unilateral exophthalmos and known Graves disease, bilateral muscle enlargement will establish the endocrine cause of the ocular symptoms. A concomitant increase in the volume of the retrobulbar fat may be manifested by protrusion of the frontal septum at the medial canthus or by indentation of the medial orbital wall.

Clinical manifestations include pronounced exophthalmos, diplopia, photophobia, increased lacrimation, and a burning, gritty sensation in the eyes. The muscle enlargement in endocrine orbitopathy mainly increases the transverse diameter of the muscle, changing its cross section from elliptical to circular. Unlike lymphoma and myositis, endocrine orbitopathy affects only the muscle bellies and spares the tendinous attachments.

Even in severe cases, the signal intensity of the extraocular muscles on T1-weighted MR images may remain unchanged. In protracted cases, however, fatty degeneration can lead to circumscribed or diffuse increases in signal intensity. The T2-weighted signal intensity of the edematous ocular muscles is very high. In protracted cases where fibrosis has occurred, the T2-weighted signal intensity is low and is often significantly below that of the retrobulbar fat.

This ability to differentiate extraocular muscle changes makes MRI the imaging modality of choice in patients with endocrine orbitopathy. The visual findings in T2-weighted images and the quantitative findings obtained by calculating T2 relaxation times correlate precisely with the stage of progression of the disease. MRI in patients with stage IV–VI endocrine orbitopathy initially shows markedly prolonged T2 relaxation times compared with normal individuals. The end stage of the disease is a completely fibrotic ocular muscle with very short T2 relaxation times.

Besides these changes, which are present in nearly all patients with stage IV–VI disease, MRI can demonstrate less common pathologic phenomena and therapeutic outcomes. It rarely shows changes in the retrobulbar fat, even though such changes are consistently seen in histologic studies of endocrine orbitopathy. T2-weighted images are almost always unremarkable. T1-weighted images may reveal patchy, hypointense infiltrate tracking between the ocular muscles within the retrobulbar fat.

Posttherapeutic changes after various types of decompressive surgery are well documented on axial and coronal MR images. While bone defects are not defined, displacement of the retrobulbar fat and extraocular muscles is clearly visualized. If ocular muscle enlargement is severe enough to cause optic nerve compression, MRI will reveal the nerve displacement. In the rare cases where atrophy develops,

MRI can document the reduction in optic nerve diameter.

Nonspecific Myositis

Orbital myositis and *orbital pseudotumor* are interpreted as manifestations of a "nonspecific inflammatory orbital syndrome," a systemic disorder that includes other fibrosing diseases such as *retroperitoneal fibrosis* and *fibrous mediastinitis* or *thyroiditis*. Orbital myositis may be unilateral or bilateral and is characterized clinically by exophthalmos, painful limitation of eye movements, and overt signs of inflammation.

CT and MRI in orbital myositis show enlargement of one, or occasionally several, eye muscles. Other cases may present as a retrobulbar mass originating from the extraocular muscles. A characteristic finding, not present in all cases, is the simultaneous involvement of the muscle belly and tendon. The exophthalmos and ocular muscle enlargement are often less pronounced than in endocrine orbitopathy, and the retrobulbar fat volume is not increased.

Involvement of the medial and lateral rectus muscles is also characteristic, with frequent sparing of the superior and inferior muscles. The affected ocular muscles show an irregular expansion that differs from the symmetric enlargement found in endocrine orbitopathy. The muscles show normal T1-weighted signal intensity and only a slight increase in T2-weighted signal intensity.

Sarcoidosis

Orbital involvement in sarcoidosis is usually manifested by involvement of the optic disk. *Papilledema* can be detected ophthalmoscopically in approximately 5% of patients. From the standpoint of differential diagnosis, it is noteworthy that ocular complaints are often the earliest clinical manifestation of sarcoidosis.

While subtle ocular changes are demonstrable in many patients with sarcoidosis, involvement of the lacrimal gland is rare. In these cases noncaseating granulomas can be found within the lacrimal gland.

There is no real indication for imaging studies in patients with known sarcoidosis. But undiagnosed cases that present initially with lacrimal gland changes should be evaluated by CT or MRI. Differentiation is required from lymphoma of the lacrimal gland, which is radiologically indistinguishable from sarcoidosis and also has a similar clinical presentation.

CT and MRI show bilateral, asymmetric enlargement of the lacrimal glands, even in cases with unilateral clinical involvement. As with all diffuse infiltrations, the shape of the lacrimal gland is unchanged. With massive enlargement, a portion of the mass extends medially along the anterior margin of the globe. Post-contrast images show pronounced enhancement.

On MRI, the lesions appear hypointense in both T1- and T2-weighted sequences.

Pseudotumor

Pseudotumor frequently presents as a *nonspecific unilateral mass* infiltrating the retrobulbar space and displacing the globe, optic nerve, or extraocular muscles. The cause of this disease is still unknown, but an immunologic cause involving an antigen-antibody reaction has been proposed.

The clinical symptoms are nonspecific, thus an accurate diagnosis relies more on morphologic imaging findings than on clinical observation.

Inflammatory pseudotumor is distinguished from infections of the orbit. The dominant clinical symptom is pain, which may be associated with various inflammatory signs, diplopia, and loss of vision.

CT and MRI reveal infiltrative processes that may affect the retrobulbar space and various orbital structures. The changes range from subtle deposits on the posterior half of the globe or optic nerve to lesions that permeate the retrobulbar space from the back of the globe to the orbital apex. Frequently there is concomitant or isolated involvement of the lacrimal gland. Inflammatory pseudotumor may also involve the extraocular muscles, usually causing a moderate degree of muscular enlargement. In typical cases the tendinous attachment to the globe is also involved, differentiating pseudotumor from endocrine orbitopathy.

On CT scans, the various forms of orbital infiltration appear hyperdense to the retrobulbar fat. A 2-mm slice thickness is required to demonstrate subtle thickening of the globe wall, and coronal scans are needed to display changes in the optic nerve sheath. Usually the lesions do not enhance after contrast administration.

On MRI, the orbital infiltrates appear isointense on T1-weighted images and may appear hyperintense on T2-weighted images. Low T2-weighted signal intensity is not always present but can help distinguish pseudotumor from metastatic lesions, which are often morphologically similar. Tendon involvement is best appreciated on parasagittal images or coronal images at a rostral level.

Traumatic Lesions

Fractures of the Orbital Margin (Fig. 8.**12**)

Direct violence to the orbit will often produce a *blowout fracture* of the orbital floor, creating a communication between the orbital cavity and maxillary sinus. A fracture of the medial lamina papyracea can establish a connection with the ethmoid labyrinth. The rare fractures of the posteriorly placed optic canal often cause damage to the optic nerve.

An orbital blowout fracture can be diagnosed on standard paranasal sinus radiographs in the occipitomental and occipitofrontal projections. Films will usually show alteration in the density of the roof of the affected maxillary sinus. With bleeding into the maxillary sinus, a fluid level may be seen as indirect evidence of a fracture. The fracture line itself can be visualized on coronal CT scans. These scans should also be obtained if there is a suspected fracture of the medial lamina papyracea.

The differential diagnosis of unilateral maxillary sinus opacification should include preexisting sinusitis. The detection of a hematoma in itself does not prove the existence of a fracture. If the diagnosis is uncertain, conventional radiographs should be followed by a CT examination.

Carotid-Cavernous Fistula

A communication between the internal carotid artery and cavernous sinus may develop spontaneously or as a late sequela to severe craniocerebral trauma. Advanced stages may be manifested by pulsating exophthalmos.

Internal and external carotid angiography is indicated whenever there is clinical suspicion of a carotid-cavernous fistula. This study can provide a simultaneous view of the internal carotid artery and surrounding cavernous sinus at the level of the carotid siphon. Today more than 80% of cases can be successfully managed by an interventional procedure in which the fistula is occluded with coils or detachable balloons. MRA can also be performed to exclude a carotid-cavernous fistula.

In many fistulas, accurate localization of the opening can be difficult because of the high flow velocities. The principal MR finding is venous enlargement without an identifiable nidus. Sites of hemorrhage or infarction may be observed as secondary signs. *Dilatation of the superior ophthalmic vein* is considered the principal sign of a carotid-cavernous fistula. MRA may also demonstrate feeding vessels and collateral channels in many cases.

Often the initial finding is an enlarged ophthalmic vein, with arterial MRA showing high flow velocities in the vein accompanied by arterial flow through the cavernous sinus. The nidus may be demonstrable by MRA in isolated cases (Fig. 8.**7**).

Imaging Criteria and Their Differential Diagnosis

The origin of an orbital lesion is of key importance in making an accurate interpretation of the lesion and its differential diagnostic criteria. The orbit can be divided into four compartments to enable the differential diagnosis of orbital masses by region. The *four compartments of the orbit* are:

- The globe.
- The optic nerve and sheath.
- The intraconal region.
- The extraconal region.

Once the origin of a lesion has been established by CT or MRI, its characteristics (morphology, enhancement, etc.) can be analyzed to further narrow the relevant differential diagnoses for that subregion.

The principal differential diagnoses for the various compartments of the orbital region are listed in Tables 8.**2**–8.**5**.

Liquid Masses

As a diagnostic category, liquid masses or structures are rarely encountered in the orbital region. Particular consideration should be given to diseases of the facial skeleton and paranasal sinuses in the evaluation of liquid masses. In CT studies, moreover, it is important to differentiate an obstructed paranasal sinus from an inflammatory or neoplastic complication.

In conventional radiography, close attention should be given to any asymmetries, density varia-

Table 8.**2** Differential diagnosis of lesions of the globe

Finding	Diagnosis
Congenital, developmental	➤ Coats disease ➤ Hypoplasia or aplasia of the globe
Tumor (Fig. 8.**5**)	➤ Uveal melanoma ➤ Retinoblastoma ➤ Metastasis ➤ Choroidal hemangioma ➤ Medulloepithelioma
Inflammatory (Fig. 8.**8**)	➤ Pseudotumor ➤ Sclerosing endophthalmitis
Trauma (Fig. 8.**12**)	➤ Frontobasal fracture ➤ Calvarial fracture ➤ Hemorrhage ➤ Hematoma ➤ Foreign body

Table 8.3 Differential diagnosis of lesions of the optic nerve and sheath

Finding	Diagnosis
Tumor	➤ Optic nerve glioma ➤ Optic nerve-sheath meningioma ➤ Optic nerve-sheath neurofibroma or schwannoma ➤ Lymphoma ➤ Metastasis ➤ Hemangioblastoma ➤ Hemangiopericytoma
Inflammatory	➤ Optic neuritis ➤ Pseudotumor ➤ Sarcoidosis ➤ Toxoplasmosis ➤ Tuberculosis ➤ Syphilis
Trauma (Fig. 8.**12**)	➤ Contusion ➤ Hematoma ➤ Foreign body
Vascular	➤ Central venous thrombosis ➤ Varix
Endocrine	➤ Graves disease
Miscellaneous	➤ Increased intracranial pressure ➤ Hydrops

Table 8.4 Differential diagnosis of intraconal lesions

Finding	Diagnosis
Tumor	➤ Cavernous hemangioma (Fig. 8.**8**) ➤ Capillary hemangioma ➤ Lymphoma ➤ Lymphangioma ➤ Metastasis ➤ Rhabdomyosarcoma ➤ Hemangiopericytoma ➤ Neurofibroma ➤ Ectopic meningioma
Inflammatory	➤ Pseudotumor ➤ Cellulitis ➤ Abscess ➤ Granulomatous disease
Trauma	➤ Hematoma ➤ Foreign body
Vascular	➤ Carotid-cavernous fistula (Fig. 8.**7**) ➤ Varix ➤ Venous thrombosis ➤ Venous angioma ➤ Arteriovenous malformation ➤ Varicocele
Endocrine	➤ Graves disease

Table 8.5 Differential diagnosis of extraconal lesions

Finding	Diagnosis
Congenital, developmental	➤ Cephalocele
Tumor	➤ Metastasis ➤ Maxillary sinus malignancy ➤ Nasal malignancy
Inflammatory	➤ Pseudotumor ➤ Sclerosing endophthalmitis
Trauma	➤ Medial blowout fracture ➤ Hematoma
Lacrimal gland	➤ Congenital –Dermoid (Fig. 8.**5**) ➤ Tumor –Adenoid cystic carcinoma –Non-Hodgkin lymphoma ➤ Inflammatory –Postviral syndrome –Sjögren syndrome –Mikulicz syndrome

tions, or morphologic disparities in adjacent bony structures. For example, the thinning of a bony sinus wall may signify a mucocele and may justify further diagnostic procedures.

The criteria for interpreting a mass lesion on noncontrast CT scans include the density of the lesion, the nature of its margins, the location of the mass in relation to other structures, and evidence of osseous involvement. Important criteria on post-contrast scans are the type of enhancement (homogeneous, nonhomogeneous, no enhancement) and the pattern of enhancement (annular, diffuse).

On MRI, the identity of a liquid orbital mass can be determined by evaluating its signal intensity in T1- and T2-weighted sequences before and after the administration of contrast medium. The T2-weighted sequence is particularly useful because of its sensitivity to tissues with a high water (proton) content. The contrast-enhanced T1-weighted sequence can further narrow the differential diagnosis. T2 weighting facilitates the identification of cystic and liquid masses because these lesions have a high signal intensity on T2-weighted images. It should be noted that ocular prostheses, which also have high T2-weighted signal intensity, can mimic a liquid intraorbital mass (Fig. 8.**2**).

Air-Containing Masses

Air-containing masses in the orbital region are most commonly a result of trauma. By analogy with the paranasal sinuses (Ch. 7), variants and lesions secondary to inflammatory or iatrogenic processes should be considered in the differential diagnosis of air-containing masses. Less common lesions with this morphology are inflammatory changes due to gas-forming organisms and tumor-associated structural defects with secondary air inclusions.

CT is the primary modality for evaluating these lesions, given the limited ability of MRI to differentiate air from bone. Also, CT can accurately define a fracture or foreign body in cases where the air-containing mass has a traumatic cause.

Tumor Masses (Figs. 8.**4**–8.**6**)

Whenever a tumor mass is detected by CT or MRI, it should be determined whether or not the lesion is associated with bone destruction. Depending on the clinical presentation, MRI is the primary modality for ophthalmologic investigations while CT is preferred for investigations of the upper facial skeleton. Besides demonstrating bone destruction by a solid mass lesion, CT aids in the detection of intratumoral calcifications and bone fragments.

The accurate differential diagnostic classification of a mass lesion of the anterior skull base requires analysis of the following criteria:

- Tumor topography: size and shape of the lesion and its relation to surrounding structures.
- Tumor morphology: predominantly cystic, solid, or calcified.
- Enhancement characteristics: intensity, homogeneity.
- Margins: well-defined, ill-defined, or infiltrative.

Besides tumor margins, topography is an essential differential diagnostic criterion, as it enables the origin of the lesion to be identified. The accurate characterization of tumor morphology also helps to advance the diagnosis. MRI is definitely superior to CT for this purpose owing to its higher soft-tissue contrast. Moreover, the signal characteristics of a solid mass lesion in various MR sequences and an analysis of its enhancement dynamics can aid in establishing its identity. MRI is also becoming an important tool for evaluating recurrent tumors and differentiating them from posttherapeutic changes (Tables 8.**6**–8.**9**).

Osseous Lesions (Fig. 8.**12**)

In evaluating osseous lesions of the orbit, *circumscribed or generalized thinning* of the bony orbital boundaries and *solitary or multiple sites of bone destruction* should be differentiated from *generalized or geographic expansion of the bone.*

Generalized or geographic *thinning of the orbit* may represent a normal variant or may denote patho-

Table 8.**6** Signal characteristics of intraconal and extraconal mass lesions on MRI

Lesion	T2-weighted SI	T1-weighted SI	Enhancement
Carcinoma, sarcoma	↗	↙	↑↑
Lymphoma	↑	↓	↑ – ↑↑
Hemangioma	↑	↓	↗
Lymphangioma	↑	↓	↗
Granuloma	↗	↗	↗
Epidermoid tumor	↑	↓	↗
Encephalocele	↑	↓	–
Lipoma	↑	↗	–
Dermoid tumor (Fig. 8.**1**)	↙	↗	↑
Tolosa–Hunt syndrome	↓	↓	↗
Pseudotumor	↓	↓	↑
Arteriovenous malformation (Fig. 8.**7**)	↓	↙	↑
Hemorrhage	↑	↑	–

↑ High SI/enhancement
↗ Isointense to hyperintense/moderate enhancement
↙ Hypointense to isointense
↓ Low SI
– No enhancement
SI Signal intensity

Table 8.7 Signal characteristics of mass lesions of the optic nerve and sheath on MRI

Lesion	T2-weighted SI	T1-weighted SI	Enhancement
Meningioma (Fig. 8.6)	↙	↙	↑↑
Optic nerve glioma	↑	↓	↑ - ↑↑
Neuritis (Fig. 8.8)	↑↑	→	↗
Metastasis	↑	↓	↑↑

↑ High SI/enhancement
→ Isointense
↗ Isointense to hyperintense/moderate enhancement
↙ Hypointense to isointense
↓ Low SI/no enhancement
SI Signal intensity

Table 8.8 Signal characteristics of mass lesions of the globe MRI

Lesion	T2-weighted SI	T1-weighted SI	Enhancement
Melanoma (Fig. 8.5)	↓	↑	↑↑
Amelanotic melanoma			↑ - ↑↑
Retinoblastoma	↓	↑	↗
Hemorrhage	↑	↑	-
Coats syndrome	↑	↑	-
Metastasis	↑	↙	↑↑

↑ High SI/enhancement
→ Isointense
↗ Isointense to hyperintense/moderate enhancement
↙ Hypointense to isointense
↓ Low SI/no enhancement
- No enhancement
SI Signal intensity

Table 8.9 Criteria for the differential diagnosis of optic nerve glioma and optic nerve-sheath meningioma

Criteria	Optic nerve glioma	Optic nerve-sheath meningioma
Age	33% are children with neurofibromatosis type I	Middle-aged women, children with neurofibromatosis type II
CT	Fusiform or eccentric enlargement of optic nerve and sheath; no calcifications	Enlargment of optic nerve and sheath; "tram track" appearance; tubular calcifications
MRT	Tumor tends to spread centrally along optic nerve	Tumor involves prechiasmatic optic nerve sheath with minimal central spread

logic change. Lesions that may be associated with the thinning of osseous structures include:

- Intracranial mass (e.g., meningioma).
- Circumscribed osteoporosis.
- Arachnoid cyst.

If solitary or multiple sites of bone destruction are found, normal anatomic features (fissures, foramina, canals) require differentiation from iatrogenic and pathologic changes. Isolated bone destruction is most commonly caused by an eosinophilic granuloma or solitary metastasis. Lesions that may cause geographic bone destruction include malignant tumors of the nasopharynx and paranasal sinuses that invade the orbit by contiguous extension—most notably nasopharyngeal or sinus carcinoma, neuroblastoma, and soft-tissue metastases. Benign osseous lesions that may cause isolated bone destruction are osteoma and bone cysts.

Less common causative lesions are epidermoid, arachnoid cyst, and meningioma. Multiple foci of bone destruction in the orbit are strongly suspicious

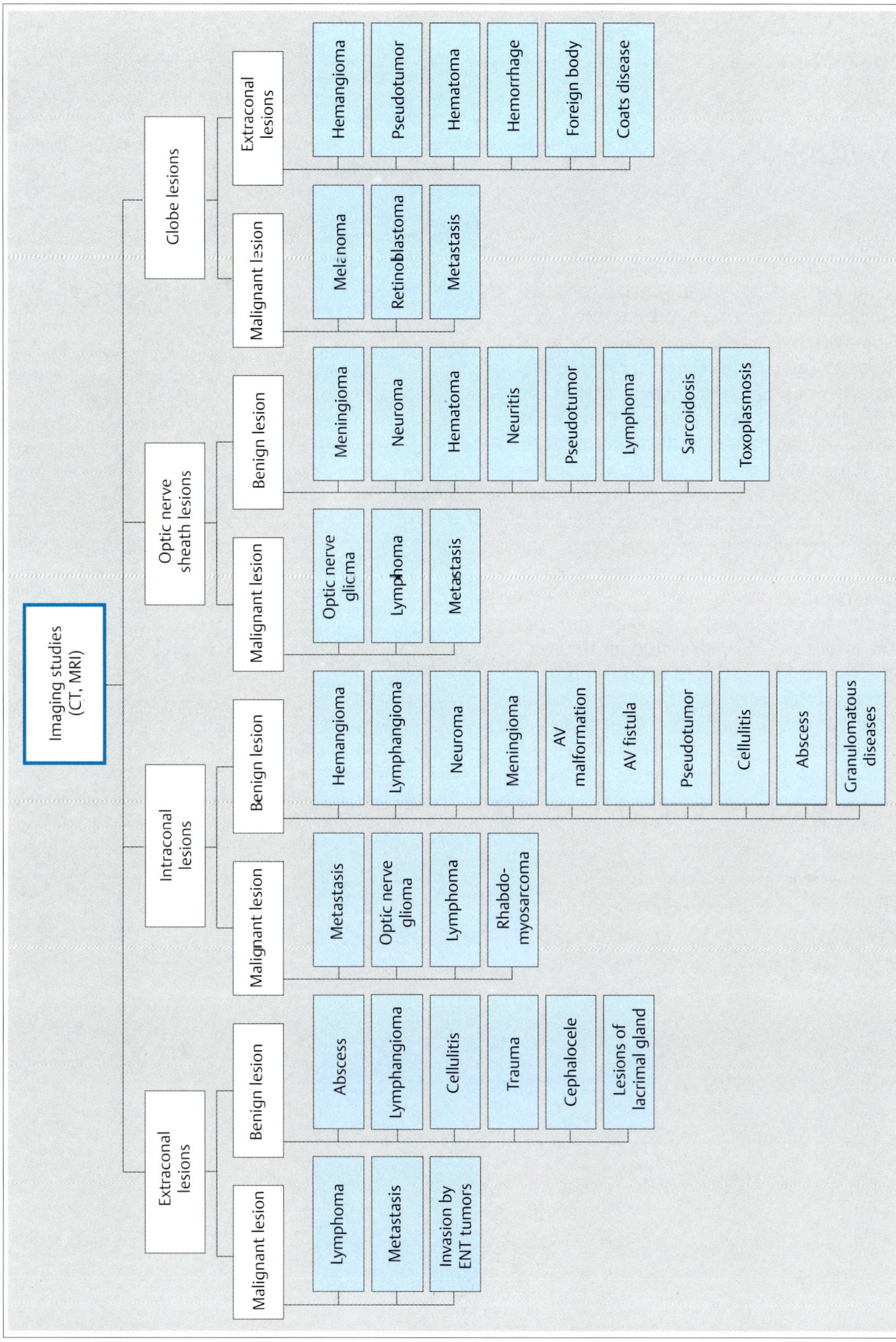

Fig. 8.14 **Differential diagnosis of orbital lesions.**

for metastases; less frequent causes are osteoporosis, myeloma, hyperparathyroidism, and osteomyelitis (Fig. 8.**14**, Table 8.**10**).

Summary and Diagnostic Strategy

Ultrasound is the primary imaging modality for the diagnosis of intraorbital soft-tissue lesions. MRI is used for the further investigation of orbital soft-tissue lesions and for excluding or confirming involvement of the cranial cavity and facial skeleton. CT is essential for evaluating areas of putative bone destruction and erosion and for detecting calcifications. CT is also an essential study in trauma patients, although classic lesions such as a blowout fracture can usually be detected on conventional radiographs. A special challenge is posed by the differential diagnosis of mass lesions involving specific orbital compartments: the globe, the optic nerve and sheath, and the intraconal and extraconal regions.

MRI, with its high soft-tissue contrast and spatial resolution, is particularly well suited for the evaluation of mass lesions in the various orbital compartments. Moreover, differences in the inherent signal intensity of a lesion and the intensity of its enhancement on post-contrast images will frequently establish the identity of the lesion.

References

1 Chapman, S., R. Nakielny: Aids to Radiological Differential Diagnosis, 3rd ed. Saunders. London 1995
2 Dähnert, W.: Radiology Review Manual, 3rd ed. Williams & Wilkins, Baltimore 1996
3 Frey, K. W., K. Mees, T. J. Vogl: Bildgebende Verfahren in der HNO-Heilkunde. Enke, Stuttgart 1989
4 Harnsberger, H. R.: Handbook of Head and Neck Imaging. 2nd ed. Mosby-Year Book, St. Louis 1995
5 Hosten, N.: Auge und Orbita: radiologische Differentialdiagnostik. Thieme, Stuttgart 1995
6 Mafee, M. F., G. E. Valvassori et al.: High resolution and dynamic sequential computed tomography. Arch Otolaryngol. 109 (1983) 691 – 696
7 Mafee, M. F., Y. Inoue, R. F. Mafee: Ocular and Orbital imaging. In: Yousem, D. M.: Head and neck imaging. Neuroimaging Clin North Am. 6 (1996): 357 – 378
8 Mödder, U., M. Lenz: Klinische Radiologie: Gesichtsschädel, Felsenbein, Speicheldrüsen, Pharynx, Larynx, Halsweichteile. Diagnostik mit bildgebenden Verfahren. Springer, Berlin 1991
9 Mödder, U., M. Lenz: Schädelbasis, Felsenbein. In Reiser, M., W. Semmler: Magnetresonanztomographie. Springer, Berlin 1992
10 Neumann, H. H.: Differentialdiagnostik in der Hals-Nasen-Ohren-Heilkunde. Thieme, Stuttgart 1990
11 Rosseau, G., A. Mark, D. O. Davis: Gd-DTPA-Enhancement Magnetic Resonance Imaging of the cavernous sinus. Acta Neurochir., Suppl. 53 (1991) 113 – 116
12 Som, P. M., R. T. Bergeron: Head and Neck Imaging, 2nd ed. Mosby Year Book, St. Louis 1991
13 Valvassori, G. E., G. D. Potter, W. N. Hanafee, B. L. Carter, R. A. Buckingham: Radiology of the Ear, Nose and Throat. Thieme, Stuttgart 1982
14 Valvassori, G. E., R. A. Buckingham, B. L. Carter, W. N. Hanafee, M. F. Mafee: Head and Neck imaging. Thieme, Stuttgart
15 Vogl, T. J.: MRI of the Head and Neck. Springer, Berlin 1991

9 Parapharyngeal Space and Adjacent Deep Compartments

The clinical and radiologic evaluation of the parapharyngeal space poses a formidable challenge to available diagnostic modalities and examiner experience. This is based on the complex anatomy of the parapharyngeal space, which is described below in some detail. The inherent difficulties of clinical examination and the fact that even large lesions may escape clinical detection underscore the importance of diagnostic radiology using modern sectional imaging techniques. In cases where a lesion of the parapharyngeal space cannot be specifically diagnosed on the basis of radiologic findings, computed tomography (CT)-guided biopsy has become an important procedure for establishing a tissue diagnosis in this region.

A knowledge of the anatomy of the parapharyngeal space is the key to understanding patterns of tumor infiltration, the origin of a lesion, and its differential diagnostic interpretation. The parapharyngeal space is the central space of the deep facial region, around which other important spaces are situated. Few lesions arise primarily in the parapharyngeal space itself; most originate in one of the surrounding spaces and either infiltrate the parapharyngeal space or cause displacement of the parapharyngeal fat and bordering spaces. Determining the true space of origin of a lesion can greatly advance the differential diagnosis.

Normal Anatomy

The parapharyngeal space (Fig. 9.**1**) is a space with irregular boundaries that is filled principally by fat. It extends from the skull base to the hyoid bone and has roughly the shape of an inverted pyramid. The *inferior boundary* of the parapharyngeal space is formed by the attachment of the posterior belly of the digastric muscle to the greater cornu of the hyoid bone. At the level of the skull base, the parapharyngeal space is bounded by the portion of the sphenoid bone around the foramen lacerum, medial to the foramen ovale, and the inferior surface of the petrous bone near the carotid canal and jugular fossa. The *medial boundary* of the parapharyngeal space is formed superiorly by the tensor veli palatini muscle and its fascia, the pharyngobasilar fascia, the levator veli palatini muscle, the superior pharyngeal constrictor muscle, and the jugular fossa. The *lateral boundary* of the space is the medial wall of the masticator space. The medial pterygoid muscle and interpterygoid fascia form the medial boundary of the masticator space, separating it from the parapharyngeal space.

The parapharyngeal space can be divided into a *prestyloid compartment* and a *poststyloid (retrostyloid) compartment.* The posterior compartment contains the neurovascular sheath. The masticator space is a separate fascial compartment enclosed by the superficial layer of the deep cervical fascia and containing the pterygoid muscles, masseter muscle, inferior temporalis muscle, and mandibular ramus.

The infratemporal fossa is an irregular space located behind the maxilla and lateral to the nasopharynx and pterygopalatine fossa. The fossa is bounded above by the zygomatic arch and below by the alveolar crest of the maxilla. Medially, the infratemporal fossa communicates with the pterygomaxillary fissure and pterygopalatine fossa. The infratemporal fossa contains the muscles of mastication, the vessels of the maxilla, and the mandibular and auriculotemporal nerves. The foramen ovale (V_3) and foramen spinosum (middle meningeal artery) form apertures in the roof of the fossa.

Prestyloid compartment of the parapharyngeal space. This compartment extends from the skull base to the superior cornu of the hyoid bone. It is bounded medially by the tensor veli palatini muscle and its fascia (which attaches to the skull base medial to the foramen ovale and passes to the styloid process and fasciae of the styloid musculature). The anteromedial boundary is formed by the medial pterygoid muscle and its fascia. The compartment is bounded posterolaterally by the medial pole of the parotid gland, posteriorly by the tensor veli palatini fascia and stylopharyngeal diaphragm, and posteroinferiorly by the styloglossus muscle.

The prestyloid compartment connects with the medial pole of the parotid gland (often there is an incomplete fascia stretching between the compartment and the parotid gland medial pole), the pterygomandibular fossa, and the submandibular space. The lingual nerve, the tensor veli palatini and tensor tympani nerves, and branches of the maxillary artery establish connections between the prestyloid compartment of the parapharyngeal space and the masticator space. The fascia of the tensor veli palatini muscle separates

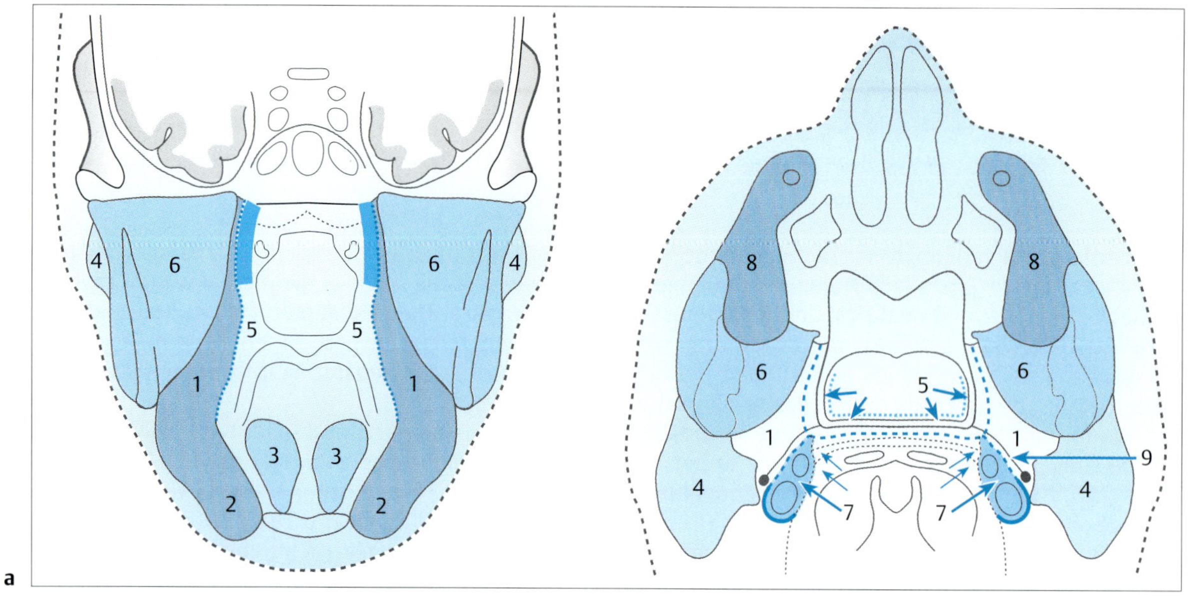

Figs. 9.**1 a, b** **Coronal and axial sections through the parapharyngeal space and bordering spaces.**
(**a**) Schematic coronal section. (**b**) Schematic axial section.
1 Parapharyngeal space
2 Submandibular space
3 Sublingual space
4 Parotid space
5 Pharyngeal mucosal space
6 Masticator space
7 Carotid space
8 Buccal space
9 Stylopharyngeal diaphragm

the prestyloid compartment from the poststyloid compartment of the parapharyngeal space.

Poststyloid compartment of the parapharyngeal space. This compartment extends from the skull base to the aortic arch. It is bounded posteriorly by the prevertebral fascia of the prevertebral muscles. Anteriorly, the styloid process and stylopharyngeal diaphragm separate the poststyloid compartment of the parapharyngeal space from the prestyloid compartment. Additionally, the stylopharyngeal diaphragm separates the poststyloid compartment from the paratonsillar space, situated between the pharyngobasilar fascia and the tensor veli palatini muscle and its fascia. The poststyloid compartment is bounded cranially by the carotid and jugular foramina. It communicates medially with the retropharyngeal space, located between the pharyngobasilar fascia and the prevertebral fascia (Table 9.**1**).

Masticator Space

The superficial layer of the deep cervical fascia splits along the inferior border of the mandible, creating a medial slip that runs along the pterygoid muscles and attaches to the skull base and a lateral slip that runs over the superficial masseter muscle to the zygomatic arch and continues cephalad over the temporalis muscle. As there is no fascia separating the temporal area from the masticator space, this cephalad extension is also termed the *suprazygomatic masticator space.*

The lateral pterygoid muscle arises by two heads from the infratemporal surface of the skull base and lateral sphenoid wing and inserts onto the medial aspect of the mandibular condyle. The medial pterygoid muscle arises in the fossa between the pterygoid plates and inserts onto the medial aspect of the angle of the mandible.

The temporalis muscle inserts on the coronoid process of the mandible. The masseter muscle descends from its origin on the zygomatic arch to the lateral surface of the ramus, angle, and posterior body of the mandible.

Table 9.1 Compartments of the deep pharynx, their contents and principal lesions

Compartment	Contents	Lesions
Pharyngeal mucosal space	➤ Mucosa ➤ Lymphatic tissue of Waldeyer ring ➤ Minor salivary glands ➤ Pharyngobasilar fascia ➤ Superior and middle pharyngeal constrictor muscles ➤ Salpingopharyngeus muscle ➤ Levator veli palatini muscle ➤ Torus tubarius ➤ Cartilaginous end of eustachian tube	Pseudomasses: ➤ Asymmetric Rosenmüller fossa (lateral pharyngeal recess) ➤ Inflammatory mucosal swelling (due to infectious or radiation-induced pharyngitis) Congenital: ➤ Tornwaldt cyst Inflammatory: ➤ Adenoidal hypertrophy ➤ Adenitis, tonsillitis ➤ Abscessation (Fig. 9.**3**) ➤ Postinflammatory dystrophic calcification ➤ Postinflammatory retention cyst Benign tumors: ➤ Benign tumor of minor salivary glands ➤ Juvenile nasopharyngeal fibroma Malignant tumors: ➤ Squamous cell carcinoma ➤ Non-Hodgkin lymphoma ➤ Minor salivary gland malignancy ➤ Melanoma ➤ Pediatric rhabdomyosarcoma
Prestyloid compartment of parapharyngeal space	➤ Fat ➤ Branch of mandibular nerve (to tensor veli palatini muscle) ➤ Ascending pharyngeal artery ➤ Branches of internal maxillary artery ➤ Pharyngeal veins ➤ Primordial salivary gland rests	Malignant tumors: ➤ Mucoepidermoid ➤ Adenoid cystic carcinoma ➤ Malignant mixed tumors of salivary gland rests ➤ Direct spread of squamous cell carcinoma Benign tumors: ➤ Benign mixed tumors of salivary gland rests ➤ Lipoma ➤ Branchial cleft cyst ➤ Schwannoma (very rare) Inflammatory: ➤ Abscess (Fig. 9.**3**) ➤ Cellulitis (Fig. 9.**2**)
Poststyloid compartment of parapharyngeal space	➤ Internal carotid artery ➤ Internal jugular vein ➤ Cranial nerves IX–XII ➤ Sympathetic chain (superior cervical ganglion) ➤ Lymph nodes (lateral pharyngeal, lateral and posterior jugular chain)	Malignant tumors: ➤ Lymph node metastasis ➤ Lymphoma ➤ Direct spread of squamous cell carcinoma Benign tumors: ➤ Paraganglioma (glomus jugulare, glomus vagale, carotid body) ➤ Neurogenic tumor (neurofibroma, schwannoma) (Fig. 9.**7**) ➤ Miscellaneous (meningioma, chordoma, etc.) (Fig. 9.**8**) Vascular: ➤ Thrombosis ➤ Aneurysms ➤ Dissection

Table 9.**1** Continuation

Compartment	Contents	Lesion
Masticator space	➤ Mandible ➤ Medial pterygoid muscle ➤ Lateral pterygoid muscle ➤ Temporalis muscle ➤ Masseter muscle ➤ Inferior alveolar nerve (V_3 sensory branch) ➤ Mandibular nerve (V_3) ➤ Inferior alveolar artery and vein	Pseudomasses: ➤ Accessory parotid gland (Fig. 9.**15**) ➤ Benign masseteric hypertrophy ➤ V_3 denervation atrophy Congenital: ➤ Hemangioma (Fig. 9.**10**) ➤ Lymphangioma Inflammatory: ➤ Odontogenic abscess ➤ Mandibular osteomyelitis Benign tumors: ➤ Osteoblastoma ➤ Leiomyoma ➤ Neurogenic tumor (neurofibroma, schwannoma) Malignant tumors: ➤ Soft-tissue sarcoma (Figs. 9.**6**, 9.**12**, 11.**27**) ➤ Chondrosarcoma ➤ Osteosarcoma ➤ Malignant schwannoma ➤ Non-Hodgkin lymphoma ➤ Squamous cell carcinoma (from oropharynx) ➤ Rhabdomyosarcoma ➤ Leiomyosarcoma ➤ Metastasis ➤ Minor salivary gland tumor
Retropharyngeal space	➤ Fat ➤ Medial retropharyngeal lymph nodes	Pseudomasses: ➤ Tortuous carotid artery ➤ Edema, lymph stasis Congenital: ➤ Hemangioma ➤ Lymphangioma Inflammatory: ➤ Reactive adenopathy ➤ Cellulitis (Fig. 9.**2**) ➤ Abscess (Fig. 9.**3**) Benign tumors: ➤ Lipoma Malignant tumors: ➤ Lymph node metastases ➤ Non-Hodgkin lymphoma ➤ Direct invasion from squamous cell carcinoma
Prevertebral space	➤ Vertebral elements ➤ Prevertebral muscles	➤ Chordoma ➤ Vertebral body metastasis ➤ Osteomyelitis with abscess
Buccal space	➤ Buccal fat ➤ Facial artery and vein ➤ Parotid duct (distal part) ➤ Buccinator muscle	➤ Usually invaded secondarily from masticator space

By connecting the mandible with the skull base, the masticator space creates an avenue by which odontogenic infections and squamous carcinoma cells from the oropharynx can reach the skull base.

The mandibular division of the trigeminal nerve (V_3) runs along the skull base and exits through the foramen ovale to enter the masticator space. It transmits both sensory and motor fibers. The motor fibers are the masticator nerve, which supplies the masseter, temporalis, and medial and lateral pterygoid muscles, and the mylohyoid nerve, which supplies the mylohyoid muscle and the anterior belly of the digastric muscle in the region of the oral floor.

The sensory branches of V_3 are the buccal, auriculotemporal, inferior alveolar, and lingual nerves. The inferior alveolar nerve enters the mandibular ramus through the mandibular foramen and runs through the mandibular canal to the mental foramen. These nerves distribute sensory fibers to the upper third of the face, the tongue, the oral floor, and the temporomandibular joint. The mandibular nerve provides a route for perineural tumor extension to the skull base and intracranial fossa. Thus, imaging evaluation of the masticator space should always cover the entire course of the mandibular nerve from the mental foramen to the lateral pons including the mandibular foramen, foramen ovale, and Meckel cavity. The parotid duct is not located within the masticator space but runs superficial to it on the masseter muscle. Lesions of the masticator space can directly infiltrate the parotid duct, and lesions of the parotid duct can apparently originate from the masticator space.

The nasopharyngeal portion of the masticator space is termed the infratemporal fossa. The portion of the masticator space above the zygomatic bone is often termed the temporal fossa or suprazygomatic fossa. However, as there is no fascia separating the temporal fossa from the infratemporal fossa, it should be considered a cephalad extension of the masticator space.

The masticator space is bounded anteriorly by the buccal space and posteromedially by the parapharyngeal space. Directly posterior to the masticator space is the parotid space.

Infratemporal Fossa

The infratemporal fossa is an irregular space located behind the maxilla and lateral to the nasopharynx and pterygopalatine fossa. The fossa is bounded above by the zygomatic arch and below by the alveolar crest of the maxilla. The infratemporal fossa communicates medially with the pterygomaxillary fissure and pterygopalatine fossa. The infratemporal fossa contains the muscles of mastication, the vessels of the maxilla, and the mandibular and auriculotemporal nerves. The foramen ovale (V_3) and foramen spinosum (middle meningeal artery) form apertures in the roof of the fossa.

The infratemporal fossa represents the nasopharyngeal portion of the masticator space.

Buccal Space

The **buccal space** does not have true fascial boundaries. With its proximity to the masticator space, it is frequently involved by infections and malignant tumors that spread from the masticator space. Since the buccal space is readily accessible to palpation and ultrasound imaging, there is often no need for any further preoperative imaging studies. Whenever the presence of a malignant tumor is suspected, however, CT or preferably magnetic resonance imaging (MRI) should be performed to analyze the relation of the tumor mass to the distal portion of the parotid duct.

Clinical Signs and Symptoms

Mass lesions of the parapharyngeal space can remain clinically silent for some time, thus it is not unusual to find a mass as large as 6 cm in diameter on initial diagnostic imaging.

As one of the deep spaces of the upper neck, the parapharyngeal space is a difficult region to examine clinically. It is nestled deeply between the mandibular ramus, the parotid gland, and the sternocleidomastoid muscle. To be clinically apparent, a mass in the parapharyngeal space must displace the lateral pharyngeal wall toward the midline or cause lateral bulging of the parotid gland.

The medial boundary of the parapharyngeal space has a soft consistency and is represented by the mucosal lining of the pharynx. The only pliable portion of the lateral boundary of the parapharyngeal space is the retromandibular portion of the parotid gland. Almost any mass can laterally displace the medial pole of the parotid gland, regardless of whether the lesion has an intraparotid or extraparotid origin.

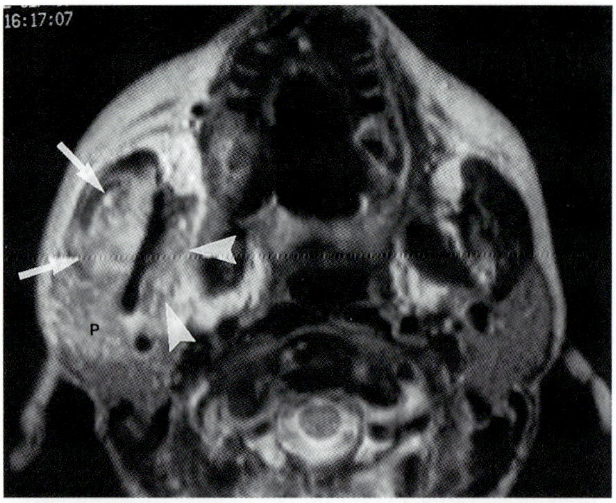

a

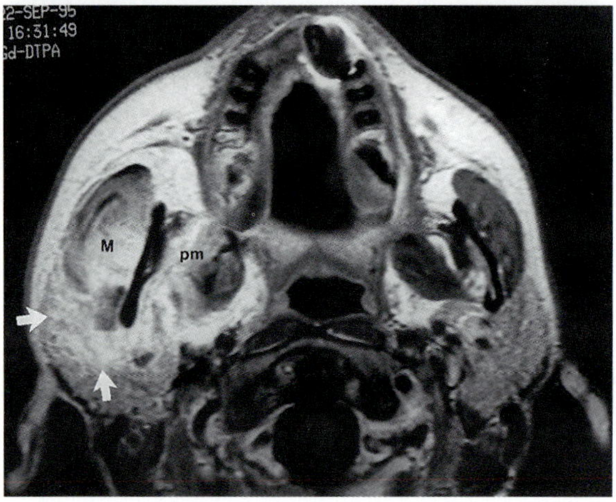

b

Figs. 9.**2a, b** **Cellulitis.**
(**a**) Axial T2-weighted MR image (TR/TE = 3000/90 ms) shows markedly increased signal intensity in the right parapharyngeal space and right masticator space. The masseter muscle (arrows) and medial pterygoid muscle (arrowheads) show marked hyperintensity. The area of increased signal intensity extends into the anterior portions of the parotid gland. Note the marked thickening of the masseter and medial pterygoid muscles in the setting of this inflammatory disease.
P Parotid gland
(**b**) Gd-enhanced axial T1-weighted image (TR/TE = 700/15 ms) shows marked contrast enhancement in the area of the right masseter and medial pterygoid muscles. A side-to-side comparison also shows marked signal enhancement in the anterior portions of the parotid gland (arrows). The cellulitis in this patient encompasses the masticator space and the prestyloid compartment of the parapharyngeal space.
M Masseter muscle
pm Medial pterygoid muscle

Imaging Evaluation and Differential Diagnosis

Before the advent of CT and MRI, the only modalities available for evaluating the parapharyngeal space were sialography and conventional angiography. Paragangliomas, for example, showed characteristic vascularity on angiograms. Despite various techniques, these conventional studies could supply a preoperative diagnosis in only 20% to 40% of cases. Prior to the late 1970's, all parapharyngeal-space masses were approached through a transparotid incision, regardless of whether or not the tumor was intraparotid in origin. By the early 1980's, however, lesions found to have an extraparotid origin could be surgically approached through a transcervical route that did not require manipulation of the facial nerve.

With the increasing refinement and differentiation of surgical techniques, MRI or CT became the standard procedure for the diagnostic evaluation of parapharyngeal space lesions. Sonography, sialography, and conventional radiography are of minor importance today in the evaluation of parapharyngeal space masses.

MRI is superior to CT in the depiction of soft-tissue contrast. T1- and T2-weighted spin-echo (SE) sequences are best for imaging the parapharyngeal space (Figs. 9.**4b, c**). A high-resolution technique using a 512 × 512 matrix has proven excellent for visualizing small anatomic structures that have an important bearing on differential diagnosis, such as the stylopharyngeal diaphragm, the ascending pharyngeal artery, and the fasciae of the tensor and levator veli palatini muscles.

Contrast-enhanced MRI (Figs. 9.**7a, b** and 9.**9**) using very rapid dynamic sequences (acquisition times ≤ 2 – 3 seconds per image) is particularly useful for investigating a suspected tumor mass in the post-styloid compartment or a tumor relating to the jugular foramen, as this will permit an optimum differential diagnostic assessment of the mass.

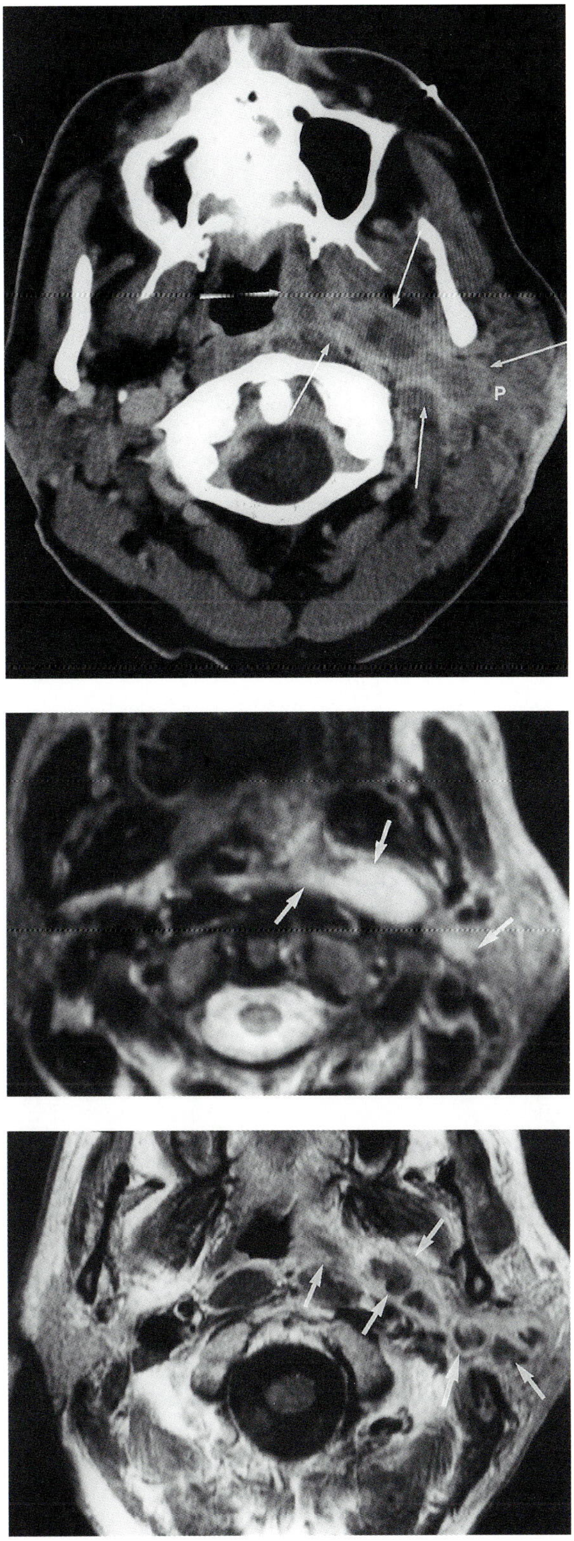

a

b

c

Figs. 9.**3 a–c** **Left parapharyngeal abscess.**
(**a**) Contrast-enhanced CT scan (soft-tissue window) shows diffuse enhancement in the left parapharyngeal space (arrows). Almost all the parapharyngeal fat on the left side is effaced. The diffuse contrast enhancement extends to the medial pole of the parotid gland, and there is swelling in the area of the left oropharynx.
P Pole of the parotid gland.
(**b**) T2-weighted MR image (TR/TE = 3000/90 ms) shows a marked increase of signal intensity in the left parapharyngeal space (arrows) involving the medial pole of the parotid gland.
(**c**) Post-contrast T1-weighted MR image shows marked contrast enhancement with central hypointense areas (arrows). The image demonstrates a loculated abscess in the left parapharyngeal space extending posteriorly to the neurovascular sheath and laterally to the medial pole of the parotid gland. The cause of this abscess collection was a peritonsillar abscess.

Imaging Findings

A variety of pathologic processes can occur in the parapharyngeal space. It is important to distinguish among congenital variations and malformations, tumors (Figs. 9.**7**–9.**9**, 9.**13**, 11.**21**), inflammatory lesions (Fig. 9.**3**), traumatic lesions, and iatrogenic lesions.

Congenital Variations and Malformations

Congenital lesions are rare in the prestyloid compartment of the parapharyngeal space, the most common being branchial cleft cysts. Other lesions such as cystic neurogenic tumors (Fig. 9.**7**), cystic hygromas, necrotic metastases, dermoid tumors, or epidermoid tumors that have similar imaging appearances are not typically found in the prestyloid compartment of the parapharyngeal space.

In the poststyloid compartment, the differential diagnosis should include a variety of vascular, neurogenic (Fig. 9.**7**), and lymphoepithelial lesions, most of which develop during postnatal life. The only congenital lesions of the poststyloid compartment are aneurysms (Fig. 14.**27**), pseudoaneurysms, and lymphangiomas (Fig. 11.**22**). The differential diagnosis should also include an ectatic, tortuous, or duplicated internal carotid artery as well as thrombosis of the internal carotid artery or internal jugular vein (Fig. 14.**29**). The MR signal characteristics of a lesion in T1- and T2-weighted sequences and its enhancement characteristics on post-gadolinium images are particularly useful for advancing the differential diagnosis.

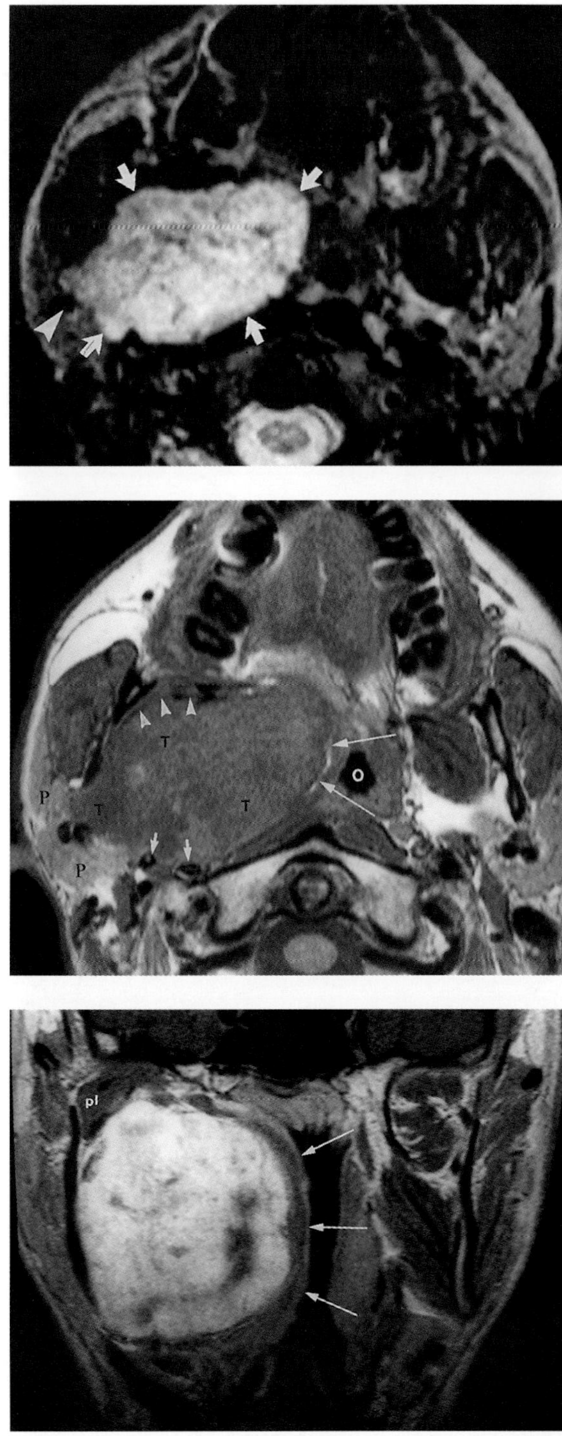

Figs. 9.**4 a–c** **Pleomorphic adenoma ("iceberg tumor") on the right side.**
(**a**) Axial T2-weighted MR image (TR/TE = 3000/90 ms) shows a pleomorphic adenoma in the right prestyloid compartment of the parapharyngeal space as a smooth-bordered mass of high signal intensity (arrows). The absence of a visible fat plane between the parotid gland and the tumor confirms that the tumor has a parotid origin.
Arrowhead: retromandibular vein.
(**b**) Axial T1-weighted MR image (TR/TE = 700/15 ms) shows a smoothly marginated tumor with a relatively homogeneous internal signal. No fat plane is seen between the parotid gland and the mass. The tumor is causing marked compression and anterior displacement of the medial pterygoid muscle (arrowheads). There is extreme medial displacement and compression of the parapharyngeal fat (long white arrows), and the carotid space (short white arrows) is displaced posteriorly. The oropharyngeal air column appears displaced toward the left. There is no evidence of destructive or infiltrative tumor growth. The tumor mass does not transgress the boundaries of the space.
O Oropharyngeal air column
P Parotid gland
T Tumor
(**c**) Gd-enhanced MR image in the coronal plane (TR/TE = 700/15 ms) shows the markedly enhancing tumor bulging the pharyngeal wall (arrows) and displacing the lateral pterygoid muscle cranially. The mass conforms strictly to the boundaries of the prestyloid compartment of the parapharyngeal space and, unlike the lesion in Fig. 9.**6**, has not infiltrated the skull base.
pl Lateral pterygoid muscle

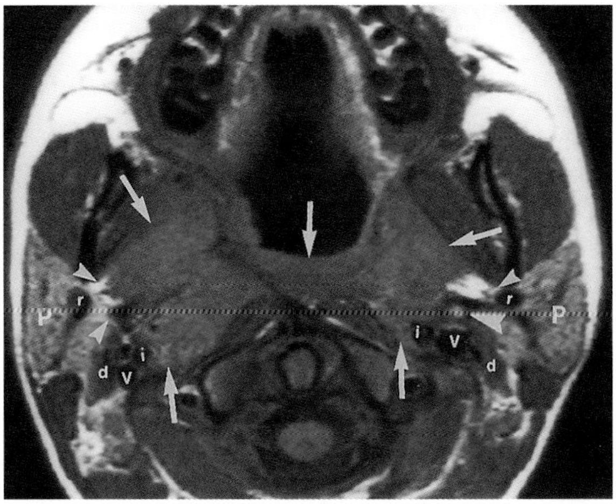

a

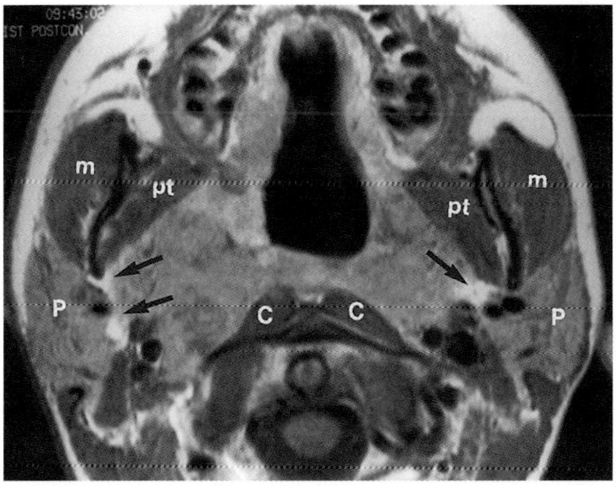

b

Figs. 9.5 a, b **Immunocytoma of the nasopharynx involving the parapharyngeal space.**
(**a**) Noncontrast T1-weighted sequence (TR/TE = 700/15 ms) shows an extensive tumor mass (arrows) involving both sides of the parapharyngeal space and the nasopharynx. The mass appears slightly hyperintense to muscle and is clearly separate from the parotid gland (fat plane = arrowheads). The neurovascular sheath is displaced posteriorly on both sides. The lesion involves both the prestyloid and poststyloid compartments.
d Posterior belly of digastric muscle
i Internal carotid artery
P Parotid gland
r Retromandibular vein
v Internal jugular vein
(**b**) Contrast-enhanced T1-weighted sequence (TR/TE = 700/15 ms) shows an intensely enhancing mass that is sharply demarcated from the pterygoid and longus capitis muscles. The markedly compressed parapharyngeal fat (arrows) confirms the extraparotid origin of the mass.
C Longus capitis muscle
m Masseter muscle
P Parotid gland
pt Medial pterygoid muscle

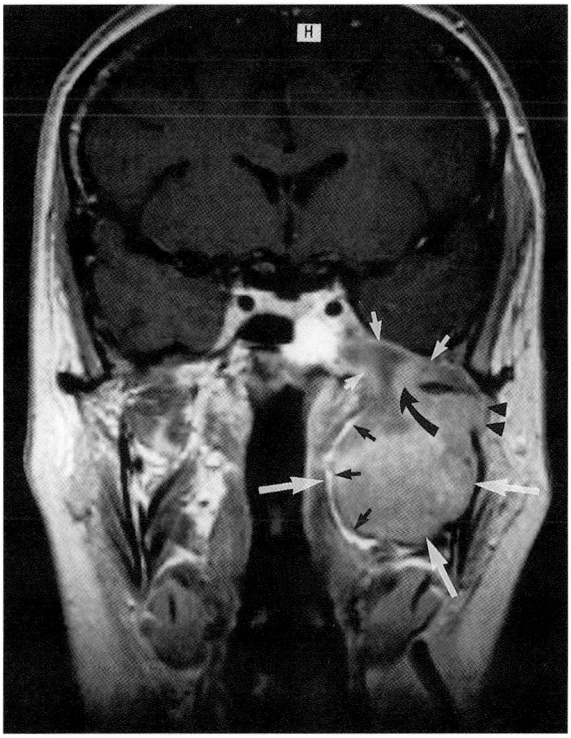

Fig. 9.6 **Leiomyosarcoma.** Axial T1-weighted image (TR/TE = 700/15 ms) after gadolinium injection (0.1 mmol/kg bw) shows relatively homogeneous contrast enhancement of the mass (large arrows). The parapharyngeal fat is markedly displaced and appears only as a thin layer (black arrows). The tumor has spread along the mandibular nerve and infiltrated the skull base through the foramen ovale (curved arrow). A thin fat plane (black arrowheads) separates the mass laterally from the parotid gland.

Tumors

Tumors of the parapharyngeal space may originate there, invade it secondarily from bordering spaces, or reach the parapharyngeal space by metastasis. *Benign parapharyngeal masses* (Fig. 9.**4**) are usually slow-growing and are often asymptomatic. When larger than approximately 3 cm in diameter, lesions typically cause medial displacement of the pharyngeal wall, tonsils, and palate and present as a retromandibular mass. These signs are consistently noted on MRI, as bony structures limit tumor growth in the cephalad and lateral directions. When these signs are present, the clinical diagnosis of a parapharyngeal mass is not difficult. It is difficult or impossible, however, to determine clinically whether the mass is primary to the parapharyngeal space or whether it originated in the masticator space or medial pole of the parotid gland. Enlargement of a parapharyngeal mass can lead to swallowing difficulties, dysphagia, and hearing loss due to involvement of the eustachian tube. A mass in the poststyloid compartment can lead to neurovascular involvement and cranial nerve dysfunction (Vernet syndrome with paralysis of cranial nerves IX–XI). Difficulties in speech and swallowing are usually caused by palatal displacement but in rare cases may result from involvement of the corresponding nerves. Involvement of the sympathetic chain can lead to Horner syndrome. Usually this occurs only with malignant tumors, however, and these typically cause pain as an early symptom.

The *most common benign tumors* of the parapharyngeal space are *salivary gland tumors.* As a group, these tumors account for 40% to 50% of all parapharyngeal space masses. Between 80% and 90% of these tumors are benign pleomorphic adenomas (Figs. 9.**4** and 10.**6**). Between 17% to 25% of parapharyngeal space masses are neurogenic tumors (Fig. 9.**7**), and 10% to 15% are glomus tumors. The rest consist of *metastases, lymph nodes, branchial cleft cysts, lipomas,* and *various other rare tumors* (Figs. 9.**6**, 9.**12**). Some 80% of all parapharyngeal space masses are benign (Fig. 9.**9**). The *most common malignant lesions* are *mucoepidermoid carcinomas, adenoid cystic carcinomas,* and *acinar cell carcinomas.*

Table 9.**1** lists the specific lesions that may occur in the various compartments of the deep pharynx.

Inflammatory Lesions

Inflammatory lesions of the prestyloid compartment most commonly result from:

- The spread of infectious material from a peritonsillar abscess (Figs. 12.**2 a, b**).
- Thrombophlebitis of the retrotonsillar vein.
- Extraction of the third molar.
- A penetrating injury of the pharyngeal wall.
- An abscess of the medial pole of the parotid gland.
- Complications of local anesthesia for a tonsillectomy or dental treatment.

Inflammation may also spread to the parapharyngeal space from the submandibular gland, branchial cleft cysts, thyroglossal duct cysts, or temporal bone infections. The pattern of spread of an inflammatory process in the parapharyngeal space (Figs. 9.**3** and 15.**3**) depends on various factors such as prior injuries, surgical procedures, radiotherapy, and individual differences in fascial anatomy. An infection in the prestyloid compartment of the parapharyngeal space can easily spread to the masticator space, parotid space, submandibular space, or to the poststyloid compartment of the parapharyngeal space. Involvement of the poststyloid compartment can lead to dysfunction of cranial nerves IX–XI or the sympathetic chain. *Infections* of the parapharyngeal space (Fig. 15.**3**) can lead to erosion of the adjacent internal carotid artery, causing a catastrophic hemorrhage, or to the development of a pseudoaneurysm. Parapharyngeal space infection can also lead to orbital involvement, intracranial extension, and osteomyelitis.

Cellulitis (Fig. 9.**2**) appears on CT scans as a soft-tissue mass that shows marked contrast enhancement, effacement of surrounding fat planes, and spread along fascial planes to the subcutaneous tissue. Affected muscles appear thickened and show enhancement on post-contrast scans. The overlying subcutaneous tissue often shows increased attenuation on CT scans.

Abscesses, which account for up to 9% of all parapharyngeal space masses (Figs. 9.**3**, 14.**5**), usually appear on imaging studies as unifocal or multifocal cystic lesions that contain air and fluid elements. On post-contrast images they show a somewhat nonhomogeneous enhancing rim (Fig. 9.**3 c**), and perifocal edema is usually present. Occasionally, purulent liquefaction is still in complete at the time of imaging or is delayed due to antibiotic therapy, causing the lesion to appear as a small, low-density abscess cavity on CT scans (Fig. 9.**3 a**) and an area of high signal intensity on T2-weighted MR images. The lesion yields little or no pus on aspiration or surgical exploration.

Both CT and MRI can accurately define the extent of the inflammatory process on axial and coronal images. The inflammatory exudate has low to moderate signal intensity on T1-weighted images

(Fig. 9.**3 c**), often appearing isointense to muscle. Cellulitis and abscesses are distinguished by their increased signal intensity on T2-weighted images (Fig. 9.**3**). Contrast-enhanced images can differentiate cellulitis from an abscess by demonstrating the enhancing abscess wall. In most cases, neither CT nor MRI can discriminate between a bacterial or granulomatous cause of the inflammatory process.

The preoperative differential diagnosis of poststyloid compartment lesions is clinically important in terms of reducing the risk of potentially fatal hemorrhagic complications during surgical intervention. The imaging modalities of CT and MRI offer significant advantages in the detection of complications and the planning of surgical drainage.

Vascular Lesions of the Parapharyngeal Space and Bordering Spaces

MRI, with its ability to depict flow voids, is superior to CT for diagnosing vascular lesions in the poststyloid compartment of the parapharyngeal space, as it can better document thrombosis of the internal carotid artery or internal jugular vein. On CT, thrombosis of the internal carotid artery or internal jugular vein is easily misinterpreted as a necrotic mass.

An *aneurysm* (Fig. 14.**27**) or *pseudoaneurysm of the internal carotid artery*, which may have the same clinical presentation as a paraganglioma, shows marked contrast enhancement on CT scans and is not clearly demarcated from the carotid artery itself. MRI frequently demonstrates a signal void on T1- and T2-weighted SE sequences. The diagnosis of an aneurysm or pseudoaneurysm is further strengthened by finding increased signal intensities on the T1-weighted image when partial thrombosis is present (Fig. 14.**27 a**). If CT or MRI cannot establish a specific diagnosis, these studies should be supplemented by angiography.

The differential diagnosis should include "vascular pseudomasses" such as an ectatic, tortuous, or duplicated internal carotid artery. This type of lesion does not require surgical treatment but may present clinically as a pulsatile parapharyngeal mass.

Thrombosis of the internal carotid artery or internal jugular vein can mimic the CT appearance of a necrotic mass in the poststyloid compartment of the parapharyngeal space. The thrombosis can be distinguished from a necrotic mass by the tubular configuration of the lesion, by its increased signal intensity on noncontrast T1-weighted MR images, or by inability to demonstrate a normal internal carotid artery or internal jugular vein.

As in the prestyloid compartment, benign lesions such as *paragangliomas* and *schwannomas* (Fig. 9.**7**) are the most common tumor masses in the poststyloid compartment of the parapharyngeal space. Paragangliomas are usually located at the carotid bifurcation but may also occur at the jugular foramen, in the middle ear cleft, or at the nodose ganglion of the vagus nerve. The most common paraganglioma of the retrostyloid compartment is the glomus vagale tumor that arises at, or just below, the nodose ganglion of the vagus nerve. Glomus jugulare tumors (Fig. 4.**29**) may infiltrate the poststyloid compartment secondarily from above, and carotid body tumors (Fig. 14.**13**) may infiltrate it from below.

Traumatic Lesions

Traumatic lesions of the parapharyngeal space are usually the result of *impalement injuries*, which in children are often caused by objects placed into the mouth. These injuries may lead to infections and abscesses of the parapharyngeal space (Fig. 9.**3**) as well as neurovascular trauma. Contrast-enhanced CT is the imaging procedure of choice in acute situations (Fig. 9.**3 a**), while MRI is preferred in subacute cases.

Iatrogenic Lesions

The most common iatrogenic lesions of the parapharyngeal space, besides those following a tumor resection, are inflammatory lesions of the prestyloid compartment due to a *complication of local anesthesia for a tonsillectomy* or *dental treatment*.

Imaging Criteria and Their Differential Diagnosis

The differential diagnostic assessment of a parapharyngeal space lesion can be significantly improved by accurately evaluating the site of the lesion (prestyloid or poststyloid compartment) and by the application of differentiating imaging criteria. This is particularly important considering that lesions originating in the salivary glands have a much greater tendency to recur in cases where biopsy was performed prior to the surgical removal of a pleomorphic adenoma (Fig. 9.**4**). Also, distinguishing a primary parapharyngeal lesion from a lesion that extends into the parapharyngeal space from the parotid gland has major therapeutic implications, as this will dictate the choice of the surgical approach.

The diagnostic superiority of MRI and CT over conventional techniques has led to the development of various MRI and CT criteria for distinguishing a lesion of parotid origin from a lesion of extraparotid origin. The main differentiating criterion is still based on visualization of the parapharyngeal fat: if fat is seen between the parotid gland and the posterolateral margin of the lesion, the mass is extraparotid in origin. MRI, with its superior soft-tissue contrast, improves our ability to demonstrate the parapharyngeal fat and thus to differentiate extraparotid from intraparotid masses (Figs. 10.**5**– 10.**7**, 10.**9**– 10.**11**).

MRI is also superior to CT in the differentiation of neurogenic tumors from minor salivary gland tumors in the parapharyngeal space. Neurogenic tumors (Fig. 9.**7**) tend to displace the internal carotid artery anteriorly, while tumors of the minor salivary glands tend to displace the artery posteriorly. Additionally, the smooth margins of a neuroma or paraganglioma, visualized most clearly on MR images, help to distinguish these tumors from the invasive growth that characterizes tumors of the minor salivary glands.

Liquid Masses (Table 9.**2**)

The differential diagnosis of a liquid lesion of the parapharyngeal space is based largely on a density analysis of the mass on plain and post-contrast CT scans and its appearance on noncontrast T1- and T2-weighted SE sequences and gadolinium(Gd)-enhanced T1-weighted sequences. The differential diagnostic analysis is based partly on a site-of-lesion assessment that assigns the lesion to the prestyloid or poststyloid compartment, and partly on determining whether the lesion is intraparotid or extraparotid in origin. Key criteria in this process are the homogeneity of the lesion, its wall structure, and its enhancement characteristics. Important differentiating points are the presence of primary (usually branchial-cleft) cyst formation, inflammatory parapharyngeal abscessation (Fig. 9.**3**), cellulitis (Fig. 9.**2**), the cystic liquefaction of a lymphoma (Fig. 14.**8**), or the cystic malignant infiltration of a parapharyngeal space lymph node. A vascular lesion such as an aneurysm (Fig. 14.**27**), even when partially thrombosed, and thrombosis of the jugular vein can usually be reliably diagnosed using the criteria of density, contrast enhancement, and signal characteristics in various MR imaging sequences.

Air-Containing Masses

Air-containing masses of the parapharyngeal space are rarely seen on imaging studies. Occasionally, small air inclusions may be seen in parapharyngeal abscesses, after trauma (especially impalement injuries), or after surgical procedures.

Tumor Masses of the Prestyloid Compartment

Most tumor masses of the prestyloid compartment (Table 9.**3**) of the parapharyngeal space are *benign tumors*. The most common of these are *salivary gland tumors*, with pleomorphic adenoma (Fig. 9.**4**) representing the most common histologic diagnosis. Most salivary gland tumors in the prestyloid compartment arise from the medial pole of the parotid gland and are found at CT or MRI to extend through the stylomandibular tunnel into the parapharyngeal space. Typically, even extensive pleomorphic adenomas ("iceberg tumors") of the parapharyngeal space do not exhibit skull base infiltration (Fig. 9.**4c**). On the other hand, tumors of the masticator space can easily infiltrate the skull base through the foramen ovale (Figs. 9.**6** and 9.**12**).

Salivary gland tumors also may originate in the prestyloid compartment when they arise from ectopic rests of salivary gland tissue. The distinction be-

Table 9.**2** Liquid masses of the parapharyngeal space

Findings	Internal structure	CT criteria	MRI criteria	Differential diagnosis	Differential diagnostic criterion
Malformation:					
➤ Branchial cleft cyst (Figs. 14.**2** – 14.**4**)	Homogeneous internal structure, smooth margins	Central fluid density, enhancing rim ↑	High T2-weighted signal, enhancing rim ↑	Cystic regressive adenoma, encapsulated abscess (Fig. 9.**3**)	Morphology, contrast enhancement
➤ Dermoid, epidermoid cyst	Usually homogeneous; smooth margins				
Tumor:					
➤ Benign (Fig. 9.**4 a**): cystic regressive adenoma	Smooth margins, nonhomogeneous internal structure	Nonhomogenous enhancement; rarely only an enhancing rim ↑	High T2-weighted signal, low T1-weighted signal on noncontrast images	Dermoid/epidermoid cyst	Density, signal, topography
➤ Malignant: Adenoid cystic carcinoma Acinar cell carcinoma (Fig. 10.**7**) Mucoepidermoid carcinoma	Indistinct margins, nonhomogeneous	Nonhomogeneous contrast enhancement ↑	Nonhomogeneous contrast enhancement ↑		
Inflammatory:					
➤ Abscess (Fig. 9.**3**)	Indistinct margins, rarely transgresses fascial boundaries	Fluid density, nonhomogeneous peripheral enhancement ↑	High T2-weighted signal, moderate T1-weighted signal, peripheral enhancement ↑, areas of liquefaction		Contrast enhancement, abscess wall
➤ Cellulitis (Fig. 9.**2 b**)	Indistinct margins, transgresses fascial boundaries		High T2-weighted signal, intense contrast enhancement ↑		
➤ Inflammatory adenopathy	Multiple definable lymph nodes, usually without involvement of adjacent structures		Hyperintense on T2-weighted images, marked contrast enhancement ↑, usually no necrotic foci		
Vascular:					
➤ Thrombosis ➤ Aneurysm (Fig. 14.**27**)	Usually homogeneous, projected onto vessels	Usually homogeneous, projected onto vessels	High signal intensity on unenhanced T1- and T2-weighted images		Density, morphology

Table 9.3 Mass lesions of the prestyloid compartment

Findings	Differential diagnostic criteria
Common:	
➤ Benign tumors:	
–Pleomorphic adenoma (origin: parotid gland, ectopic salivary gland rests)	Topography homogeneity, contrast enhancement
–Lipoma	Density, signal intensity, homogeneity
–Complicated branchial cleft cyst	Density, signal intensity, contrast enhancement ↑
➤ Inflammatory lesions:	
–Chronic abscess (Fig. 9.**3**)	Density, topography
➤ Vascular lesions:	
–Chronic jugular vein thrombosis (Fig. 14.**27**)	Topography, signal intensity
–Thrombosed or partially thrombosed aneurysm of internal carotid artery	
Rare:	
➤ Malignant tumors:	Infiltration, destruction, homogeneity
–Adenocarcinoma	
–Adenoid cystic carcinoma	
–Mucoepidermoid carcinoma	

tween tumors of the parotid gland and tumors derived from salivary rest cells is important for surgical planning, since tumors that arise from the medial pole of the parotid gland generally require surgical control of the facial nerve, whereas an extraparotid lesion of the prestyloid compartment can be excised with very little risk of injury to the facial nerve.

On CT, benign salivary gland tumors usually appear as an oval soft-tissue mass. Typically they appear homogeneous when small, but larger tumors may contain areas of low density representing sites of cystic degeneration or collections of seromucous fluid. Lesions occasionally contain foci of increased density caused by small calcifications.

On MRI, benign salivary gland tumors (Figs. 9.**4** and 10.**6**) appear as smoothly marginated masses with low to moderate signal intensity on T1-weighted images (Fig. 9.**4b**) and proton-density images, and they show moderate to high signal intensity on T2-weighted images (Fig. 9.**4a**). Smaller lesions up to approximately 2.5 cm in diameter usually have a homogeneous internal structure and show marked contrast enhancement after Gd-DTPA (0.1 mmol/kg bw). Larger lesions usually appear heterogeneous in all SE sequences, containing hypointense areas of calcification or fibrosis. Also, small areas of intratumoral hemorrhage can produce signal increases in unenhanced T1-weighted and proton-density images.

Lipomas are rare in the prestyloid compartment of the parapharyngeal space. They are readily identified by their isointensity to fat on all MR imaging sequences. They show characteristic low attenuation values on CT scans.

Branchial cleft cysts are also rarely found in the prestyloid compartment. Uncomplicated cysts have low signal intensity on T1-weighted images and high signal intensity on T2-weighted images. Infected cysts may demonstrate increased T1-weighted signal intensity.

Malignant tumors of the prestyloid compartment are far less common than benign tumors. Most are salivary gland malignancies such as *mucoepidermoid carcinomas, adenoid cystic carcinomas*, and *acinar cell carcinomas*. Malignancies may also *infiltrate the prestyloid compartment secondarily* from bordering spaces. It may be difficult to distinguish malignant from benign lesions, since approximately two-thirds of prestyloid compartment malignancies have smooth margins and, like larger benign masses, may show nonhomogeneous internal signal intensity. Thus, the heterogeneity of a mass is not a reliable criterion for differentiating benign and malignant lesions. A more useful indicator appears to be the presence of small calcifications in pleomorphic adenomas, seen most clearly on CT scans, or the appearance of a smooth, lobulated mass on MR images. Irregular or infiltrative margins are suggestive of malignancy (Figs. 9.**11 a–c**), although an inflammatory perifocal reaction associated with a benign tumor or cellulitis (Fig. 9.**2**) may have a similar imaging appearance.

A lesion in the prestyloid compartment of the parapharyngeal space is assumed to have an extraparotid origin if an intact fat plane can be seen between the posterolateral margin of the lesion and the medial pole of the parotid gland (Figs. 9.**5 a, b**). High-resolution, unenhanced, thin-section T1-weighted images on axial planes are best for identifying this tissue band, which often is quite thin. With a very large mass (> 4 cm), it is sometimes difficult or impossible to determine whether the lesion is of intraparotid or extraparotid origin, since compression of the parapharyngeal structures may cause poor delineation of the intervening fat.

The principal *indirect signs* of a tumor mass in the prestyloid compartment of the parapharyngeal space are as follows:

- Medial displacement of nasopharyngeal soft-tissue structures, lateral displacement of the masticator space.
- Extension of tumor posteriorly with expansion of the stylomandibular tunnel.
- Extension of tumor into the submandibular space.

➤ Tumor extension cephalad is limited by the convergent fasciae that attach medial to the foramen ovale.

Tumor Masses of the Poststyloid (Retrostyloid) Compartment

The diagnosis of a mass lesion in the poststyloid compartment of the parapharyngeal space is based on the relation of the lesion to the styloid process and internal carotid artery, and on the displacement of fat in the prestyloid compartment of the parapharyngeal space.

CT demonstrates the *glomus vagale tumor* (Fig. 4.**30**) as a well-circumscribed mass in the poststyloid compartment that almost always displaces the internal carotid artery anteriorly. The tumor shows marked, usually homogeneous enhancement on postcontrast scans. Nonenhancing foci are occasionally seen within the mass and usually represent small areas of intratumoral hemorrhage or necrosis. For *paragangliomas* that arise in the jugular foramen, CT using a high-resolution bone algorithm can demonstrate osseous changes and define the relation of the tumor to the middle ear. The rest of the head and neck region should also be carefully surveyed to exclude multiplicity.

The MR appearance of paragangliomas is that of a smooth-contoured, slightly lobulated mass that is well demarcated from the surrounding tissue. MRI can also document the anterior displacement of the internal carotid artery (Fig. 14.**3**). Paragangliomas appear isointense or slightly hyperintense to surrounding muscle on T1-weighted images and show increased signal intensity on T2-weighted images.

A characteristic MR finding is the presence of linear areas of signal void similar to those seen in hemangiomas. These signal voids may not be visible in every section, but every tumor larger than 1.5–2 cm in diameter should exhibit flow voids on high-resolution T1-weighted MR images so that a confident diagnosis of a paraganglioma can be made. Unless a dynamic enhancement study is performed after the bolus injection of Gd-DTPA (0.3 mmol/kg bw), paragangliomas are difficult to distinguish from schwannomas, which also show intense contrast enhancement. Paragangliomas differ from neuromas (Fig. 9.**7**) and meningiomas (Fig. 9.**8**) by showing significantly more rapid contrast appearance and an early "dropout effect" following a high-dose application (0.3 mmol/kg bw) (Fig. 9.**9**). If necessary, the diagnosis of parapharyngeal space tumors can be confirmed by biopsy, preferably using the subzygomatic approach (Fig. 9.**13**).

Table 9.**4** Mass lesions of the poststyloid compartment

Findings	**Differential diagnostic criteria**
Common:	
➤ Tumors:	
–Paraganglioma (Figs. 4.**29**, 4.**30**, 14.**13**)	Signal intensity, vascularity, internal structures
–Neuroma (Fig. 9.**7**)	Morphology, contrast enhancement
–Meningioma (Fig. 9.**8**)	Morphology, topography
➤ Vascular lesions:	
–Aneurysm of internal carotid artery (Fig. 14.**27**)	Density, morphology
–Thrombosis of internal jugular vein	Density, morphology
–Kinking/elongation of the internal carotid artery	Topography
Rare:	
➤ Lymphadenopathy (inflammatory, neoplastic)	
➤ Benign and malignant mesenchymal tumors	
➤ Inflammatory masses	

Tumor Masses of the Masticator Space

The following questions should be addressed in the imaging analysis of a masticator space mass:

➤ Is the mass primary to the masticator space?
➤ Is there perineural tumor spread along cranial nerve V_3?
➤ Has the tumor infiltrated the skull base or suprazygomatic masticator space?
➤ Has the tumor infiltrated the mandible?
➤ Has the tumor infiltrated the parotid duct?

The most common lesion seen in the masticator space is the *odontogenic abscess*. Most patients report a history of chronic dental problems or a recent dental extraction. CT demonstrates a mass of fluid density. On MRI, T2-weighted sequences show markedly increased signal intensity in the region of the masticator space with marked swelling of surrounding soft tissues. Bone destruction due to *osteomyelitis of the mandible or skull base* is best visualized by CT. Given the frequent difficulty of palpating the affected region due to pain, it is imperative that the extent of the odontogenic abscess be accurately defined by CT or MRI. Osteomyelitis of the skull base or mandible, involvement of other spaces, and involvement of the suprazygomatic masticator space are important ques-

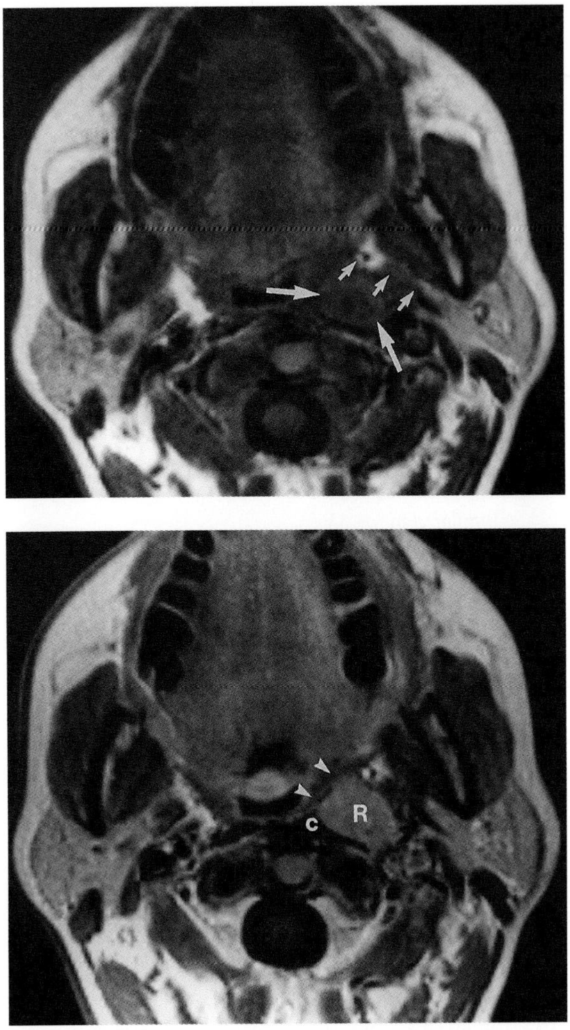

a

b

Fig. 9.**7 a, b Glossopharyngeal neuroma.**
(**a**) Axial noncontrast T1-weighted MR image (TR/TE = 700/15 ms) shows a smooth, rounded mass (large arrows) in the left parapharyngeal space displacing the neurovascular sheath posterolaterally and the parapharyngeal fat anteriorly (small arrows). There is some indentation of the left pharyngeal constrictor muscle.
(**b**) Contrast-enhanced T1-weighted image (TR/TE = 700/15 ms) shows marked contrast enhancement of the mass and more clearly delineates the mass (R) from the longus capitis muscle (c) and pharyngeal constrictor muscle (arrowheads).
c Longus capitis muscle
R Mass

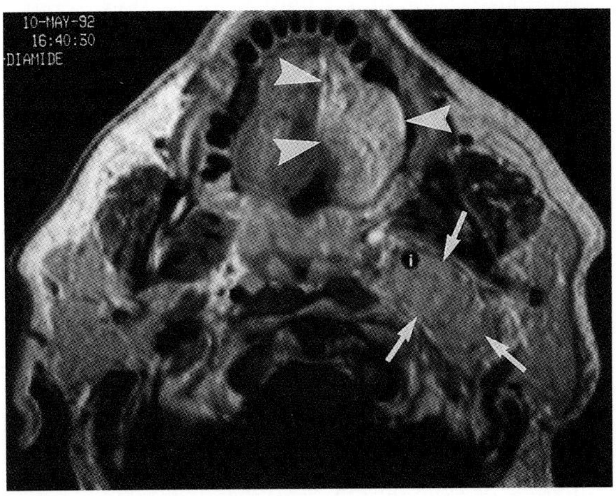

Fig. 9.**8 Meningioma that has spread down through the jugular foramen into the left parapharyngeal space.** Contrast-enhanced T1-weighted image shows the markedly enhancing tumor mass (arrows) in the left parapharyngeal space. Unlike the glossopharyngeal neuroma (see Fig. 9.**7**), this tumor is displacing the internal carotid artery anteromedially. The image also shows a marked increase of signal intensity in the left half of the tongue (arrowheads). This signal increase, caused by tumor compression of the hypoglossal nerve, is confined strictly to the left half of the tongue and is typical of hypoglossal nerve palsy.
i Internal carotid artery

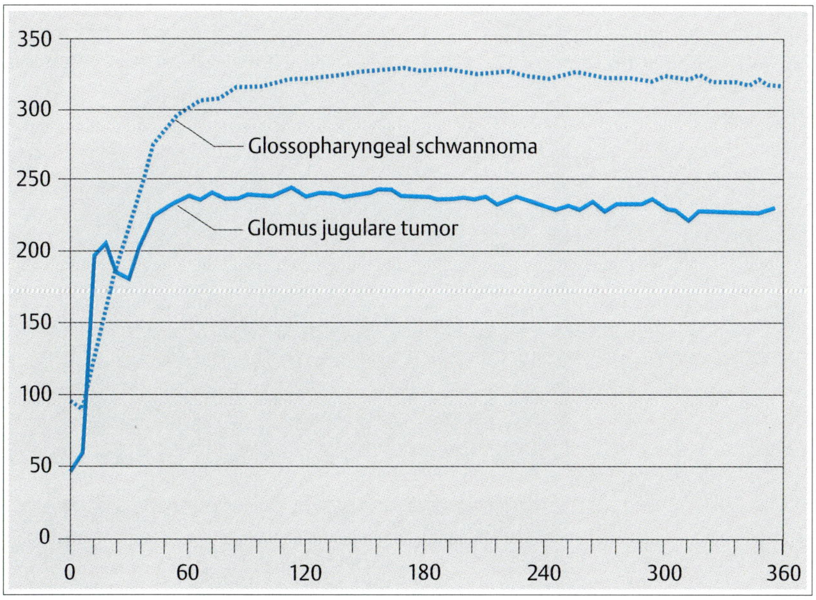

Fig. 9.**9** **Time-signal intensity curve for a glomus jugulare tumor (Fig. 4.29) and a glossopharyngeal schwannoma** (Fig. 9.**7 b**). A turbo FLASH sequence is needed to demonstrate the "dropout effect" in the glomus jugulare tumor (TR/TE/TI = 7/300 ms, 128 × 128 matrix, acquisition time 2 s with 2 s interval between acquisitions).

tions to be resolved in the differential diagnosis of these lesions.

Malignant tumors. Because the principal structures of the masticator space are muscles and the mandible, primary malignant tumors of this space are often sarcomas (soft-tissue sarcoma [Figs. 9.**6** and 9.**12**], chondrosarcoma, osteosarcoma). These tumors usually arise from the region of the temporomandibular joint. Osteosarcomas can arise from any portion of the mandible. At imaging, osteosarcomas show neoplastic new bone formation on CT scans, while chondrosarcomas tend to show chondroid calcifications within the mass. Both MRI and CT can demonstrate an infiltrating mass in the masticator space, usually associated with some degree of mandibular destruction. Frequently, however, these masses are indistinguishable from other malignancies of the masticator space.

Malignant schwannoma, known also as neurogenic sarcoma or fibrosarcoma, usually arises from the inferior alveolar nerve or masticator nerve in the masticator space. CT or MRI will often demonstrate a mass along the course of cranial nerve V_3. The tumor may spread along the main trunk of V_3 through the foramen ovale to infiltrate the skull base, and it may spread perineurally to the gasserian ganglion in the Meckel cavity.

Non-Hodgkin lymphoma can likewise be difficult to distinguish radiologically from other malignant tumors of the masticator space. An important aid to differential diagnosis is the presence of enlarged lymph nodes outside the masticator space. The demonstration of multiple pathologically enlarged lymph nodes that show nonhomogeneous, ground-glass enhancement on post-contrast images is strongly suggestive of lymphomatous disease. A single focus of non-Hodgkin lymphoma in the masticator space has the same imaging appearance as any other malignant mass.

An infiltrating *squamous cell carcinoma* may enter the masticator space by direct extension from the oropharynx via the tonsillar fossa or by perineural tumor spread along the inferior alveolar nerve involved by mandibular invasion from the oral cavity.

In evaluating a lesion of the masticator space, it is imperative to examine the entire course of cranial nerve V_3 (Figs. 9.**6** and 9.**12**) and all of the masticator space, including the suprazygomatic fossa. When a lesion is detected, it must be differentiated from a pseudomass such as an asymmetric accessory parotid gland, benign hypertrophy of the masseter muscle, or muscular atrophy due to cranial nerve V_3 denervation. An accessory parotid gland is normally found at the surface of the masseter muscle, outside the masticator space. The differentiation of an accessory parotid gland (Fig. 9.**15**) from a tumor mass should rely on MRI, that permits evaluation of the mass on various sequences. If the signal characteristics of the pseudomass are identical to those of the parotid gland on all plain and contrast-enhanced sequences, the mass may be identified as an accessory parotid gland. Also, MRI can clearly differentiate benign hypertrophy of the masseter muscle from malignant and benign (Fig. 9.**10**) tumor masses. In cases of bilateral masseteric hypertrophy, CT or MRI can easily establish the diagnosis. A frequent cause of bilateral masseteric hypertrophy is bruxism (nocturnal grinding of the teeth). Coexisting hypertrophy of the medial and lateral pterygoid muscles and temporalis muscle allow a confident diagnosis of benign masseteric

Figs. 9.**10 a, b** **Cavernous hemangioma.**
(**a**) Axial T2-weighted image (TR/TE = 3979/93 ms) shows a very hyperintense, cystic-appearing mass in the area of the right masseter muscle (black and white arrows). The tongue is displaced to the left by the endotracheal tube.
(**b**) Axial Gd-enhanced T1-weighted image (TR/TE = 690/15 ms) shows nonhomogeneous enhancement of the cavernous hemangioma (black and white arrows) in the right masticator space. The nonenhancing areas represent cystic components. There is no evidence of mandibular bone destruction (arrowheads). The hemangioma is displacing the parotid duct (open arrow) but, being confined to the masticator space, has not infiltrated it.

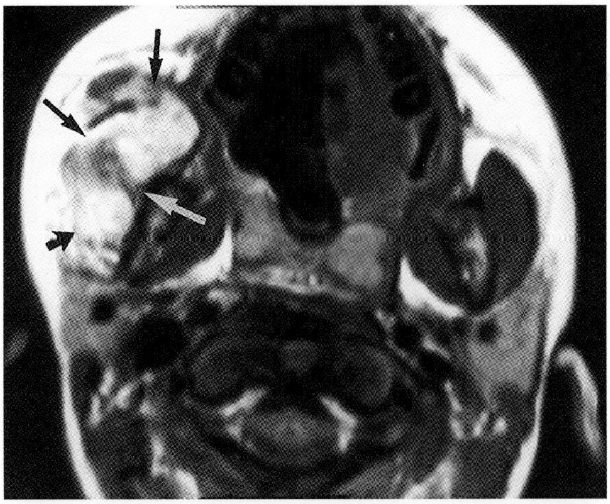

a

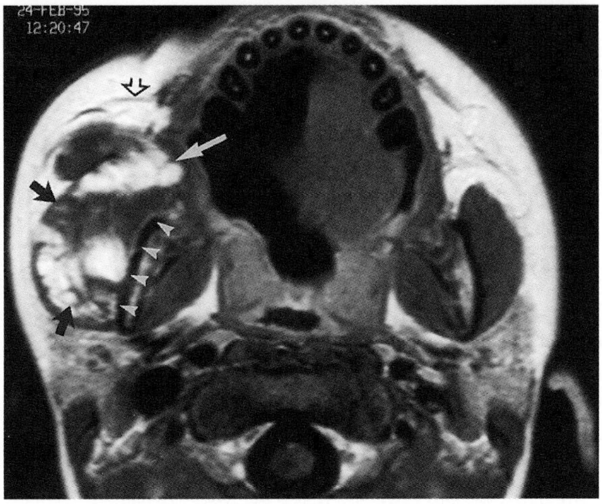

b

hypertrophy. In cases of unilateral masseteric hypertrophy, MRI, with its superior tissue discrimination, should be performed to exclude a neoplasm. Indistinct muscle contours should always raise suspicion of a neoplastic mass.

The motor branch of the trigeminal nerve courses with the mandibular nerve to supply the masticatory muscles, the anterior belly of the digastric muscle, the mylohyoid muscle, and the tensor tympani and tensor veli palatini muscles. Injury to this nerve leads to atrophy of the corresponding muscles with subsequent fatty infiltration. Ordinarily this change is seen only on one side. Fatty infiltration becomes evident approximately 6 weeks after the nerve injury, marked by the appearance of fat-equivalent signal intensities in all MR imaging sequences.

Caution: there is a danger of misinterpreting the normal contralateral side as a tumor mass.

Very rarely, lymph node metastases or tumors arising from the parotid duct may be encountered in the masticator space (Figs. 9.**14 a, b**).

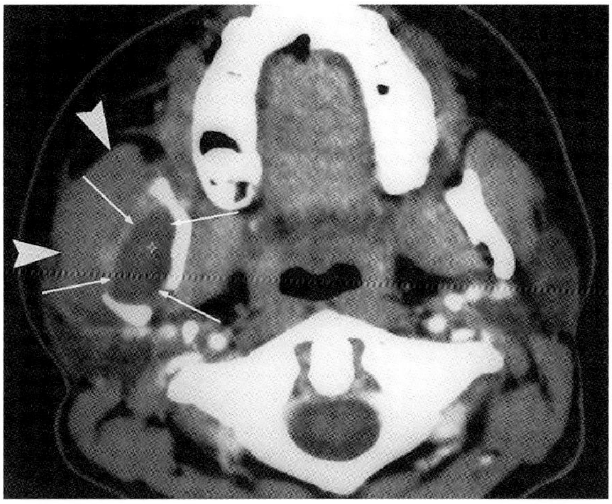

a

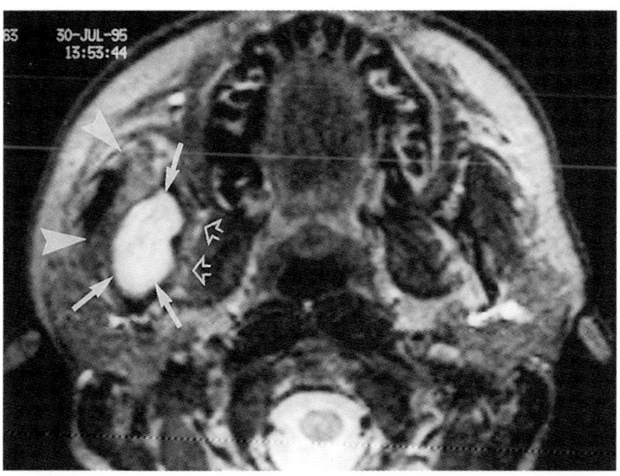

b

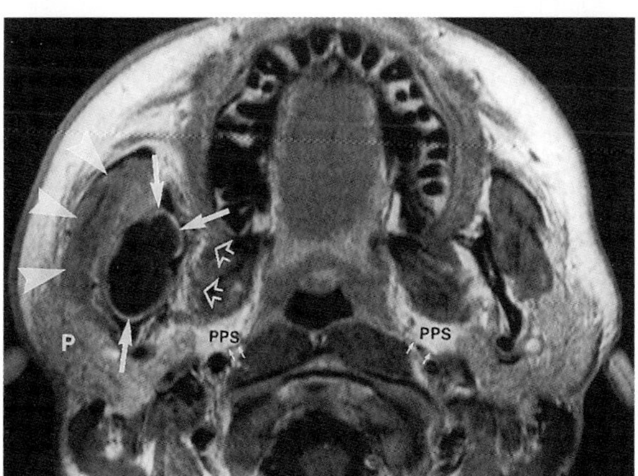

c

Figs. 9.**11 a–c** **Infected keratocyst of the mandible.**
(**a**) Axial CT scan with a soft-tissue window shows expansion and partial destruction of the right mandible (arrows) along with subtle soft-tissue swelling in the area of the right masseter muscle (arrowheads).
(**b**) Axial T2-weighted image (TR/TE = 3000/90 ms) shows a smoothly marginated mass of high signal intensity (arrows) in the right side of the mandible. The signal characteristics in the T2-weighted sequence are consistent with a cystic mass. The image also shows an accompanying inflammatory reaction involving the masseter muscle (arrowheads) and, to a lesser degree, the medial pterygoid muscle (open arrows).
(**c**) Gd-enhanced axial T1-weighted image (TR/TE = 700/15 ms) shows a cystic mass of the mandible with an enhancing wall (arrows). The masseter muscle (arrowheads) and medial pterygoid muscle (open arrows) also show marked enhancement. The mass does not involve the parotid gland or the prestyloid compartment of the parapharyngeal space.

Small arrows	Stylopharyngeal diaphragm
P	Parotid gland
PPS	Prestyloid compartment of parapharyngeal space

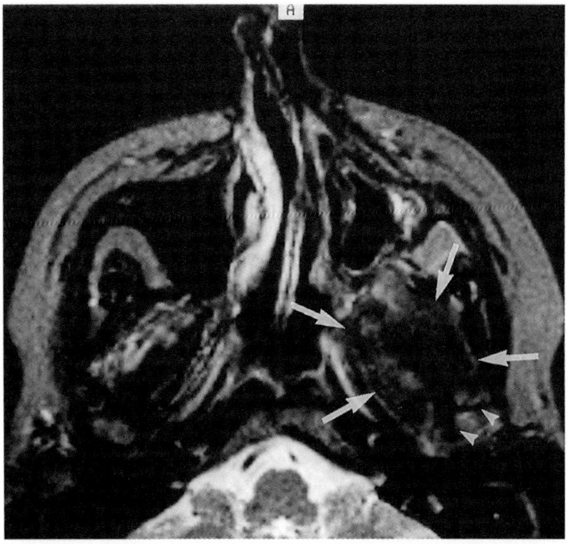

Fig. 9.**12** **Leiomyosarcoma.** Axial T2-weighted image (TR/TE = 3000/90 ms) shows a hypointense mass in the left masticator space (arrows) that has caused marked posteromedial displacement of the parapharyngeal space. A thin fat plane (arrowheads) is still visible between the mass and the parotid space. The mass appears markedly hypointense relative to pleomorphic adenoma (see Fig. 9.**3 a**).

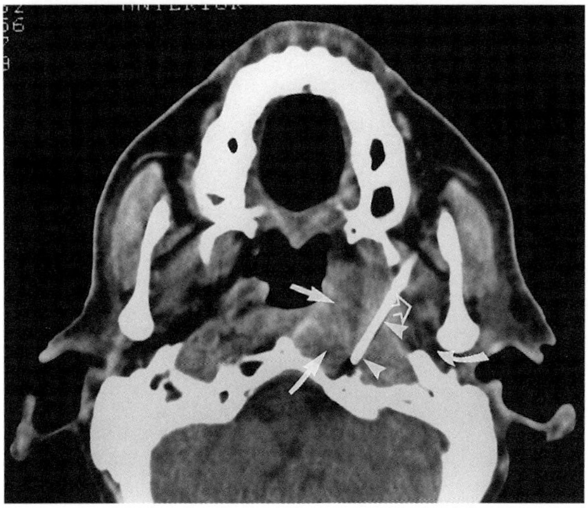

Fig. 9.**13** **CT-guided needle biopsy of a parapharyngeal space mass.** CT scanning with a soft-tissue window shows a tumor mass in the left parapharyngeal space (arrows). The mass is biopsied under CT guidance through a subzygomatic approach (arrowheads = needle). Histologic evaluation confirmed a recurrence of squamous cell carcinoma. Note that the parapharyngeal fat has been displaced far anterolaterally by the mass, appearing only as a thin layer (open arrow). There is no apparent infiltration of the stylomandibular tunnel on the left side (curved arrow).

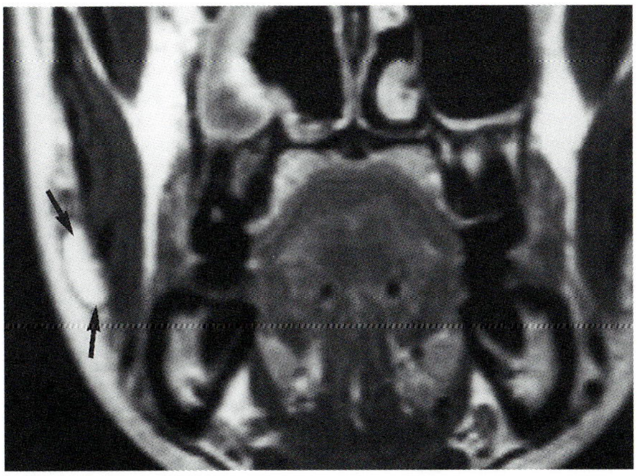

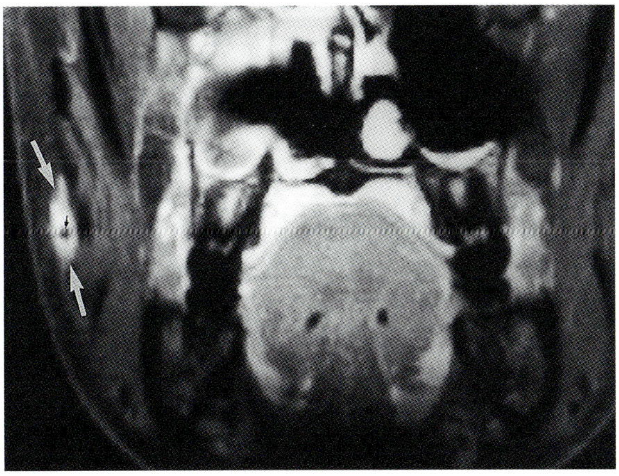

Figs. 9.**14a, b** **Extraglandular, paraductal recurrence of adenoid cystic carcinoma.**
(**a**) Post-contrast T1-weighted SE sequence in the coronal plane demonstrates a smoothly marginated mass with a high signal intensity and homogeneous internal structure located lateral to the masseter muscle and the ascending ramus of the mandible (arrows).
(**b**) Post-contrast FATSAT sequence in the coronal plane. This fat-suppressed sequence demarcates the mass (white arrows) from the central, low-signal parotid duct (small black arrow) that the tumor encases. The tumor infiltration is confined to the paraductal space and has not yet caused complete ductal obstruction. Histologic examination confirmed local invasion by a recurrence of adenoid cystic carcinoma.

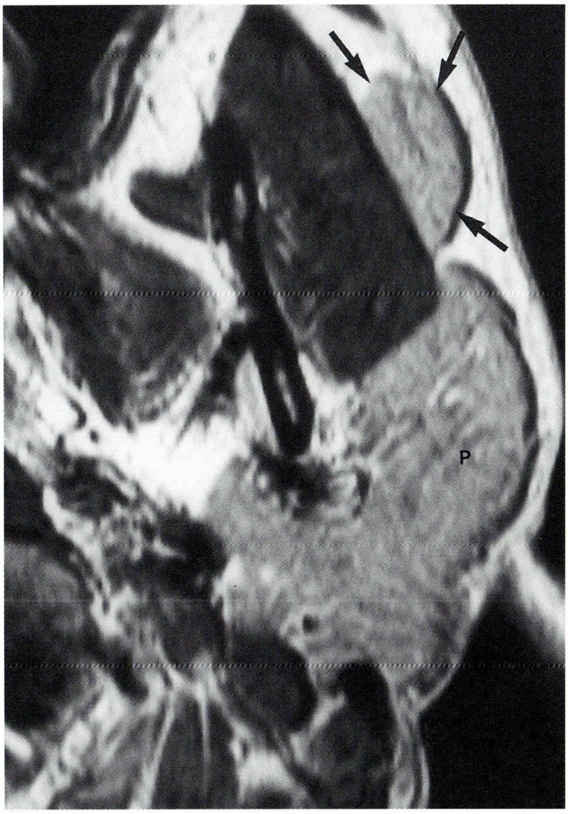

Fig. 9.**15** **Accessory parotid gland.** Gd-enhanced axial T1-weighted image (TR/TE = 690/15 ms) reveals a mass about 1 cm in diameter lateral to the left masticator space in the area of the subcutaneous connective tissue. The accessory parotid gland (arrows) shows the same signal characteristics as the parotid gland in all imaging sequences.
P Parotid gland

Summary and Diagnostic Strategy

Given the complex anatomy of the parapharyngeal space and the diversity of soft-tissue structures in and around the space, imaging studies will usually enable a very precise differential diagnosis to be made following a rigorous analysis of key landmarks. Plain and contrast-enhanced MRI has become the method of choice for this type of analysis. After the lesion has been localized on a T2-weighted SE sequence, pre- and post-gadolinium images are obtained to identify the appropriate landmarks (e.g., the parapharyngeal fat and tensor veli palatini muscle) and define the relation of the mass to surrounding structures.

In cases where MRI and CT do not allow a confident, precise differential diagnosis, the parapharyngeal mass should be biopsied under imaging guidance after a vascular lesion such as an aneurysm of the internal carotid artery (Fig. 14.**27**) or arterial pseudomass has been excluded.

References

1 Aspestrand, F., M. Boysen: CT and MR Imaging of primary tumors of the masticator space. Acta Radiol. 33 (1992) 518–522
2 Braun, I. F., W. E. Torres, J. A. Landmann et al: Computed Tomography of benign masseteric hypertrophy. J Comput Assist Tomogr. 9 (1985) 167–170
3 Curtin, H. D.: Seperation of the masticator space from the parapharyngeal space. Radiology 163 (1987) 195–204
4 Durrant, T. J., R. J. Sevick, C. Lauryssen, M. E. MacRae: Parapharyngeal branchial cleft cyst presenting with cranial nerve palsies. Can Assoc Radiol J. 45 (1994) 134–136
5 Elango, S.: Parapharyngeal space lipoma. Ear Nose Throat J. 74 (1995) 52–53
6 Guneri, A., M. U. Gunbay, E. A. Guneri, K. Ceryan, S. Sutay: Management of parapharyngeal space cysts. J Laryngol Otol. 108 (1994) 795–797
7 Harnsberger, H. R., A. G. Osborn: Differential diagnosis of head and neck lesions based on their space origin. 1. The suprahyoid part of the neck. AJR 157 (1991) 147–154
8 Pensak, M. L., J. L. Gluckman, K. A. Shumrick: Parapharyngeal space tumors: an algorithm for evaluation and management. Laryngoscope 104 (1994) 1170–1173
9 Saing, H., W. F. Lau, Y. F. Chan, F. L. Chan: Parapharyngeal teratoma in the newborn. J Pediatr Surg. 29 (1994) 1524–1525
10 Silver, A. J., M. E. Mawad, S. K. Hilal et al.: CT of the nasopharynx and related space. II Pathology. Radiology 147 (1983) 733–738
11 Som, P. M., I. F. Braun, M. D. Shapiro et al.: Tumors of the parapharyngeal space and upper neck: MR Imaging characteristics. Radiology 164 (1987) 823–829
12 Yousem, D. M., M. J. Sack, K. A. Scanlan: Biopsy of parapharyngeal space lesions. Radiology 193 (1994) 619–622

10 Salivary Glands

The major salivary glands consist of three paired glandular bodies: the serous *parotid glands*, the *submandibular glands*, and the predominantly mucus-secreting *sublingual glands*. The salivary glands have a highly differentiated parenchyma and are subject to involvement by numerous pathologic processes. Functional disorders, inflammatory diseases, and primary and secondary neoplasms should all be considered in the rational differential diagnosis of salivary gland disorders. Most neoplasms of the salivary glands are of epithelial origin, but mesenchymal and metastatic tumors can also occur.

Normal Anatomy (Fig. 10.1)

In imaging studies of the salivary glands, a variety of anatomic structures are visualized within a relatively small area. The essential landmarks about the *parotid gland* are the buccal fat pad, which is closely related to the masseter muscle and glandular parenchyma, the facial artery and vein, and the retromandibular vein. Other structures that may appear on imaging studies of the parotid gland are the facial nerve and the parotid duct. The facial nerve, cushioned by a fat pad, exits the temporal bone at the stylomastoid foramen and enters the substance of the parotid gland lateral to the posterior portion of the digastric muscle. The parotid gland is bounded anteriorly by the masseter muscle and medially by the pterygoid muscles, styloid process, external and internal carotid arteries, and internal jugular vein. It is bounded posteriorly by the sternocleidomastoid muscle and the posterior belly of the digastric muscle.

The sublingual and submandibular glands are located in the region of the oral floor. The more cranial *sublingual* soft-tissue space is separated from the lower *submandibular* (Fig. 10.**2**) and *submental* space (Fig. 10.**4**) by the transversely oriented mylohyoid muscle, the only communication between the spaces occurring posterior to the free border of the mylohyoid (Fig. 10.**4**). Lateral to the digastric muscle on each side is the *submandibular fossa* (Fig. 10.**2**), which contains the submandibular gland and submandibular lymph nodes. The paired *sublingual fossae* are bounded medially by the extrinsic muscles of the

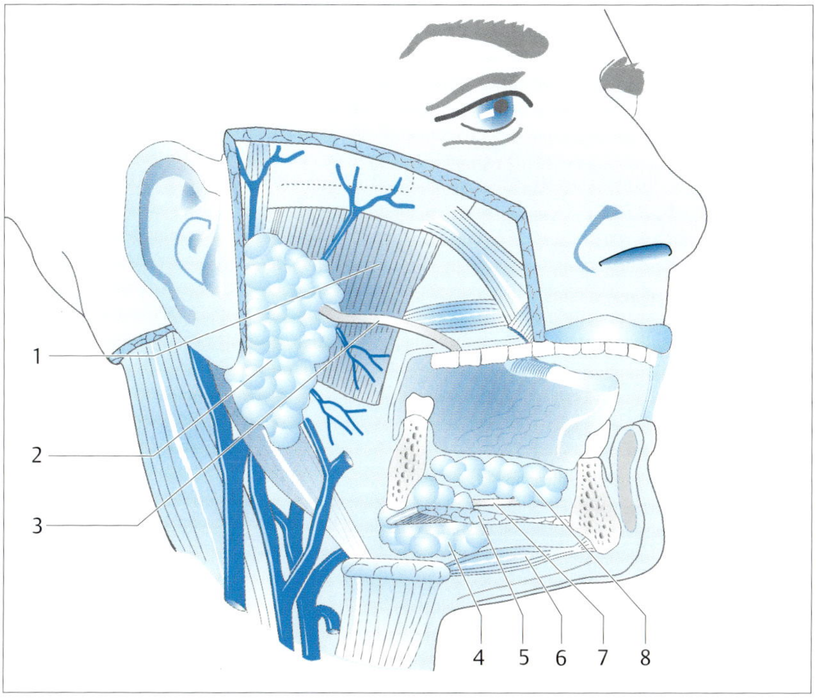

Fig. 10.**1** **Relation of the salivary glands to the surrounding muscles.**
1 Masseter muscle
2 Parotid gland
3 Parotid duct
4 Submandibular gland
5 Mylohyoid muscle
6 Anterior belly of digastric muscle
7 Submandibular duct
8 Sublingual gland

tongue and laterally by the mandible. Each fossa contains the sublingual gland, submandibular duct, lingual artery and vein, and hypoglossal and lingual nerve.

Clinical Signs and Symptoms

The symptoms most commonly associated with salivary gland disorders are:

- Unilateral or bilateral pain.
- Enlargement or swelling of the gland.
- Salivary gland dysfunction.

The symptoms of pain and swelling often coincide and are usually referable to an inflammatory process such as acute sialadenitis, the stasis of salivary secretions, or malignant neoplasms. Chronic inflammations and benign tumors, on the other hand, cause a painless hypertrophy of the affected glands. In cases of secretory dysfunction, deficient salivary secretion is more common than sialorrhea and may be due to Sjögren disease with primary sialopenia or xerostomia (Fig. 10.**14**) or a decrease in salivary secretion during and after radiation therapy. Another type of salivary gland dysfunction is dyschylia, referring to an abnormal biochemical composition of the secretions.

Imaging Evaluation and Differential Diagnosis

Sialography

Rarely performed today, sialography can demonstrate sites of ectasia, stenosis, or luminal obstruction in the *parotid duct* secondary to inflammatory or neoplastic disease. A water-soluble contrast medium is injected into the excretory duct, and radiographic films are taken in standard projections (lateral, anteroposterior, oblique). Radiopaque calculi can be directly visualized, and nonradiopaque calculi are seen as filling defects.

Ultrasound imaging with a 7.5-MHz linear transducer is a rapid, noninvasive procedure that has largely replaced sialography for imaging studies of the parotid gland. Ultrasonography can demonstrate the parenchymal structure of the glandular tissue and is superior to sialography in the detection of *sialoliths*.

Magnetic Resonance Imaging (MRI)

MRI should be the primary sectional imaging study in patients with a suspected salivary gland neoplasm. After the administration of gadolinium (Gd)-DTPA, the normal glandular parenchyma always shows a significant degree of enhancement. Because the facial nerve and its main branches do not enhance with Gd-DTPA, they appear as contrasting areas of low signal intensity within the gland. Images should always be acquired on axial and coronal planes. Axial images are useful for evaluating superficial structures and the relation of the lesion to its surroundings, while coronal images can document the extension of the mass toward the skull base and its relation to major blood vessels. The recommended clinical protocol consists of T1- and T2-weighted spin-echo (SE) sequences and contrast-enhanced (0.1 mmol/kg bw Gd-DTPA) T1-weighted sequences. T1-weighted sequences with fat suppression yield added information on the vascularity of pathologic processes.

Computed Tomography (CT)

CT scanning has only a minor role in the differentiation of parenchymatous changes because of its limited soft-tissue resolution.

Imaging Findings

Congenital Variations and Malformations

Unilateral or bilateral aplasia of the salivary glands or duct system is a rare anomaly. Most cystic lesions are acquired, but there are instances in which a ranula occurs as a developmental anomaly (Fig. 10.**3**).

Tumors

Cystic Lesions

Cystic lesions of the salivary glands (Fig. 10.**5**) are generally slow-growing lesions that may cause submental or intraoral swelling, dysphagia, dyspnea, or speech impediment, depending on their size and location. There are cases in which rupture or superinfection of the cyst will require differentiation from an oral floor abscess or cellulitis.

Cystic lesions arising from the salivary glands are found mainly in the oral floor (Figs. 10.**2** and 10.**4**) and present a broad differential diagnostic spectrum. The majority of cysts arise from the *salivary glands.* Inflammatory processes have been cited as the leading cause of intraglandular duct obstruction with cyst formation, predominantly affecting the submandibular gland (Fig. 10.**2**). A special type of cystic lesion is the *ranula*, caused by the obliteration of one of the small excretory ducts of the sublingual gland (Fig. 10.**3**). It presents clinically as a cyst below the lateral portion of the tongue that, in severe cases, shows more medial extension. Rarely, the cyst may extend into the submental area through a gap in the mylohyoid muscle to form an "hourglass" ranula (Fig. 12.**5**).

Differentiation is required from oral floor lesions that do not arise from the salivary glands. *Epidermoid cysts* (Fig. 12.**4**) have a keratinizing squamous epithelial lining surrounded by a mantle of connective tissue. The contents consist of keratin debris. *Dermoid cysts* (Fig. 10.**4**) are similar, except that adnexal structures such as hair, sweat glands, and sebaceous glands are embedded in the epidermal wall. Both lesions are classified as dysontogenetic cysts caused by a persistence of pluripotent epithelial cells during embryonic closure of midline body clefts. Nestled in the soft-tissue compartment between the mylohyoid and geniohyoid muscles, these lesions can grow to enormous size. *Ectopic colloid cysts* most commonly occur in the base of the tongue and along the path of thyroid descent. *Odontogenic cysts* are fixed to the mandible and typically occur on the lingual aspect of the alveolar process.

Cystic lesions of the parotid gland usually develop in the setting of an underlying infectious disease. *Lymphoepithelial cysts* (Fig. 10.**5**), for example, are a common occurrence in HIV-infected patients. Most of these cysts are bilateral, and large solitary cysts may cause clinical complaints requiring excision. This type of cystic lesion does not arise in the submandibular or sublingual glands.

Benign Salivary Gland Tumors

Common benign tumors of the salivary glands are pleomorphic adenoma and cystadenolymphoma (Warthin tumor). Hemangiomas, lymphangiomas, and lipomas rarely occur in the salivary glands.

Pleomorphic Adenoma (Fig. 10.6)

Pleomorphic adenoma is a firm, fleshy mass that usually arises from the parotid gland and most commonly occurs in middle-aged individuals. Generally these tumors do not affect salivary secretion or facial nerve function.

Morphologically, pleomorphic adenomas are sharply marginated masses that occasionally have a lobulated surface. On ultrasound imaging, small tumors appear moderately echogenic while larger tumors show a complex, nonhomogeneous echogenicity caused by cystic elements and calcifications. On MRI, the overall signal intensities are low on T1-weighted images (Figs. 10.**6a, b**) and high on T2-weighted images (Fig. 10.**6c**). Contrast-enhanced images frequently show nonhomogeneous areas of liquefaction and necrosis.

A special form is the "iceberg tumor" (Fig. 9.**4**), a dumbbell-shaped adenoma of the parapharyngeal space whose intraoral component is palpable within the tonsillar fossa.

Cystadenolymphoma (Warthin Tumor) (Fig. 10.11)

Cystadenolymphoma occurs chiefly in the parotid gland and is usually bilateral. The clinical presentation is that of a soft, mobile mass that is generally asymptomatic. The appearance of a Warthin tumor on MR images is similar to that of pleomorphic adenoma. The tumor remains confined to the parotid compartment, showing no evidence of infiltration. On sonography, the mass shows a more homogeneous, hypoechoic internal structure with no evidence of cystic or regressive changes.

Malignant Salivary Gland Tumors

There are four main histologic types of malignant salivary gland tumor:

- Squamous cell carcinoma.
- Mucoepidermoid carcinoma.
- Adenocarcinoma.
- Adenoid cystic carcinoma.

Uncommon types are acinar cell carcinoma (Fig. 10.**7**), malignant lymphoma (Fig. 10.**10**), and mesenchymal and mixed tumors (Fig. 10.**9**).

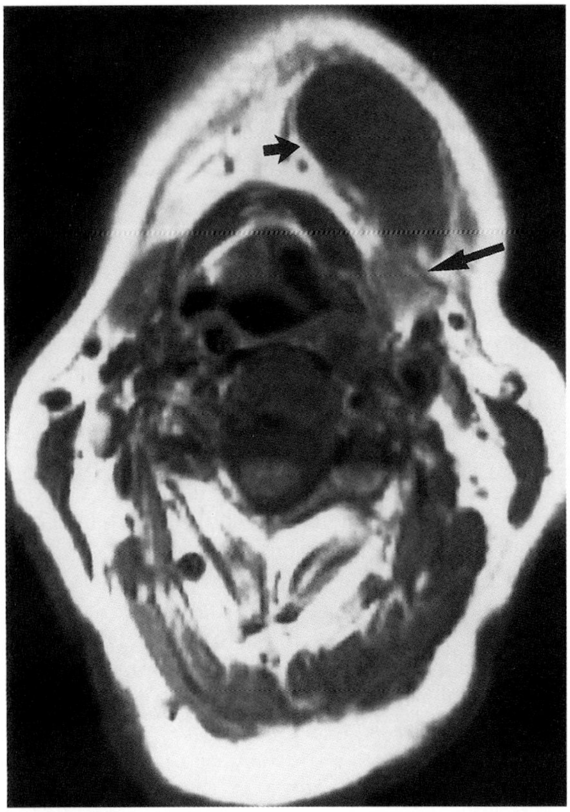

a

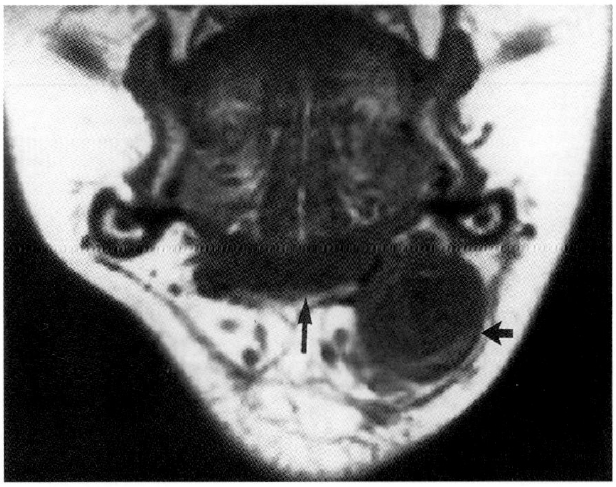

b

Figs. 10.**2 a, b** **Cyst of the submandibular gland.**
(**a**) T1-weighted MR sequence shows a hypointense mass (short arrow) in contact with the left submandibular gland (arrow). This smoothly marginated, homogeneous lesion is a salivary gland cyst.
(**b**) In the coronal plane, the caudal location of the cyst (short arrow) relative to the mylohyoid muscle (arrow) means that a cervical approach should be used if surgical resection of the cyst is required.

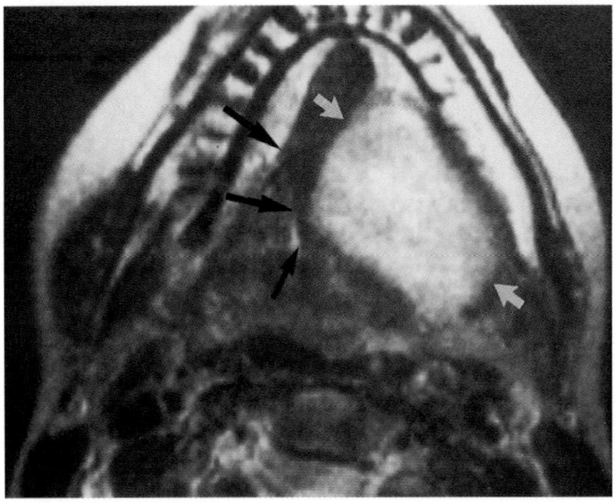

Fig. 10.**3** **Ranula.** T2-weighted MR image shows a hyperintense mass (white arrows) arising from the left sublingual gland and displacing the geniohyoid muscles (black arrows) toward the opposite side. The high signal intensity (consistent with a fluid-filled cyst) and typical location identify the lesion as a ranula.

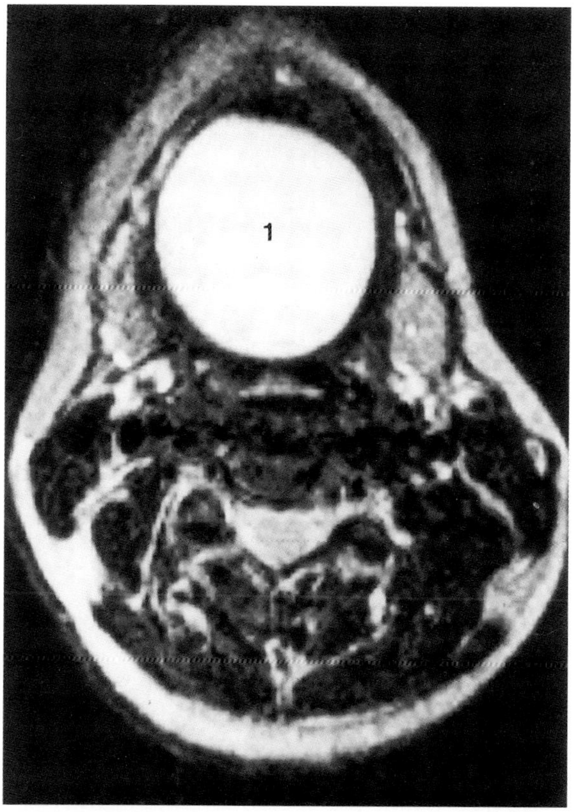

a

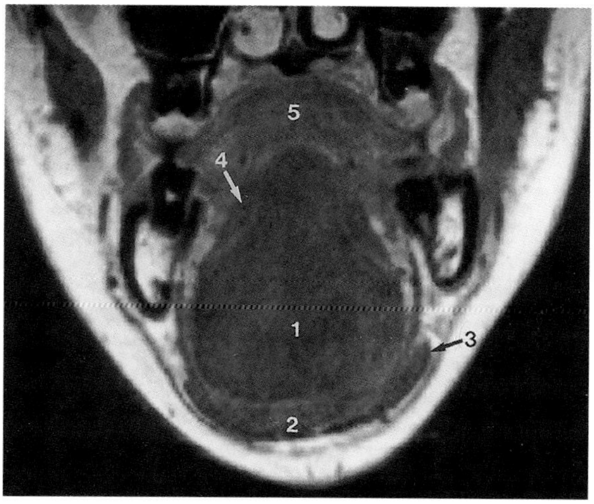

b

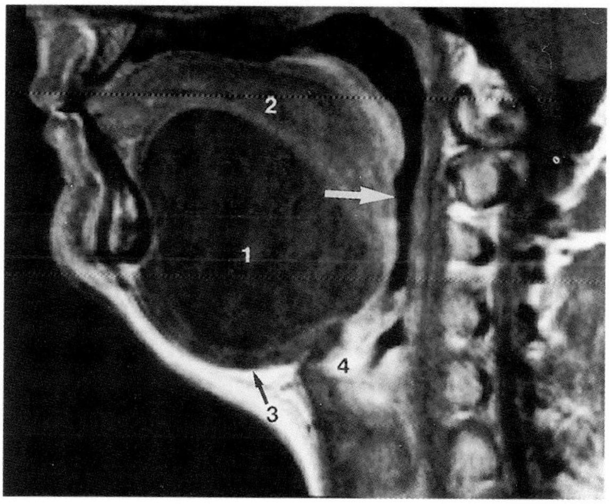

c

Figs. 10.**4 a – c** **Sublingual dermoid cyst.**
(**a**) Axial noncontrast T2-weighted SE sequence (TR/TE = 3000/90 ms) shows high signal intensity consistent with a cystic mass. Surrounding oral floor structures cannot be evaluated further.
1 Cystic mass
(**b**) The cyst appears uniformly hypointense on a coronal, Gd-enhanced T1-weighted SE sequence (TR/TE = 700/15 ms). The mylohyoid and digastric muscles are seen caudal to the cyst. The geniohyoid muscle and intrinsic lingual muscles are displaced superolaterally.
1 Cyst
2 Mylohyoid muscle
3 Digastric muscle
4 Geniohyoid muscle
5 Intrinsic lingual muscles
(**c**) The large cystic mass is displacing the intrinsic tongue muscles superiorly and the mylohyoid muscle inferiorly. It is also causing marked indentation of the oropharynx (white arrow).
1 Cystic mass
2 Intrinsic lingual muscles
3 Mylohyoid muscle
4 Preepiglottic fat

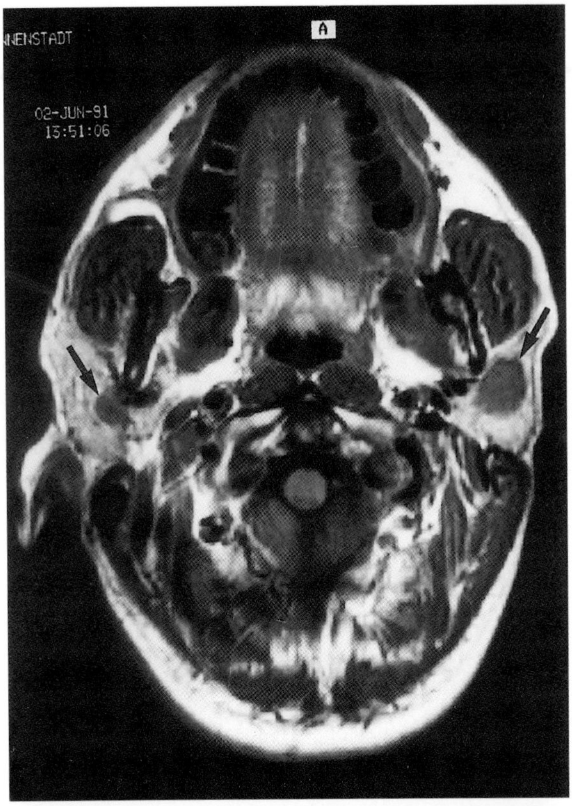

a

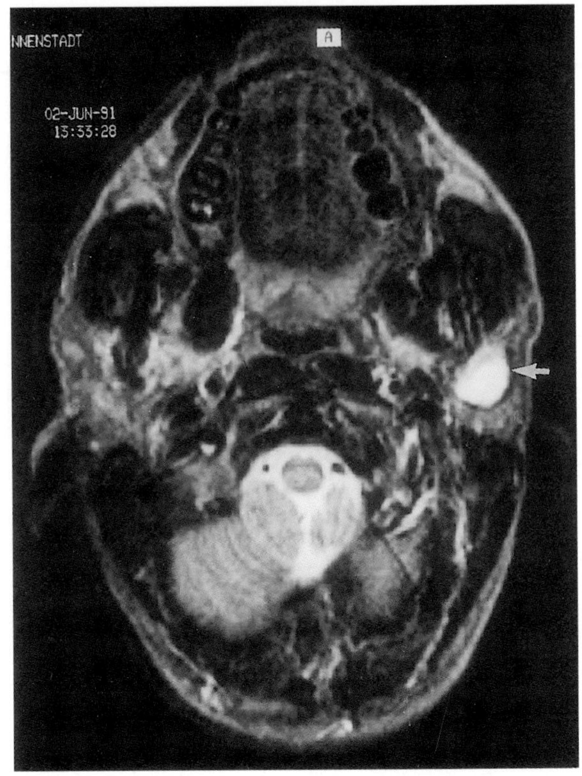

b

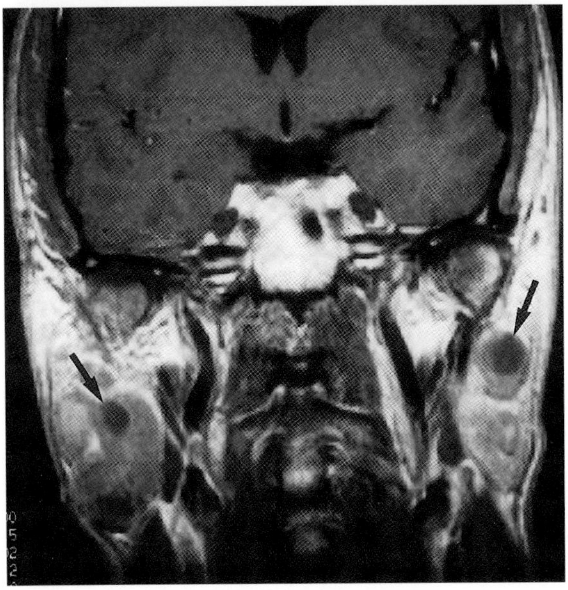

c

Figs. 10.**5 a – c** **Bilateral lymphoepithelial cysts of the parotid gland.**

(**a**) Axial noncontrast T1-weighted SE sequence (TR/TE = 600/17 ms) in this patient shows a 1.5-cm intraparenchymal cystic mass on the left side and a 1-cm lesion on the right side (arrows). Neither lesion produces a mass effect.

(**b**) The cyst (arrow) appears hyperintense on T2-weighted SE sequences (TR/TE = 3000/90 ms) because of its liquid contents and is easily differentiated from a solid tumor. The lesion was identified as a lymphoepithelial cyst in a patient with known HIV infection.

(**c**) The coronal image reveals concomitant cystic changes in the opposite parotid gland (arrows).

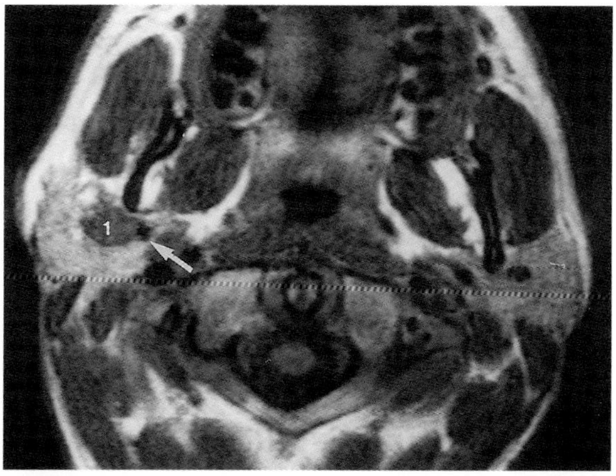

a

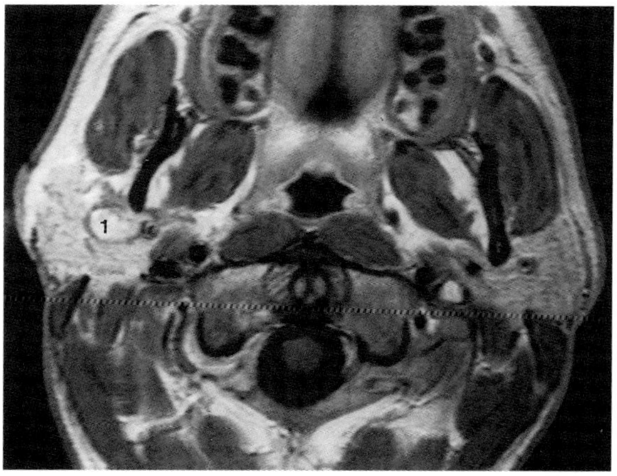

b

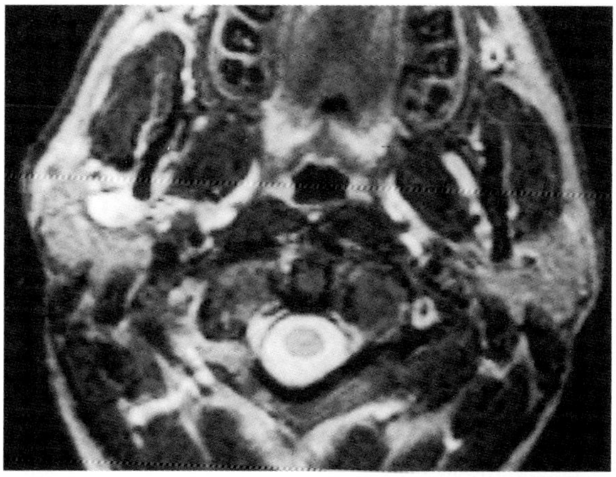

c

Figs. 10.**6 a – c** **Pleomorphic adenoma.**
(**a**) T1-weighted SE sequence (TR/TE = 600/17 ms) shows a hypointense mass in the right parotid gland abutting on the medial retromandibular vein (arrow).
1 Hypointense mass
(**b**) Post-contrast image shows homogeneous enhancement of the adenoma. The smooth, capsule-like border is consistent with the benign nature of the mass. The parenchymal texture of the surrounding parotid gland is unchanged.
1 Homogeneous enhancement of the adenoma.
(**c**) The T2-weighted sequence shows the typical high signal intensity from the fluid-equivalent internal tissues of the pleomorphic adenoma.

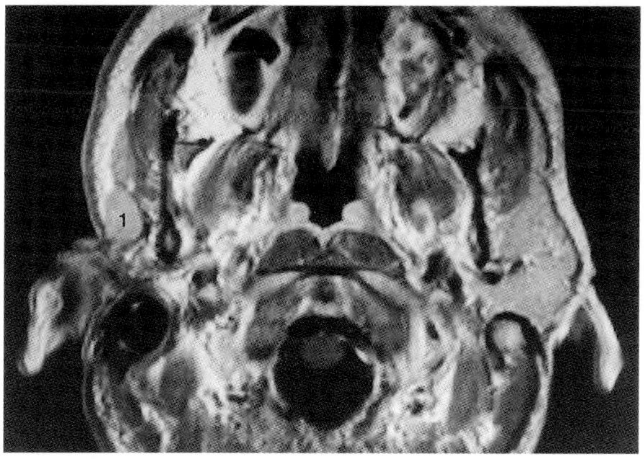

Fig. 10.**7** **Recurrence of an acinar cell tumor.** At follow-up MRI in a patient who underwent complete resection of an acinar cell tumor, a markedly enhancing tumor mass was found anterior to the surgical defect. This should create a very high index of suspicion for a recurrent tumor.
1 Tumor mass

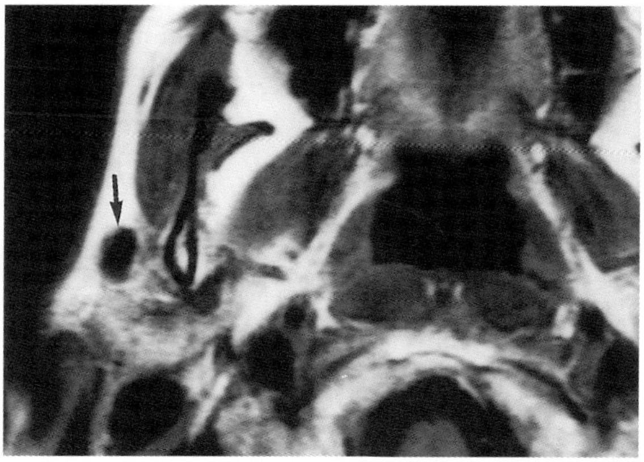

Fig. 10.**8** **Sialolithiasis in the parotid gland.** Unlike the previous tumors, this salivary stone (arrow) in the parotid gland appears as a signal void on MRI and does not enhance with contrast medium.

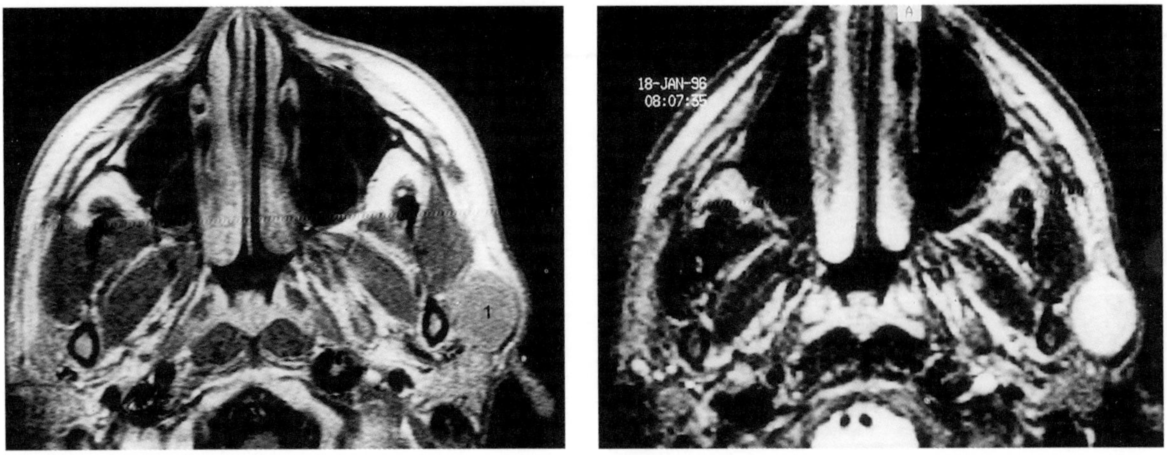

a b

Figs. 10.**9a, b** **Histiocytosis.**
(**a**) T1-weighted MR image (TR/TE = 600/17 ms) shows a clinically palpable mass in the area of the left parotid gland. The mass shows smooth margins and homogeneous contrast enhancement.
1 Smooth margins

(**b**) In a T2-weighted sequence, the lesion appears hyperintense and is well demarcated from surrounding structures. Histologic examination identified the lesion, with its nonspecific imaging features, as histiocytosis.

Adenocarcinoma

Adenocarcinoma is the most common malignant salivary gland tumor. The site of predilection is the parotid gland. Gadolinium(Gd)-enhanced MR images invariably show a marked, diffuse, infiltrative pattern of tumor spread. This diffuse infiltration makes the facial nerve difficult to identify, and facial nerve palsy is an early clinical feature. These tumors usually cause compression or erosion of the retromandibular vein, and advanced lesions infiltrate the pterygoid muscles, internal carotid artery, and internal jugular vein.

Adenoid Cystic Carcinoma

Adenoid cystic carcinoma (Figs. 9.**4a, b**) is a highly aggressive malignancy. Tumors of the parotid gland tend to spread diffusely toward the parapharyngeal space and laterally, infiltrating the cervical muscles, the masseter muscle, and the mandible. Adenoid cystic carcinomas also are frequently diagnosed in the minor salivary glands of the oral floor. In many cases, normal glandular parenchyma can no longer be identified on the affected side. While the musculature often appears intact on unenhanced T1- and T2-weighted sequences, contrast-enhanced images will frequently disclose infiltration of the surrounding muscle tissue. Infiltrative growth along neurovascular tracts is common, leading to paralysis of other cranial nerves and early distant metastasis.

Squamous Cell Carcinoma

Primary squamous cell carcinomas may arise in the parotid, submandibular, and sublingual glands, but they are less common than the malignancies described above. They display typical malignant features on imaging studies: indistinct margins, nonhomogeneous internal structure, and low-signal areas on Gd-enhanced MR images representing sites of necrosis. Patients present clinically with pain, facial nerve palsy, and extensive regional lymphadenopathy.

Mucoepidermoid Carcinoma

Mucoepidermoid carcinomas occur mostly in the parotid gland and show a female predominance. The tumors are divided into two types: the more common, slow-growing *low-grade malignancy*, which is usually associated with mild clinical symptoms, and the less common, more aggressive *high-grade malignancy*, which grows rapidly and undergoes early lymphogenous spread. The imaging appearance of mucoepidermoid carcinoma is largely nonspecific, and histologic examination is necessary for a definitive diagnosis.

Lymphoma (Fig. 10.**10**)

The parotid gland is the most frequent site of salivary gland involvement by lymphoma, which usually coexists with Sjögren disease. Histologically, lymphomas are usually assigned to the category of non-Hodgkin lymphomas. Morphologically, the involved nodes appear as large conglomerate masses that completely displace the normal glandular tissue and typically show small parapharyngeal extensions. The degree of contrast enhancement corresponds to that of squamous cell carcinoma. The lymphoma capsule appears as a bright rim of enhancement surrounding a homogeneous core of less intense enhancement.

Mikulicz syndrome refers to diffuse swelling of the parotid gland and lacrimal glands in the setting of chronic lymphadenosis.

Secondary Tumors

Even when there is no evidence of an immunologic disease such as Sjögren syndrome (Fig. 10.**14**), the parotid gland may be involved by a Hodgkin or non-Hodgkin type of systemic lymphatic disease. Additionally, the salivary glands may harbor metastatic deposits from other malignant epithelial and mesenchymal tumors. In particular, it is not unusual for malignant melanoma to metastasize to the salivary glands. These secondary tumors cannot be diagnosed by imaging studies and require histologic differentiation from a second carcinoma in patients with a known primary tumor.

Inflammatory Lesions

Acute Sialadenitis

Acute sialadenitis may be caused by sialoliths, ascending infection, and in rare cases by hematogenous dissemination. The parotid gland is most commonly affected (Figs. 10.**12** and 10.**13**). Acute sialadenitis is diagnosed on the basis of clinical and radiologic criteria. Causative sialoliths in the excretory ducts can be visualized on plain radiographs (calcifications) and ultrasound images (Fig. 10.**16**). Sialography is contraindicated in the acute stage of sialadenitis, as it may exacerbate the inflammation. The MRI of acute parotitis demonstrates an enlarged gland showing marked contrast enhancement and high signal intensity on T2-weighted sequences. The buccal fat pad, subcutaneous fat, and masseter muscle often show edematous expansion and indistinct margins due to inflammatory infiltration, which also may compress the retromandibular vein.

A special form is viral epidemic parotitis (mumps), principally a childhood disease that presents with bilateral swelling of the parotid glands. Mumps is indistinguishable from bacterial parotitis on imaging studies unless the bacterial inflammation has caused liquefaction or abscess formation.

Sjögren Syndrome (Fig. 10.**14**)

Chronic inflammation commonly develops in patients with recurrent bouts of acute sialadenitis or as an immunologic process in the setting of Sjögren syndrome ("dry eye, dry mouth, dry synovia"). Chronic inflammation of the parotid gland is manifested as atrophy and smallness of the gland, which acquires a nonhomogeneous internal structure. Particularly in Sjögren syndrome, this change is marked by a small to medium-size nodularity and honeycombing of the parenchyma. The differential diagnosis should include neoplasms as well as noninflammatory sialadenosis (Fig. 10.**15**), which can mimic the radiologic features of chronic sialadenitis. Sialography in the chronic stage can demonstrate ectatic and/or stenotic changes in the parotid duct. Sonography permits evaluation of the parenchymal structure, which in chronic cases exhibits fibrotic changes and nonhomogeneous echogenicity. On MRI, the regionally distributed intact residual parenchyma shows intense enhancement on post-gadolinium images, contrasting with the slight enhancement that occurs in fibrosed tissues. Contrast-enhanced MRI is also useful for staging, as the intensity of contrast enhancement in the affected parenchyma correlates with the clinical activity of the disease process.

Systemic and Degenerative Lesions

Sarcoidosis (Boeck Disease)

Another form of chronic sialadenitis occurs in the setting of sarcoidosis, which is mainly characterized by thoracic manifestations with hilar lymph node enlargement and fibrotic changes. The changes in the parotid gland resemble those seen in Sjögren syndrome and nonspecific chronic sialadenitis. Heerfordt syndrome refers to concomitant enlargement of the lacrimal glands.

Sialadenosis (Fig. 10.**15**)

Sialadenosis is a noninflammatory condition marked by bilateral, usually painless swelling of the parotid glands. Generally the amount and composition of the saliva is normal. The diagnosis is suggested by the appearance of a narrowed, rarefied ductal system at sialography ("leafless tree" pattern). MRI may show an enlarged gland with a mostly homogeneous parenchyma.

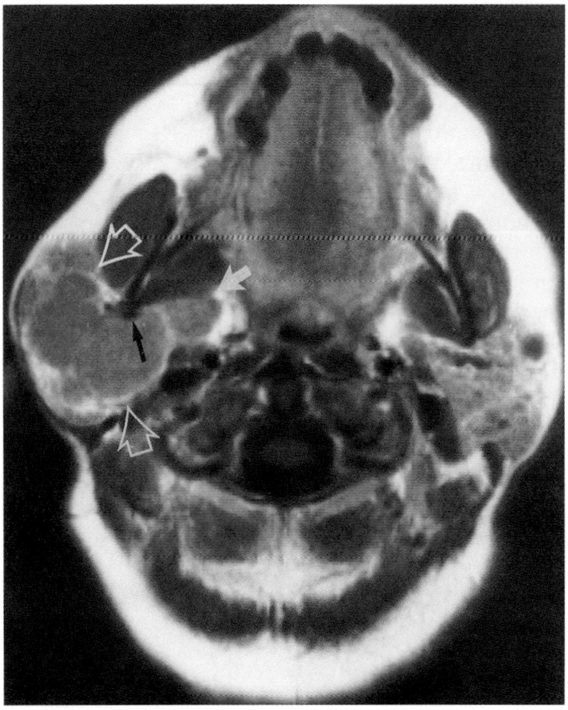
a

Figs. 10.**10a–c** **Involvement of the parotid gland by lymphoma.** MR and sonographic findings.
(**a**) Contrast-enhanced T1-weighted MR image shows several homogeneous, intraparenchymal lymph nodes (white arrow and open arrows) that are expanding the right parotid gland. The lymph nodes extend into the right parapharyngeal space and compress the retromandibular vein (black arrow). The glandular parenchyma on the left side shows changes typical of Sjögren disease.
(**b**) Sonographic appearance of a solitary lymph node with a nonhomogeneous internal structure (arrow) within the edematous glandular tissue.
(**c**) Multiple hypoechoic lymph nodes appear within a very echogenic right parotid gland and in the parapharyngeal space outside the glandular parenchyma (arrows).

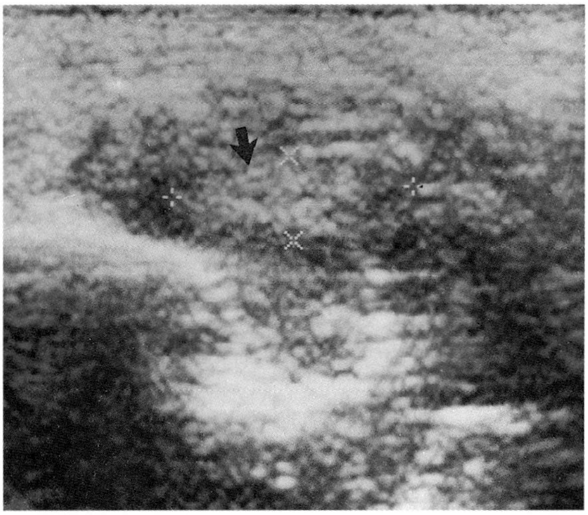
b

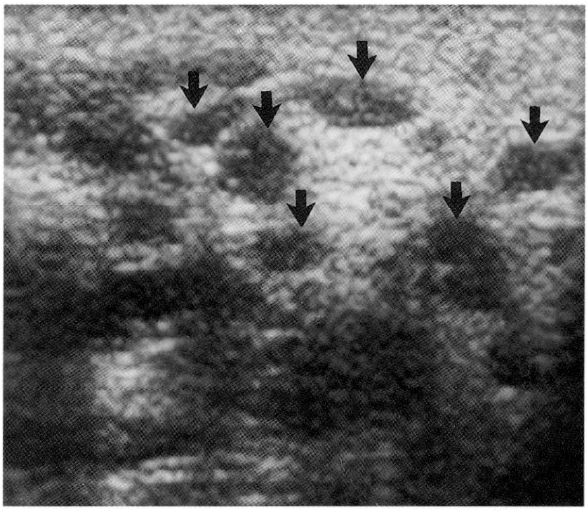
c

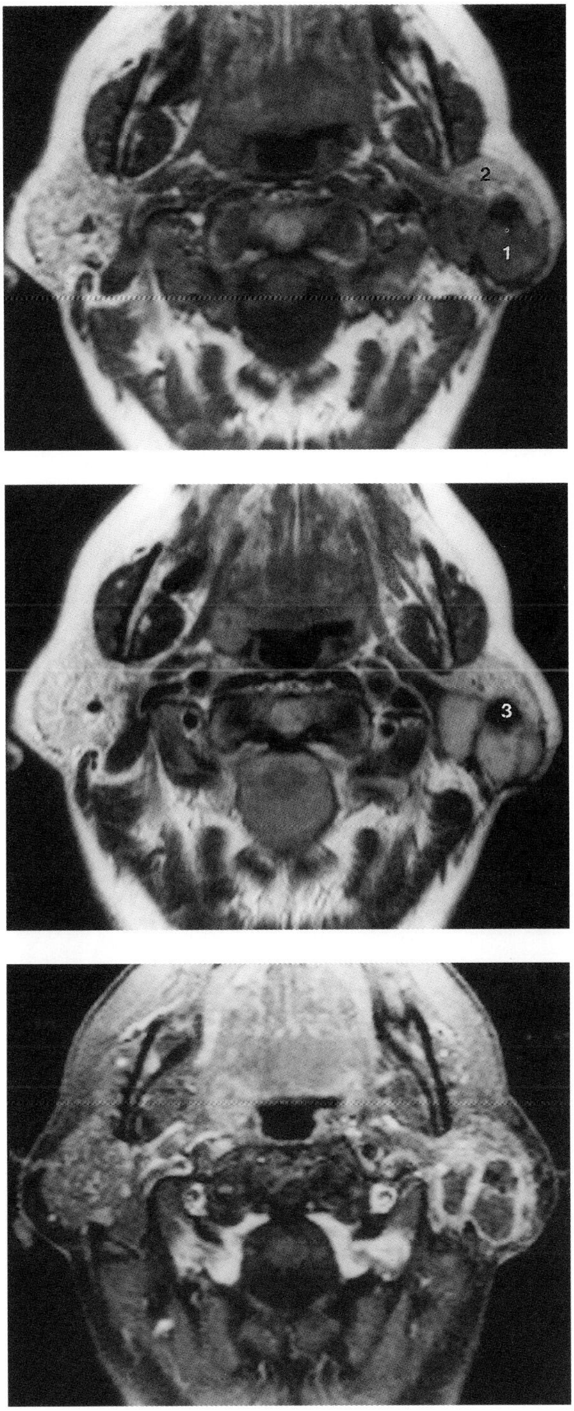

a b c

Figs. 10.**11 a – c** **Cystadenolymphoma (Whartin tumor).**
(**a**) Precontrast T1-weighted MR image shows a mass lesion of low signal intensity arising from the posterior part of the parotid gland. The lesion has smooth margins and is clearly demarcated anteriorly from the hyperintense, compressed glandular parenchyma.
1 Tumor mass
2 Parenchyma
(**b**) The post-contrast image shows marked enhancement in the posterior, tumorous portions of the gland with a central area of low signal intensity and several radial septations.
3 Hypointense area
(**c**) The fat-suppressed T1-weighted image shows three smooth-bordered cystic masses with a hypointense internal structure and a brightly enhancing wall.

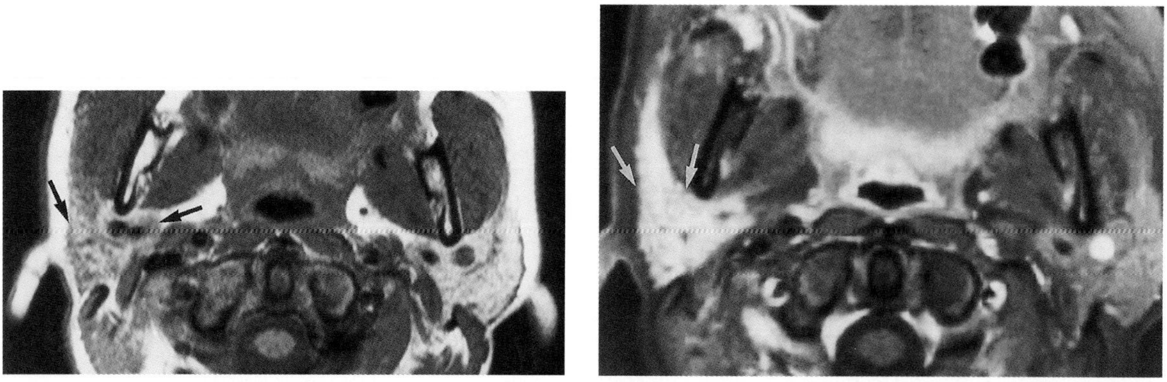

Figs. 10.**12 a, b** **Acute parotitis.**
(**a**) Precontrast T1-weighted SE sequence (TR/TE = 600/17 ms) shows several low-signal areas in a nonhomogeneous parotid gland on the right side (arrows).

(**b**) The post-contrast sequence shows asymmetric enhancement with markedly greater signal intensity on the right side than on the left. The affected gland presents sharp overall boundaries and a homogeneous internal structure consistent with acute, unilateral, right-sided parotitis (arrows).

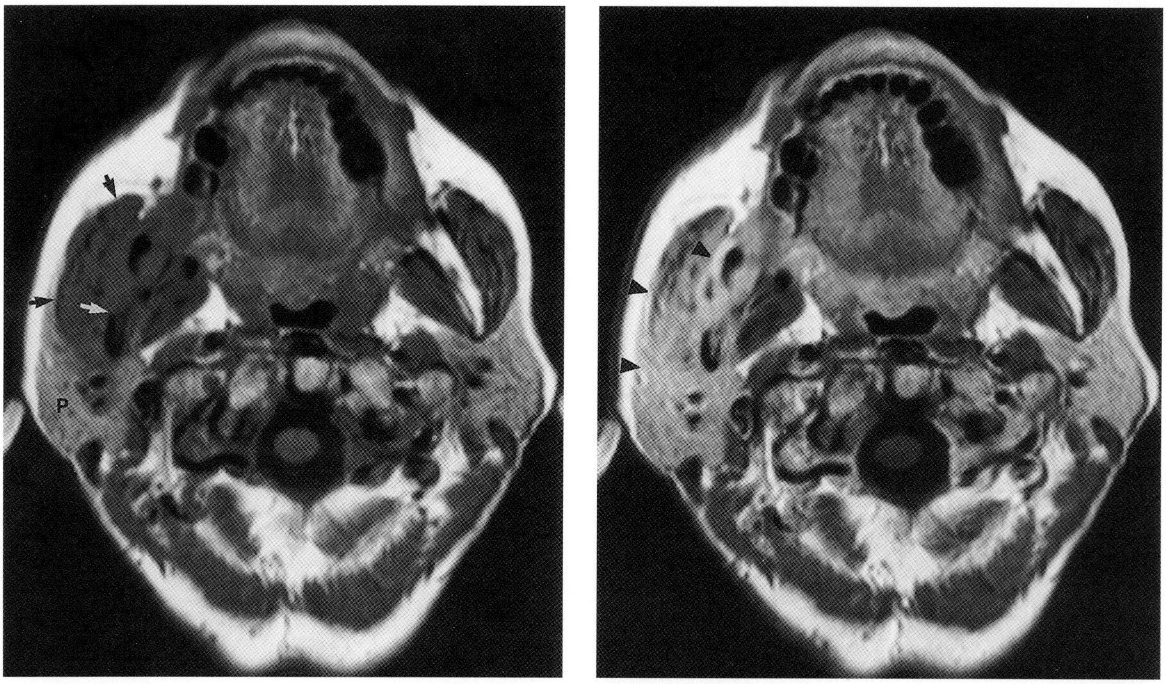

Figs. 10.**13 a, b** **Parotitis and myositis in a patient with actinomycosis.**
(**a**) Precontrast T1-weighted SE sequence (TR/TE = 600/17 ms) shows inflammatory expansion of the right masseter muscle (black arrows) and scattered hypointense areas caused by destruction of the mandible with loss of signal from the medullary space (white arrow).
P Parotid gland

(**b**) Post-contrast image shows diffuse enhancement of the right parotid gland and rostral muscles with obscured parenchymal boundaries (arrowheads). This lesion represents an acute, liquefying parotitis bordered by myositis and osteomyelitis in a patient with actinomycosis.

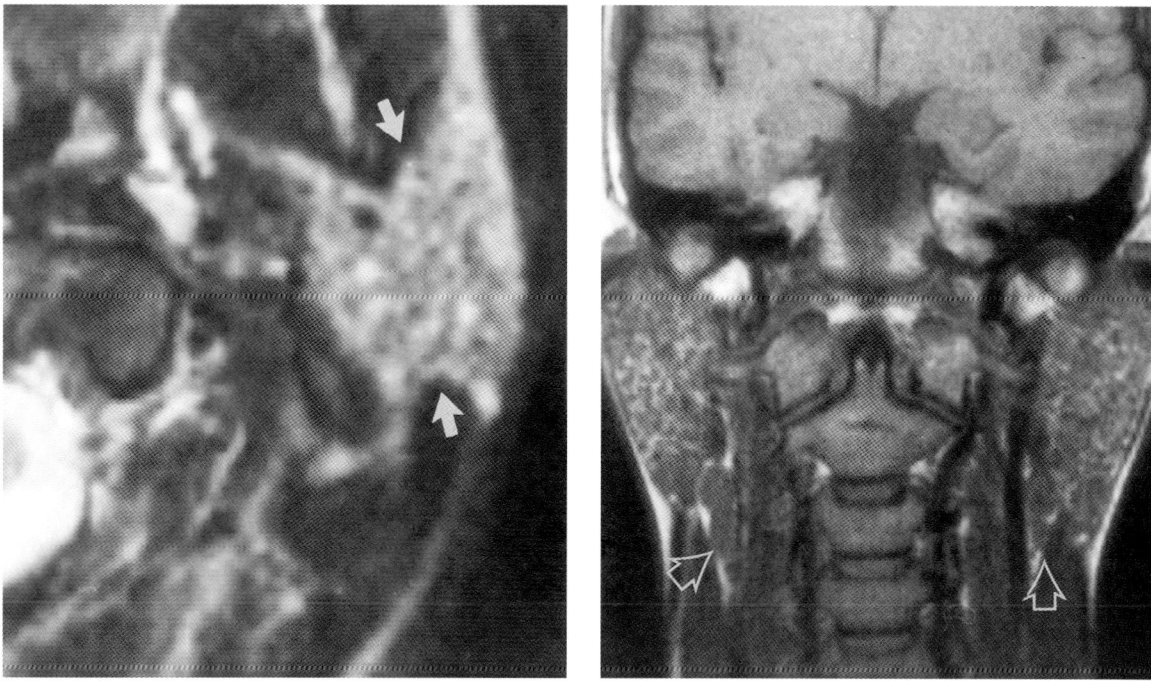

a b

Figs. 10.**14 a, b** **Sjögren syndrome.**
(**a**) This T2-weighted SE sequence (TR/TE = 3000/90 ms) shows typical MR features of Sjögren syndrome: a reticulo-nodular pattern in the glandular parenchyma (arrows) with smooth overall delineation of the glandular tissue.
(**b**) Coronal imaging shows marked parotid enlargement accompanied by enlargement of the lower accessory lymph nodes on each side (arrows).

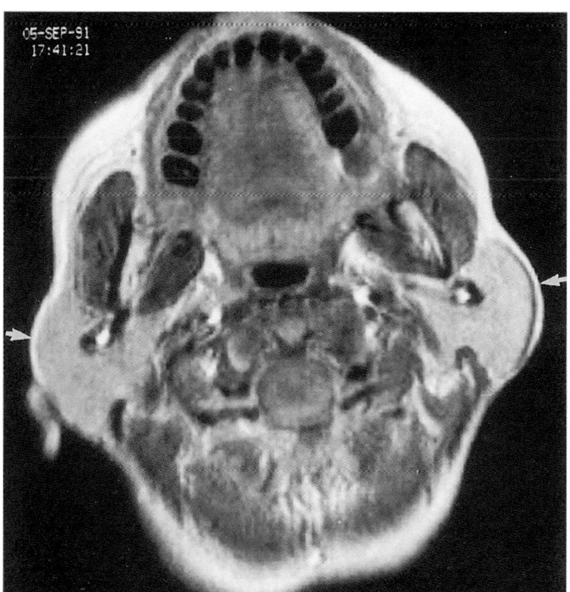

Fig. 10.**15** **Sialadenosis.** T1-weighted SE sequence MR image shows marked bilateral parotid hypertrophy (arrows), but the homogeneous parenchymal structure of the glands and the absence of infiltrative changes are consistent with a benign sialadenosis.

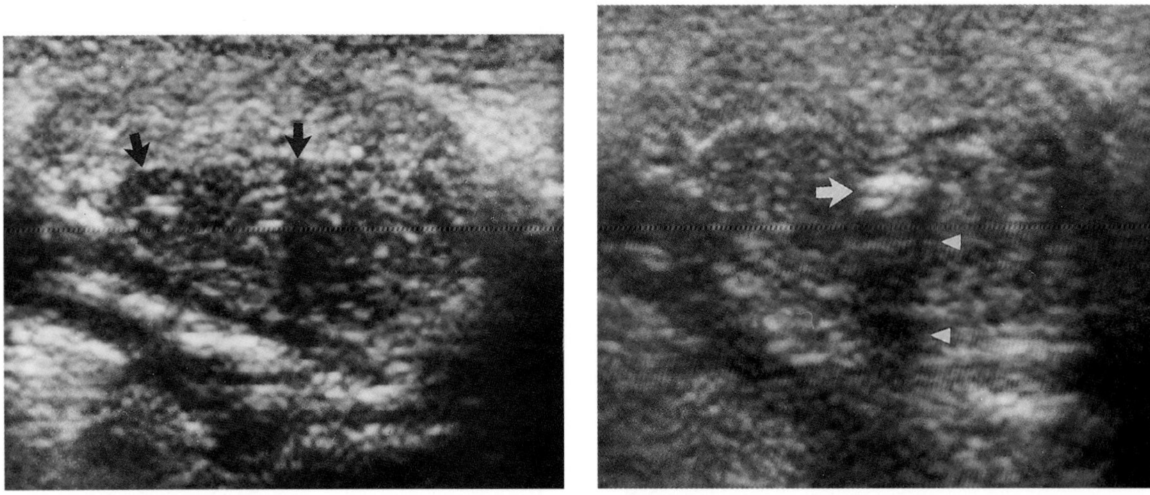

Figs. 10.**16 a, b** **Sialolithiasis.**
(**a**) The inflammatory focus (arrows) appears sonographically as a sharply defined area of low echogenicity within the submandibular gland.
(**b**) Slight angulation of the transducer reveals a hyperechoic salivary stone (arrow) with a characteristic acoustic shadow (arrowheads) as the cause of the inflammatory process.

Sialolithiasis

Local pain and swelling of a salivary gland due to lithiasis most commonly affect the parotid gland and tend to worsen at mealtimes. The causes include electrolyte disorders (calcium) and foreign bodies. The most important complication of sialolithiasis is acute sialadenitis. Stones in the excretory ducts can be demonstrated by radiography (calcifications) and by sonography (Fig. 10.**16**). Sialography documents a circumscribed duct obstruction but is contraindicated in the acute inflammatory stage.

Iatrogenic and Posttherapeutic Lesions

Radiation therapy induces a partial or complete arrest of salivary secretion from the glands in the irradiated field. The resulting xerostomia and intraoral burning pain are managed by treatment with saliva substitutes. In many patients, salivary secretion resumes within a few weeks after the termination of radiotherapy. The chronic phase of radiogenic salivary gland irritation is marked by the presence of fibrotic and atrophic changes, which are best demonstrated by MRI. Awareness of these changes is mainly important in follow-up evaluations for malignant tumor recurrence, when intravenous paramagnetic contrast should be used to differentiate fibrotic connective tissue from intensely enhancing recurrent tumor.

Imaging Criteria and Their Differential Diagnosis

Cystic Masses

All primary cystic lesions of the salivary glands are distinguished by a liquid internal structure with smooth peripheral walls and an expansile type of growth with no signs of infiltration. Often it is difficult to make an accurate differential diagnosis of individual cystic lesions on the basis of morphologic criteria. Important differentiating features include the presence of solid components in a dermoid cyst and the typical appearance of cystic liquefaction in tumors or lymph nodes with central necrotic foci and thick, irregular margins. The differential diagnosis of cystic lesions in the oral floor region can be significantly advanced by giving attention to topographic criteria, which can distinguish cysts arising from the lesser major salivary glands from several other types of lesion (Tables 10.**1** and 10.**2**).

The primary imaging study for salivary gland cysts is sonography. Fluid density on CT scans (from 0 to 20 HU), high signal intensity on T2-weighted MR sequences, and rim enhancement on Gd-enhanced scans are the typical imaging criteria of these lesions. Nevertheless, it is usually necessary to combine morphologic and topographic criteria before a more specific diagnosis can be made.

Table 10.**2** Cystic masses of the salivary glands

Findings	Differential diagnostic criteria
Variation:	
➤ Primary cyst formation (Fig. 10.**2**)	Morphology
Mass lesion:	
➤ Dermoid cyst (Fig. 10.**4**)	Solid components
➤ Cystic lymphoma	Solid components
➤ Necrotic tumor or lymph node	Intense contrast enhancement
Inflammatory lesion:	
➤ Abscess (Fig. 10.**13**)	Contrast enhancement
➤ Lymphoepithelial cysts (HIV) (Fig. 10.**5**)	Only in parotid gland, morphology
Traumatic lesion:	
➤ Hematoma	Morphology

Tumor Masses of the Parotid Gland

Solid tumor masses of the parotid gland may represent any of a number of benign or malignant histologic types (Figs. 10.**6** – 10.**13**, 10.**17**), and a definitive diagnosis requires histologic evaluation. The criteria listed in Table 10.**3** are useful for narrowing the radiologic differential diagnosis.

Table 10.**1** Cystic masses of the oral floor and their relations to other structures

Lesion	Relation to mylohyoid muscle	Relation to midline
Sublingual cyst	Cranial	Lateral
Odontogenic cyst	Cranial	Lateral
Ranula (Fig. 10.**3**)	Cranial	Lateral
Submandibular gland cyst (Fig. 10.**2**)	Caudal	Lateral
Lateral cervical cyst (Figs. 14.**2**, 14.**4**)	Caudal	Lateral
Median cervical cyst (Fig. 14.**3**)	Caudal	Midline
Colloid cyst	Caudal	Midline
Hourglass ranula	Caudal	Midline
Dermoid cyst (Fig. 10.**4**)	Variable	Midline
Epidermoid cyst (Fig. 12.**4**)	Variable	Midline
Abscess, cellulitis	Variable	Variable
Cystic lymphoma	Variable	Variable
Lymph node metastasis (Fig. 12.**3**)	Variable	Variable
Cystic lymphangioma	Variable	Variable
Cystic hemangioma	Variable	Variable

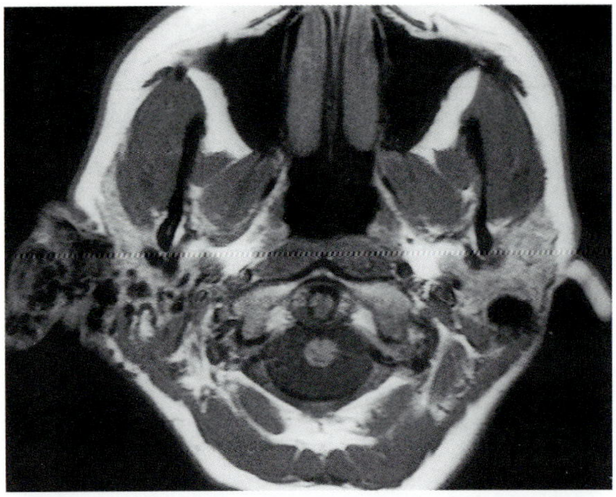
a

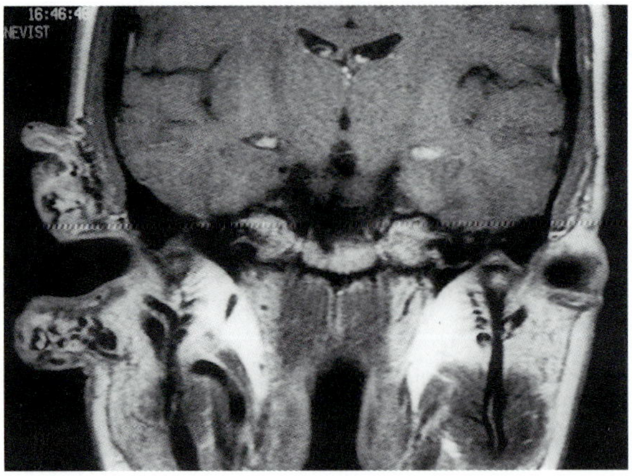
b

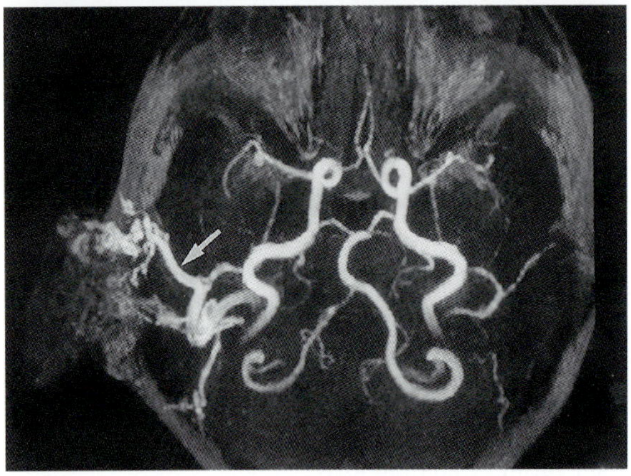
c

Figs. 10.**17 a – c** **Arteriovenous malformation.**
(**a**) A T1-weighted MR sequence (TR/TE = 600/17 ms) shows multiple structures of low signal intensity in the right parotid gland and a mass of soft-tissue density in the area of the right ear. Otherwise the parenchyma of the parotid gland displays a normal signal intensity.
(**b**) Coronal MRI shows expansion of the right ear by the arteriovenous malformation, that abuts upon, and partially permeates, the parotid gland.
(**c**) MR arteriography confirms perfusion of the arteriovenous malformation and defines a feeding vessel from the external carotid artery (arrow).

Tumor Masses of the Sublingual and Submandibular Glands

The differential diagnosis of sublingual and submandibular gland masses should include malignant tumors, which are relatively common in this region. Adenoid cystic carcinoma, for example, is more common in the lesser major salivary glands than in the parotid gland. These glands also show more frequent involvement by cystic lesions arising from the glandular parenchyma (except for lymphoepithelial cysts in AIDS patients [Fig. 10.**5**]) and more frequent sialolithiasis due to the mucinous secretions of the glands (Fig. 10.**16**).

Reticular Parenchymal Changes

A diffuse reticular appearance of the glandular parenchyma can provide a very useful criterion for differential diagnosis (Fig. 10.**14** and Table 10.**4**).

Summary and Diagnostic Strategy

Given the variety of histologic tumor types that may involve the major salivary glands, the radiologist can often do no more than evaluate the extent of the lesion and provide a descriptive diagnosis. The ability of ultrasound to differentiate solid and cystic masses is amply documented. Contrast-enhanced MRI has become the imaging procedure of choice for further elucidating the pattern of infiltration and advancing the differential diagnosis of solid masses.

Table 10.3 Differential diagnosis of tumor masses of the parotid gland

Findings	Differential diagnostic criteria
Common:	
➤ Variation:	
–Parotid gland hyperplasia	Morphology
–Pseudomass	Morphology
➤ Tumor:	
–Pleomorphic adenoma (Fig. 10.**6**)	Nonhomogeneity
Whartin tumor (Fig. 10.**11**)	Homogeneity
–Adenocarcinoma	Infiltration
–Mucoepidermoid carcinoma (low grade)	Homogeneity
➤ Inflammatory:	
–Acute sialadenitis (Fig. 10.**12**)	Edema
–Sialolithiasis (Fig. 10.**16**)	Direct visualization
–Mumps	Homogeneity
–Abscess	Abscess membrane
–Sjögren syndrome (Fig. 10.**14**)	Nonhomogeneity
Rare:	
➤ Tumor:	
–Squamous cell carcinoma	Infiltration
–Mucoepidermoid carcinoma (high grade)	Infiltration
–Adenoid cystic carcinoma (Fig. 9.**14 a**)	Infiltration
–Lymphoma (Figs. 10.**10**)	Homogeneity
–Metastasis	Homogeneity
➤ Systemic:	
–Sialadenosis	Homogeneity
➤ Trauma:	
–Internal hemorrhage	History

Table 10.4 Reticular parenchymal changes in the parotid gland

Findings	Differential diagnostic criteria
Common:	
➤ Inflammation:	
–Sjögren syndrome (Fig. 10.**14**)	Bilateral, nodular
➤ Iatrogenic:	
–Postirradiation	Nonhomogeneity, atrophy
Rare:	
➤ Inflammation:	
–Chronic sialadenitis	Nonhomogeneity
➤ Systemic:	
–Sialadenosis (Fig. 10.**15**)	Homogeneity, hypertrophy

References

1 Casselmann, J. W., A. A. Mancuso: Major salivary gland masses: comparison of MR imaging and CT. Radiology 165 (1987) 183–189

2 Dillon, W. P., H. R. Harnsberger: The impact of radiologic imaging on staging of cancer of the head and neck. Semin Oncol. 18 (1991) 64–79

3 Naumann, H. H.: Differentialdiagnostik in der Hals-Nasen-Ohren-Heilkunde. Thieme, Stuttgart 1990

4 Som, P. M., J. M. A. Shugar, M. Sacher, A. L. Stallmann, H. F. Biller: Benign and malignant parotid pleomorphic adenomas: CT and MR studies. J Comput Assist Tomogr. 12 (1988) 65–69

5 Teresi, L. M., R. B. Lufkin, D. G. Warthan, E. Abemayor, W. N. Hanafee: Parotid masses: MR Imaging. Radiology 163 (1987) 405–409

6 Vogl, Th.: Kernspintomographie der Kopf-Hals-Region. Springer, Heidelberg 1991

7 Vogl, Th., S. Dresel, M. Juergens, J. Assal, J. Lissner: MR Imaging with Gd-DTPA in lesions of the head and neck. J Otolaryngol. 22 (1993) 4–9

8 Vogl, T., S. Dresel, M. Späth, G. Grevers, C. Wilimzig: Parotid gland: plain and gadolinium-enhanced MR Imaging. Radiology 177 (1990) 667–674

11 Temporomandibular Joint

The clinical incidence of disorders of the temporomandibular joint (TMJ) has been climbing in recent years, and these diseases have become an important issue in differential diagnosis. While clinical methods of examination are based largely on function testing, inspection, and palpation, diagnostic imaging provides much greater accuracy in the diagnosis and differential diagnosis of TMJ abnormalities. In particular, the advent of surface coil technology in magnetic resonance imaging (MRI) has created a reproducible tool for making detailed evaluations of the TMJ.

An optimum evaluation of the normal or diseased TMJ must, however, be based on the combined analysis of clinical information, conventional radiography, MRI, and topographic principles. It is essential, therefore, that the radiologist become familiar with the principles of TMJ function as well as TMJ pathology. Our goal in this chapter is to explore the basic aspects of TMJ diagnosis and the various differential diagnostic possibilities that need to be considered.

The list of common and rare TMJ disorders in Table 11.**1** can serve as an introduction to differential diagnosis.

Table **11.1** Disorders of the TMJ that are accessible to diagnostic imaging

Common:

- Degenerative diseases (Fig. 11.**10**)
- Rheumatoid arthritis
- Internal derangement (Figs. 11.**15** – 11.**18**, 11. **30**)

Rare:

- Accompanying diseases:
  —Paget disease
  —Fibrous dysplasia
- Ankylosing spondylitis
- Gout (Fig. 11.**20**)
- Iatrogenic (steroids)
- Juvenile rheumatoid arthritis
- Infectious arthritis (Fig. 11.**19**)
- Loose bodies
- Neoplasms (osteochondroma)
- Osteochondrosis dissecans, pigmented villonodular synovitis, psoriatic arthritis

Normal Anatomy

The articulation between the cranium and lower jaw in humans is formed by the apposition of two originally separate temporal membrane bones. The shape of the articular structures of the temporal bone and mandible is closely related to the evolution and function of the bite. Two other developmental and functional features make the TMJ unique among the joints of the human body. First, the articular surfaces are covered not with hyaline cartilage but with a very vascular fibrous layer composed of a predominantly collagenous material. Second, a mobile articular disk subdivides the joint into two compartments that, while spatially separate, interact to create a functional unit (Figs. 11.**1** and 11.**2**).

The *mandibular condyle* (the head of the condylar process) is a rounded eminence that shows significant individual variations in size, shape, and position. The axis of the joint is directed medially backward, forming an angle of 15° to 33° with respect to the coronal plane. The articular surface of the temporal bone is elliptical to quadratic in shape. It is raised anteriorly to form the articular tubercle and hollowed posteriorly to form the glenoid fossa.

The *articular disk* (Fig. 11.**1 b**) sits atop the mandibular condyle like a baseball cap, dividing the TMJ into an *upper (discotemporal) compartment* and *lower (discocondylar) compartment*. Several ligaments strengthen the joint and limit its range of motion in certain directions. A knowledge of the normal anatomy of the joint is essential for understanding its functions. Jaw movements are not only for mastication (chewing and swallowing) but also participate in nonmasticatory functions such as speaking, singing, yawning, and facial expressions. *Functional movements of the mandible* are always a combination of several of the following basic movements (Figs. 11.**2** – 11.**5**):

- Opening and closure (depression/elevation, abduction/adduction; Fig. 11.**4**).
- Protrusion and retraction (Fig. 11.**2**).
- Lateral movements (Fig. 11.**3**).

Opening the mouth from the occlusal position proceeds in two phases. As the tonus of the elevator muscles decreases, gravity and the oral floor muscles produce a slight rotation of the mandibular condyles in the lower joint compartment. The inferior head of the lateral pterygoid muscle then pulls the condyles forward and downward in the upper joint compartment (Fig. 11.**4b**).

During *closure of the mouth*, the articular disk and condyle slide upward and backward over the articular tubercle. During protrusion and retraction of the mandible, the condyles glide along the sagittal condylar track (Fig. 11.**5**).

The great importance of clinical MRI in evaluations of the TMJ is based on its ability to give highly detailed anatomic and topographic views of the joint and associated structures (Figs. 11.**13**– 11.**17**). Sagittal MR images (Fig. 11.**13**) are used mainly to document the relation of the articular disk to the glenoid fossa and condyle (Fig. 11.**1** and Table 11.**2**).

Figures 11.**1** and 11.**2** show the relationship of the articular disk to the temporal and mandibular articular surfaces in the resting position (teeth slightly separated) and with the mouth opened 4 cm. The posterior band of the articular disk is on the summit of the condyle, roughly on line with the long axis of the condylar process. This relationship of the disk to the condylar process is termed the 12 o'clock position. In the normal TMJ this position ranges between 10 o'clock and 12 o'clock. In abnormal joints the disk may occupy an anterior or posterior position relative to the condyle. Figure 11.**3** shows the typical condyle-disk relationship in the coronal plane.

Table 11.**2** Normal appearance of the articular disk and mandibular condyle on MRI (T1-weighted SE sequence)

Articular disk:
- Signal intensity
  - Hypointense: anterior band, posterior band, pole of articular disk (Fig. 11.**4**)
  - Hyperintense: bilaminar zone, retrocondylar tissue (Fig. 11.**4**)
- Morphology: posterior boundary of the posterior band: shape of biconcave disk

Mandibular condyle:
- Cancellous bone appears hyperintense on T1-weighted images due to fat content of bone marrow. Cortical structures appear dark (Fig. 11.**4**).
- Full congruence of mandibular condyle, glenoid fossa, and articular disk

Figs. 11.**1 a, b** **Appearance of the TMJ on MRI compared with its gross morphology.**
(**a**) Sagittal MR image shows marked differences in signal intensity between the dark posterior pole of the articular disk and the bilaminar zone. The discontinuities along the posterior aspect of the mandibular condyle (arrows) probably represent partial volume artifacts.
C Mandibular condyle
f Glenoid fossa
t Articular tubercle
(**b**) Contralateral joint sections comparing in vitro MRI with gross morphology. MRI documents the differences in signal intensity between the bilaminar zone and the rest of the articular disk.
C Mandibular condyle
d Articular disk
f Glenoid fossa
p Bilaminar zone
t Articular tubercle
3 Temporal bone

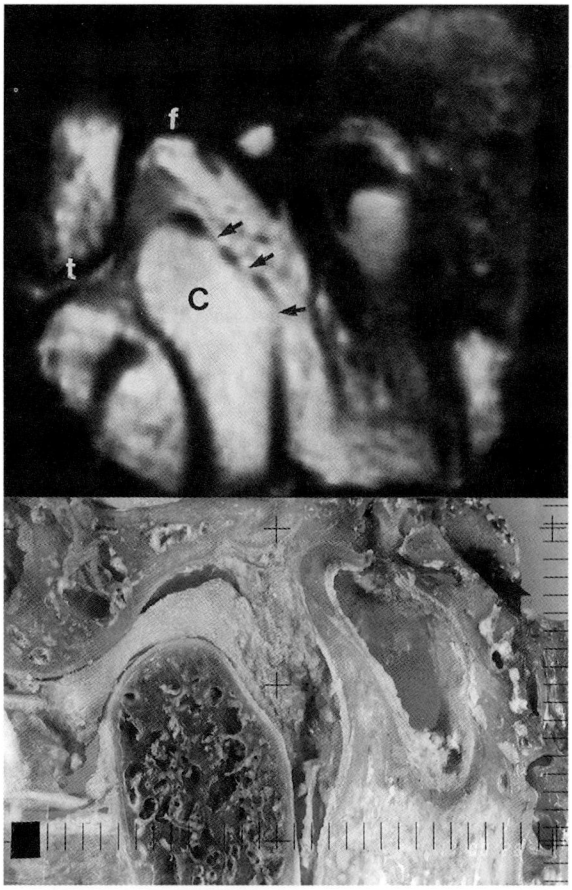

a

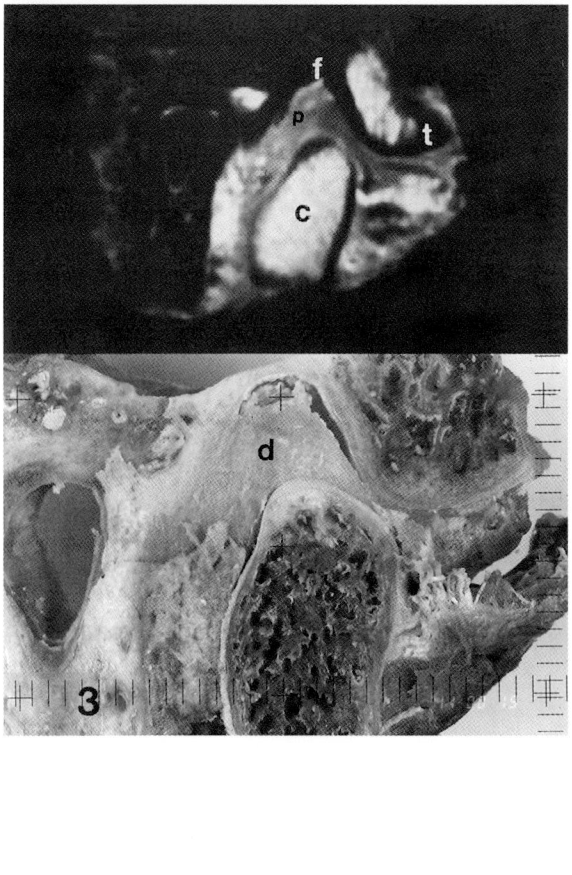

b

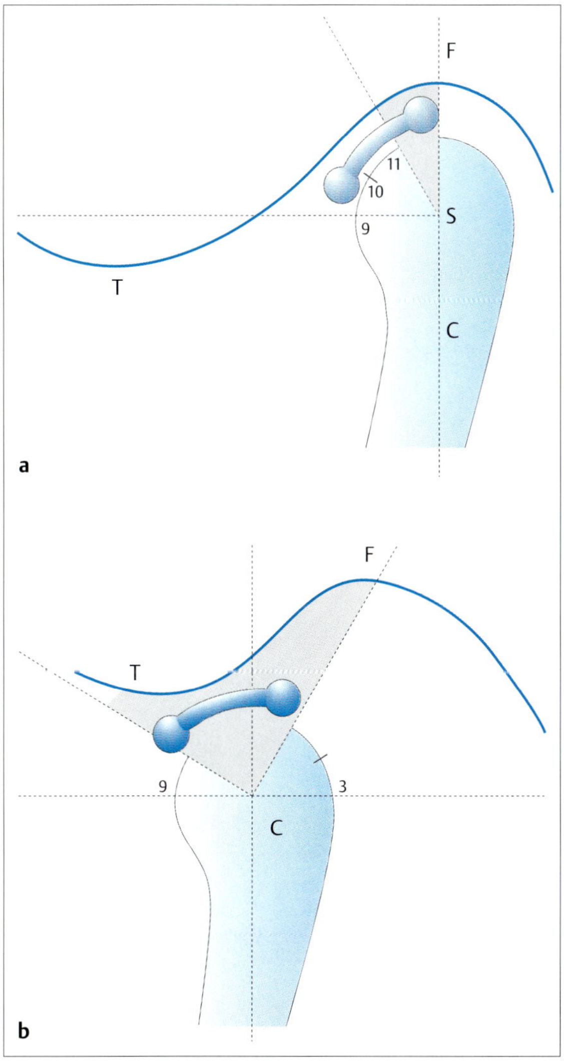

Figs. 11.2 a, b **Changing relationship of the articular disk to the temporal and mandibular surfaces of the TMJ.**
(**a**) Resting position.
(**b**) Mouth opened 4 cm. Note the dumbbell configuration of the articular disk over the mandibular condyle.
C Mandibular condyle
F Glenoid fossa
S Center of rotation
T Articular tubercle

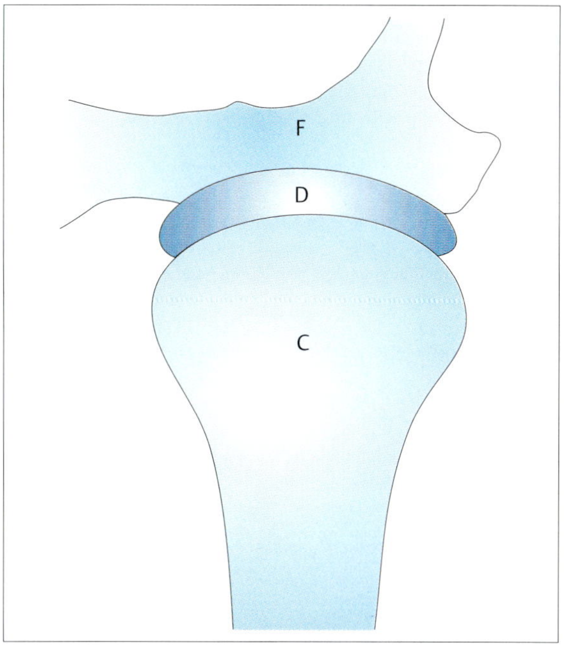

Fig. 11.3 **Normal relationship of the articular disk to the mandibular condyle in coronal section.**
C Mandibular condyle
D Articular disk
F Glenoid fossa

Figs. 11.**4 a, b** **TMJ of a healthy subject.**
(**a**) MRI in the resting position shows a normal condyle-disk relationship with the condyle centered in the TMJ. The posterior band of the articular disk (arrow and arrowhead) is in the 11 to 12 o'clock position relative to the condyle.
C Mandibular condyle
F Glenoid fossa
T Articular tubercle
(**b**) With the mouth opened 4 cm, the condyle has moved below the apex of the articular tubercle and is centered under the articular disk (arrow and arrowhead).
C Mandibular condyle
F Glenoid fossa
T Articular tubercle

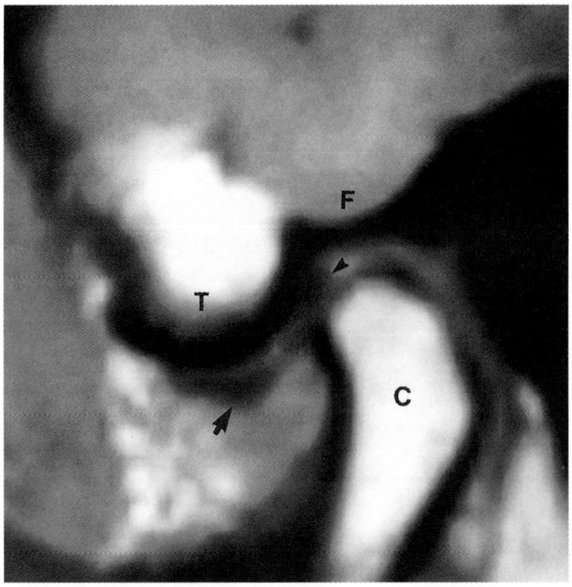

a

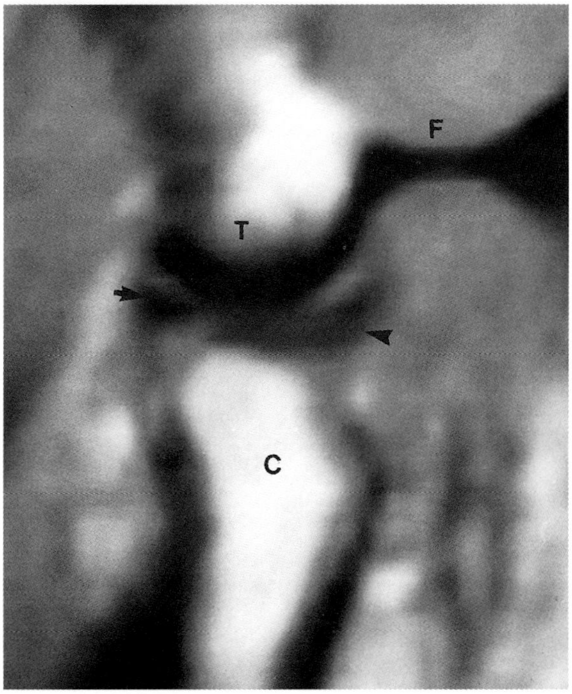

b

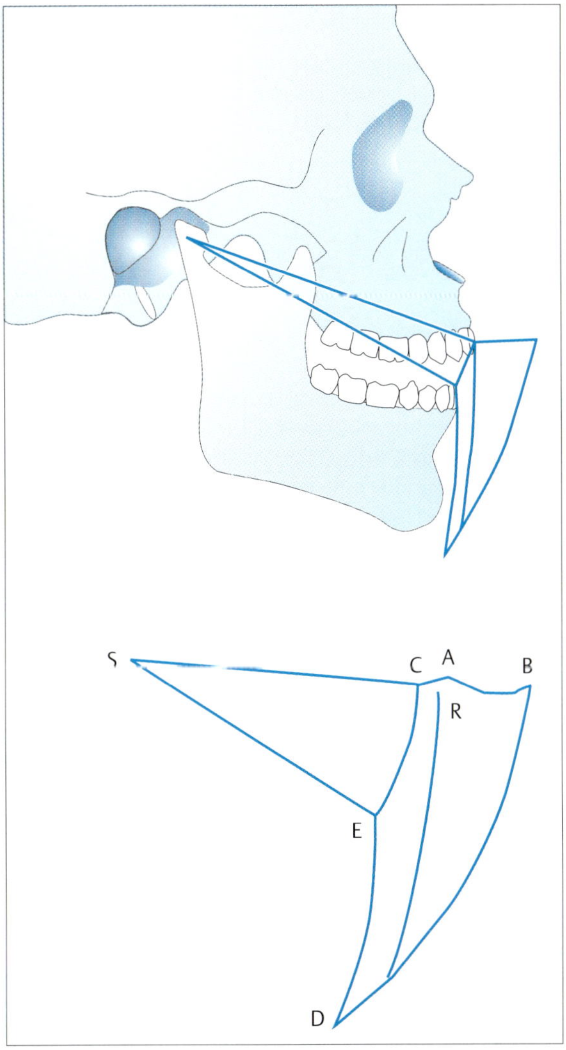

Fig. 11.5 **Schematic drawing of the limits of mandibular movements in the sagittal plane.**
A Habitual occlusion
B Maximum protrusion
C Maximum retraction
C–E Hinge motion
E–D Gliding
D Maximum mandibular opening
R Resting position
S Terminal hinge point

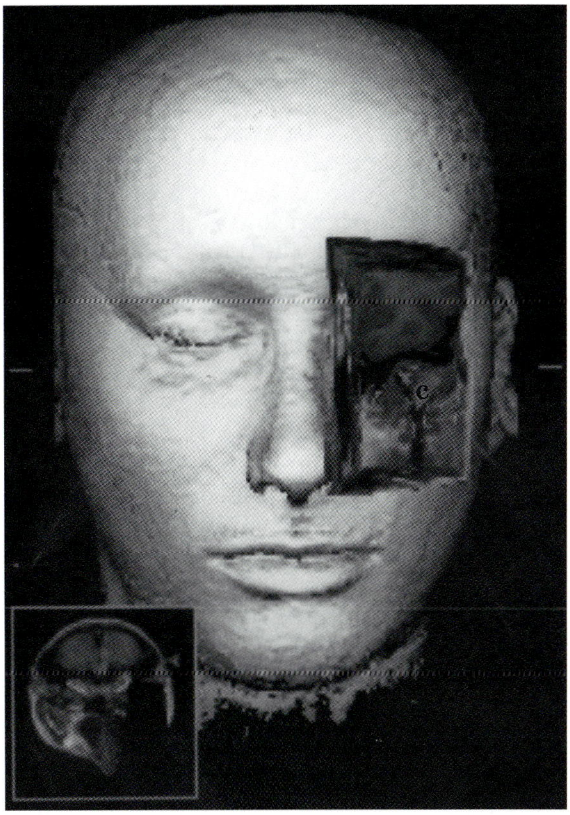

Fig. 11.6 **3-D reconstruction** (3-D magnetization-prepared rapid-acquisition gradient-echo [MP-RAGE] sequence) demonstrates the symmetric relationship of the condyles to the facial skeleton.
C Mandibular condyle

Clinical Signs and Symptoms

Clinical manifestations are based on the complex interaction of the various structures of the human masticatory system including the maxilla and mandible, the TMJ, the periodontium, the masticatory muscles, the mimetic muscles, and the tongue and surrounding soft tissues. *Primary TMJ disorders* belong to several basic categories:

- Arthritis (Fig. 11.**19**).
- Osteoarthritis having a specific or nonspecific (Fig. 11.**10**) cause.
- Tumors.
- Malformations and growth disturbances (Fig. 11.**7**).

The TMJ, like any other joint, may be affected by arthritis that is unrelated to functional demands. Typical manifestations of TMJ arthritis are local swelling, tenderness to pressure, lateral deviation of the jaw (Fig. 11.**19**), and constitutional symptoms. The cause may be a hematogenous or contiguous bacterial infection (e.g., from otitis media), mandibular osteomyelitis, or trauma (Fig. 11.**11**). Less common are specific forms of arthritis occurring in the setting of a gonorrheal or tuberculous disease, for example. The differential diagnosis should also include nearby suppurative processes such as a post-injection abscess or acute parotitis (Figs. 10.**12**, 10.**13**). *Rheumatic diseases* of the skeletal system can lead to TMJ involvement in 5% to 86% of cases. The underlying disease may be any of the true rheumatic disorders:

- Rheumatoid arthritis.
- Juvenile rheumatoid arthritis (Still disease).
- Bekhterev disease.
- Other systemic diseases such as psoriasis and metabolic disorders (Fig. 11.**20**).

Tumors of the TMJ are extremely rare and may be malignant or benign (Figs. 11.**8**, 11.**23**). The great majority arise from articular structures (e.g., osteoma, chondroma, myxoma, hemangioma), but rare bone metastases (e.g., from renal or breast carcinoma) may occur.

Malformations and growth disturbances of the TMJ (Fig. 11.**7**) occur in association with congenital mandibulofacial and mandibulocranial dysostoses and in numerous syndromes. Clinical attention should also be given to disorders of the masticatory muscles, which may include splinting, myeloses, spasms, and systemic muscular diseases such as myotonia, myasthenia gravis, and other forms of myositis.

The main clinical manifestations of TMJ disorders include *symptomatic functional disturbances*. Limitation of mandibular movement, or trismus, can have various causes. Trismus is distinguished from locking, in which the condyle is displaced forward from the glenoid fossa and becomes locked in front of the articular tubercle, causing limitation of jaw movement. The myarthropathy syndrome includes pain, joint noises, and tenderness.

Table 11.3 Etiologic factors in TMJ disorders

Idiopathic, traumatic: ➤ Acute injuries, whiplash (Fig. 11.**11**) ➤ Irregular sleeping habits
Iatrogenic: ➤ Arthritis ➤ Orthopedic ➤ Odontogenic ➤ Emotional, psychogenic, etc.

Another class of TMJ disorders is the *discopathies* (Table 11.**3**). The following diseases can lead to discopathies and eventual disk displacement:

- Hyperextension.
- Trauma.
- Occlusal interferences.
- Muscular imbalance.
- Dysplasias of the articular components.
- Psychogenic factors.

The clinical manifestations of these discopathies include function-dependent TMJ pain and joint sounds such as snapping and crepitation.

Imaging Evaluation and Differential Diagnosis

Depending on the clinical problem and the severity of the disease, the modern staged diagnostic workup of the TMJ is based on the procedures set out below.

Conventional Radiography

Conventional radiographs are usually based on Schüller projections (in three different functional positions), which may be supplemented as needed by an orthopantomogram or panoramic radiograph. Essential criteria include an analysis of symmetry and an evaluation of the essential structures of both TMJs.

Invasive Arthrography

Invasive arthrography involving the direct injection of contrast medium into the upper or lower TMJ space has become largely obsolete. The procedure may be necessary in rare instances to document a communication between the joint spaces, but today only a few centers still practice the technique.

Computed Tomography (CT)

Axial and coronal CT scans (Figs. 11.**10**, 11.**11**, 11.**20**) are used mainly for the evaluation of trauma. Axial scans should be directed parallel to the X-axis or orbitomeatal line. The slice thickness should not exceed 4 mm, and 2 mm is recommended for the optimum definition of fine bony details. Coronal or sagittal reconstructions can be added to facilitate the evaluation.

Magnetic Resonance Imaging

MRI of the TMJ should generally be performed with dedicated coils and sequences. A dual coil system is advantageous, as it permits the simultaneous examination of both joints in one acquisition. The quality of the MR image depends critically on the ratio of the acquired signal to the background noise (the signal-to-noise ratio). It also depends directly on the sensitivity of the high-frequency coils and on parameters such as coil geometry, size, and volume (which directly affect coil sensitivity). The simultaneous imaging of both TMJs is best accomplished with a dual coil system using bilateral receiving coils. These coils provide a field of view of 3 to 4 cm, with smaller coils offering a superior signal-to-noise ratio. Accurate patient positioning is of key importance when dual coils are used (Fig. 11.**6**).

The sequences listed in Table 11.**4** have proven effective for TMJ examinations.

Assessment of Mandibular Opening

MRI, with its short data acquisition times, can evaluate both the morphology and the function of the TMJ by imaging the joint in various phases of mandibular movements. The standard protocol for a dynamic study of the TMJ involves the acquisition of static images in closed-mouth and open-mouth positions. Various mechanical devices are used to achieve a standard degree of mouth opening. Simple Lego blocks or syringes make satisfactory occlusal stops, or special positioning devices can be purchased commercially. We developed a system composed of two nested Plexiglas cylinders connected by a rubber tube. This creates a plunger mechanism that allows the patient to actively control the degree of mandibular opening.

Table 11.**4** MR sequences for TMJ investigations

T1-weighted SE sequences:
- Optimum resolution of anatomic details
- Accurate delineation of muscles and intra-articular structures
- Short TR and TE
- Accurate delineation of the articular disk

T2-weighted SE sequences:
- Poorer anatomic resolution
- Good tissue discrimination: fluid, mass, edema (Fig. 11.**19**)
- Long TR
- Long TE (Fig. 11.**19**)

Gradient-echo sequences:
- Short acquisition time (Fig. 11.**16**)
- Susceptible to artifacts
- Good delineation of articular disk
- Poor delineation of surrounding structures

Cine-MRI:
- Optional sequence for studying phases of mandibular movements

3-D MRI:
- Visualization of mass lesions (Fig. 11.**6**)

Movie MRI:
- Using echoplanar techniques

Contrast Agents

Paramagnetic contrast agents are unnecessary for primary MRI of the TMJ spaces. The intravenous injection of contrast agents does offer advantages, however. It increases the sensitivity of the study by enhancing small mass lesions that are isointense to surrounding tissues on noncontrast images (Fig. 11.**9b**). This increases specificity for better characterization of pathologic processes and aids in the diagnosis of articular disk perforation. All intravenous contrast agents in current use are paramagnetic and are well tolerated. They are used mainly in the diagnosis of neoplasms and disk perforations.

Imaging Findings

Congenital Variations and Malformations

The growth of the mandible is a function-dependent process that proceeds from various growth centers. *Disturbances of the chondro-osseous junction* in the TMJ can affect the growth of the entire hemimandible, especially if there is significant associated dysfunction. The time at which an injurious agent acts upon growth critically influences the severity of the developmental anomaly. The result may be aplasia or hypoplasia of the condyle or a shortened or elongated mandibular ramus causing obliquity of the masticatory plane (Fig. 11.**7**). There may be associated otologic anomalies (auditory canal atresia, auricular appendages) or orofacial dysmorphias (facial asymmetry, bird face, microgenia). A great many etiologic factors have been postulated in these developmental defects, but only a few have been established. These include hereditary disorders, teratogenic insults during embryonic development, mandibular trauma, and X-ray exposure during childhood. Endocrine disturbances such as acromegaly can also play a role. Condylar aplasia or hypoplasia (Fig. 11.**7**) may accompany various congenital mandibulofacial or mandibulocranial dysostoses, including Franceschetti syndrome (slanted palpebral fissures, coloboma of lower lid, maxillary hypoplasia, auricular deformity, auditory canal atresia) and Pierre Robin syndrome (microgenia, cleft palate, glossoptosis).

Condylar hyperplasia is unilateral in most cases. A special form of hyperplasia is unilateral hemihypertrophy of the facial skeleton. Various disease groups should be considered in the differential diagnosis of these enlargements.

Paget disease of bone (osteitis deformans) in adults also leads to expansion of the condylar process. *Acromegaly* presents with mandibular deformity and enlargement. *Recklinghausen disease* (neurofibromatosis) is often associated with hypoplasia of the mandibular coronoid process and elongation of the condylar process. *Craniofacial dysplasia* with maxillomandibular disproportion can occur in various syndromes:

- Otomandibular dysostosis.
- Cleidocranial dysostosis.
- Craniofacial dysostosis (Conn syndrome).
- Mandibulofacial dysostosis (Franceschetti–Zwahlen syndrome).
- Maxillofacial dysostosis (Peters and Hoeve syndrome).
- Oculoauricular dysplasia (Goldenhar syndrome).
- Robin syndrome.
- Down syndrome.
- Facial hemihypertrophy.
- Condylar hypoplasia and hyperplasia.
- Trauma.

Tumors

Besides a palpable mass about the TMJ, limitation of mouth opening provides an important differentiating clinical sign. Normal mouth opening, measurable by the interincisal distance, should be at least 40 mm, and limitations are graded on a three-point scale. Most limitations of mandibular movement have an inflammatory-reflex cause (Fig. 11.**9**) in which the masticatory muscles are infiltrated by inflammatory cells from an odontogenic abscess, cellulitis, surgical wound, etc. Myopathies, tetanus infections, and benign or malignant tumors can also cause limitation of jaw movement (Figs. 11.**21** – 11.**26**, 11.**28**, 11.**29**).

Benign Tumors

Cysts

By definition, a cyst is a pathologic cavity that has a specific lining and usually contains liquid or semisolid material. The diagnosis is based on the combination of clinical features, radiologic findings, and in some cases histologic analysis. Cysts are relatively common in the mandible and may involve the condyle as well as the coronoid process. An etiologic distinction is drawn between odontogenic and nonodontogenic forms. *Odontogenic cysts* arise from derivatives of the developing teeth. *Nonodontogenic cysts* form along the zone of fusion of various bones or may result from embryologic processes.

Odontogenic cysts of the maxilla and mandible can attain a large size and may extend to the skull base. On MRI, the contents of the cyst show high signal intensity on T2-weighted images and low to intermediate signal intensity on T1-weighted images. Other forms of odontogenic cysts are periodontal cysts and odontogenic keratocysts, but they are of minor importance in TMJ evaluations. A pneumatized bone cavity or aneurysmatic bone cyst are rare possibilities that should be considered in the differential diagnosis of localized areas of low signal intensity in bone.

Other benign tumors are described based on their site of occurrence and histologic features. They are classified histologically as epithelial, mesodermal, or mixed-cell tumors.

Figs. 11.**7 a, b** **Hypoplasia of the right TMJ.**
(**a**) Sagittal 2-D FLASH sequence (TR/TE = 36/10 ms, flip angle = 60°) in the resting position demonstrates the hypoplastic right mandibular condyle. The articular disk is faintly defined. Panel **b** documents normal mandibular opening despite the condylar hypoplasia.

Arrow	Anterior pole of articular disk
Arrowhead	Posterior pole of articular disk
T	Articular tubercle
F	Glenoid fossa
A	External acoustic meatus
c	Mandibular condyle

(**b**) Same MR sequence in the open-mouth position.
A External acoustic meatus
c Mandibular condyle
F Glenoid fossa
T Articular tubercle

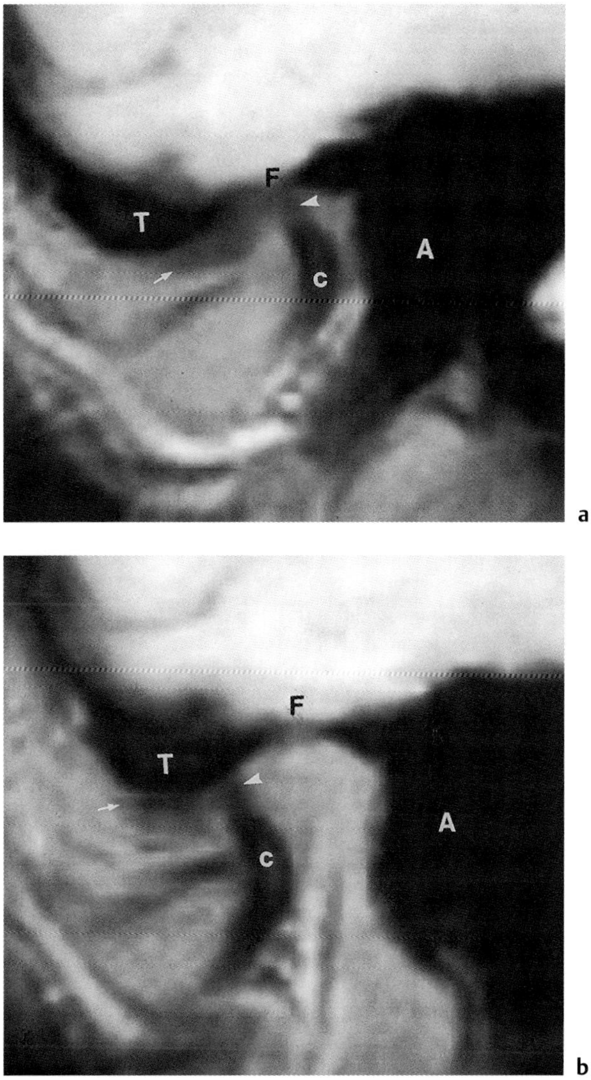

Ameloblastoma (Fig. 11.**23**)

Ameloblastoma is defined as a benign epithelial odontogenic tumor that arises from ameloblasts. Some 81% of ameloblastomas occur in the mandible, and the remaining 19% involve the maxilla. Conventional radiographs depict ameloblastoma as a unilocular or multilocular lucency. MRI reveals expansile lesions in the body and ramus of the mandible, varying in size from small cystic masses to an extensive area of mandibular destruction. The tumor tends to become locally invasive as extensive soft-tissue components break through the cortical bone. The signal intensity is intermediate on T1-weighted images and high on T2-weighted images.

Pindborg Tumor (Fig. 11.**24**)

This is a calcifying epithelial odontogenic tumor, characterized on plain radiographs by marked bone expansion with loss of cortical bone structures. MRI reveals hypointense calcifications within the lesion. Generally the tumor shows ill-defined margins with signs of aggressiveness. Its signal characteristics closely resemble those of ameloblastoma, from which it is indistinguishable by MRI.

Benign Nonodontogenic Tumors

The same criteria apply to benign nonodontogenic tumors as to tumors occurring at other skeletal sites, and their radiologic features are essentially the same. The morphology and MRI criteria of specific lesions are described below.

Exostoses

Exostoses appear as flat nodular or pedunculated bony excrescences on the cortical surface of the mandible or maxilla. They appear as areas of increased bone density on conventional radiographs and as hypointense areas on MR images. Location, topography, and soft-tissue changes should be documented by MRI on all planes.

Osteoma

Osteoma is a benign neoplasm of cortical bone occurring at an endosteal or periosteal site. The tumors are extremely variable in size and predominantly affect women. The mandible is involved more frequently than the maxilla.

Conventional radiographs of osteoma show a dense, well-circumscribed mass with a sclerotic internal structure. If multiple lesions are found, the differential diagnosis should include Gardner syndrome, in which multiple osteomas are combined with multiple colonic polyps, epidermoids, cysts, and dermoid tumors of the skin. MRI can accurately diagnose these lesions based on their low signal intensity in T1- and T2-weighted sequences.

Histiocytosis X

Three forms of histiocytosis X are distinguished:

- Abt–Letterer–Siwe disease.
- Hand–Schüller–Christian disease.
- Benign form of eosinophilic granuloma.

Eosinophilic granulomas of the mandible appear as sharply circumscribed "punched-out" osteolytic defects. Areas of cortical destruction have low signal intensity on MR images, and the soft-tissue component is optimally demonstrated in T1- and T2-weighted spin-echo (SE) sequences. These lesions consistently show marked enhancement after the injection of paramagnetic contrast medium.

Articular Tumors

The various tissues that constitute the TMJ, such as the synovial membrane, fibrous capsule, articular disk, and articular cartilage, may give rise to a benign or malignant mesenchymal tumor of the TMJ. These articular tumors present clinically with pain, swelling, and increasing limitation of jaw movement. Given the close physical proximity of the mandibular condyle, glenoid fossa, articular tubercle, zygomatic process, and tympanic plate, some degree of bone destruction is generally present even in early cases. Bone destruction about the TMJ is most commonly caused by primary malignant tumors of the external auditory canal, middle ear, or buccal mucosa, which may spread to involve the joint. The second most common cause is hematogenous metastasis, which produces regular or irregular osteolytic areas. Benign or semimalignant tumors cause circumscribed bone destruction (Fig. 11.**20**) that may be cystic or loculated. Intraosseous lesions may cause expansion of the affected bone segment, depending on their type and rate of growth. The differential diagnosis is aided by noting the presence of periosteal reactions and circumscribed calcifications in the tumor area. It is noteworthy that tumors arising from articular surface tissues tend to erode the bone on both sides of the joint space, while tumors that arise from adjacent bone tend to destroy only the bony joint compartment on one side of the joint space. Soft-tissue tumors such as carcinoma of the buccal mucosa do not obey this rule.

Clinical MR examination of the TMJ requires a thorough knowledge of benign and malignant mass lesions. In some cases the examination technique may have to be modified to accurately define the routes of tumor infiltration.

Fibro-osseous Lesions

*Fibrous Dysplasia (Fig. 11.**8**)*

Fibrous dysplasia has major significance in the diagnosis of TMJ pathology. This etiologically obscure disease is more common in the maxilla than in the mandible, where it usually affects the posterior segments of the bone. The lesion is often diagnosed in the first three decades of life. Three forms are distinguished:

- Monostotic dysplasia.
- Polyostotic fibrous dysplasia.
- Albright syndrome.

The clinical symptoms of monostotic fibrous dysplasia are swelling and fullness of the mandible with displacement and protuberance of the maxilla. Albright syndrome is an etiologically obscure developmental defect that is associated with cutaneous pigmentation and multiple skeletal lesions.

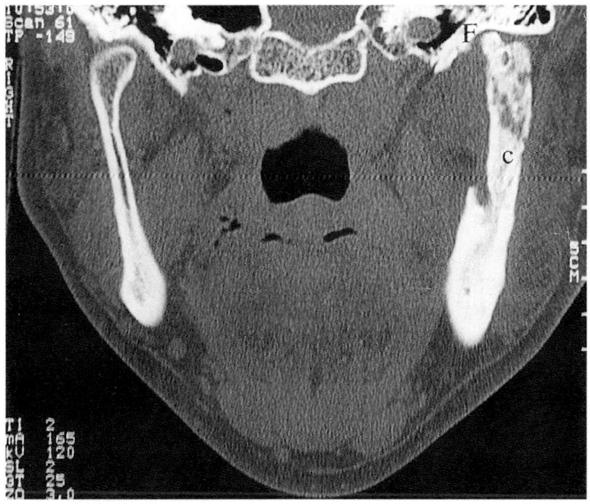

a

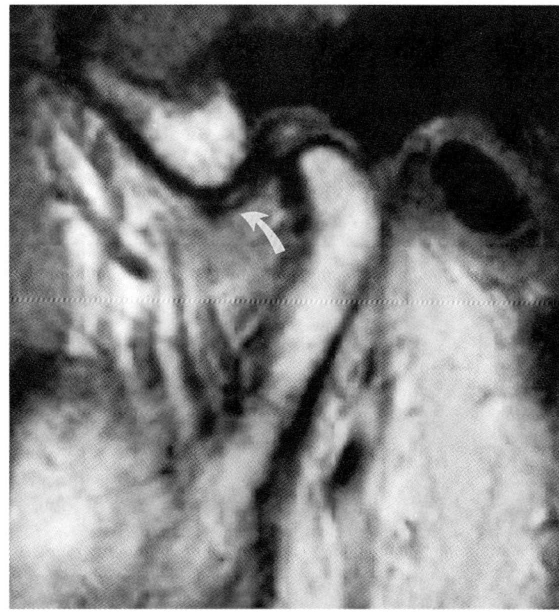

c

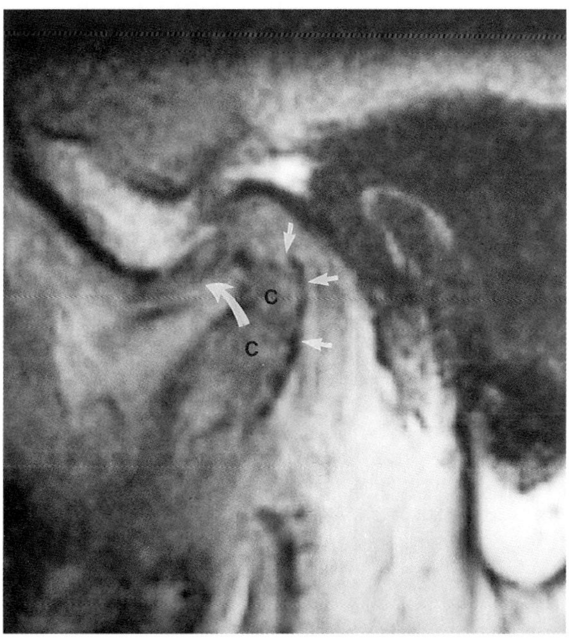

b

Figs. 11.**8 a – c** **Fibrous dysplasia.** Comparative CT and MRI views of the right and left TMJs in the same patient.

(**a**) Coronal CT scan with a 2-mm slice thickness shows a condyle and TMJ of normal appearance on the right side. On the left side, the glenoid fossa is shallow and the head and neck of the condylar process are expanded. The entire left mandibular ramus shows a patchy, nonhomogeneous structure with areas of very dense sclerosis, considered pathognomonic for fibrous dysplasia.

c Condylar process of mandible

F Glenoid fossa

(**b**) Sagittal unenhanced MR image (TR/TE = 500/15 ms) helps resolve the question of articular involvement. The condylar process shows a mixed, nonhomogeneous signal pattern in which only peripheral cortical structures are well defined (arrows). The image also shows a moderate increase of soft tissue in the joint space and nonhomogeneous delineation of the articular disk (curved arrow).

C Condylar process of mandible

(**c**) Comparative MR image of the normal right side shows a condylar process of normal appearance and a normal position of the articular disk (curved arrow).

The radiographic appearance of fibrous dysplasia is extremely variable, ranging from well-defined unilocular or multilocular lucencies to a circumscribed, homogeneous increase in bone density with expansion of osseous structures. The latter form is characterized histologically by bony trabeculae interspersed with scant connective tissue. Cystic lesions are associated with cortical thinning and expansion, but perforation is rare. On MRI, the sclerotic components of fibrous dysplasia show low signal intensity in both T1- and T2-weighted SE sequences. Active areas that still have a vascular supply tend to occur at the periphery of these expansile processes and also appear hypointense to muscle on noncontrast MR images. Paramagnetic contrast can significantly improve the diagnosis of these soft-tissue processes, with areas of vascularized connective tissue generally showing intense enhancement.

Ossifying Fibroma

Ossifying fibroma is a benign neoplasm composed of connective tissue and irregular bony trabecular structures. The ossified areas become more extensive as the lesion matures. The most common site of occurrence is the mandible. Conventional radiographs and CT scans show a sharply circumscribed lesion that appears as a lucent feature during the early growth period. On MRI, the tumor is consistently found to have two components:

- Hypovascular bony areas.
- Enhancing soft-tissue elements.

Hemangioma

Hemangiomas, while common in the skull and vertebral bodies, are rare in the mandible (Fig. 9.**10 b**). Radiographs and CT demonstrate the lesion as a lucent area with fine trabeculations. Large hemangiomas cause thinning and expansion of cortical structures. The tumor can be specifically diagnosed by its prolonged T2 relaxation time on MR images. It consistently shows intense enhancement with paramagnetic contrast.

Neurogenic Tumors

Benign neurogenic tumors include neuromas, neurofibromas, and traumatic neuromas. Radiographs demonstrate these lesions as solitary lucencies that expand in the alveolar canal or as multilocular lesions with a marked destructive component. On MRI, the lesions display low signal intensity on T1-weighted images and show marked enhancement after the administration of gadolinium(Gd)-DTPA.

Malignant Tumors

There are three pathogenic mechanisms by which malignant tumors can involve the TMJ:

- They may invade the mandible or maxilla secondarily from adjacent soft tissues of the oropharynx or paranasal sinuses.
- They may originate from the mandible or maxilla.
- They may metastasize to that region.

The goal of diagnostic imaging is to differentiate malignant tumors from primary benign tumors and cysts and accurately determine the extent of the lesion. A routine evaluation is generally based on high-resolution CT scans. Soft-tissue structures are better delineated by MRI, however, and this study is also useful for evaluating infiltration of the joint compartments and monitoring response to therapy.

Carcinoma

Most carcinomas that invade the mandible originate from the oral cavity and paranasal sinuses and are classified histologically as squamous cell carcinomas. These tumors may spread to the mandible and maxilla along vascular channels or by direct erosion due to tumor infiltration.

Radiographically, invasion of the bone by carcinoma is manifested by an irregular "moth-eaten" appearance of the cortical boundary. CT is excellent for defining the cortical structures but gives little information on concomitant involvement of the cancellous bone and adjacent soft tissues. The tumor can be identified on MRI by its moderately prolonged T1 and T2 relaxation times compared with surrounding muscle tissue. An advantage of MRI is its ability to document cancellous bone involvement in the mandibular ramus and condyle, with tumor invasion causing a definite loss of signal intensity relative to the opposite side. Following paramagnetic contrast administration, the infiltrated area shows marked enhancement in T1-weighted sequences, the signal intensity approximating that of normal fatty tissue.

Another type of carcinoma that may involve the mandible is mucoepidermoid carcinoma (Figs. 11.**26**, 11.**27**), which arises from aberrant salivary gland tissue within the maxilla or mandible. The lesion appears radiologically as an ill-defined lytic area or multilocular cystic mass that is usually associated with greater tissue destruction than squamous cell carcinoma. Embryonic mixed tumors may also be encountered in this region.

Figs. 11.**9a, b** **Trismus and soft-tissue swelling in the right masticator space and parotid gland with a parotid soft-tissue mass involving the masseter muscle and causing limitation of jaw movement.**
(**a**) Unenhanced axial T1-weighted SE sequence (TR/TE = 500/15 ms) shows a hypointense mass (arrows) anterior to the parotid gland with involvement of the masseter muscle (open arrow).
(**b**) Gd-enhanced axial T1-weighted SE sequence (TR/TE = 500/15 ms) shows marked enhancement about the anterior pole of the parotid gland (arrow), confirming parotitis with involvement of the masseter muscle.

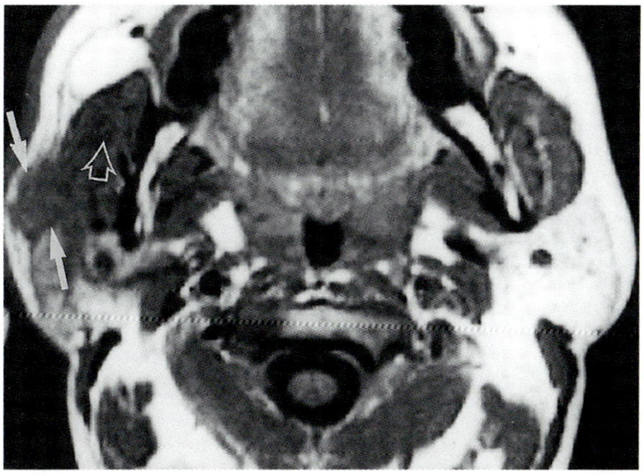

a

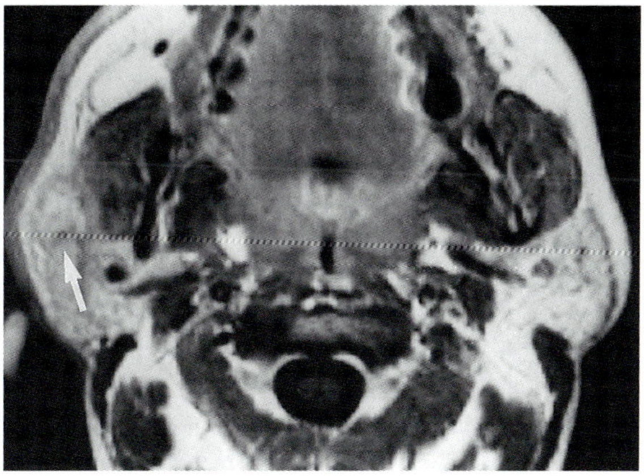

b

Arthritis

The TMJ is like other joints in that it may be affected by arthritis that is unrelated to functional demands. *Nonspecific* arthritis of the TMJ presents with local swelling, tenderness, and lateral deviation of the jaw. Joint effusion may widen the space between the condyle and glenoid fossa on the affected side, causing deviation of the mandibular midline to the unaffected side. The arthritis may be caused by a hematogenous or contiguous bacterial infection (Fig. 11.**19**) due to otitis media or mandibular osteomyelitis, or it may have a traumatic cause (Fig. 11.**11**). *Specific* arthritis of the TMJ is less common and may result from a specific infectious disease such as gonorrhea or tuberculosis. Arthritis can also result from a nearby suppurative processes caused, for example, by unerupted maxillary wisdom teeth, a post-injection abscess, or acute parotitis (Fig. 11.**9**).

Rheumatic diseases of the skeletal system lead to TMJ involvement in 5% to 86% of cases. The underlying disease may be a true rheumatic disorder such as rheumatoid arthritis, juvenile rheumatoid arthritis (Still disease), Bekhterev disease, Reiter disease, and other systemic diseases such as psoriasis and metabolic disorders that are associated with crystal deposition (gout [Fig. 11.**20**], pseudogout). Prolonged rheumatoid arthritis of the TMJ can lead to severe joint destruction culminating in the clinical and radiologic features of degenerative arthritis (Table 11.**5**).

Diseases of the masticatory muscles (*myopathies*) should be considered in the differential diagnosis of inflammatory and reactive changes in the TMJ. Basically, the demonstrable forms of TMJ myopathy represent a response of the muscle to general pathologic stimuli or a disturbance of muscle tonus. Myopathies can occur in the setting of various metabolic and rheumatic diseases (Table 11.**6**).

Table 11.**5** Primary disorders of the TMJ

Arthritis:
➤ Nonspecific, specific (Fig. 11.**19**)
➤ Rheumatic, gout (Fig. 11.**20**)

Table 11.6 Myopathies of the masticatory muscles

- Muscle splinting
- Myogelosis
- Muscle spasm
- Contracture
- Muscular hypertrophy
- Myalgia
- Forms of myotonia
- Myasthenia gravis
- Fibrous myositis, ossifying myositis
- Myoarthropathy syndrome

Degenerative Diseases

Ankylosis

While trismus (Fig. 11.**9**) refers only to the symptom of limited mouth opening, ankylosis denotes the complete or almost complete immobility of the joint itself. Fibrous union of the articular surfaces (fibrous ankylosis) usually allows a slight residual degree of opening, whereas bony ankylosis generally prohibits mandibular opening. Ankylosis is caused by processes that destroy the articular cartilage and articular disk, most notably trauma (Fig. 11.**11**) and infections (Fig. 11.**19**). Suppurative otitis media in children, for example, may spread to involve the TMJ. Infected fractures are also associated with an increased risk of TMJ ankylosis, as are central fracture dislocations in which the condyle is impacted into the glenoid fossa. A severe deforming arthropathy of the TMJ may progress to ankylosis with complete immobility of the mandible (Fig. 11.**10**).

Joint Trauma

Despite its protected position, the TMJ is susceptible to injury by forces acting directly or indirectly on the lower jaw. The traumatizing force may, depending on its magnitude, cause subluxation or dislocation of the mandibular condyle (Figs. 11.**13** – 11.**16**), articular disk displacement, or an impacted fracture. If the mandible is injured during growth phase in small children, this can cause severe developmental disturbances of the mandible resulting in facial asymmetry. Most injuries of the TMJ result in a traumatic arthritis incited by damage to the articular surfaces, joint capsule, and suspensory structures. Possible causes include extreme mouth opening during general endotracheal anesthesia or dental procedures. Other symptoms relate to intra-articular effusion. Trauma to the joint can also cause fractures through the neck or head of the condylar process, marked clinically by tenderness to preauricular palpation and pressure on the tip of the chin. Treatment planning relies on radiographic findings (panoramic radiographs of the mandible, occipitofrontal skull film, and CT) (Fig. 11.**11**) and, in selected cases, on MRI.

Disk Displacement

Various hypotheses have been advanced on the cause of disk displacements (Figs 11.**11** and 11.**12**). Hyperextension of the TMJ is caused by excessive excursion of the mandible due, for example, to yawning, general endotracheal anesthesia, or opening the mouth widely during dental procedures. Hyperextension of the joint causes excessive stretching of the attached ligamentous structures. Traumatic events such as joint compression and whiplash trauma lead to intra-articular soft-tissue injuries.

The main clinical symptoms of discopathies are function-dependent pain and joint sounds such as clicking and crepitation. Causes may include muscular imbalances, dental instabilities, occlusal interferences, traumatic lesions, changes in the shape of the articular surfaces, and psychogenic causes. Clinically important forms of anterior disk displacement are illustrated in Figure 11.**12**.

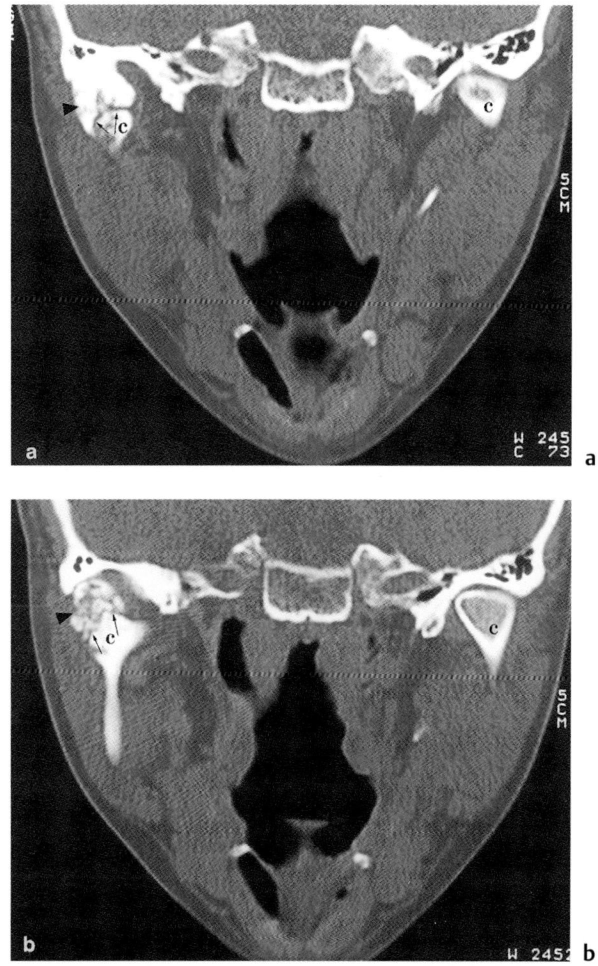

Figs. 11.**10 a, b** **Degenerative arthritis of the right TMJ.** (**a**) Coronal CT scan (2-mm slice thickness) shows degenerative changes in the right TMJ with osteophyte formation due to osteochondrosis and areas of lytic resorption in the right condylar process. These findings are specific for degenerative arthritis (small arrows).

c	Mandibular condyle
Arrowhead	Degenerative-sclerotic intra-articular material

(**b**) Adjacent coronal section.

Arrowhead	Sclerotic osteophytosis
Arrows	Degenerative deformity of condylar process
c	Condylar process

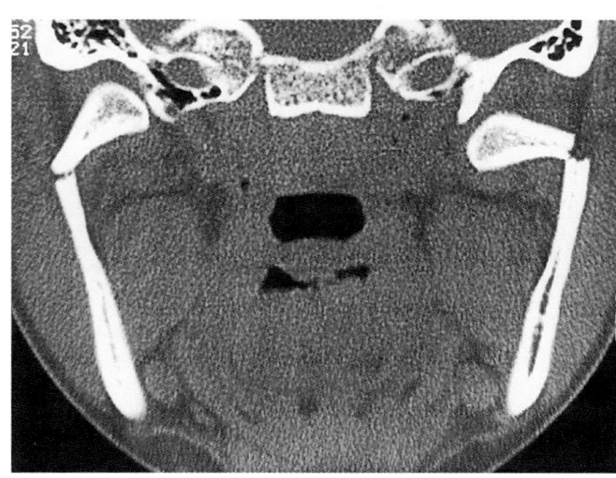

Fig. 11.**11** **Bilateral fractures of the condylar process.** Coronal CT scan (4-mm slice thickness) in a patient with soft-tissue swelling and limited mouth opening reveals bilateral subcondylar fractures through the base of the condylar process.

Figs. 11.**12 a – c** **Schematic diagram of disk displacement.**
(**a**) Grade 1 partial anterior disk displacement.
(**b**) Grade 2 partial anterior disk displacement.
(**c**) Complete reducible anterior disk displacement.
A Anterior pole of condyle
S Superior pole of condyle

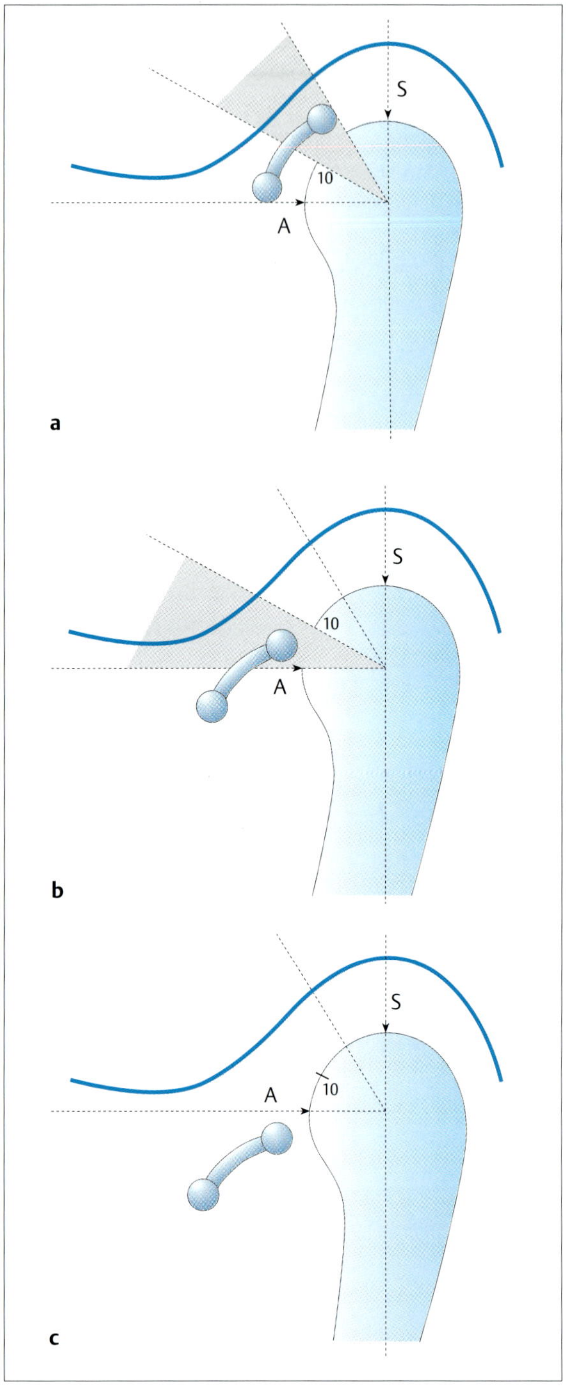

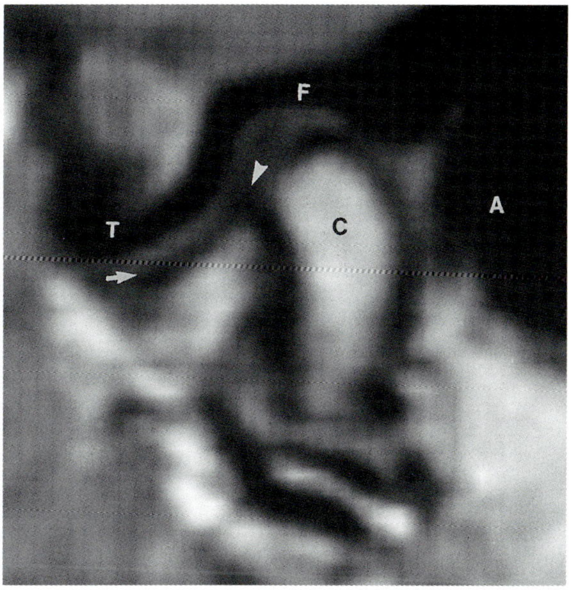

a

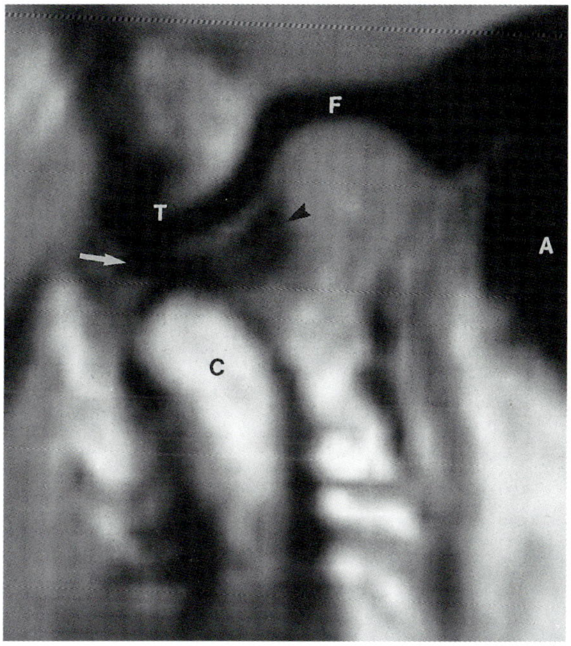

b

Figs. 11.**13 a, b** **Grade 2 reducing partial anterior disk displacement.**
(**a**) Sagittal SE sequence (TR/TE = 600/15 ms) in the resting position shows a uniform disk contour with the posterior pole of the disk apposed to the anterior pole of the condyle. The condyle occupies a high posterior position.

A	External acoustic meatus
C	Mandibular condyle
F	Glenoid fossa
T	Articular tubercle
Arrow	Anterior pole of disk
Arrowhead	Posterior pole of disk

(**b**) Same MR sequence in the open-mouth position shows the condyle positioned immediately anterior to the apex of the articular tubercle, with reduction of the disk. The posterior band is thickened.

A	External acoustic meatus
C	Mandibular condyle
F	Glenoid fossa
T	Articular tubercle
Arrow	Anterior pole of disk
Arrowhead	Posterior pole of disk

Imaging Criteria and Their Differential Diagnosis

Disk Displacement

Today the radiologic diagnosis of discopathies and disk displacements is based largely on morphologic findings in MRI, where disk position and disk morphology are evaluated in the closed-mouth and open-mouth positions using T1-weighted SE sequences (Fig. 11.**13**). In evaluating disk displacements, various authors have analyzed the relation of the intermediate zone of the disk to the anterior and superior poles of the mandibular condyle and to the center of rotation for mandibular movements. The posterior pole of the articular disk, the greatest superior circumference of the mandibular condyle, and its greatest anterior circumference are identified as anatomic reference points on the MR image. The disk position can be uniquely specified by reference to these landmarks. The disk displacements that can be diagnosed with MRI are summarized in Table 11.**7**. In the model that we use, the superior pole of the condyle corresponds to the 12 o'clock position and the

Table 11.7 Disk displacements diagnosable on MR images

Findings	Differential diagnostic criteria
Anterior disk displacement (Fig. 11.**16**) that reduces on mouth opening	
Partial:	
➤ Grade 1	Posterior pole of disk is between 10 and 11 o'clock positions
➤ Grade 2	Posterior pole of disk is between 9 and 10 o'clock positions
➤ Complete MR findings	Disk is anterior to condyle; its posterior pole has no contact with condylar articular surface (Fig. 11.**16**)
Nonreducing anterior disk displacement	Disk is anterior to the posterior inferior articular surface of the articular tubercle
Posterior disk displacement	
➤ Grade 1	Posterior pole of disk is between 9 and 10 o'clock positions
➤ Grade 2	Disk has slid completely onto secondary articular surface of condyle; anterior pole of disk is on or behind superior pole of condyle
Transverse disk displacement (pure medial or lateral)	Diagnostic criterion: medial or lateral disk attachment to mandibular condyle is displaced
Anteromedial or anterolateral displacement plus rotation	All of the disk cannot be visualized in one section

anterior pole to the 9 o'clock position (Fig. 11.**12**, Table 11.**8**).

Anterior Disk Displacement
(Figs. 11.**13** – 11.**18**)

Anterior disk displacement is the most clinically significant intra-articular functional derangement of the TMJ. The disk usually relates anteromedially to the condyle in this type of displacement. A *partial* anterior disk displacement is differentiated from a *complete* displacement. With a partial disk displacement, the posterior pole of the disk is between the 11 and 9 o'clock positions relative to the condyle. The 11 o'clock position has been cited as the threshold for diagnosing an unstable disk position on MRI. In our group, we diagnose a grade 1 partial disk displacement if the posterior pole of the disk is between the 10 and 11 o'clock positions (Figs. 11.**12 a** and 11.**13 b**); a grade 2 displacement is diagnosed if the posterior pole is between the 9 and 10 o'clock positions (Fig. 11.**12 b**). With a complete anterior disk displacement, the disk is anterior to the mandibular condyle and its posterior band has lost contact with the condylar articular surface. The reducibility of the articular disk is a critical issue in the diagnosis of discopathies. It is assessed by evaluating the mobility of the disk, the functional status of the suspensory apparatus of the disk, and posterior recoil. Static MR images in the open- and closed-mouth positions can accurately establish the position of the disk but are of little value in assessing its reducibility. An anterior disk displacement may incite a progressive intra-articular functional derangement with increasing damage to the articular disk.

Table 11.**8** Diagnostic criteria for articular disk displacement

Clock face model:
- ➤ Articular disk:
  - —Reference point is the posterior pole of the disk
- ➤ Mandibular condyle:
  - —Reference point is the greatest superior circumference
  - —Superior pole of condyle at 12 o'clock position
  - —Anterior pole of condyle at 9 o'clock position

Anterior disk displacement (Figs. 11.**13** – 11.**18**)
- ➤ Partial anterior disk displacement
- ➤ Complete anterior disk displacement

Posterior disk displacement:
- ➤ Posterior pole of disk

Transverse disk displacement:
- ➤ Pure medial
- ➤ Pure lateral
- ➤ Anteromedial
- ➤ Anterolateral
- ➤ Pure anterior rotation

A *nonreducing anterior disk displacement* can take various forms depending on the cause of the displacement. It may involve an excessive anterior displacement of the disk or a disk avulsion. The latter condition can be accurately diagnosed by MRI.

Posterior Disk Displacement

Posterior disk displacement is less common than anterior displacement. It exhibits two grades of severity on MR images. The diagnostic reference points are the greatest superior circumference of the mandibular condyle and the relation of the anterior and posterior poles of the disk to the temporal articular surface. With a grade 1 posterior disk displacement, the posterior pole of the disk is displaced past the superior pole of the condyle to the 1 o'clock position. With a grade 2 posterior disk displacement, the anterior pole of the disk has also moved behind the superior pole of the condyle. These cases usually present clinically with limitation of jaw movement.

Transverse Disk Displacement

Transverse disk displacements may be classified as purely medial or lateral, anteromedial, or anterolateral. There may also be a rotational component that hampers MRI evaluation.

Table 11.**10** Pathologic disk shapes in sagittal MRI

Disk shape	Features	MRI criteria
Normal (Figs. 11.**1** – 11.**5**)	Normal morphology	ap, pp, iz clearly identifiable; ap and pp are of equal size
Thickening of posterior band		ap, pp, iz clearly identifiable; pp > ap
Thickening of anterior band		ap, pp, iz clearly identifiable; ap > pp
Linear, uniform disk structure, elongated and thinned		ap, pp, iz not identifiable
Concave		Thickened iz
Convex		Shortened iz
S-shaped		Elongated iz
C-shaped		Short, thick iz
Y-shaped		ap, pp, iz not identifiable; complete destruction

ap Anterior pole of disk
pp Posterior pole of disk
iz Intermediate zone

Shape and Structural Changes in the Articular Disk

Besides disk displacement, it is important to consider possible changes in the shape and structure of the articular disk. Degenerative changes with thinning and tearing usually commence in the lower portion of the upper lamina of the disk.

As the ground substance is broken down, changes occur in the MRI signal characteristics of the disk in T1- and T2-weighted SE sequences. As a rule, disk remodeling must be fairly well advanced before a definite increase in signal intensity is observed on T2-weighted images. Severe forms of TMJ arthritis are the most frequent cause of these changes (Table 11.**9**).

Table 11.**9** Differential diagnosis of structural changes in the articular disk in T1-weighted SE sequences

Hypointense areas:
- Degenerative microcalcifications

Hyperintense areas:
- Mucoid degeneration and increasing hydration

Structural Changes in the Articular Disk and Bilaminar Zone

The imaging findings listed in Table 11.**10** can be interpreted as differential diagnostic criteria for the presence of degenerative or posttraumatic changes (Figs. 11.**15** – 11.**18**).

Differential Diagnosis of Internal Derangement

"Internal derangement" is a term applied to intra-articular functional disturbances of the TMJ based on changes in the shape, position, or structure of the joint components. Excessive or unphysiologic loading of the TMJ can lead to alterations in the shape of these components. Since the articular disk must accommodate to the incongruent articular surfaces of the glenoid fossa and mandibular condyle (Figs. 11.**1** – 11.**4**), it must also absorb any pathologic shear stresses and compressive loads that develop within the joint. MRI of the disk and soft-tissue structures can detect the early stages of degenerative arthritis even before changes in the width of the joint spaces can be seen radiographically. In all, *six stages of internal derangement* can be defined and differentiated on MR images (Table 11.**11**).

Clinically, patients complain of joint sounds such as snapping or clicking as the jaw opens and closes.

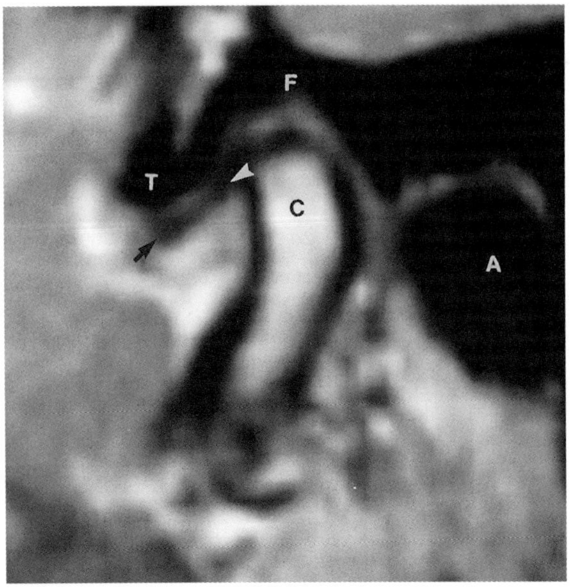

a

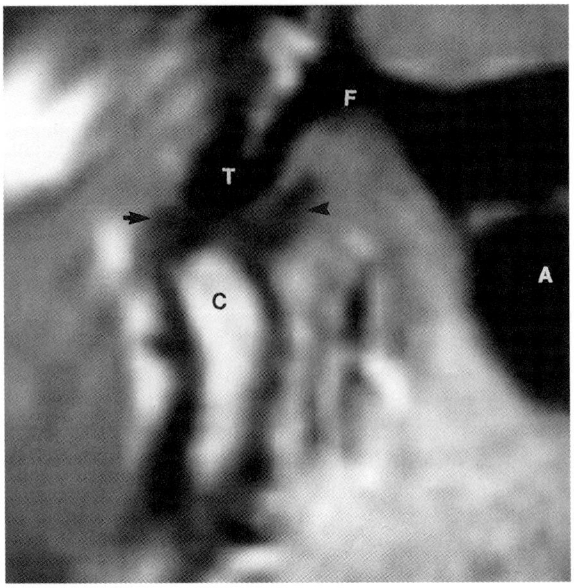

b

Figs. 11.**14 a, b** **Reducing complete anterior disk displacement.**
(**a**) Sagittal SE sequence (TR/TE = 600/15 ms) in the resting position shows the posterior pole of the disk in front of the anterior pole of the condyle. The condyle shows physiologic distraction and a slightly posterior position.

A	External acoustic meatus
C	Mandibular condyle
F	Glenoid fossa
T	Articular tubercle
Arrow	Anterior pole of disk
Arrowhead	Posterior pole of disk

(**b**) Same sequence with the mouth opened 3.5 cm (interincisal distance) shows a thickened contour of the disk, which is in a reduced position. The condyle is below the articular tubercle.

A	External acoustic meatus
C	Mandibular condyle
F	Glenoid fossa
T	Articular tubercle
Arrow	Anterior pole of disk
Arrowhead	Posterior pole of disk

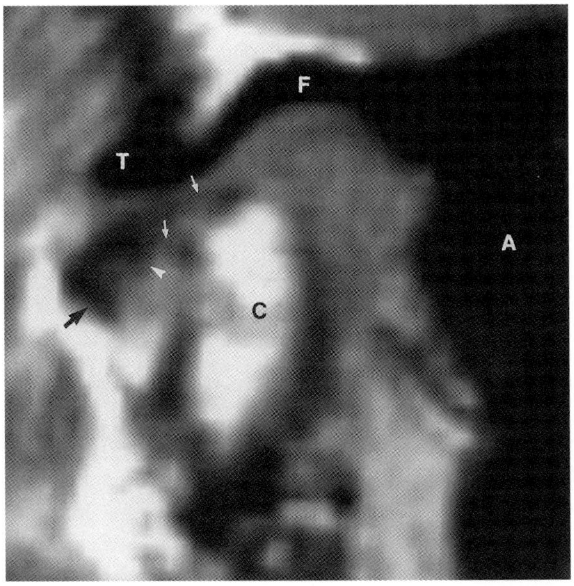

Fig. 11.**15** **Nonreducing complete anterior disk displacement with a C-shaped disk.** Sagittal SE sequence (TR/TE = 600/15 ms) shows complete, nonreducing anterior displacement of the C-shaped disk (arrows). The mandibular condyle exhibits marked degenerative changes.

A External acoustic meatus
C Mandibular condyle
F Glenoid fossa
T Articular tubercle

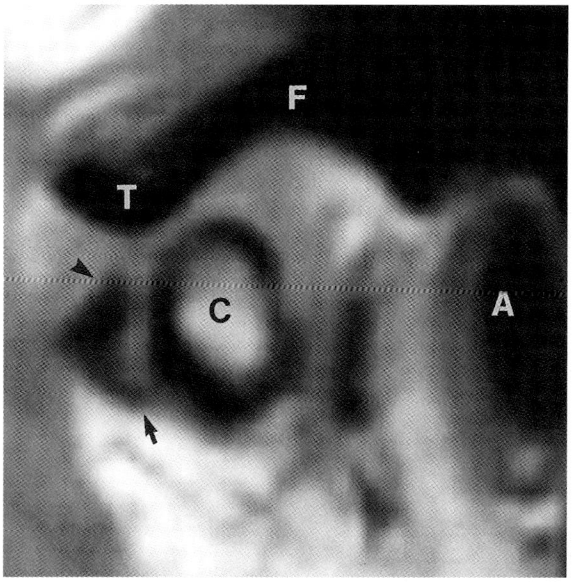

Fig. 11.**16** **Complete anterior disk displacement with a triangular disk shape** (arrow and arrowhead). Sagittal MR image (TR/TE = 100/15 ms) shows a typical triangular shape of the completely displaced articular disk.

A External acoustic meatus
C Mandibular condyle
F Glenoid fossa
T Articular tubercle

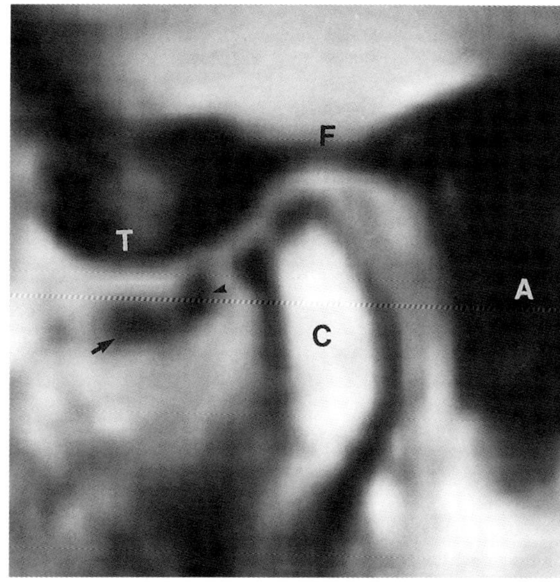

Fig. 11.**17** **Displaced articular disk with a concave shape.** Sagittal T1-weighted SE sequence (TR/TE = 1000/15 ms) demonstrates the concave shape (arrow and arrowhead) of the displaced articular disk.

A External acoustic meatus
C Mandibular condyle
F Glenoid fossa
T Articular tubercle

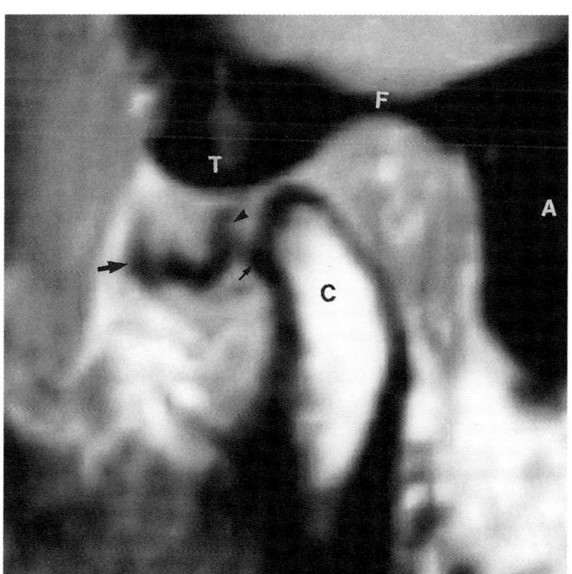

Fig. 11.**18** **Anterior disk displacement with a sigmoid disk shape.** Sagittal T1-weighted MR image (TR/TE = 1000/15 ms) shows the displaced, sigmoid-shaped disk with its anterior (large arrow) and posterior (small arrow) zone.

A External acoustic meatus
C Mandibular condyle
F Glenoid fossa
T Articular tubercle
Arrowhead Superior pole of disk

Table 11.**11** Diagnostic criteria for internal derangement of the TMJ

Stage 1:
➤ Early phase with mild, partial, reducing disk displacement
Stage 2:
➤ Reducing disk displacement (Figs. 11.**13**–11.**18**) and disk deformity
Stage 3:
➤ Intermediate stage with nonreducing disk displacement and adhesion
Stage 4:
➤ Progressive changes in osseous shape and structure (Fig. 11.**16**)
Stage 5:
➤ Disk avulsion, perforation
Stage 6:
➤ Destruction of mandibular condyle (Fig. 11.**18**)

Stages 1 and 2 cover the early phase of internal derangement. Stage 3 is a nonreducing disk displacement, while stages 4, 5, and 6 denote advanced stages of internal derangement.

The *early phase* on MRI is marked chiefly by disk changes that in *stage I* are associated with a reducing partial displacement, usually anterior and unaccompanied by alterations of disk shape. *Stage 2* is marked by clinical manifestations and TMJ nonhomogeneities that include an alteration of disk shape.

An important diagnostic criterion is the hypointense posterior band, which serves as a landmark for detecting anterior, posterior, and transverse (medial or lateral) disk displacements.

Stages 3 through 6 are basically characterized by nonreducing disk displacements. The cause may be a disk adhesion or an excessive anterior disk position. If the distal suspensory apparatus becomes stretched and lax, deficient posterior recoil results. *Stage 3* is commonly associated with fascial thickening in the pterygoid muscles. *Stage 4* is characterized by pronounced disk deformity and osteophytic changes, *stage 5* by a change in the condylar outline with progressive destructive changes, usually followed by massive disk perforation and disk avulsion.

Other changes such as degenerative arthritis have very distinctive features on MRI and present no difficulties in terms of differential diagnosis.

Altered Signal Intensity of the Mandibular Condyle on MRI

The differential diagnosis of altered signal intensity in the mandibular condyle starts with an awareness of its normal signal characteristics in T1- and T2-weighted SE sequences. Thus, the condyle consistently shows variable signal intensity in T2-weighted sequences, high signal intensity in T1-weighted sequences, and low signal intensity in gradient-echo sequences.

A condyle affected by acute avascular necrosis displays high signal intensity on T2-weighted images and low signal intensity on T1-weighted images as a result of edematous changes in the cancellous bone. With further progression of the avascular necrosis, the condyle shows a decline in T2-weighted signal intensity.

Effusion and Soft-Tissue Proliferation in the TMJ (Tables 11.**13**–11.**15**)

The differential diagnosis of effusions in the TMJ is as wide-ranging as that of joint effusions in other skeletal regions.

The most likely cause of TMJ effusion is *reactive or inflammatory arthritis* (Figs. 11.**19**, 11.**20**). Acute inflammation of the TMJ presents clinically with local pain, swelling, and an acute arthrogenic trismus. The jaw reflexly assumes an antalgic, slightly open position.

Pyogenic arthritis (Fig. 11.**19**) is a clinically important form that may result from local trauma or hematogenous spread or may develop as a complication of acute otitis media, an auditory canal furuncle, bacterial parotitis, or osteomyelitis of the mandibular ramus.

Chronic arthritis of the TMJ may occur in the setting of rheumatoid arthritis, ankylosing spondylitis, or psoriatic arthritis. Other chronic bacterial

Table 11.**12** Changes in the signal intensity of the mandibular condyle

	T2-weighted signal intensity	T1-weighted signal intensity	Gradient-echo sequence
Normal condyle	Variable	High signal	Low signal
Acute avascular necrosis	High signal	Low signal	Variable
Late avascular necrosis	Low signal	Low signal	Low signal
Osteochondrosis dissecans	Variable	Low signal	Variable

Table 11.13 Differential diagnosis of TMJ arthritis

- Hematogenous
- Pyogenic
- Chronic bacterial
- Psoriatic
- Gouty
- Spondylarthrosis
- Parotitis
- Otitis
- Osteomyelitic
- Reactive-neurogenic
- Traumatic
- Rheumatoid
- Chronic polyarthritic

Table 11.14 Differential diagnosis of TMJ effusion

Common:
- Inflammatory manifestations
- Specific or nonspecific arthritis (Figs. 11.**19**, 11.**20**)
- Degenerative changes: internal derangement (Fig. 11.**10**)

Uncommon:
- Neoplasms (lymphoma) (Fig. 11.**22**)
- Posttraumatic sequelae (Figs. 11.**11**, 11.**30**)

Table 11.15 Pathology of the articular disk

MRI signal intensity:
- Hypointense: degenerative remodeling with microcalcifications
- Hyperintense: mucoid degeneration, hydration

Site of degenerative changes:
- Early form: thickening of the anterior and posterior bands
- Advanced degeneration: thinning of intermediate zone

Resorptive forms:
- Late forms: concave, convex
- S-shaped, C-shaped, Y-shaped, triangular
- Resorptive forms

changes can result from a suppurative cholesteatoma or chronic mandibular myelitis. The TMJ may also be affected by gout (Fig. 11.**20**) and by rheumatoid disorders such as Still disease, Bekhterev disease, psoriasis, and Reiter syndrome.

Many of these conditions are associated with deposits in the bone marrow of the mandibular condyle.

On the whole, radiologic findings are not specific enough to differentiate the above disorders.

Acute Nonspecific Arthritis

The principal MR finding is an intra-articular fluid collection visible on T2-weighted images (Fig. 11.**19**). There may also be isolated cases of specific arthritis triggered by a gonorrheal or tuberculous infection. Post-contrast images show slght but definite enhancement of the synovium. Chronic or recurrent abscesses are also found in cases of craniocervical involvement by actinomycosis.

Chronic Polyarthritis

This disease is often manifested initially by a serous inflammation of the synovium. Further progression leads to an inflammation that spreads to the subchondral bone and culminates in avascular necrosis and erosive changes in the TMJ.

Mass Lesions

In the radiologic diagnosis of mass lesions of the TMJ, it is important to determine the location of the mass, accurately define its locoregional topography, and make an accurate differential diagnosis (Fig. 11.**8**).

The differential diagnostic strategies for TMJ masses are presented below for specific morphologic presentations:

- Lesions that invade the mandible and maxilla from adjacent soft-tissue structures of the oropharynx and paranasal sinuses.
- Lesions that originate from the mandible or maxilla.
- Lesions that metastasize to that region.

Cystic Masses

This type of mass may or may not be associated with volume expansion in the TMJ. The mass appears on CT scans as a low-density area with a moderately attenuating rim.

On MRI, cysts display high signal intensity in T2-weighted sequences and low signal intensity in T1-weighted sequences.

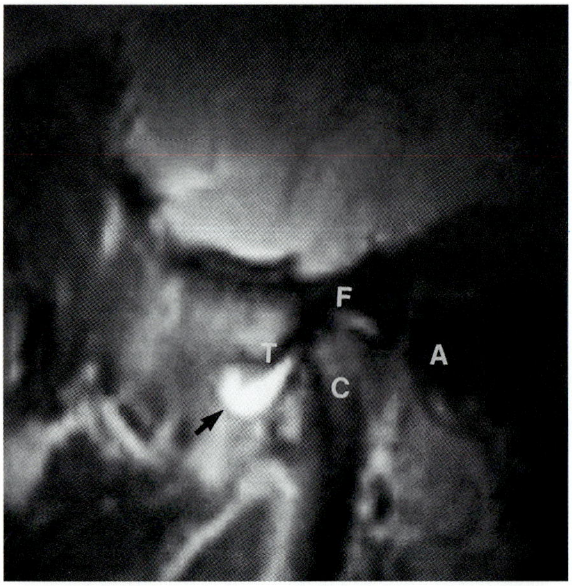

Fig. 11.**19** **Acute bacterial arthritis of the TMJ.** Sagittal T2-weighted SE sequence (TR/TE = 2500/90 ms) demonstrates the effusion (arrow) as a hyperintense fluid collection in the right anterior joint space.
A External acoustic meatus
C Mandibular condyle
F Glenoid fossa
T Articular tubercle

Masses of the Masticator Space (Fig. 11.**21**)

In the diagnostic imaging of the masseter muscle and its bordering spaces, an analysis of morphologic and topographic relationships often allows a precise pretherapeutic diagnosis. Contrast-enhanced MRI is particularly rewarding, as its high soft-tissue resolution permits the examiner to identify the etiologic substrate of a lesion.

In the evaluation of pseudotumors, for example, areas of muscular hypertrophy can be differentiated from accessory glandular structures and from benign and malignant neoplasms (Figs. 9.**6**, 9.**10**, 9.**13**).

The entities that can cause mass lesions in the masseter muscle are listed in order of frequency in Table 11.**16**.

The imaging analysis should cover the following points:

Masses That Do Not Cause Architectural Disruption:

- Benign masseter hypertrophy.
- Accessory salivary glands.

Masses That Cause Architectural Disruption and Show Signs of Infiltration:

- Benign and malignant tumors (Figs. 11.**22** – 11.**27**).
- Non-Hodgkin lymphoma.
- Inflammation with abscessation or cellulitis.

Table 11.**16** Entities responsible for mass lesions in the masseter muscle region

Malformations:
- Congenital craniofacial malformations

Tumor masses:
- Pseudotumors:
  - —Benign masseter hypertrophy
  - —Accessory parotid gland
- Malignant tumors:
  - —Sarcoma (soft-tissue [Fig. 11.**27**], chondrosarcoma, osteosarcoma)
  - —Malignant schwannoma (Fig. 11.**25**)
  - —Non-Hodgkin lymphoma (Fig. 11.**22**)

Inflammatory masses:
- Odontogenic abscess

Masses That Show Intense Peripheral Enhancement

Rim enhancement is most commonly observed in benign or malignant recurrent tumors (Fig. 11.**29**) and in various inflammatory processes ranging from abscesses to foreign-body reactions with granulomatous infiltrates (Fig. 11. **30**):
- Odontogenic abscess.
- Malignant schwannoma.
- Benign or malignant recurrent tumor.
- Granulomatous reaction (e.g., foreign body).

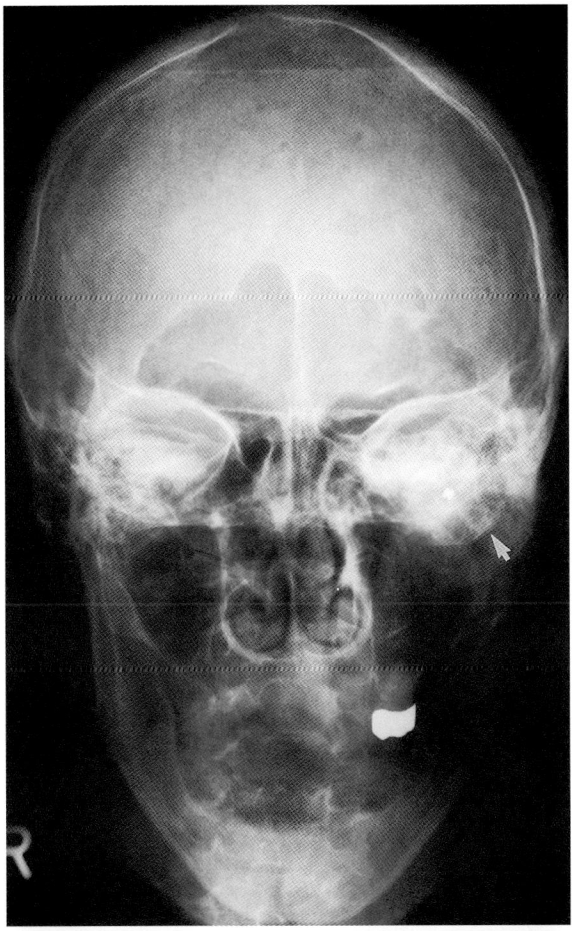

a

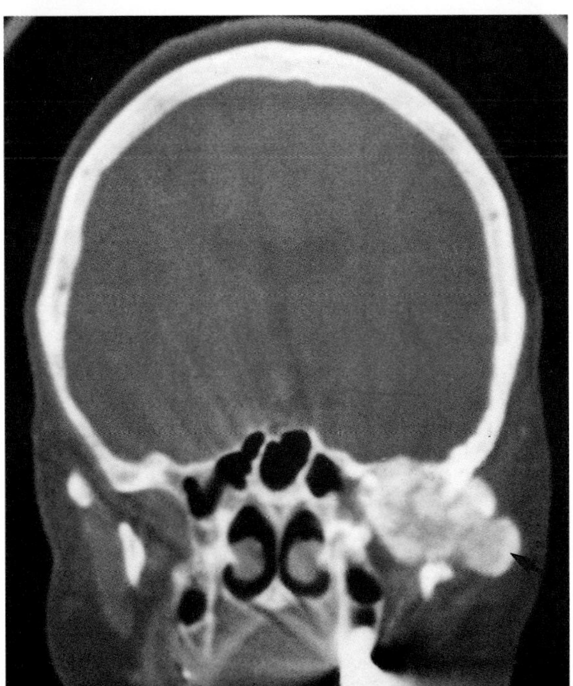

b

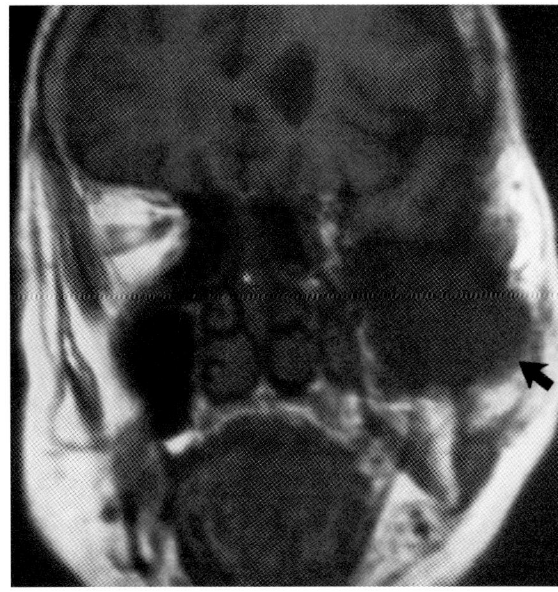

c

Figs. 11.**20 a – c** **Gouty involvement of the TMJ with joint destruction.**
(**a**) Skull radiograph shows increased density in the area of the left petrous bone (arrow).
(**b**) Coronal CT scan shows deposition of urate crystals about the left TMJ extending from the skull base to the masticatory muscles (arrow).
(**c**) Coronal T1-weighted MRI reveals the gouty tophus (arrow) as a hypointense mass with a peripheral inflammatory reaction.

Figs. 11.**21 a, b** **Masticatory space mass showing high T1-weighted signal intensity and marked contrast enhancement.**
(**a**) T1-weighted SE sequence shows a hyperintense mass (arrows) in the masseter compartment arising from the mandibular condyle. The smooth margins and moderate nonhomogeneity are consistent with an ameloblastoma containing lipid components or zones of intratumoral hemorrhage.
C Mandibular condyle
m Masseter compartment
(**b**) Sagittal MP-RAGE reconstruction shows the intact mandibular condyle (C) above an extensive, enhancing mass.

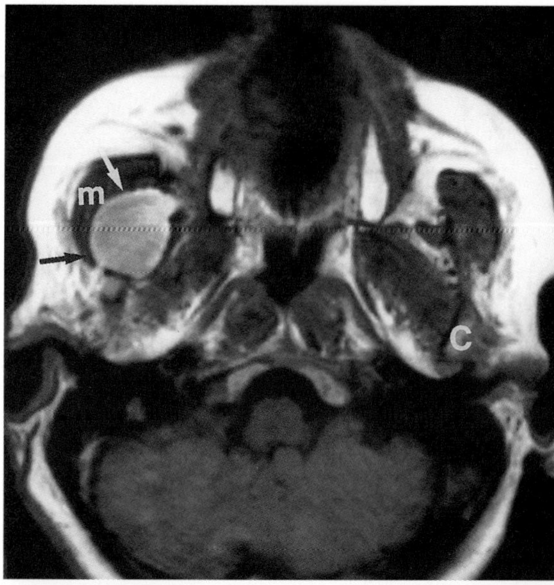

a

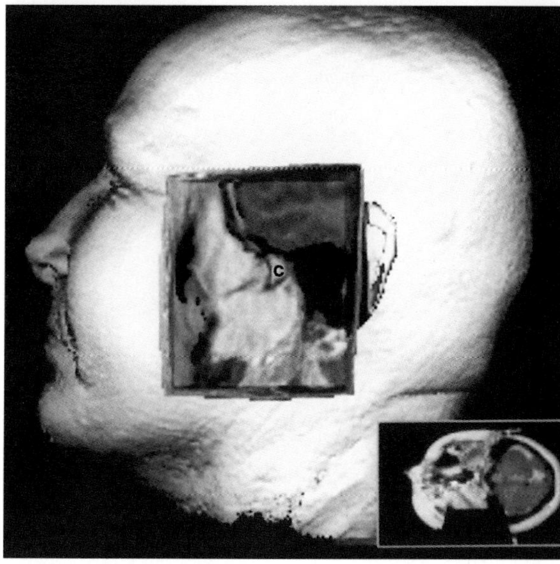

b

Condylar Hyperplasia

Hyperplasia of the condylar process is unilateral in most cases. A special form of hyperplasia is *unilateral hemihypertrophy* of the facial skeleton. Various disease groups should be considered in the differential diagnosis of these enlargements.

Expansion of the Mandibular Condyle and Articular Structures

Paget disease of bone (osteitis deformans) in adults also leads to expansion of the mandibular condyle. *Acromegaly* is associated with deformity and enlargement of the mandible. *Recklinghausen disease* (Fig. 14.**12**) is frequently associated with hypoplasia of the coronoid process and elongation of the condylar process.

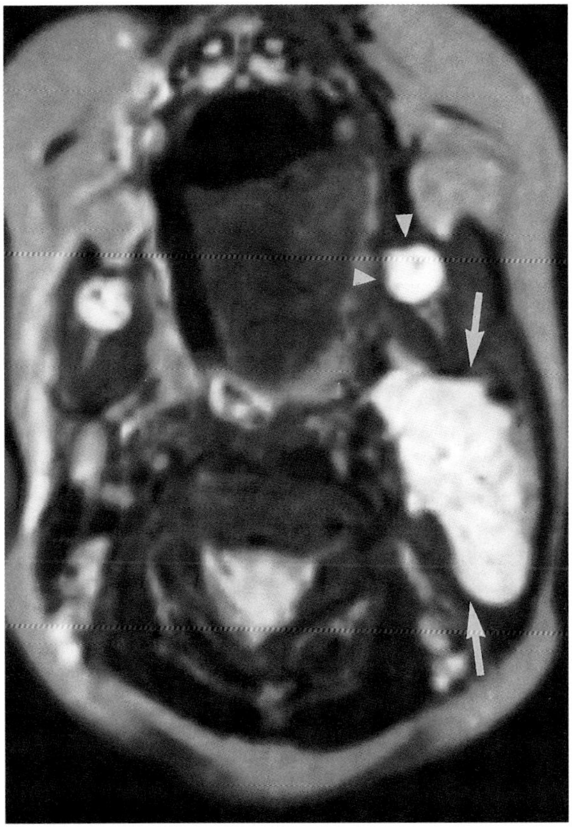

a

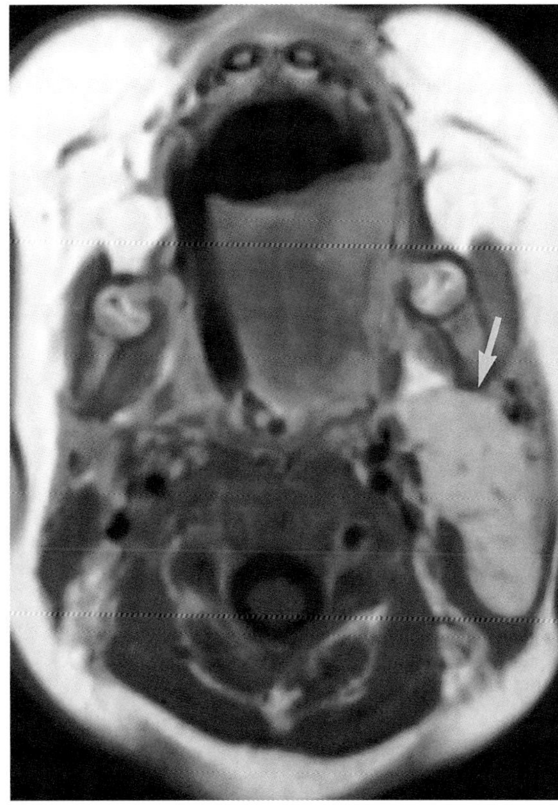

b

Figs. 11.**22 a, b** **Lymphangioma involving the left parotid gland and posterior portions of the masseter muscle.** Comparison of T1- and T2-weighted SE sequences.
(**a**) Axial T2-weighted SE sequence (TR/TE = 2500/90 ms) shows a huge, irregular, septated mass of the parotid gland (arrows) with typical hypointense internal structures. The image also documents the hyperintense epiphyseal plate (arrowheads) of the mandibular ramus in this infant patient.
(**b**) In the comparative T1-weighted SE sequence, the mass (arrow) appears hyperintense to the muscles. The age of the patient and the signal intensity of the mass are consistent with lymphangioma.

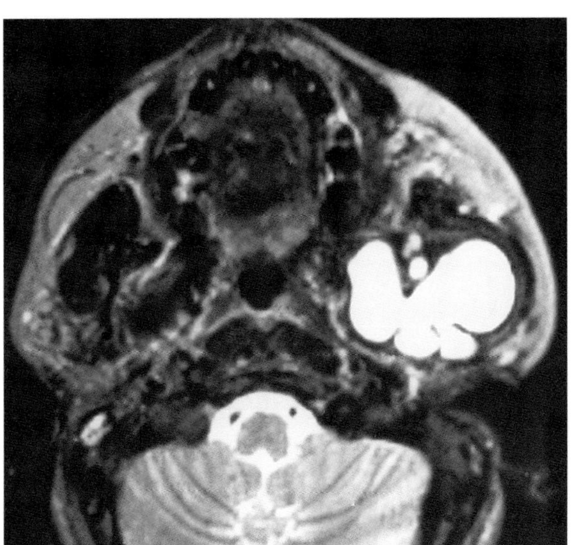

Fig. 11.**23** **Ameloblastoma.** Axial T2-weighted sequence (TR/TE = 3000/90 ms) shows a hyperintense septic mass with well-defined margins and a honeycomb structure in the left mandibular ramus. The morphology is characteristic of ameloblastoma.

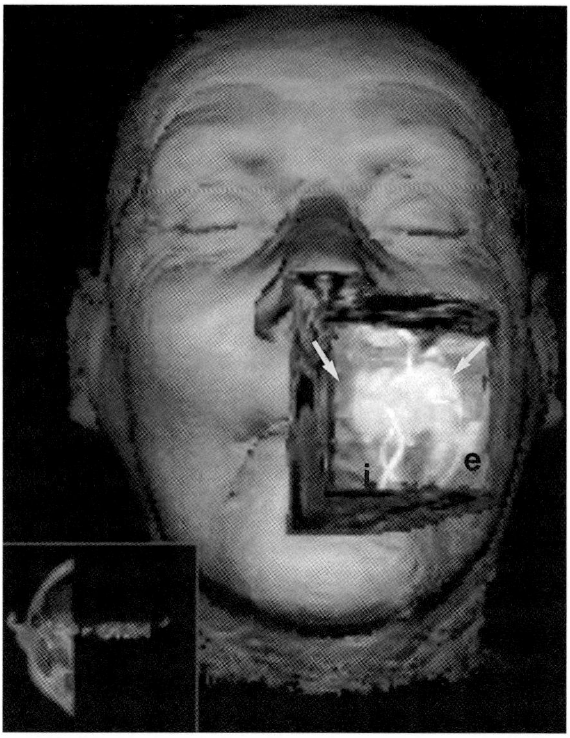

Fig. 11.**24** **Pindborg tumor.** Gd-enhanced 3-D MP-RAGE sequence with frontal cutout shows an intensely enhancing nodular mass with smooth margins (arrows) measuring 5 × 3 × 6 cm in the left parapharyngeal space.
C Mandibular condyle
e External carotid artery
i Internal carotid artery

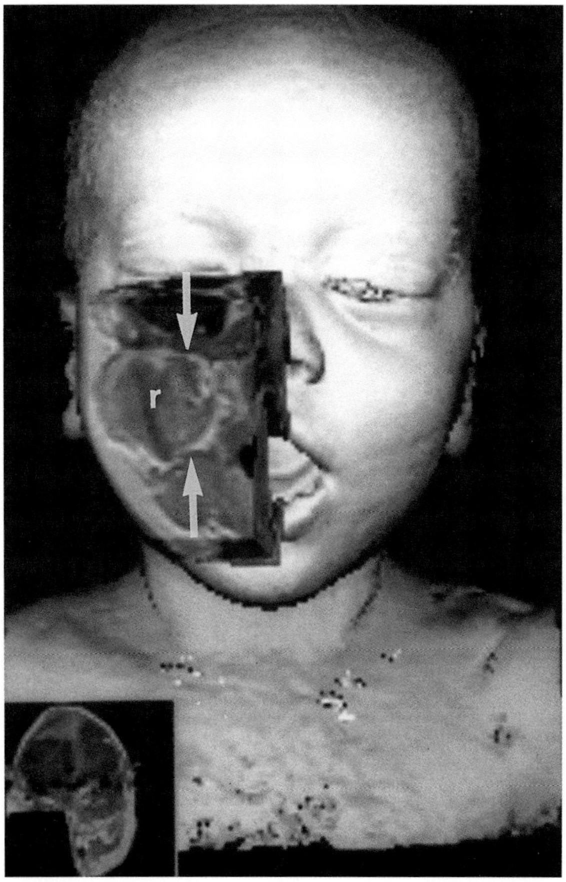

a

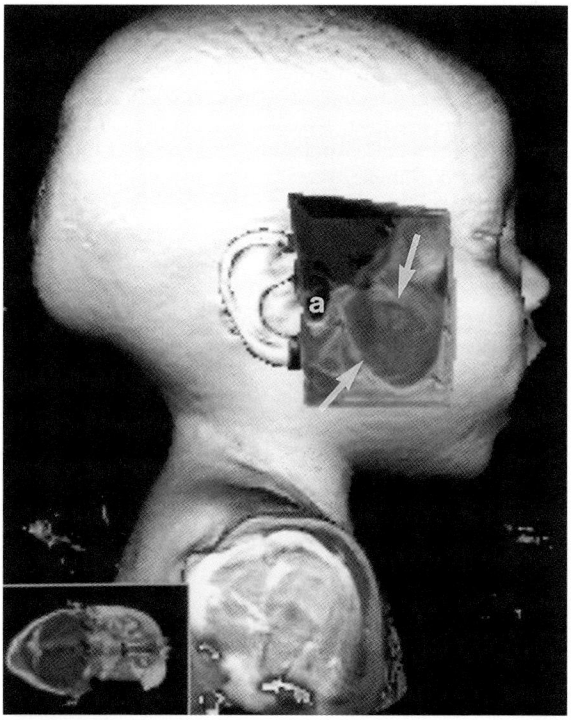

b

Figs. 11.**25**

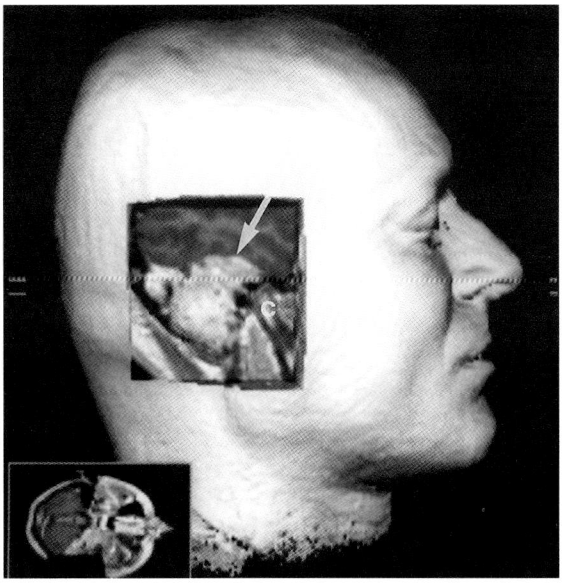

Fig. 11.**26** **Mucoepidermoid carcinoma.** Gd-enhanced 3-D MP-RAGE reconstruction with sagittal cutout shows a destructive tumor (arrow) infiltrating the petrous bone and middle skull base with extension toward the temporal lobe. The tumor has invaded the retrocondylar space.
C Condylar process of mandible

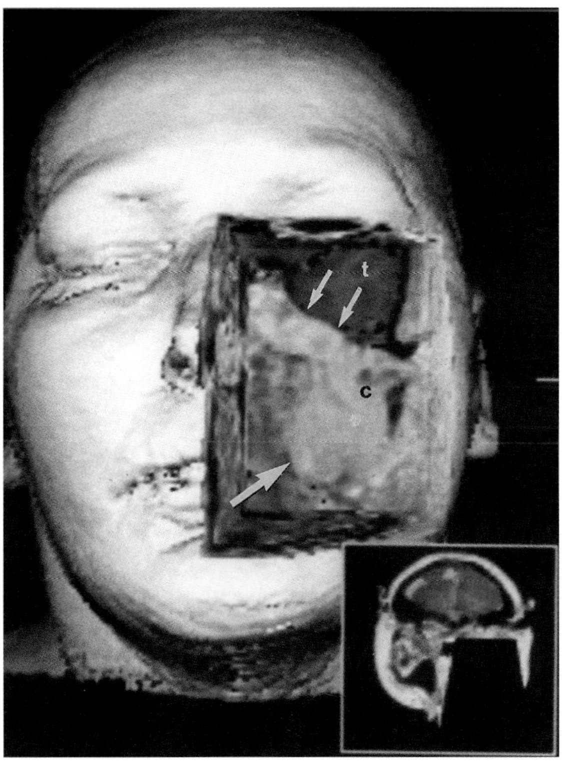

Fig. 11.**27** **Leiomyosarcoma.** Coronal Gd-enhanced 3-D MP-RAGE reconstruction with frontal cutout shows an enhancing, infiltrative 7 x 6 x 5-cm mass (arrows) filling the left infratemporal fossa and extending downward into the parapharyngeal space. There is obvious involvement of the petrous bone, retromaxillary space, and parotid compartment, and tumor has encased the mandibular condyle. Note the increased separation of the mandibular condyle from the glenoid fossa.
c Mandibular condyle
t Temporal lobe

◁ Figs. 11.**25 a, b** **Neuroblastoma.** MP-RAGE sequences show a diffusely spreading neuroblastoma infiltrating the orbit, zygoma, and right mandibular ramus and condylar process. The mandible is expanded and shows loss of signal from the cancellous bone.
(**a**) 3-D reconstruction with frontolateral cutout.
r Mandibular ramus
(**b**) 3-D reconstruction with sagittal cutout.
a External acoustic meatus

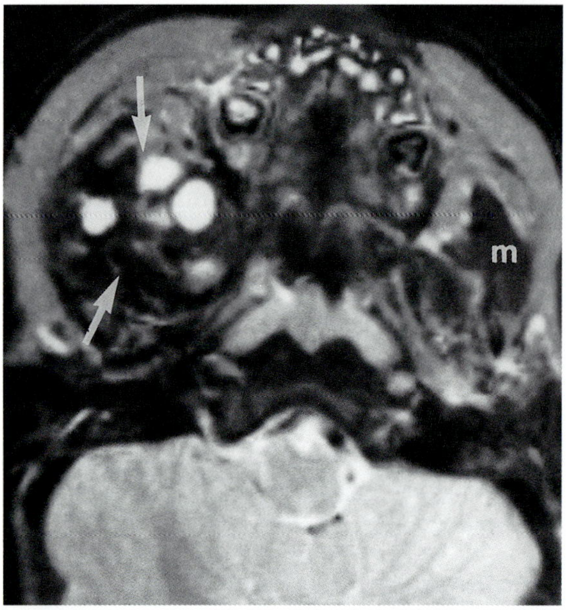

a

Figs. 11.**28 a–c** **Teratoma of the masticator space.** MR sequences demonstrate a multicystic, nonhomogeneous mass (arrows) in the right half of the face. Tumor tissue has invaded the retromaxillary space and completely fills the infratemporal fossa.
(**a**) Axial T2-weighted sequence (TR/TE = 3000/90 ms).
m Masseter muscle
(**b**) Axial Gd-enhanced T1-weighted sequence (TR/TE = 500/17 ms).
(**c**) Coronal Gd-enhanced T1-weighted sequence (TR/TE = 500/17 ms).

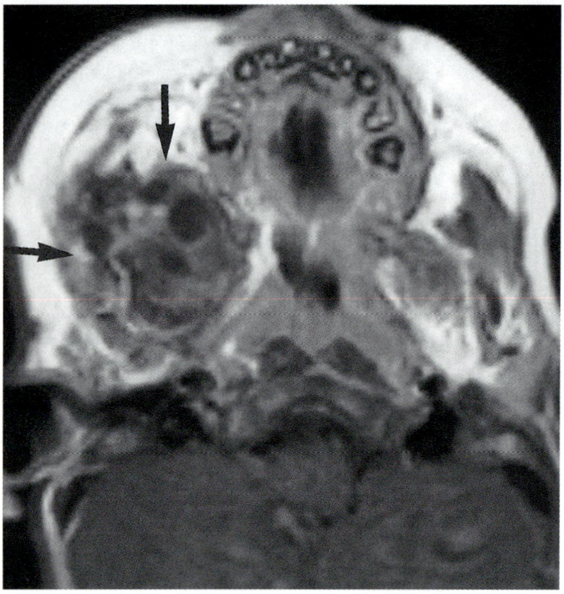

b

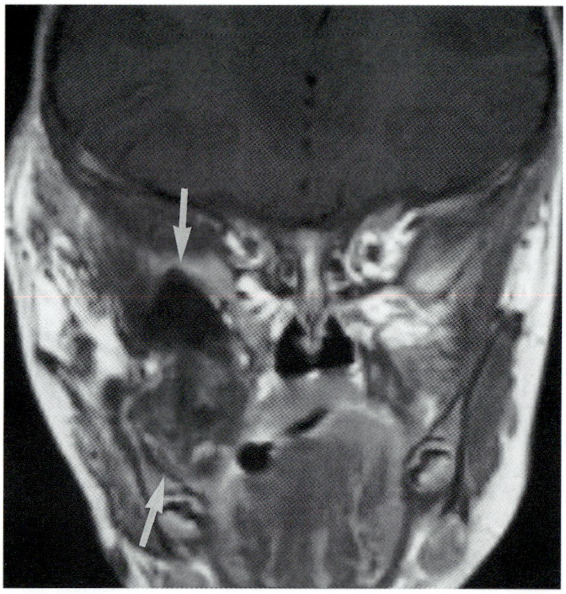

c

Summary and Diagnostic Strategy

CT and especially MRI are mainstays in the differential diagnosis of TMJ pathology. CT evaluations follow basically the same imaging criteria and differential diagnostic guidelines as were presented in Chapter 7. Primary osseous lesions are a definite indication for CT. For example, thin-section CT scans with subsequent 3-D reconstruction are essential for the evaluation of *dysostoses* and *primary craniofacial malformations* and for planning and executing therapeutic procedures. If the investigation of these congenital variations and malformations raises specific questions about the status of the articular disk and ligaments of the TMJ, the CT study should be followed by an optimal MR examination that includes bilateral coils and functional views.

Contrast-enhanced CT is also used for the primary evaluation of *mass lesions* of the TMJ (Figs. 11.**22**–11.**27**), but increasingly it is being superseded by multiplanar MRI. In investigations of *inflammatory lesions* of the TMJ (Figs. 11.**19** and 11.**20**), it is appropriate to follow conventional radiographic studies (Schüller projections, panoramic view) with MRI before and after the administration of a paramagnetic contrast

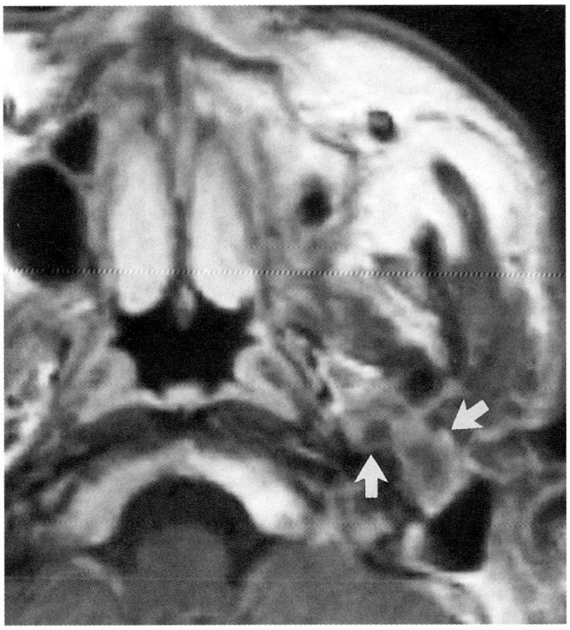

Fig. 11.**29** **Recurrent carcinoma of the parotid gland with invasion of the infratemporal fossa, parapharyngeal space, and parotid gland region.** Axial Gd-enhanced T1-weighted sequence (TR/TE = 500/17 ms) shows two peripherally enhancing lesions in the infratemporal fossa (arrows). The large defect in the left mastoid is from previous resective surgery.

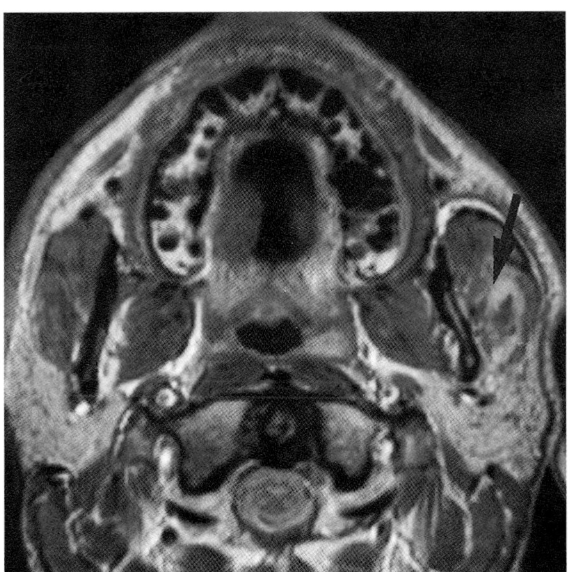

a

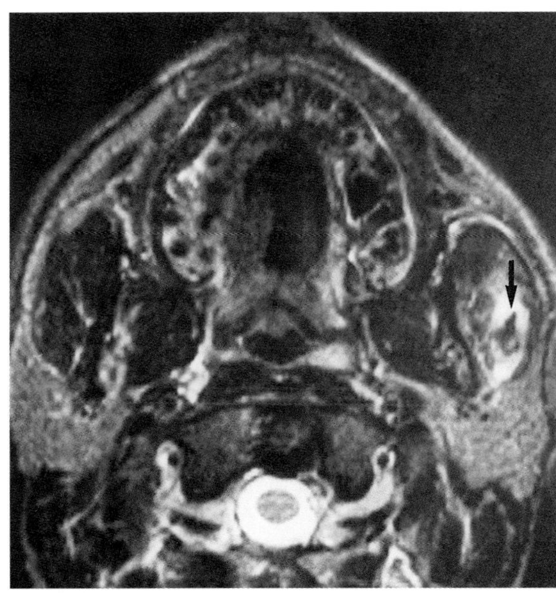

b

Figs. 11.**30 a, b** **Foreign-body reaction with grade 2 trismus following a fracture of the left auditory canal.** Evaluation for possible scarring of the left masseter muscle revealed a glass sliver (hypointense) with an associated foreign-body reaction (arrow). The T2-weighted image also demonstrates inflammatory muscle edema with fluid.

(**a**) Axial proton-density sequence (TR/TE = 3000/22 ms).
(**b**) Axial T2-weighted sequence (TR/TE = 3000/90 ms).

medium. The same strategy applies to the investigation of *degenerative processes* ranging from disk displacements to the diagnosis of preosteoarthritic changes, osteoarthritis, and ankylosis.

References

1 Minomi, M., A. Yamamoto et al.: Ameloblastoma in the maxillomandibular region: MR Imaging. Radiology 184 (1992) 389–393
2 Nokes, S. R., C. E. Spritzer, J. B. Vogler, E. Dolan et al.: Assessment of the temporomandibular joint meniscus perforation with MR Imaging. Radiology 169 (1988) 99–103
3 Schellhas, K. P., Ch. Wilkes, K. B. Heithoff et al.: Temporomandibular joint: diagnosis of internal derangements using magnetic resonance imaging. Minn Med. 69 (1986) 516–520
4 Schellhas, K. P., Ch. Wilkes: Temporomandibular joint inflammation: comparison of MR fast scanning with T1- and T2-weighted imaging techniques. AJR 153 (1989) 93–97
5 Vogl, Th. J., D. Eberhard, J. Randzio et al.: MR-Diagnostik des „Internal derangement" des Temporomandibulargelenks. Radiologe 31 (1991) 537–544
6 Vogl, Th. J., D. Eberhard: MR des Temporomandibulargelenks. Thieme, Stuttgart 1993
7 Wilkes, Ch.: Internal derangements of the temporomandibular joint: pathologic variations. Arch Otolaryngol. 115 (1989) 469–473

12 Oral Cavity, Oropharynx, and Oral Floor

The diagnosis and differential diagnosis of lesions of the oral cavity, oropharynx, and oral floor are basically limited to determining the topography of a lesion that in many cases has already been detected clinically. As a rule, imaging procedures must address the clinical questions of the deep tissue extent of the lesion and what vital neurovascular and other soft-tissue structures it involves. Following an initial ultrasound examination, which is done mainly to assess lymph-node status, the mainstays of modern diagnostic imaging are computed tomography (CT) (especially with spiral technique) and magnetic resonance imaging (MRI). While it is true that the clinical features of a lesion can significantly advance the differential diagnosis in many patients, imaging studies provide information that is crucial for analyzing key differential diagnostic criteria and identifying the lesion as accurately as possible so that appropriate treatment can be provided.

Normal Anatomy

The *oral cavity* extends from the lips and oral fissure (rima oris) to the oropharyngeal isthmus. It is bounded anteriorly and laterally by the lips and cheeks. The roof of the oral cavity consists of the hard and soft palate, and its floor is formed by the muscular oral floor and the structures it supports.

The tongue occupies almost all of the oral cavity when the mouth is closed, its upper surface lying against the palate. The tongue consists of a tip, body, and root (tongue base). The foramen cecum and vallate papillae form the boundary between the body of the tongue and its root. The valleculae separate the tongue base from the epiglottis. The musculature of the tongue consists of intrinsic muscles as well as extrinsic muscles that are inserted into the tongue—the genioglossi, hypoglossi, palatoglossi, and styloglossi. Raising the tip of the tongue from the oral floor exposes the sublingual fold on each side, each fold bearing a sublingual papilla with the opening of the excretory ducts of the sublingual and submandibular glands (Wharton duct). The musculature of the oral floor is composed of the genioglossus, geniohyoid, and mylohyoid muscles. The hyoid bone is supported by muscles that insert on the mandible and the inferior surface of the temporal bone: the geniohyoid, digastric, and stylohyoid muscles.

The *oropharynx* extends from the uvula to the margin of the epiglottis and communicates with the oral cavity via the oropharyngeal isthmus. Within the oropharynx, the palatine tonsils are situated between the faucial pillars. The anterior and posterior pillars converge superiorly at a sharp angle to form the supratonsillar fossa. Portions of the tongue base and valleculae belong to the oropharynx.

The principal *superficial structures* are the paired palatine tonsils. They are surrounded by a thin outpouching of the pharyngobasilar fascia, which appears hypointense on MRI. The tonsils are approximately isointense to muscle tissue on T1-weighted images and are hyperintense on T2-weighted images.

Arterial and venous vessels appear hypointense due to the vascular flow-void effect. Branches of the lingual artery can always be identified in the body of the tongue. Marrow-containing bone structures such as the mandible and hard palate appear as hyperintense zones surrounded by hypointense cortical bone.

From the standpoint of differential diagnosis, it is important to differentiate the oral cavity from the oropharynx due to the distinctive ways in which lesions of these two regions may spread. The oral cavity is anterior to the oropharynx and is separated from it by a ring of diverse structures that include the soft palate, vallate papillae, and anterior pillars.

The mylohyoid muscle separates the sublingual space from the submandibular space, except along its posterior margin, where the spaces communicate.

The *mandible*, the only cranial bone that is freely mobile, develops as a paired set of membrane bones lateral to the Meckel cartilage. Each hemimandible initially has a syndesmotic attachment to the mental symphysis, which undergoes synostosis during the 1st year of life. As the mandibular arch fuses, it differentiates into a *body* (horizontal ramus) and a *ramus* (vertical ramus).

Accurate differential diagnosis and preoperative planning require an analysis of the various spaces in the region of the oral cavity, oropharynx, and oral floor. The principal spaces within the oral cavity are the mucosal area, the sublingual space, and the submandibular space.

The *mucosal area* lines the entire oral cavity, oral floor, and oropharynx. The mucosal area within the oral cavity is only a few millimeters deep. Neither CT nor MRI can define a boundary between the mucosal area and adjacent oropharyngeal structures.

The *sublingual space* is located superomedial to the mylohyoid muscle and, like the mucosal area, lacks a true fascial boundary. Because there is no fascia separating the posterior sublingual space and the submandibular space, tumors can easily spread from one space to the other.

The *submandibular space* is located inferolateral to the mylohyoid muscle and superior to the hyoid bone. There is no fascial barrier between the posterior submandibular space and the inferior parapharyngeal space, so tumors of one space can easily invade the other.

Clinical Signs and Symptoms

Patients usually present clinically with oropharyngeal pain and swelling or a disturbance of taste sensation. Burning throat pain with an acute onset that radiates to the ear and is later associated with difficult swallowing and fever suggests an *inflammatory cause* such as tonsillitis, infectious mononucleosis, or pharyngitis. Severe unilateral complaints are more consistent with a *peritonsillar abscess* or *tumor*. Pain accompanied by blood in the saliva may signify a *malignancy* or may result from *trauma* or *corrosive ingestion* in patients with a corresponding history.

Most inflammatory lesions can be diagnosed clinically and do not require radiologic evaluation.

Imaging Evaluation and Differential Diagnosis

Diagnostic imaging of the oral cavity and oropharynx should always be preceded by thorough *inspection* and *palpation* to detect any mucosal irregularities and direct the use of imaging procedures. The *history* is also essential and should include specific questions about symptoms such as swallowing difficulties, globus sensation, breath odor, and the characteristics and radiation of pain.

Imaging procedures should always be deferred until the history has been taken and the patient has been examined by inspection and palpation. The following modalities are available for imaging the oral cavity and oropharynx:

- Conventional radiographs including function studies.
- Ultrasonography (percutaneous and intraoral).
- CT.
- MRI.
- Digital subtraction angiography (DSA).
- Radionuclide imaging.

Conventional Radiography

Conventional radiographs have a minor role in the oral cavity and oropharynx except in the diagnosis of radiopaque salivary stones and dental diseases or to verify an elongated styloid process.

Ultrasound

The ultrasound examination generally precedes CT and MRI. B-mode imaging is definitely superior to A-scans in examinations of the oral cavity, tongue, and oropharynx. Ultrasound is most useful for evaluating the deep tissue extent and midline transgression of tongue and oral-floor tumors and detecting areas of liquefaction due to inflammatory processes. For percutaneous imaging, a coupling gel is applied to the skin, and the region of interest is scanned with a 5-MHz sector probe (or a 7.5-MHz linear probe for small volumes) using the hyoid bone and bony mandible as landmarks. "Fingertip probes" are available for intraoral scanning.

Computed Tomography (CT)

The role of CT has been declining in recent years compared with that of MRI. The reasons for this include the poor soft-tissue contrast of CT, its low specificity in tissue characterization, and the limitation of direct CT scans to the axial plane. CT is still the modality of choice, however, for confirming or excluding osseous involvement by tumors of the oropharynx, oral cavity, and oral floor.

Today MRI has become the primary imaging modality for lesions of the oral cavity, oral floor, and oropharynx, provided there are no contraindications to the study. CT is the primary modality of choice only in patients with a suspected inflammatory process such as a peritonsillar abscess or submandibular abscess (Fig. 12.**3**).

Digital Subtraction Angiography (DSA)

DSA, which is far superior to conventional angiography (less radiation exposure, shorter examination time), is only occasionally indicated for the evaluation of a suspected hypervascular tumor (e.g., hemangioma). At present, contrast-enhanced MRI combined with magnetic resonance angiography (MRA) has replaced diagnostic DSA in virtually all applications.

Radionuclide Imaging

The only current application for radionuclide scanning in the oral region is for the evaluation of a suspected lingual goiter. In this study the tongue base and neck are scanned 10 minutes after the intravenous injection of 500 μCi of ^{99m}Tc pertechnetate or 24 hours after the oral administration of 10 to 50 μCi of ^{131}I to document radiotracer uptake and check for the presence of thyroid tissue at its normal location.

Magnetic Resonance Imaging (MRI)

A neck coil is used for most MR examinations of this region. A head coil can be used on patients with a long, slender neck and will provide a better signal-to-noise ratio than a Helmholtz neck coil.

Although T2-weighted imaging of the tongue is occasionally hampered by motion artifacts, it should still be used in cooperative patients because of its high sensitivity to pathologic changes. T2-weighted turbo spin-echo (TSE) sequences can reduce the problem of motion artifacts by shortening the acquisition time. T1-weighted sequences after the administration of gadolinium(Gd)-DTPA show a moderate to intense increase in signal intensity. For tumors in the body of the tongue, Gd-enhanced T2-weighted imaging is superior to unenhanced imaging for accurately defining the depth of invasion. Necrotic areas and tumor vascularization are particularly well demonstrated on Gd-enhanced images. T2-weighted sequences are necessary in some cases for the differential diagnosis of cystic and inflammatory processes.

An axial T2-weighted sequence is excellent for initial screening, as it is the most sensitive sequence for detecting lesions of the oral cavity, oropharynx, and oral floor. The T1-weighted spin-echo (SE) sequence is also recommended for the accurate delineation of lesions. For example, the low signal intensity of an oral floor lesion in the T1-weighted sequence clearly distinguishes it from surrounding structures, which have a high primary signal intensity because of their fat content.

Multiplanar images are essential for the accurate assessment of tumor invasion. With a standard axial series, the radiologist can analyze the muscle groups of the oral floor and evaluate important structures such as the submandibular and sublingual glands. Axial views are effectively supplemented by coronal images, which can evaluate for invasion of the intrinsic and extrinsic muscles and involvement of the submandibular space. Coronal images are also useful for defining and evaluating all the cervical lymph-node groups.

Since tumors and cervical lymph nodes are often seen more clearly on unenhanced sequences, coronal imaging should always be performed without contrast medium. Coronal images can yield additional information on lesions of the tonsillar fossa and processes distant from the midline. Combined axial and sagittal imaging is recommended for tumors that involve the body and base of the tongue with extension to the preepiglottic space. Gd-enhanced images should be obtained routinely, as they can critically influence the differential diagnosis owing to the specific enhancement characteristics of different lesions.

Imaging Findings

Congenital Variations and Malformations

Most congenital variations and malformations involving the oral cavity, oral floor, and oropharynx are readily detected clinically, but they can be difficult to assign to a specific group or syndrome, particularly since many of these conditions are quite rare. It is not unusual for these malformations to coexist with anomalies in other body regions.

The principal types of malformation include *cleft anomalies* (Fig. 12.**1**), *hyperplasias*, *hypoplasias*, and *heterotopias* (Table 12.**2**). Other congenital lesions that may involve the oropharynx and oral cavity are *congenital hemangiomas*, *lymphangiomas*, and *cystic hygromas*.

Tumors

Whenever CT or MRI is performed to evaluate a mass lesion, these principal questions should be addressed:

- How deeply does the mass extend into adjacent tissues?
- What neurovascular structures are involved?

Morphologic changes in the oral cavity, oral floor, and oropharynx usually lead quickly to functional impairment (ingestion, mastication, respiration, speech). Inflammatory soft-tissue swelling is often difficult to distinguish clinically from a neoplasm, since inflammation and neoplasia may coexist. Most tumors of this region are malignant (Fig. 12.**10**). The more common tumors of the oral cavity, oral floor, and oropharynx are listed in Table 12.**3**.

Oral Cavity and Body of the Tongue

Squamous cell carcinoma of the body of the tongue that is diagnosed in an advanced stage (T2 or higher) tends to be particularly invasive and destructive and often undergoes central necrosis. On the other hand,

T1 tumors involving the mucosa of the tongue and oral floor are not consistently detected by MRI. Even extensive tumors may cause little mass effect as the original musculature undergoes replacement by tumor tissue.

While carcinomas tend to infiltrate soft-tissue structures at an early stage, considerable time passes before they cause detectable erosion of the bony mandible and hyoid bone. T1- and T2-weighted sequences are advantageous for detecting tumor erosion of cortical and cancellous bone in the mandible.

These tumors usually appear hypointense to the tongue muscles on *T1-weighted images*. If the tumor has invaded the intrinsic tongue muscles, noncontrast MRI is best for demonstrating the internal architectural destruction that results (Fig. 12.**12a**).

The tumor may appear hyperintense to the muscles on *T2-weighted images*, depending on its proton content.

Vallecula and Tongue Base

Carcinoma of the vallecula and tongue base tends to invade the tongue base first and must reach a fairly advanced stage (T3) before spreading to the intrinsic tongue muscles, epiglottis (Fig. 12.**13**), and supraglottic portions of the larynx. Initially the tumors grow by expansion and displace surrounding structures, but more advanced lesions become locally invasive. An individually adjustable neck coil should be used for all MR examinations.

T1-weighted sequences show the best contrast between the tumor and its surroundings. T2-weighted sequences are also advantageous for differentiating tumor from the lymphatic tissue of the tongue base. In typical cases, lymphatic tissue is similar to tumor tissue in its T1 characteristics but shows a markedly prolonged T2.

Tumor and lymphatic hyperplasia enhance markedly after the intravenous administration of Gd-DTPA. Lymphatic hyperplasia is, however, distinguished by its relatively homogeneous internal structure with markedly enhancing linear septa and noninfiltrating margins.

Classification of Tumors of the Oropharynx, Oral Cavity, and Oral Floor

The classification of malignant tumors of the oropharynx, oral cavity, and oral floor follows the *TNM system* of the *UICC*, which is based on the size of the tumor and the extent of its spread. Tumor size is staged as follows:

- *Stage T1* tumors are smaller than 2 cm in their greatest diameter and are confined to their site of origin.
- *Stage T2* tumors are between 2 cm and 4 cm in diameter.
- *Stage T3* tumors are larger than 4 cm in diameter but have not invaded adjacent structures.
- *Stage T4* signifies the invasion of adjacent structures.

Squamous cell carcinoma is the most common of all mass lesions of the oropharynx, oral cavity, and oral floor (Figs. 12.**11** and 12.**14**).

Approximately 80% of *oropharyngeal carcinomas* are tonsillar. Smaller numbers arise from the palate (approximately 15%) and posterior pharyngeal wall (approximately 4%). The most common primary site for tonsillar cancers is the anterior pole of the tonsils, followed by the posterior pole and adjacent posterior pharyngeal wall. These tumors tend to spread upward into the soft palate, downward into the lateral pharyngeal wall and tongue base, and laterally into the parapharyngeal space, mandible, and vascular sheath.

Besides invading the parapharyngeal space, small mucosal tumors will infiltrate the body of the tongue in more than 70% of cases. With an extensive lesion, 40% of cases will show invasion of the longus colli muscle with indentation of the pharyngeal wall. These tumors metastasize early to regional lymph nodes, and distant metastasis (to lung, skeleton, or liver) is not uncommon (Tables 12.**4** and 12.**5**).

Inflammatory Lesions

Most inflammatory lesions of this region (cheilitis, gingivostomatitis, aphthae, pharyngitis, tonsillitis, etc.) are diagnosed and treated clinically.

Diagnostic imaging is indicated only in more advanced stages of inflammatory disease. Especially in patients with *peritonsillar* and *oral floor abscesses*, MRI or CT can yield valuable information and can accurately document the extent of the lesion. Typically, abscess formation occurs in the loose tongue muscles or connective-tissue spaces of the oral floor as a result of minor foreign-body injuries (fish bones, bone fragments) to the sublingual gland, lingual tonsil, or dental tissues.

Infections of the submandibular or sublingual space are common and can easily spread to an adjacent space. Most infections of the submandibular space arise from the dental tissues, oral floor, or from buccal infections that drain into the submandibular lymph nodes. Infections that originate from the submandibular gland are usually caused by a stone lodged in the excretory duct. Cellulitis and abscesses can easily spread posteriorly into the prestyloid compartment of the parapharyngeal space. Odontogenic infections most commonly arise from the roots of the second or third molar next to the attachment of the mylohyoid muscle and can lead to direct involvement of the submandibular space. Root infections anterior

Table 12.1 Compartments of the oral cavity and oropharynx—contents and potential lesions

Compartment	Contents	Lesions
Mucosal area	➤ Mucosa ➤ Squamous epithelium ➤ Minor salivary gland remnants (especially on inner surface of lip, buccal mucosa, and palate)	Congenital: ➤ Hemangioma, lymphangioma ➤ Cystic hygroma ➤ Lingual thyroid tissue Malignant tumors: ➤ Squamous cell carcinoma ➤ Minor salivary gland malignancies Benign tumors: ➤ Benign mixed tumors of minor salivary glands Inflammatory: ➤ Abscess (Fig. 12.**3**) ➤ Cellulitis, Ludwig angina ➤ Odontogenic infection
Sublingual space	➤ Hyoglossus muscle ➤ Lingual nerve ➤ Cranial nerves IX–XII ➤ Lingual artery and vein ➤ Sublingual gland ➤ Submandibular gland (deep portion) ➤ Excretory duct of submandibular gland (Wharton duct)	Pseudotumor: ➤ Hypoglossal nerve motor atrophy Congenital: ➤ Hemangioma, lymphangioma ➤ Cystic hygroma ➤ Epidermoid/dermoid ➤ Lingual thyroid tissue Inflammatory: ➤ Ludwig angina/cellulitis ➤ Abscess ➤ Dilated excretory duct of submandibular gland ➤ Ranula (simple or diving) (Fig. 12.**5**) Benign tumors: ➤ Benign mixed tumors of minor salivary glands Malignant tumors: ➤ Squamous cell carcinoma (Figs. 12.**11**, 12.**12**) ➤ Adenoid cystic carcinoma, mucoepidermoid carcinoma, acinar cell carcinoma of sublingual gland
Submandibular space	➤ Anterior belly of digastric muscle ➤ Submandibular gland (superficial portion) ➤ Submandibular lymph nodes ➤ Submental lymph nodes ➤ Facial artery and vein ➤ Fat ➤ Hypoglossal nerve	Pseudotumor: ➤ Motor atrophy due to cranial nerve damage (mylohyoid muscle, anterior belly of digastric) Congenital: ➤ Branchial cleft cyst ➤ Thyroglossal duct cyst ➤ Cystic hygroma/ lymphangioma ➤ Hemangioma Inflammatory: ➤ Ludwig angina secondary to abscess or cellulitis ➤ Reactive adenopathy ➤ Submandibular gland inflammation ➤ Diving ranula (Fig. 12.**5**) Benign tumors: ➤ Lipoma ➤ Epidermoid/dermoid ➤ Benign tumors of submandibular gland ➤ Salivary calculus (Fig. 12.**17**) Malignant tumors: ➤ Lymph-node metastasis ➤ Adenoid cystic carcinoma, mucoepidermoid carcinoma, acinar cell carcinoma of submandibular gland ➤ Direct invasion by squamous cell carcinoma (Fig. 12.**11**)

Table 12.**1** Continuation

Compartment	Contents	Lesions
Mandible		Fractures: ➤ Simple linear fracture ➤ Fracture involving the alveolar ridge ➤ Comminuted fracture ➤ Complicated fracture involving the alveolar artery or nerve ➤ Pathologic fracture Infections: ➤ Osteomyelitis (Figs. 12.**19 a–c**, 12.**21**) Benign tumors: ➤ Ameloblastoma (Fig. 12.**18**) ➤ Various other benign odontogenic tumors ➤ Bone cyst ➤ Odontogenic cyst ➤ Nonodontogenic cyst Malignant tumors: ➤ Secondary invasion by carcinoma ➤ Sarcoma ➤ Myeloma

Table 12.**2** Congenital variations and malformations of the oral cavity, oral floor, and oropharynx

Cleft anomalies (dysraphias):
- Cleft upper lip (cheiloschisis) (Fig. 12.**1**)
- Alveolar cleft (gnathoschisis)
- Cleft palate (palatoschisis)
- Combinations of the above
- Bifid uvula
- Oblique facial cleft (meloschisis)
- Transverse facial cleft or buccal cleft

Hypoplasias and hyperplasias:
- Of the lips, tongue, maxilla, and mandible

Heterotopias:
- Goiter of tongue or tongue base
- Glandular cheilitis
- Fordyce disease (ectopic sebaceous glands)
- Dermoid cyst

Miscellaneous anomalies:
- Palatolingual atresia
- Ankyloglossia
- Palatal fistulae
- Cysts (nasopalatine, oronasal, nasoalveolar)
- Median and lateral neck cysts (Figs. 14.**2**, 14.**3**)

Table 12.3 Common tumors of the oral cavity, oral floor, and oropharynx

Benign tumors:
- Papilloma
- Keratocanthoma
- Pleomorphic adenoma
- Fibroma
- Lipoma
- Histiocytoma
- Rhabdomyoma
- Leiomyoma
- Myxoma
- Hemangioma and lymphangioma (Fig. 12.**6**)
- Neuroma
- Neurofibroma
- Granular cell tumor
- Chondroma
- Osteoma
- Giant cell tumor (osteoclastoma)
- Myoblastic myoma (Abrikossoff tumor)

Malignant tumors:
- Squamous cell carcinoma (Figs. 12.**11** – 12.**13**)
- Anaplastic carcinoma (lymphoepithelial tumor, Schmincke tumor)
- Adenoid cystic carcinoma
- Malignant lymphoma
- Melanoma
- Adenocarcinoma
- Plasmacytoma (extramedullary)
- Malignant chordoma
- Mucoepidermoid tumors
- Sarcoma
- Ewing sarcoma

Pseudotumors:
- Ossifying fibroma
- Lingual goiter (ectopic tissue)
- Fibrous dysplasia
- Cysts (dermoid and epidermoid cyst [Fig. 12.**22**], dentogenic cyst, Tornwaldt cyst, salivary gland cyst)
- Hamartoma
- Giant cell granuloma
- Brown tumor (hyperparathyroidism)
- Xanthogranuloma
- Plasma cell granuloma
- Epulis
- Foreign body granuloma
- Lethal midline granuloma
- Exostosis
- Pyogenic granuloma
- Gouty tophus
- Sarcoidosis
- Wegener granulomatosis (Fig. 13.**14**)
- Torus palatinus
- Paget disease

Table 12.4 Disease groups associated with mass lesions of the mandible

Primary neoplastic:
- Benign
- Malignant

Congenital:
- Follicular cyst
- Primordial cyst, etc.

Inflammatory:
- Osteomyelitis
- Periodontitis

Table 12.5 Benign and malignant tumors of the mandibular region

Benign tumors:
- Arising from the bony mandible:
  - —Osteoma
  - —Osteoblastoma
  - —Osteochondroma
  - —Chondroma
  - —Chondroblastoma
  - —Myxoma (Fig. 12.**23**)
- Arising from the dental system:
  - —Odotoma
  - —Ameloblastoma (Fig. 12.**18**)
  - —Adamantinoma
  - —Dentinoma
  - —Odontogenic fibroma
  - —Ameloblastic fibroma (Fig. 12.**22**)
  - —Cementoma (Fig. 12.**20**)
  - —Etc.

Malignant tumors:
- —Sarcoma
- —Secondary: invasion by squamous cell carcinoma (Fig. 12.**16**)

to the second molar tend to spread above the mylohyoid muscle, leading to infection of the sublingual space. Most are streptococcal or staphylococcal infections; mixed infections are also common.

Special note should be taken of a potentially lethal form of acute sublingual space infection known as *Ludwig angina*. Defined as a cellulitis of the oral floor, Ludwig angina most commonly results from a dental infection, trauma, or tooth extraction. By definition, the cellulitis always involves both sublingual glands and spreads rapidly through the suprahyoid soft tissues of the neck, leading to edema with posterior and superior displacement of the tongue. Untreated cases swiftly progress to concomitant involvement of the pre- and poststyloid compartments of the parapharyngeal space, the retropharyngeal space, and occasionally the mediastinum and subphrenic region. Imaging studies reveal expansion of the soft tissues with cellulitic changes permeating the subcutaneous tissue.

Traumatic Lesions

Scalds are common in children who accidentally ingest hot liquids, and adults may sustain *caustic injuries* of the lips, oral cavity, and oropharynx as a result of confusion or attempted suicide. Radiologic evaluation of the esophagus may consist of chest films to exclude esophageal damage (e.g., mediastinal widening due to perforation) and static or dynamic X-ray examinations of the esophagus using a water-soluble contrast medium.

Foreign bodies are generally less common in the oral cavity and oropharynx than in the hypopharynx. In most cases they do not require diagnostic imaging and are easily removed clinically.

Gunshot and stab injuries generally require immediate treatment. Imaging studies may be performed to detect bony injuries and locate projectiles.

Iatrogenic Changes (Fig. 12.**2a**)

This group includes changes in the oropharynx, oral cavity, and oral floor that may be seen in patients who undergo periodic radiologic examinations as part of their follow-up for head and neck cancer. The main indications for imaging in these patients are to investigate complications and exclude recurrent disease. Reconstructive surgery of the head and neck has made substantial progress in recent years. Various flap procedures can be used to repair the soft-tissue defects left by tumor resections, including swinging flaps, free flaps, and interpositional small-bowel transfers with microvascular anastomosis. Even an uncomplicated tissue transfer exhibits diverse morphologic features in the various sectional imaging modalities.

Changes induced by radiotherapy or chemotherapy may also appear on posttherapeutic images and will require a correct morphologic interpretation.

Attention should also be given to posttherapeutic changes following the operative treatment of benign conditions such as congenital anomalies (Fig. 12.**1**) or lesions resulting from a prior tonsillectomy (Fig. 12.**2**).

Staging of Nodal Disease

Because nodal metastases (Table 12.**1**) are commonly found in patients who present with a primary tumor of the head and neck region and imply a reduction of approximately 50% in life expectancy, it is essential that involved lymph nodes be accurately described and staged prior to initial treatment. Som reports that 86% to 90% of all malignant tumors of the nasopharynx have already spread to the lymph nodes by the time of initial diagnosis (Table 6.**1**).

Lymph-node involvement is staged according to TNM system of the UICC:

- *Stage N1* denotes involvement of a single ipsilateral node 3 cm or less in diameter.
- *Stage N2a* denotes involvement of a single ipsilateral node between 3 cm and 6 cm in diameter.
- Stage *N2b* denotes involvement of multiple ipsilateral nodes not more than 6 cm in diameter.
- *Stage N2c* denotes involvement of ipsilateral and contralateral nodes not more than 6 cm in diameter.
- *Stage N3* denotes involvement of one or more nodes larger than 6 cm in diameter.

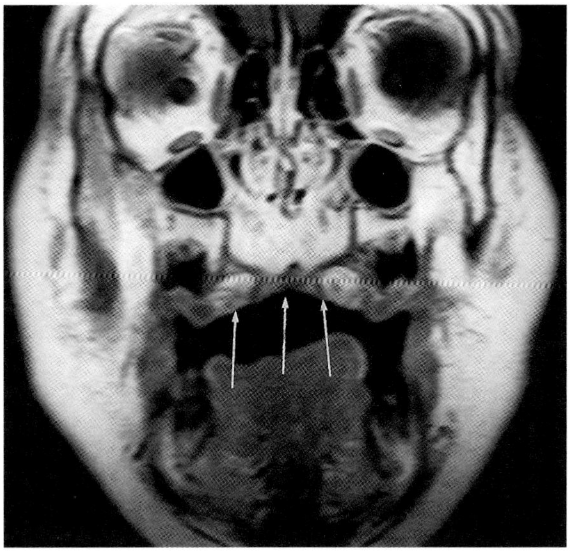

Fig. 12.**1** **Surgically repaired cleft lip and palate.** Coronal Gd-enhanced T1-weighted image (TR/TE = 690/15 ms) demonstrates the surgically repaired hard palate (arrows), which shows typical deformation of the palatal shelf and scar tissue in the area of the repaired palatal cleft.

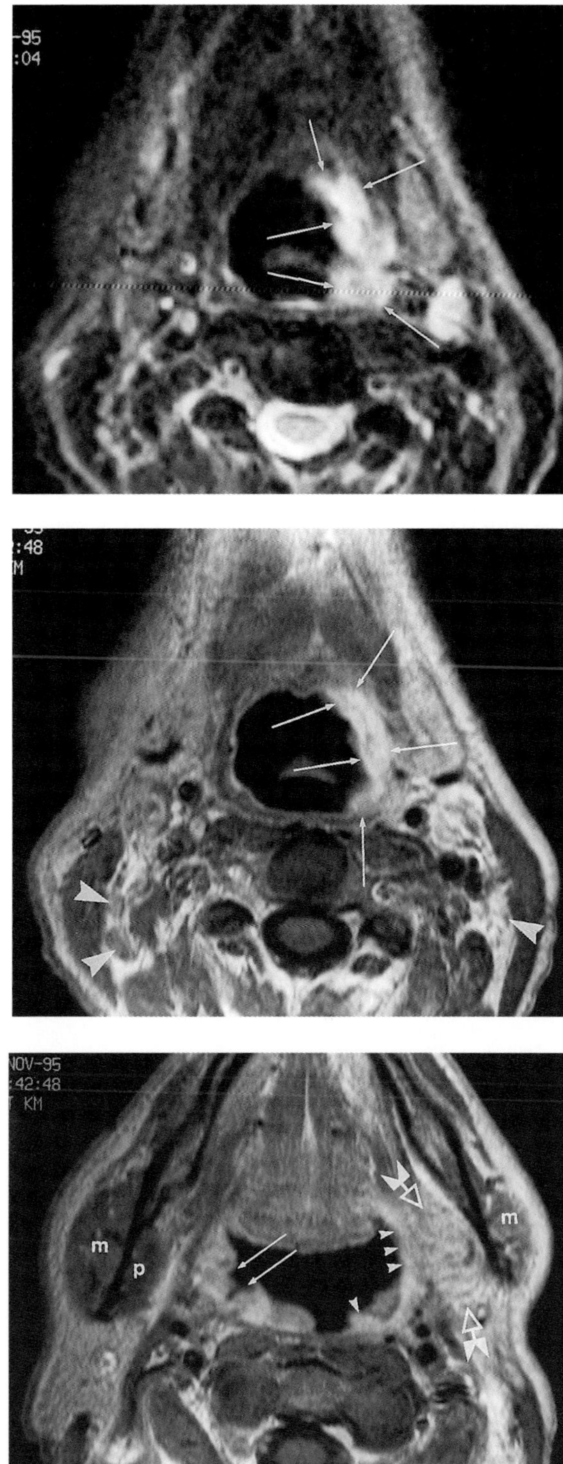

a

b

c

Fig. 12.**2 a–c** **Left-sided pharyngitis in an HIV-positive patient who previously underwent left tonsillectomy.**
(**a**) Axial unenhanced T2-weighted image (TR/TE = 3000/90 ms) shows an area of increased signal intensity in the left pharyngeal wall (arrows) indicating an inflammatory reaction.
(**b**) Gd-enhanced T1-weighted image (TR/TE = 700/15 ms) shows marked enhancement along the left pharyngeal wall consistent with an acute inflammatory reaction (arrows). Multiple lymph nodes of the internal jugular group show reactive enlargement (arrowheads).
(**c**) Gd-enhanced T1-weighted image (TR/TE = 700/15 ms) shows marked ulcerative lesions in the right tonsillar fossa (arrows). The left tonsillar fossa shows post-tonsillectomy inflammatory changes involving the mucosa (arrowheads), pterygomandibular fossa (open arrows), and adjacent soft-tissue structures, with markedly greater enhancement on the left side than on the right.
m Masseter muscle
p Medial pterygoid muscle

Table 12.**6** Incidence of lymph-node metastases in squamous cell carcinoma of the head and neck region (see Figs. 12.**11** and 12.**12**) (after Som PM. Radiology. 1987; 165: 593–600)

Primary tumor	Incidence of lymph node metastasis (%)
Nasopharynx	86–90
Oropharynx	50–71
Oral cavity	30–65
Hypopharynx	50–72
Supraglottic larynx	31–54
Glottic larynx	< 10
Paranasal sinuses	< 10

Affected lymph nodes may be described by groups or levels (Tables 12.**7** and 12.**8**). The level terminology adopted by the New American Joint Committee on Cancer (AJCC) is based on the fact that the extent and level of cervical nodal involvement by metastatic tumor seem to be an important prognostic indicator.

Table 12.**8** Lymph node classification by levels based on the guidelines of the NJCC

Level I nodes:
- Submental nodes
- Submandibular nodes

Level II nodes:
- Upper deep cervical chain nodes

Level III nodes:
- Middle deep cervical chain nodes

Level IV nodes:
- Lower deep cervical chain nodes

Level V nodes:
- Spinal accessory nodes
- Transverse cervical chain nodes

Level VI nodes:
- Pretracheal nodes
- Prelaryngeal nodes
- Paratracheal nodes

Level VII nodes:
- Superior mediastinal nodes

Imaging Criteria and Their Differential Diagnosis

The following questions should be addressed in evaluations of the oropharynx, oral cavity, and oral floor:
- What is the deep tissue extent of the lesion?
- What is the relation of the lesion to neurovascular structures?
- What is the stage of the lesion?
- In the oral cavity: has the tumor invaded the lingual septum, the mandible, the tongue base?
- What is the lymph node status in the submental and submandibular spaces?

An analysis of the deep cervical lymph nodes is also essential.

Table 12.**7** Classification of lymph nodes

Common terms	Alternative terms
Jugulodigastric nodes	Upper group of internal jugular chain
Internal jugular nodal chain	Deep cervical chain
Virchow nodes	Lower group of internal jugular chain
Parotid nodal group	–
Submandibular nodal group	–
Submental nodal group	–
Facial nodal group	–
Transverse cervical nodal chain	Supraclavicular chain
Spinal accessory nodal chain	Posterior triangle chain
Anterior cervical nodal chain	Includes prelaryngeal, pretracheal, and paratracheal nodal groups
Pretracheal nodal group	Delphian nodes
Retropharyngeal nodal group	Lateral group are nodes of Rouviere
Mastoid nodal group	–
Occipital nodal group	–

Liquid Masses or Lesions of the Oropharynx and Oral Cavity

Most liquid masses of the oropharynx and oral cavity originate from the salivary glands. In patients with corresponding clinical symptoms, the differential diagnosis should also include abscesses and metastatic lymph nodes that have undergone necrotic liquefaction. The imaging criteria for differentiating these lesions are described below.

Cystic masses consist primarily of *lesions of embryonic origin* (dermoid and epidermoid cysts [Fig. 12.**4**], medial and lateral neck cysts [Figs. 14.**2** and 14.**4**], colloid cysts), *lymphangiomas* (Figs. 12.**6** and 12.**7**), and *hemangiomas*.

Cystic lesions of the oropharynx, oral cavity, and oral floor tend to enlarge slowly and remain asymptomatic until they reach considerable size. Assigning the cyst to a site of origin and determining its relation to the muscles of the oral floor are essential for sound preoperative planning.

A *colloid cyst* can be identified radiologically by its central position and by its high signal intensity on T1-weighted MR images due to the protein-rich contents of the cyst and the frequent presence of a hemorrhagic component.

A *submandibular cyst* can usually be diagnosed by its location and MRI signal characteristics. It appears as a mass of fluid attenuation on CT scans and as a uniformly hyperintense mass on T2-weighted MR images. It enhances peripherally after the administration of contrast medium (Gd-DTPA). Rarely, a submandibular cyst is difficult to distinguish from a diving ranula (Fig. 12.**5**).

A *ranula* is a postinflammatory retention cyst of the sublingual gland that generally results from stenosis or occlusion of the excretory duct. A *simple ranula* is a cystic mass that is confined strictly to the sublingual space, so it does not transgress the fascial boundaries of the submandibular space. If the cyst ruptures through its capsule into the submandibular space, it is termed a *diving ranula* (Fig. 12.**5**). A ranula at this stage is usually confined to the boundaries of the submandibular space but may spread into the prestyloid compartment of the parapharyngeal space.

A diving ranula typically displays a narrow fluid track extending around the posterior border of the mylohyoid muscle into the sublingual space. This fluid track, which runs between the mylohyoid muscle and the hyoglossus or geniohyoid muscle, serves to distinguish the ranula from an epidermoid cyst (Fig. 12.**4**) or lymphangioma (Fig. 12.**6**). Very rarely, a simple ranula with an unbroken capsule may grow so large that it projects into the submandibular space and closely resembles a diving ranula. Wall thickening is commonly seen as a result of inflammatory change or previous surgery.

Air-Containing Masses or Lesions of the Oropharynx and Oral Cavity

The main lesions to be considered in the differential diagnosis of air-containing masses are inflammatory complications, posttraumatic lesions, and iatrogenic changes. The most common inflammatory lesions are abscesses and cellulitic inflammation; the latter may be caused by anaerobic or aerobic organisms (Table 12.**9**).

Tumor Masses

It is important to differentiate *lymphatic tissue* in the tonsillar fossa and tongue base from areas of possible tumor invasion. *Lymphatic hyperplasia* is distinguished from *lymphomatous infiltration* using the same criteria as in the nasopharynx. Unlike carcinoma, lymphatic hyperplasia (tonsillar hyperplasia) is generally painless. It is most common in children and adolescents and is characterized by nasal airway obstruction with increased oral respiration. The cause is an excessive reactive proliferation of immunocompetent lymphoepithelial tissue. The MRI appearance of tonsillar hyperplasia is that of a mostly symmetric hyperplasia affecting both palatine tonsils and/or both adenoids. Hypervascular septa are consistently seen on T2-weighted images and contrast-enhanced T1-weighted images. Lymphomatous involvement (Figs. 12.**8** and 12.**9**) usually affects only one tonsil and is typically associated with high T2-weighted signal intensity and marked, homogeneous enhancement on T1-weighted images. The absence of hypervascular septa in lymphoma aids in distinguishing that lesion from lymphatic hyperplasia. On post-contrast images, tonsillar lymphoma shows a ground-glass appearance similar to that of nasopharyngeal lymphoma. Unlike lymphatic hyperplasia, involvement by carcinoma

Table 12.**9** Air-containing masses or lesions

Findings	**Differential diagnostic criteria**
➤ Inflammatory: —Abscess (submucous) (Fig. 12.**3**) —Cellulitis (deep compartments)	Morphology, topography
➤ Iatrogenic: —Biopsy —Operation	Topography
➤ Posttraumatic: —Emphysema	Spread

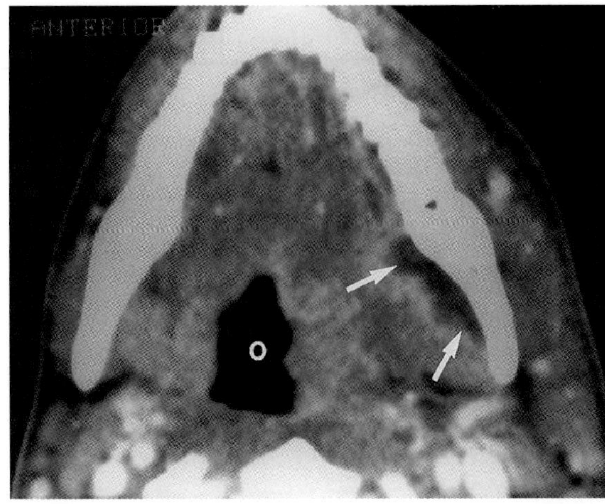

Fig. 12.**3** **Submandibular abscess.** Axial CT scan with a soft-tissue window shows an area of fluid density in the left pterygomandibular fossa (arrows) causing distortion of the oropharyngeal air column. The demarcation of the abscess from the tonsillar fossa is not consistent with a peritonsillar abscess, thus CT findings warrant surgical removal of the abscess through an external approach. With a peritonsillar abscess, intraoral drainage would be indicated.
O Oropharyngeal air column

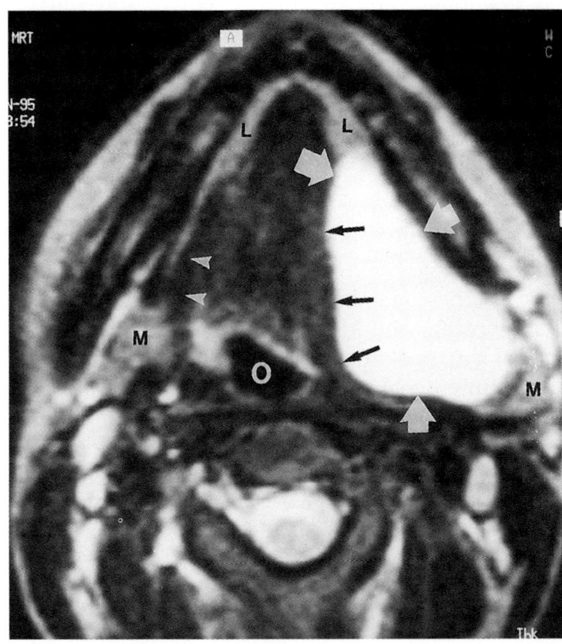

Fig. 12.**4** **Left-sided epidermoid cyst.** The T2-weighted image (TR/TE = 2500/80 ms) shows a well-circumscribed mass of very high signal intensity (thick white arrows) in the left submandibular space. The mylohyoid muscle is displaced medially (black arrows), and the oropharyngeal air column is displaced to the right. This definitely localizes the mass to the submandibular rather than the sublingual space. The lesion is clearly demarcated from the diving ranula, that lies medial to the mylohyoid muscle (see Fig. 12.**5**).

L	Sublingual gland
M	Submandibular gland
O	Oropharyngeal air column
Arrowheads	Hyoglossus muscle

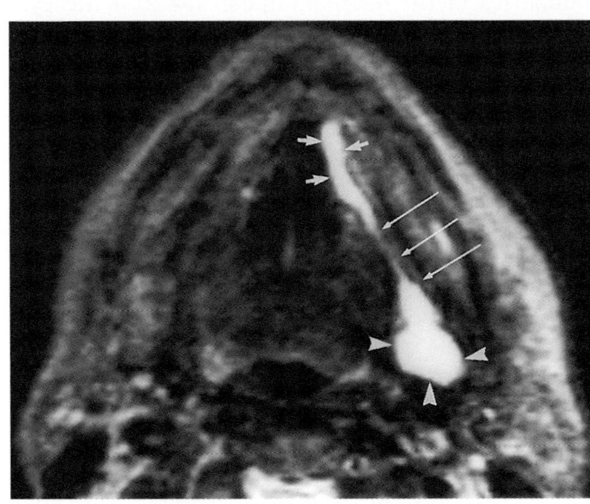

Fig. 12.**5** **Diving ranula on the left side.** The T2-weighted image (TR/TE = 2500/80 ms) shows a hyperintense mass extending from the sublingual space (short arrows) into the submandibular space (arrowheads). Note the lateral position of the mylohyoid muscle (long arrows) in relation to the mass.

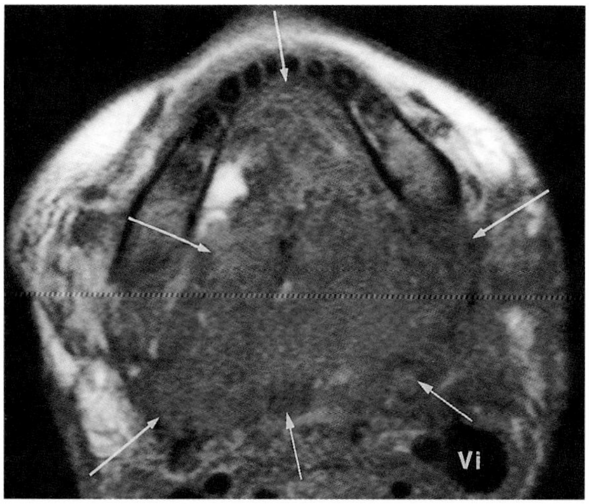

a

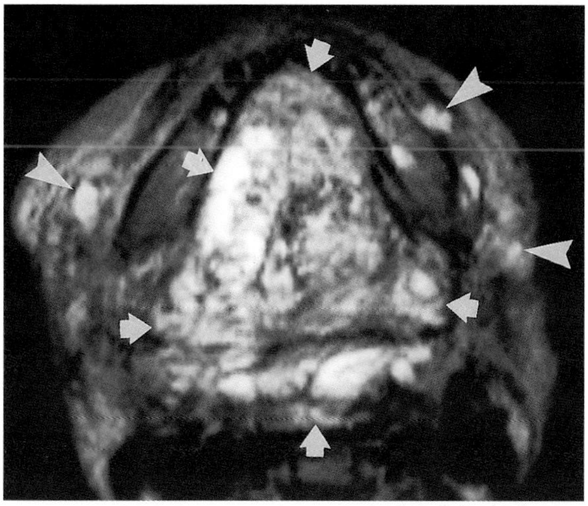

b

Figs. 12.**6a, b** **Lymphangioma.**
(**a**) Axial unenhanced T1-weighted image (TR/TE = 700/15 ms) shows an extensive oropharyngeal mass (arrows) with involvement of the parapharyngeal space. The mass is isointense to muscle tissue in the plain T1-weighted sequence.
(**b**) Axial T2-weighted image (TR/TE = 3000/80 ms) demonstrates the lymphangioma (arrows) as a hyperintense mass involving the parapharyngeal space, submandibular space, oropharynx, oral cavity, and subcutaneous tissue (arrowheads).

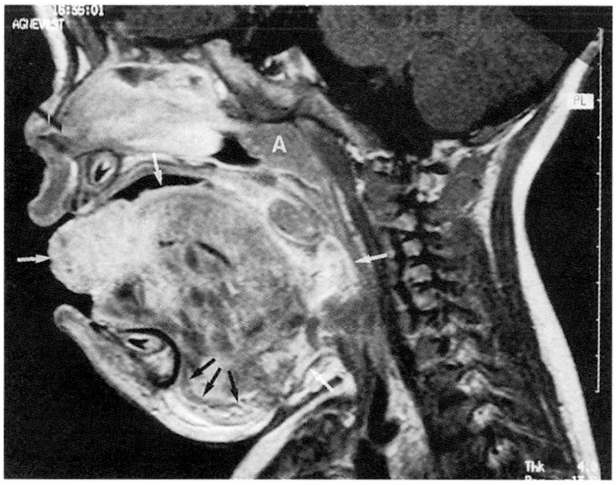

Fig. 12.**7** **Lymphangioma of the tongue.** Sagittal Gd-enhanced T1-weighted image shows an extensive mass lesion (white arrows) occupying the oral cavity and oropharynx. The mass involves all of the tongue and is so extensive that it prevents closure of the mouth. It is also causing marked downward displacement of the mylohyoid muscle (black arrows).
A Adenoid hyperplasia

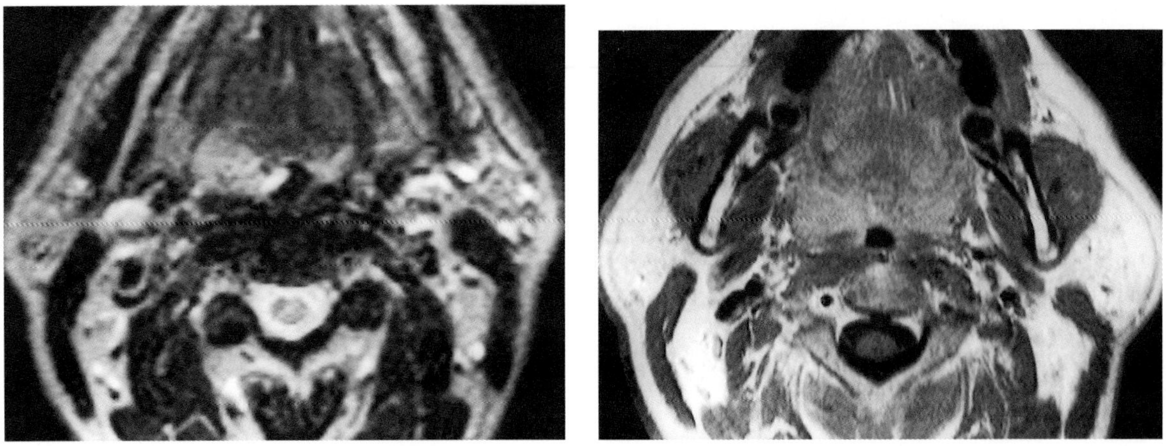

a b

Figs. 12.**8 a, b** **Right-sided tonsillar lymphoma.**
(**a**) T2-weighted image shows markedly increased signal intensity in the right tonsillar area (arrows) consistent with tonsillar lymphoma.

(**b**) Gd-enhanced T1-weighted image (TR/TE = 700/15 ms) shows homogeneous ground-glass enhancement in the right tonsillar area. Histologic evaluation confirmed tonsillar lymphoma.

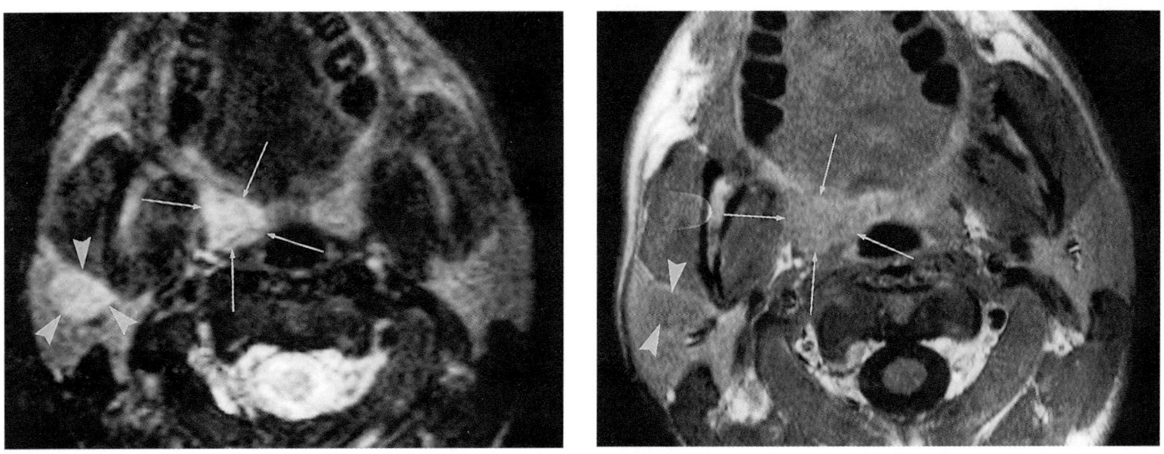

a b

Figs. 12.**9 a, b** **Lymphoma of the right tonsil and parotid gland.**
(**a**) Axial T2-weighted image (TR/TE = 3000/90 ms) shows increased signal intensity in the right tonsil (arrows) and a hyperintense elliptical mass in the right parotid gland (arrowheads).

(**b**) Axial Gd-enhanced T1-weighted image (TR/TE = 700/15 ms) shows nonhomogeneous ground-glass enhancement of the enlarged right tonsil (arrows) and homogeneous ground-glass enhancement of an elliptical intraparotid mass (arrowheads) following the administration of 0.1 mmol/kg bw Gd-DTPA.

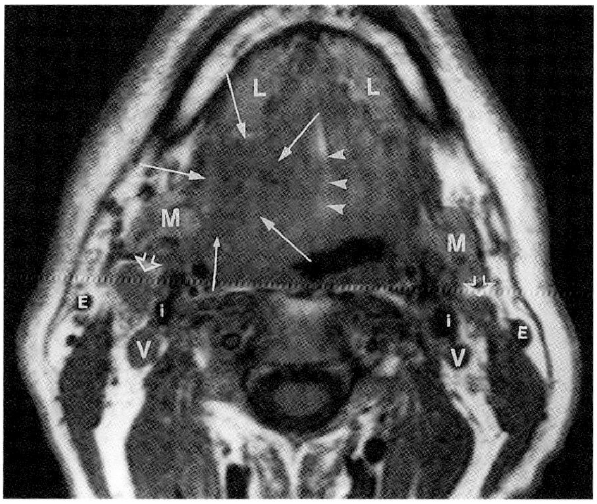

a

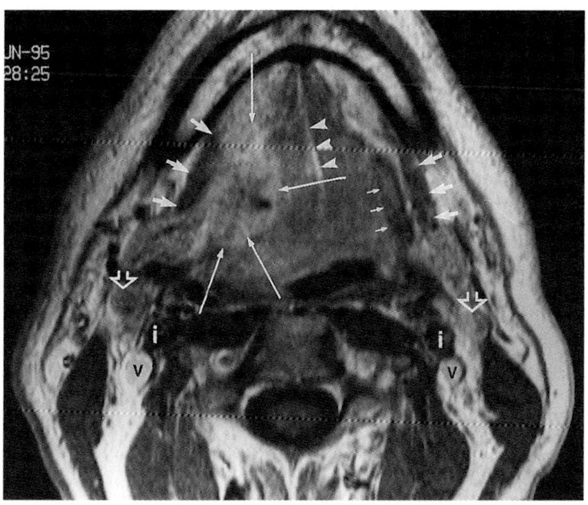

b

Figs. 12.**10 a, b** **Right-sided oropharyngeal carcinoma.**
(**a**) Axial unenhanced T1-weighted image shows an extensive mass (arrows) that extends to the mylohyoid muscle and sublingual gland and is invading the geniohyoid, genioglossus, and hyoglossus muscles on the right side. The mass extends posteriorly into the right tonsillar fossa. The lingual septum (arrowheads) is displaced to the right. Metastatic jugulodigastric nodes are visible on both sides (open arrows). Tumor stage T3 N2 c.

E External jugular vein
i Internal carotid artery
L Sublingual gland
M Submandibular gland
V Internal jugular vein

(**b**) Axial T1-weighted image (TR/TE = 700/15 ms) after the administration of 0.1 mmol/kg bw Gd-DTPA demonstrates marked tumor enhancement (long arrows).

i	Internal carotid artery
V	Internal jugular vein
Arrowheads	Displaced lingual septum
Open arrows	Metastatic lymph nodes
Short thick arrows	Mylohyoid muscle
Short thin arrows	Hyoglossus muscle

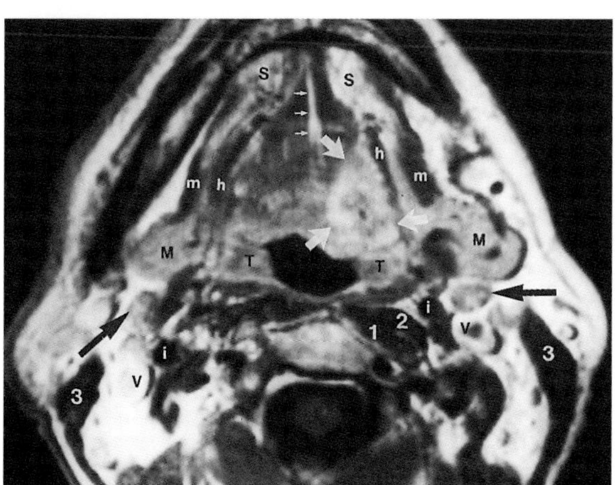

Fig. 12.**11** **Squamous cell carcinoma of the left oral floor.** Axial Gd-enhanced T1-weighted image (TR/TE = 700/15 ms) shows a markedly enhancing lesion (large white arrows) of the left oral floor with no apparent involvement of the ipsilateral tonsil or sublingual gland. The mass is medial to the hyoglossus muscle. There is evidence of bilateral involvement of the jugulodigastric nodes (level II) (black arrows). Tumor stage T2 N2 c.

1 Longus colli muscle
2 Longus capitis muscle
3 Sternocleidomastoid muscle
h Hyoglossus muscle
i Internal carotid artery
m Mylohyoid muscle
M Submandibular gland
S Sublingual gland
T Tonsil
V Internal jugular vein

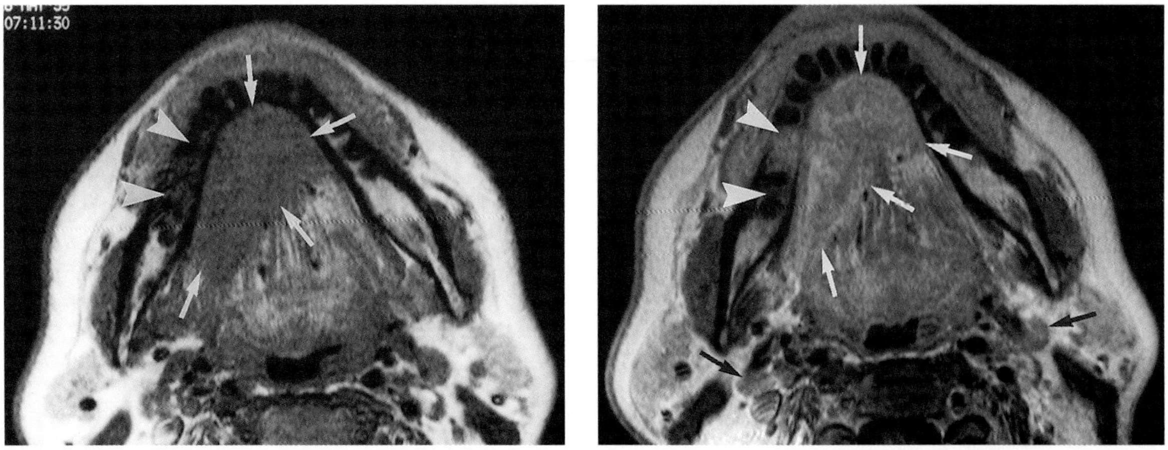

Figs. 12.**12 a, b** **Oral floor carcinoma.**
(**a**) Axial unenhanced T1-weighted image (TR/TE = 700/15 ms) shows an extensive oral floor mass (arrows) that replaces the normal signal texture of the oral floor with high signal intensity due to the fat content of the mass. The scan also shows a marked reduction of signal intensity in the mandibular cancellous bone on the right side (arrowheads).

(**b**) Post-contrast T1-weighted image shows marked, nonhomogeneous enhancement of the oral floor carcinoma (white arrows). Marked enhancement also appears in the right side of the mandible (arrowheads), signifying mandibular invasion. Note the accompanying bilateral enlargement of the jugulodigastric nodes (black arrows). Tumor stage T4 N2 c.

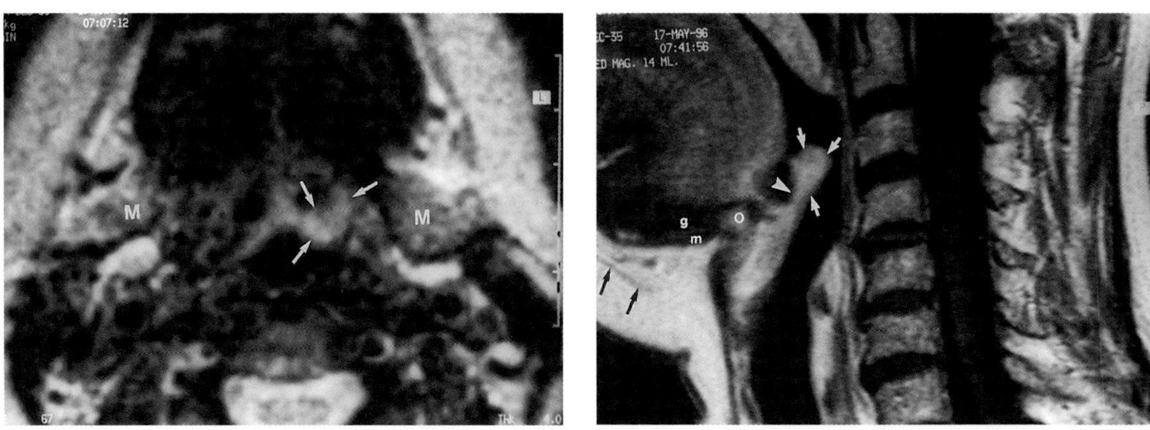

Figs. 12.**13 a, b** **Left-sided epiglottic carcinoma.**
(**a**) Axial T2-weighted image (TR/TE = 3000/90 ms) shows increased signal intensity along the left epiglottic margin (arrows), consistent with the clinical diagnosis of epiglottic carcinoma. There is no apparent invasion of the preepiglottic fat.
M Submandibular gland

(**b**) Sagittal Gd-enhanced T1-weighted image (TR/TE = 700/15 ms) demonstrates the markedly enhancing epiglottic mass (white arrows). The small indentation in the anterior surface of the epiglottis (arrowhead) is a biopsy defect.

g	Geniohyoid muscle
m	Mylohyoid muscle
O	Hyoid bone
Black arrows	Platysma

a 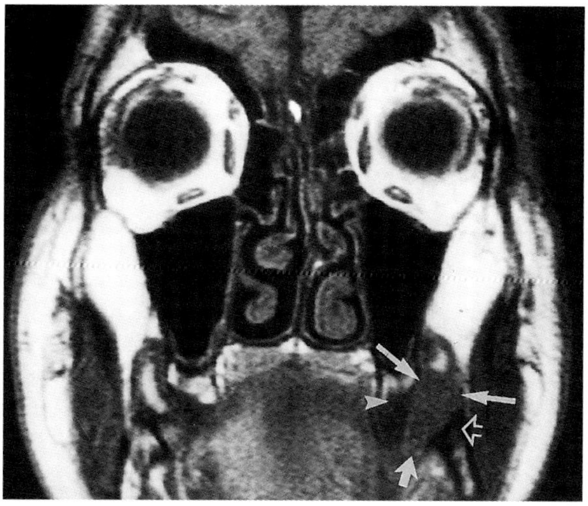

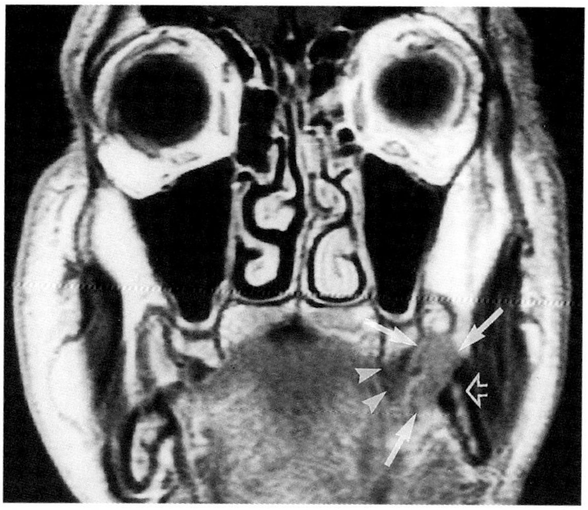 b

Figs. 12.**14 a, b** **Squamous cell carcinoma of the left palatoglossal arch.**
(**a**) Unenhanced coronal T1-weighted image (TR/TE = 700/15 ms) shows involvement of the left palatoglossal arch by a mass (long arrows) that is slightly hyperintense to muscle. The low signal intensity of the cancellous bone in the left maxilla (arrowhead and short arrow) and left mandibular ramus (open arrow) is consistent with tumor invasion.
(**b**) Gd-enhanced coronal T1-weighted image demonstrates marked enhancement of the tumor mass (arrows). Nonhomogeneous enhancement is visible in the left maxilla (arrowheads) and left mandibular ramus (open arrow).

(Fig. 12.**17**) or lymphoma is usually unilateral. When carcinoma of the oropharynx or oral floor has reached stage T2 or T3 (Figs. 12.**10** and 12.**12**), hypointense areas frequently appear at the center of the mass due to necrosis. Normally these areas are not seen in lymphatic hyperplasia or tonsillar lymphoma.

Combined coronal and sagittal MR imaging has proven effective for evaluating lesions of the tongue, epiglottis (Fig. 12.**13**), and palatoglossal arch (Fig. 12.**14**).

In HIV-positive patients, Kaposi sarcoma should always be considered in the differential diagnosis of intraoral and oropharyngeal masses (Fig. 12.**15**).

MRI is superior to CT for distinguishing post-therapeutic changes from residual or recurrent tumor, but this assessment can be difficult in some cases (Fig. 12.**16**).

Benign Tumors

Benign tumors of this region are uncommon, but a specific diagnosis can often be made from MR findings. T2-weighted sequences are useful for differentiating cystic lesions from solid tumors. Spontaneous and postoperative hemorrhage can be distinguished from tumor masses by the combined analysis of T1 and T2 relaxation times.

Benign tumors appear on CT and MRI as a uniformly enhancing mass with well-defined margins. Salivary stones are nonenhancing lesions that appear hypointense in all MR sequences and very dense on CT scans. Benign tumors arising from the minor salivary glands constitute the largest group of benign mass lesions.

Lingual Thyroid Tissue

Lingual thyroid tissue appears on CT and MRI as a mass extending from the mucosal surface of the tongue base on the midline into the medial sublingual space. The mass appears hyperdense on plain and post-contrast CT scans. It should always be evaluated by radionuclide imaging, both to confirm the presence of functioning ectopic thyroid tissue and to show that a normal thyroid gland is present. It is noteworthy that removal of the lingual thyroid tissue induces permanent hypothyroidism in approximately 80% of cases.

Inflammatory Lesions of the Oropharynx and Oral Cavity

CT is the primary imaging modality for diagnosing inflammatory lesions of the oropharynx, oral cavity, and oral floor (Fig. 12.**3**). It is faster and more accurate than MRI for identifying small calcifications and detecting mandibular osteomyelitis (Figs. 12.**19** and 12.**21**).

T2-weighted and contrast-enhanced T1-weighted MR sequences are best for differentiating an inflammatory lesion from a tumor mass (Fig. 12.**2**).

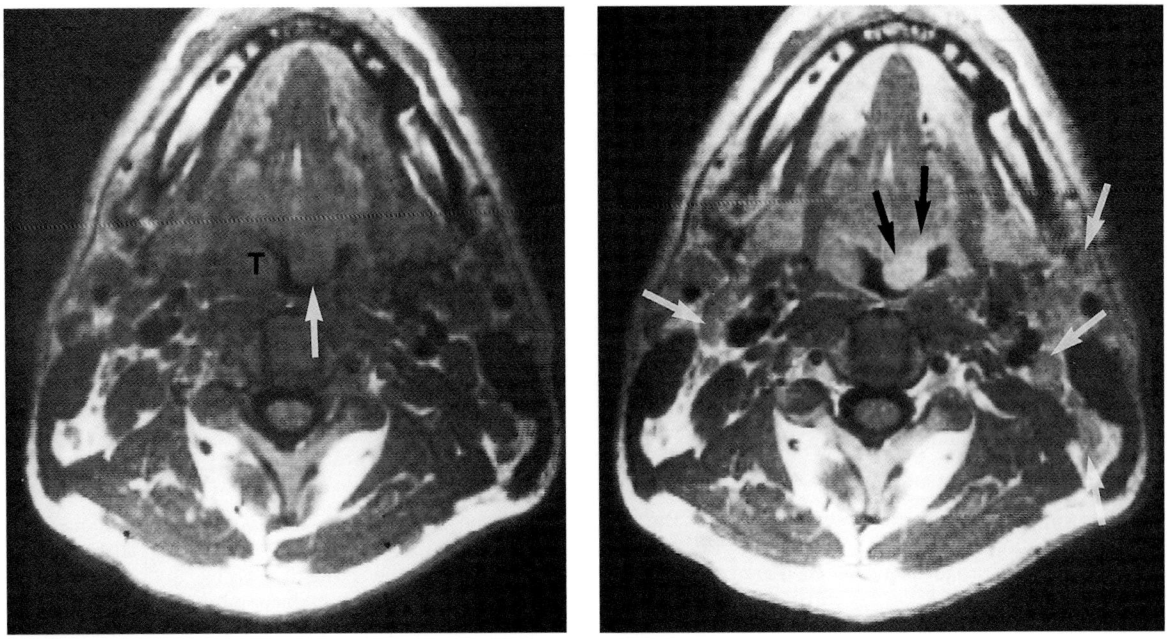

a b

Figs. 12.**15a, b** **Kaposi sarcoma in the posterior half of the tongue.**
(**a**) Unenhanced axial T1-weighted image (TR/TE = 500/25 ms) show a mass lesion extending into the pharynx from the tongue base but showing no apparent invasion of the posterior tongue (arrow). The mass is not clearly demarcated from the intrinsic tongue muscles on the plain image. A hyperplastic right palatine tonsil is noted as an incidental finding.
T Palatine tonsil

(**b**) Postcontrast T1-weighted image (TR/TE = 500/25 ms) shows homogeneous enhancement of the Kaposi sarcoma, which displays high signal intensity. The tumor is more clearly demarcated from the tongue muscles on the post-Gd-DTPA image (black arrows). The hyperplastic right tonsil also shows marked contrast enhancement. Multiple enlarged jugulodigastric and deep cervical lymph nodes (white arrows) are documented on each side.

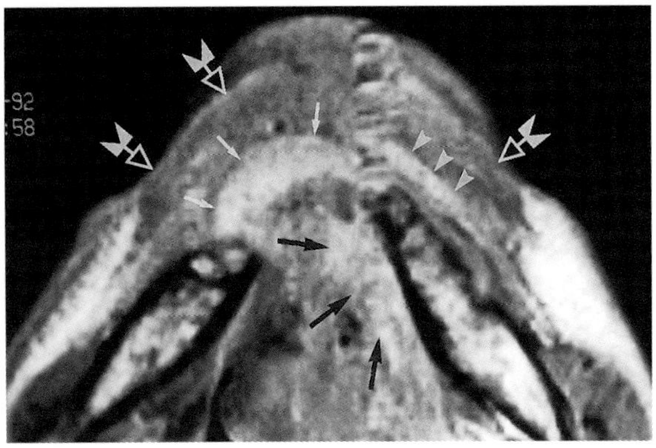

Fig. 12.**16** **Recurrence of squamous cell carcinoma.** Axial Gd-enhanced T1-weighted image (TR/TE = 700/15 ms) shows intensely enhancing premandibular lesions on the right (white arrows) and left sides (arrowheads), interpreted as recurrent carcinoma of the oral floor. Marked enhancement also appears in the oral floor and sublingual gland on the left side (black arrows). Histologic examination confirmed recurrent carcinoma at all three sites. Note also the conspicuous postirradiation changes in the skin and subcutaneous tissue (open arrows).

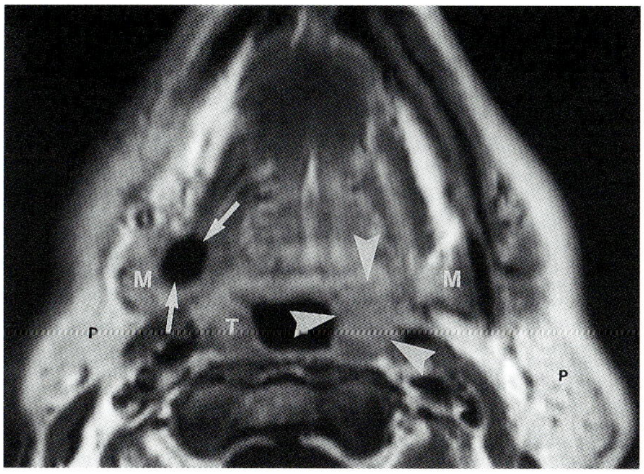

Fig. 12.**17** **Stone in the right submandibular gland and left tonsillar carcinoma.** Axial T1-weighted image (TR/TE = 700/15 ms) shows a circumscribed area of signal void (arrows) in the right submandibular gland. This area appears markedly hypointense in T1- and T2-weighted sequences and shows osseous density on CT scans. The image also shows a markedly enhancing soft-tissue mass in the left tonsillar fossa (arrowheads) consistent with tonsillar carcinoma.
M Submandibular gland
P Parotid gland
T Tonsil

This is particularly important considering that localized inflammatory processes (e.g., from a tongue bite) can mimic a tumor. Morphologically, inflammatory processes tend to have ill-defined margins and rarely displace adjacent structures. Small lingual carcinomas that do not cross the midline often cause displacement of the lingual septum, while an inflammatory lesion (e.g., a tongue bite) tends to involve the tongue diffusely and increase the signal intensity of the tongue muscles on T2-weighted images. A tumor mass is usually well demarcated on T1-weighted images and is markedly hypointense to the normal tissues of the oral cavity and oral floor.

Bone Destruction

The cortical and cancellous bone of the mandible should be closely scrutinized as part of the routine workup of tumors involving the oral floor and lateral portions of the tongue. Axial and coronal T1-weighted images can disclose subtle cortical bone changes, which appear as areas of increased signal intensity. Areas of cancellous bone invasion show a reduction in signal intensity.

Imaging of the mandible. Conventional radiographic studies, especially panoramic tomograms, are still the primary modality for analyzing traumatic lesions of the mandible. Conventional radiographs have no role in diagnosing mandibular invasion by squamous cell carcinoma. CT should be used to evaluate mandibular osteomyelitis (Fig. 12.**19**) and invasion of the bone by a malignant tumor (usually squamous cell carcinoma). Both soft-tissue and bone reconstructions should be analyzed in the CT study, and contrast medium can be administered by intravenous bolus injection to help differentiate vascular structures from tumor masses and lymph nodes. In selected cases, such as patients with dental implants, dental CT scans can provide secondary reconstructed views of the alveoli.

There are only a few indications for MRI in patients with mass lesions or infections of the mandible. Mandibular infiltration can be evaluated with plain and post-contrast T1-weighted sequences and fat-suppressed T1-weighted sequences. Noncontrast T1-weighted sequences are the most sensitive for this application.

The principal MRI criteria and their differential diagnostic implications are reviewed in Table 12.**10**.

T2-weighted sequence:

The T2-weighted sequence can contribute greatly to the differential diagnosis of mandibular masses:

- Circumscribed mass of high signal intensity: cyst.
- Circumscribed mass of intermediate signal intensity: cementoma, adamantinoma, carcinoma, myxoma (Fig. 12.**23**), plasmacytoma.
- Circumscribed mass of low signal intensity: ameloblastoma (Fig. 12.**18**), odontoma, osteoma.
- Diffuse increase in signal intensity without a circumscribed mass: e.g., osteomyelitis.

Fig. 12.**18** **Ameloblastoma of the mandible.** Axial CT scan with a soft-tissue window demonstrates the mixed cystic and solid components of the ameloblastoma (arrows).

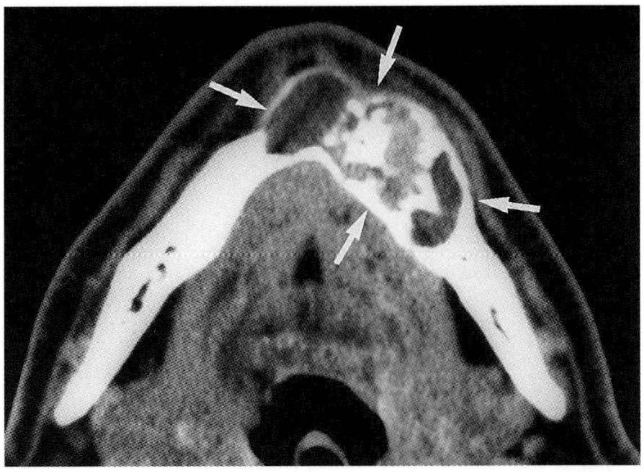

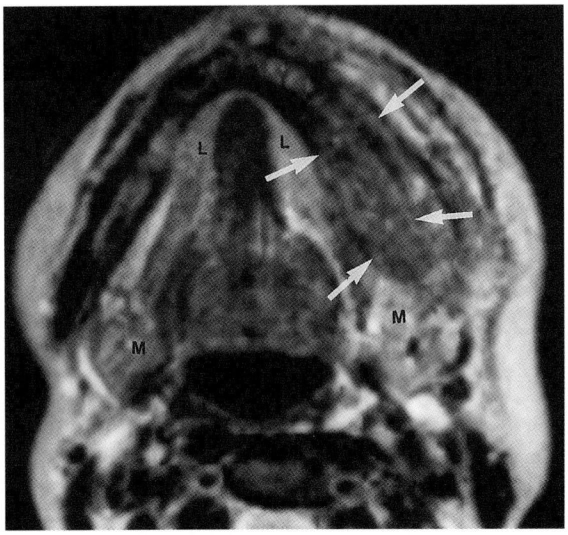

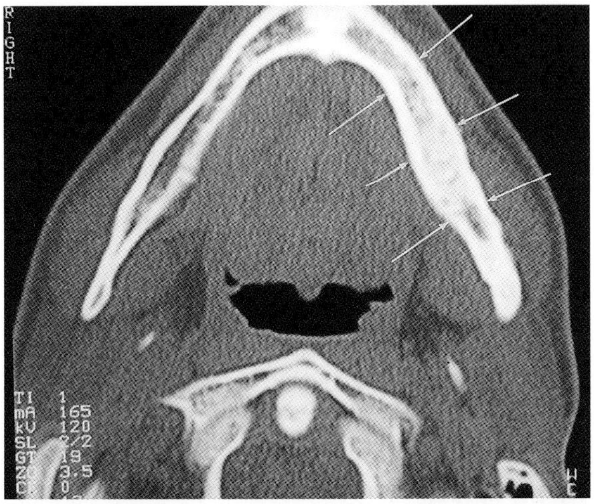

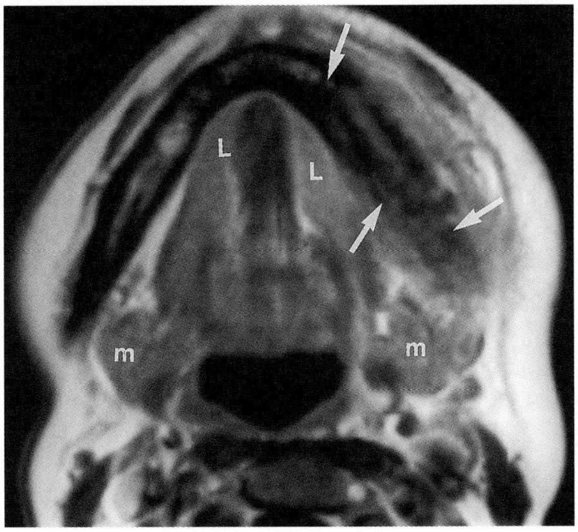

Figs. 12.**19 a–c** **Osteomyelitis.**

(**a**) Unenhanced T2-weighted image (TR/TE = 2500/90 ms) reveals a diffuse area of increased signal intensity in the left mandibular body (arrows) relative to the right side. The cortical structures in that area are poorly defined.

L Sublingual gland

M Submandibular gland

(**b**) CT scan with a bone window shows the osteomyelitis-induced osseous structural changes (arrows) in the left mandibular body.

(**c**) T1-weighted image (TR/TE = 700/15 ms) after the administration of 0.1 mmol/kg bw Gd-DTPA shows nonhomogeneous enhancement of cortical and cancellous bone areas in the left mandibular body (arrows), contrasting with the normal-appearing right side.

L Sublingual gland

m Submandibular gland

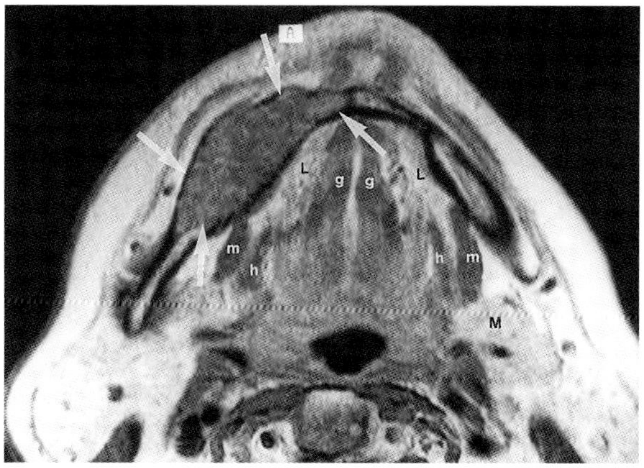

a

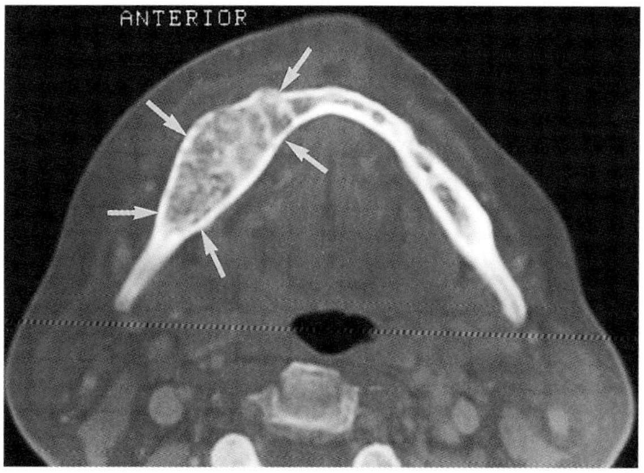

b

Figs. 12.**20 a, b** **Fibrosing cementoma.**
(**a**) Post-contrast T1-weighted image (TR/TE = 700/15 ms) shows a moderately enhancing mass in the right mandibular body. The cortical bone is greatly thinned in places, but its overall continuity is preserved.
g Geniohyoid muscle
h Hyoglossus muscle
L Sublingual gland
M Submandibular gland
m Mylohyoid muscle

(**b**) CT scan (bone window) documents the fusiform expansion of the right mandibular body (arrows).

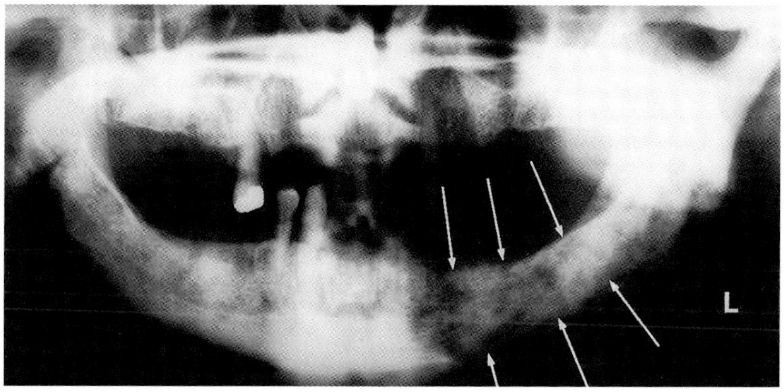

Fig. 12.**21** **Osteomyelitis.** Panoramic tomogram documents rarefying osteomyelitis of the mandible (arrows) on the left side. Irregular, ill-defined lucencies permeate the left mandible in a moth-eaten pattern. The process has destroyed the contours of the mandibular canal and the basal cortical plate. Since the osteomyelitis is chronic, osteolytic processes are accompanied by new bone formation, which appears as cloudy, marble–like areas of sclerosis.

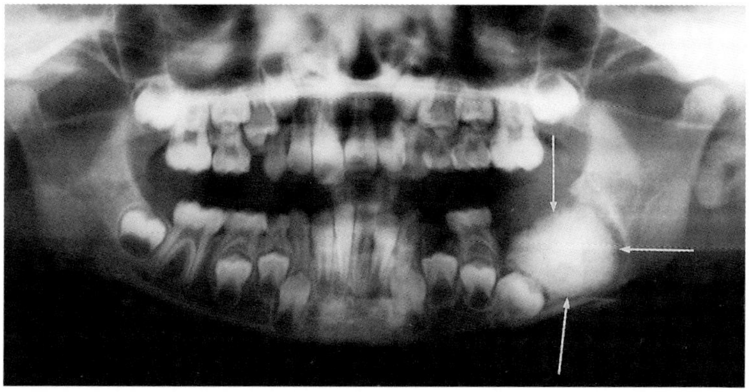

Fig. 12.**22** **Ameloblastic fibroma.** Panoramic tomogram demonstrates the mass (arrows) in the left mandibular body. The tumor displays prominent sclerotic areas and a surrounding lucent zone.

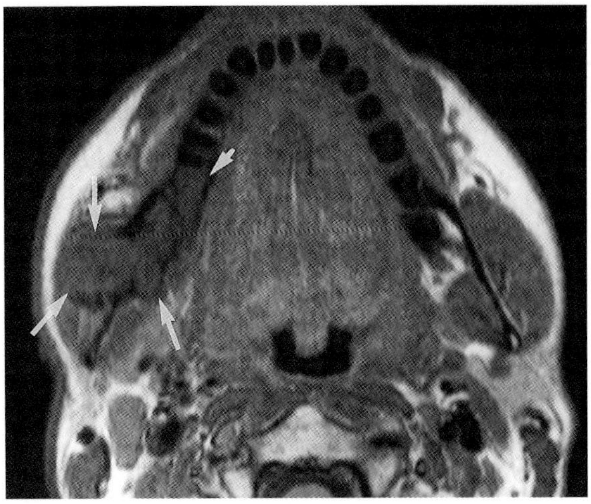
a

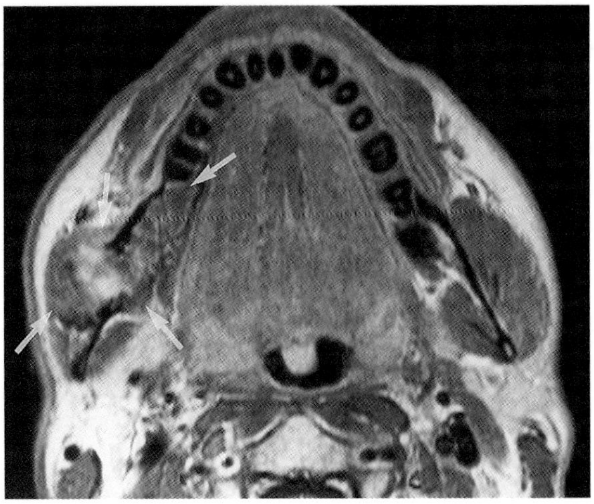
b

Figs. 12.**23 a, b** **Myxoma of the right mandible.**
(**a**) Unenhanced T1-weighted image (TR/TE = 700/15 ms) shows a mass in the right mandible (arrows) that is isointense to muscle. There is concomitant involvement of the masseter muscle and pterygomandibular fossa.

(**b**) T1-weighted image (TR/TE = 700/15 ms) after the administration of 0.1 mmol/kg bw Gd-DTPA demonstrates nonhomogeneous enhancement of the myxoma.

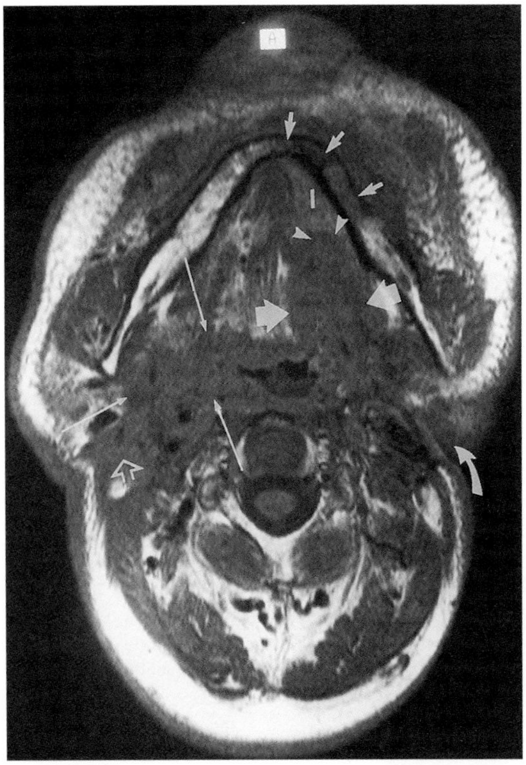

Fig. 12.**24** **Recurrence of oral floor carcinoma.** Unenhanced T1-weighted image (TR/TE = 700/15 ms) shows a recurrence of oral floor carcinoma (thick arrows) on the left side. The mass extends anteriorly to the sublingual gland (I) (arrowheads) and displaces the geniohyoid muscle to the right. The tumor is well demarcated from normal tissues, which appear hyperintense due to their fat content. The image also documents a jugulodigastric nodal metastasis (open arrow) on the right side. Additional tumor masses are visible in the right tonsillar fossa (long thin arrows). There is marked bilateral swelling of the subcutaneous tissues due to lymphedema. The low signal intensity of the cancellous bone in the left mandibular body signifies invasion of this segment by carcinoma (short thin arrows). Postoperative changes including scar contractures of the skin and subcutaneous tissue are visible on the left side (curved arrow).

Table 12.**10** Signal characteristics of various common tumors of the oropharynx, oral cavity, and oral floor

Findings	Unenhanced T2-weighted signal intensity relative to surrounding tissue	Unenhanced T1-weighted signal intensity relative to surrounding tissue	Gd-enhanced T1-weighted signal intensity relative to surrounding tissue	Margins	Internal structure, pattern of infiltration
Malignant tumors:					
➤ Squamous cell carcinoma (Figs. 12.**10** – 12.**14**)	Iso- to hyperintense	Hypointense	Iso- to hyperintense, moderately intense enhancement ↑	Ill-defined	Nonhomogeneous, sometimes with central necrosis; tends to be locally invasive, occasionally infiltrates bony structures
➤ Lymphoma (Fig. 12.**9**)	Markedly hyperintense	Hypointense	Hyperintense, intense enhancement ↑	Smooth	Homogeneous, ground-glass appearance
➤ Minor salivary gland tumors	Iso- to hyperintense	Hypointense	Slightly hyperintense, moderately intense enhancement ↑	Ill-defined	Nonhomogeneous, sometimes with central necrosis
Benign tumors:					
➤ Neuroma	Hyperintense	Hypointense	Slightly hyperintense, intense enhancement ↑	Smooth	Homogeneous
Inflammatory diseases				Indistinct margins; diffuse surrounding reaction; may not appear as circumscribed mass	
➤ Abscess	Very hyperintense	Isointense	Intense rim enhancement, hypointense center	Smooth margins; a capsule is often defined	Nonhomogeneous
➤ Tonsillitis	Hyperintense with indistinct margins	Hypointense	Hyperintense, moderate enhancement ↑; frequent reactive involvement of adjacent soft tissues	Diffuse tonsillar enlargement with minimal surrounding reaction	Nonhomogeneous, frequent
➤ Odontogenic inflammation	Hyperintense, arises from dental tissues	Hypointense	Hyperintense, moderate enhancement ↑	Indistinct margins	Nonhomogeneous

Summary and Diagnostic Strategy

In differential diagnostic evaluations of the oral cavity, oropharynx, and oral floor, the primary imaging modality that should follow the clinical examination is MRI. If this modality is unavailable or if there is clinical suspicion of bone invasion or abscess formation, contrast-enhanced CT (preferably with spiral technique) can also be performed. The MR examination should start with axial T2- and T1-weighted images followed by coronal T1-weighted images. Axial T1-weighted imaging should then be repeated after the intravenous administration of Gd-DTPA. Morphologic changes that suggest a tumor mass are increased signal intensity in the T2-weighted sequence and areas of decreased signal intensity that show enhancement on post-contrast images. An accurate diagnosis relies on a precise description of the mass in relation to anatomic landmarks and associated spaces and the differentiation of benign from malignant disease. Except for abscesses and cystic masses, benign lesions are rarely subjected to a detailed imaging evaluation.

References

1 Aspestrand, F., M. Boysen, V. Engh: Prognostic significance of contrast enhancement and tumor demarcation at CT of squamous cell carcinomas of the oral cavity and oropharynx. Acta Radiol. 35 (1994) 217 – 221

2 August, M., M. Nguyen: Evaluation of metastatic neck disease by computed tomography. Int J Oral Macillofac Surg. 23 (1994) 290 – 293

3 Avrahami, E., M. Englender: Relation between CT axial cross-sectional area of the oropharynx and obstructive sleep apnea syndrome in adults. AJNR 16 (1995) 135 – 140

4 Coit, W. E., H. R. Harnsberger, A. G. Osborn, W. R. K. Smoker, M. H. Stevens, R. B. Lufkin: Ranulas and their mimics: CT evaluation. Radiology 163 (1987) 211 – 216

5 Held, P., A.: Breit: MRI and CT of tumors of the pharynx: comparison of the two imaging procedures including fast and ultrafast MR sequences. Eur J Radiol. 18 (1994) 81 – 91

6 Minami, M., T. Kaneda, H. Yamamoto, et al.: Ameloblastoma in the maxillomandibular region: MR Imaging. Radiology 184 (1992) 389 – 393

7 Muraki, A. S., A. A. Mancuso, H. R. Harnsberger et al.: CT of the oropharynx, tongue base, and floor of the mouth: normal anatomy and range of varations, and applications of staging carcinoma. Radiology 148 (1983) 725 – 731

8 Nguyen, V. D., J. L. Potter, M. Hersh-Schick: MR: Ludwig angina: an uncommon and potentially lethal neck infection. AJNR 13 (1992) 215 – 219

9 Som, P. M., M. L. Urken, H. Biller, M. Lidov: Imaging the postoperative neck. Radiology 187 (1993) 593 – 603

10 Underhill, T. E., J. O. Katz, T. L. Pope et al.: Radiologic findings of diseases involving the maxilla and mandible. AJR 159 (1992) 345 – 350

11 Vogl, T. J., W. Steger, S. Ihrler, P. Ferrera, G. Grevers: Cystic masses in the floor of the mouth: value of MR imaging in planning surgery. AJR 161 (1993) 183 – 186

13 Hypopharynx and Larynx

The primary diagnostic evaluation of diseases of the hypopharynx and larynx is based on clinical procedures such as inspection and indirect examination, followed by endoscopic procedures such as microlaryngoscopy and other types of direct laryngoscopy with a self-supporting instrument. These procedures are adequate for evaluating the mucosae and taking tissue samples for histologic examination. Phonetic studies and quantitative procedures such as stroboscopy and electromyography can yield valuable information on the mobility of the vocal cords. Deglutition can be evaluated with conventional oral contrast studies using barium or a water-soluble contrast medium, supplemented by video cinematography or high-speed cinematography.

The sectional imaging modalities of computed tomography (CT) and magnetic resonance imaging (MRI) are mainly indicated for the evaluation of traumatic lesions, inflammatory masses, and tumor masses in these regions. MRI is of major value in the diagnosis of recurrent tumors owing to its high soft-tissue contrast. Below we shall review the essential diagnostic and differential diagnostic criteria that are applied in conventional radiography, CT, and MRI of the hypopharynx and larynx.

Normal Anatomy

The main subdivisions of the larynx are the supraglottis, glottis, and subglottis. The *supraglottis* extends from the ventricular folds (false vocal cords) above to the true vocal cords (vocal folds) below. It is bounded anteriorly by the thyroid cartilage, laterally and posteriorly by the aryepiglottic folds. The glottis includes the vocal cords, vocal muscles, and laryngeal ventricles (sinus of Morgagni). The anterior and posterior attachments of the vocal cords are termed the anterior and posterior commissures. The inferior borders of the thyroid and cricoid cartilages define the topographic boundaries of the *subglottis*, which is the laryngeal segment below the glottis and above the trachea.

The *hypopharynx* extends from the oropharynx to the supraglottic portion of the larynx. It is bounded superiorly by the free margin of the epiglottis and the lateral pharyngoepiglottic folds that form the valleculae. Anterior to the epiglottis is the fat-filled preepiglottic space. The left and right piriform sinuses and the esophagus form the posterior boundaries of the hypopharynx. The aryepiglottic folds extend from the arytenoid cartilages to the epiglottis, forming a triangular airway. The apex of this triangle is formed by the anterior commissure, its basal angles by the paired posterior commissures.

The vocal cords and vocal muscles display low signal intensity on MR images (Fig. 13.**3**), while the more superiorly placed ventricular folds show a higher signal intensity because of their fat content. (Coronal images are best for comparing these structures.) The mucosa lining the larynx is less than 1 mm thick, and diffuse or circumscribed thickening of the laryngeal mucosa is suggestive of disease. The preepiglottic and paralaryngeal spaces are occupied mostly by fat. The medial preepiglottic space extends from the hyoid bone to the anterior commissure and is continuous laterally with the paralaryngeal space.

The musculature appears hypointense on MRI and contrasts sharply with the hyperintense fat. The superior muscle group, consisting of the aryepiglottic and thyroepiglottic muscles, protects the respiratory tract by causing the epiglottis to close off the laryngeal airway during deglutition. The conus elasticus is a fibrous membrane set between the cricoid and arytenoid cartilages, its medial free edge forming the vocal ligament of the true vocal cords. This gives the conus elasticus an important role in the limitation of lateral, supraglottic, and subglottic tumor spread.

Clinical Signs and Symptoms

The three main *clinical manifestations* of diseases of the hypopharynx and larynx are as follows:

- Swallowing difficulties (dysphagia).
- Hoarseness.
- Respiratory impairment (dyspnea).

A variable degree of nonspecific pain may also be present. Dysphagia tends to be the dominant complaint in patients with mass lesions of the hypopharynx (Figs. 13.**7** – 13.**11**), while hoarseness and dyspnea are more characteristic of laryngeal disease. Hoarseness may result from tumor invasion of neural structures, usually the recurrent laryngeal nerve, or from a direct limitation of motion of the intrinsic laryngeal muscles, adjacent ligaments, or cartilage structures. Imaging in these cases will often document the paramedian position of a vocal cord. Consequent narrowing of the respiratory tract at this site can lead to respiratory difficulties and inspiratory stridor.

Imaging Evaluation and Differential Diagnosis

Computed Tomography (CT)

CT imaging of the hypopharynx (Figs. 13.**8** and 13.**9**) and larynx is done mainly to evaluate tumors, traumatic lesions (Fig. 13.**6**), and postoperative complications. CT is better than MRI for demonstrating erosive and destructive changes in bone and cartilage caused by tumor invasion. Moreover, CT is a less lengthy examination that is better tolerated by uncooperative patients. Image quality in MRI can be seriously compromised by motion artifacts, especially in patients with stage T4 disease; CT in these cases can provide acceptable results in less time.

The CT examination may employ single-slice scanning or spiral technique. The advantages of spiral CT (with a 5-mm slice thickness and table increment) are a shorter examination time, less contrast medium, and various postprocessing options. The administration of 100 mL of an iodinated contrast medium by pressure injection (Figs. 14.**5** and 14.**20**) (e.g., 1.0 mL/s with 30 s delay time) helps to delineate vessels and tumors and distinguish them from surrounding soft tissues. Generally there is no need for unenhanced scans. A suitable window can be selected to match the reconstruction algorithm (bone or soft-tissue) to the specific inquiry.

CT examinations of the mandibular region may be compromised by metallic artifacts due to dental work. Because of this problem and the limited capacity of CT for soft-tissue discrimination, MRI often must be added to resolve issues of malignant invasion (Fig. 12.**23**) or inflammatory infiltration. Approximately 5% of patients are unable to tolerate the requisite hyperextension of the head during a complete MR examination. High-resolution, thin-slice CT scanning can be used for selected investigations of the laryngeal cartilages.

Magnetic Resonance Imaging (MRI)

Unenhanced T1-weighted MR sequences do not permit an adequate evaluation of glottic (Fig. 13.**3**) and hypopharyngeal lesions (Figs. 13.**10** and 13.**11**), but they are very useful for differentiating tumor from fatty tissue in the supraglottic area. Optimum image quality is achieved with T1-weighted images and the paramagnetic contrast agent gadolinium(Gd)-DTPA, which greatly improves the contrast between tumor tissue and muscle (Figs. 13.**10 b**, 13.**11 b**, 13.**18 b**). Following intravenous contrast administration, all heavily vascularized tumors show significant enhancement in relation to surrounding structures. One difficulty, however, is that the normal mucosa that lines the larynx and hypopharynx to a thickness of several millimeters (Fig. 13.**10 b**) also enhances after contrast administration, making it difficult to appreciate small mucosal lesions. Central necrosis in tumors and fluid-filled laryngoceles (Fig. 13.**2**) show low signal intensity on noncontrast images, and intravenous contrast enhances only the periphery of the tumor or the cyst wall. In some cases MRI can overestimate tumor size due to the signal from inflammatory granulation tissue surrounding the mass.

T2-weighted and proton-density MR sequences are advantageous for evaluating cartilage invasion. Also, lymphatic and glandular tissues and fluid-filled cysts (Figs. 13.**2 a** and 14.**3**) show high signal intensity in T2-weighted sequences. But these sequences involve long acquisition times and often yield poor-quality images, since patients with laryngeal tumors often have dyspnea and dysphagia that cause motion artifacts due to coughing and respiratory movements.

MRI is superior to CT in its capacity for soft-tissue discrimination, its ability to define physiologic and pathologic structures in multiple planes without repositioning the patient, and the lack of radiation exposure, which allows multiple follow-up examinations to be scheduled without concern.

Imaging Findings

Congenital Variations and Malformations

Morphologic Anomalies

Clinically important congenital anomalies are the *laryngeal web*, a thin membranous connection between the vocal cords; a *laryngeal cleft* due to defective fusion of the cartilage laminae; and *laryngomalacia*, an immaturity of the laryngeal cartilages leading to dyspnea and stridor. In all of these conditions, endoscopic evaluation takes precedence over diagnostic imaging.

Laryngocele, Pharyngocele

A laryngocele (Figs. 13.**1** and 13.**2**) is caused by *dilatation of the laryngeal ventricle*, which may be congenital or acquired in adulthood (common in horn players and glass blowers). An analogous saccular protrusion of the pharyngeal wall is called a pharyngocele. Either lesion may be filled with air or fluid and displays well-defined margins. The sac appears on CT as a cystic mass of variable attenuation, depending on its degree of fullness. The combined use of T1- and T2-weighted MR sequences (Fig. 13.**2**) can differentiate intracystic air and fluids with varying protein contents. It is clinically significant that laryngoceles often coexist with malignant tumors or tuberculosis.

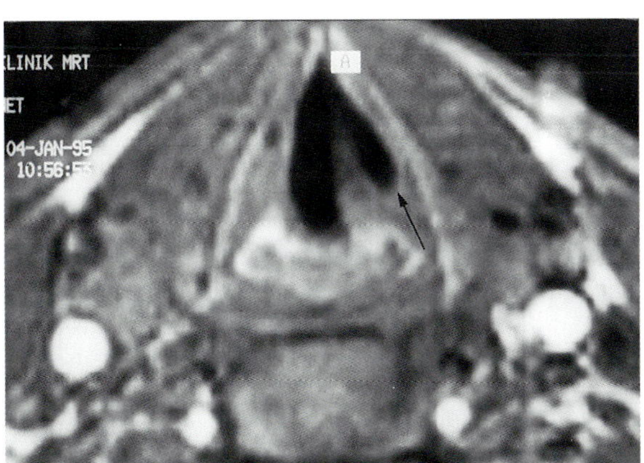

Fig. 13.**1** **Air-filled laryngocele.** Axial MRI of the larynx in a patient who attempted suicide by hanging shows a post-traumatic laryngocele on the left side (arrow) that communicates anteriorly with the laryngeal air column at the level of the cricoid cartilage.

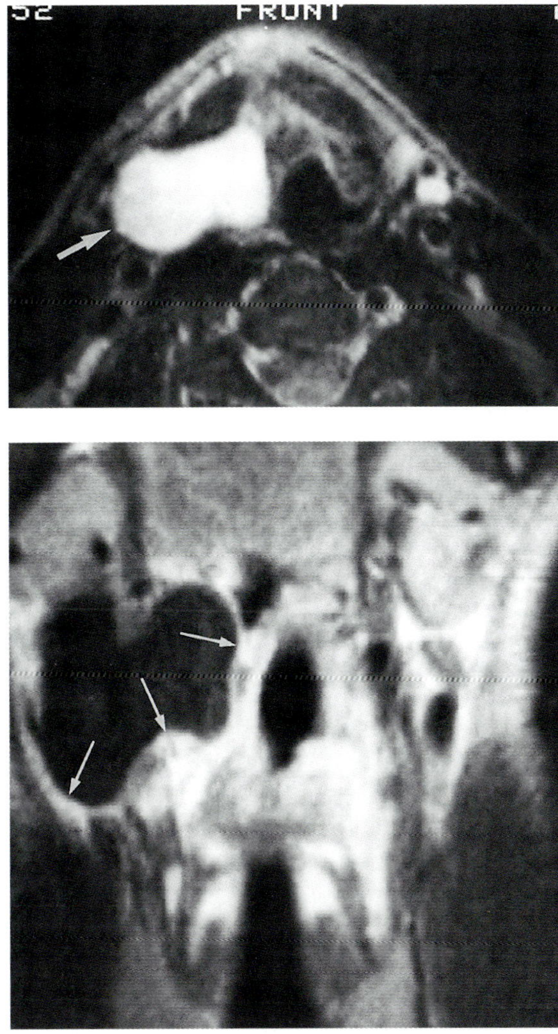

a

b

Figs. 13.**2 a, b** **Fluid-filled laryngocele.**
(**a**) Axial T2-weighted image of the larynx (TR/TE = 3000/90 ms) shows a well-circumscribed mass of high signal intensity. The axial view confirms its connection with the respiratory tract. The high signal intensity of this laryngocele results from its liquid contents.
(**b**) Coronal MRI demonstrates the full extent of the laryngocele and its expansile growth (arrows). The fluid contents appear hypointense on the T1-weighted image (TR/TE = 500/17 ms).

Tumors

Benign Tumors

Papilloma, Polyp

These lesions are commonly found in children. Radiologically they are well circumscribed, may present a cauliflower-like appearance, and typically involve the anterior part of the vestibular or vocal fold with subglottic extension. In papillomatosis, the larynx is diffusely lined with papillomatous lesions.

Chondroma

Most commonly arising from the cricoid cartilage (Figs. 13.**5** and 13.**15**), chondroma shows a characteristic amorphous calcified matrix that is best demonstrated by CT. Other imaging features are smooth margins, airway encroachment, and scant contrast enhancement.

Amyloidosis

Laryngeal amyloidosis is a rare disorder characterized by a circumscribed absence of contrast enhancement with inflammatory thickening of the surrounding mucosa (Fig. 13.**16**).

Adenoma

The basic imaging features of adenomas are smooth margins, a homogeneous internal structure, slow expansile growth, and moderate contrast enhancement.

Endolaryngeal Cyst

This lesion presents as a mucosa-lined cystic mass on the true or false vocal cords or aryepiglottic folds that shows low attenuation on CT scans and high signal intensity on T2-weighted MR images.

Malignant Tumors

Squamous Cell Carcinoma

The staging of squamous cell carcinoma is based on the *TNM system* of the *UICC*. Current TNM staging criteria define a *stage T1* tumor as being confined to one subsite, i.e., the supraglottis, glottis, subglottis, or hypopharynx. Glottic tumors are subclassified as *T1 a* when confined to one vocal cord and *T1 b* when both vocal cords are involved.

Stage T2 tumors have spread to an adjacent site but are still confined to the larynx or hypopharynx (Fig. 13.**10**). Thus, a supraglottic or subglottic tumor has reached the glottic plane while a glottic tumor has spread to the supraglottis or subglottis. The vocal cords (Fig. 13.**3**) may have normal or limited mobility. T2 lesions of the hypopharynx are not fixed to the larynx (Fig. 13.**10**).

Stage T3 tumors are more advanced, with supraglottic lesions involving the piriform sinus or preepiglottic tissue. Glottic tumors are associated with unilateral or bilateral vocal cord fixation.

Stage T4 tumors have already spread to adjacent regions such as the oropharynx or the infrahyoid muscles and other soft tissues of the neck. Glottic and supraglottic tumors involve the thyroid cartilage, cricoid cartilage, or both. Hypopharyngeal tumors have invaded the epiglottis.

The imaging criteria for a malignant tumor are asymmetric, infiltrative growth with ill-defined margins and a heterogeneous internal structure (Figs. 13.**10** and 13.**18**). CT may disclose bone and cartilage destruction. Malignant tumors show significant enhancement on post-contrast CT and MRI (Figs. 13.**3 b**, 13.**10 b**, 13.**11 b**, 13.**18 b**) and may cause airway constriction (Figs. 13.**3** and 13.**18**).

Many hypopharyngeal, supraglottic, and subglottic carcinomas are diagnosed only after cervical nodal metastasis has been detected (Figs. 14.**9 a–e**). Glottic carcinomas rarely present initially with regional lymph node involvement, and most are signaled clinically by hoarseness.

Rhabdomyosarcoma, Fibrosarcoma, Adenoid Cystic Carcinoma

Generally these tumors are indistinguishable from squamous cell carcinoma by their radiologic morphology. An atypical site of occurrence or lesional spread from and along muscular structures or tendon attachments may suggest the correct diagnosis.

Semimalignant Tumors

Kaposi Sarcoma

Kaposi sarcoma is a nodular tumor that grows en plaque and does not cause bone destruction. The lesions enhance intensely on CT and MRI due to their rich blood supply (Fig. 13.**12**). They do not cause regional nodal involvement or distant metastases. They are also characterized by relatively well-defined margins, rapid growth, and an association with HIV.

Inflammatory Lesions

Acute Epiglottitis

Acute epiglottitis is manifested clinically by massive swelling of the epiglottis with thickening of the mucosa and airway constriction (Fig. 13.**13**). Often these changes are visible on standard lateral radiographs. Because acute cases may require urgent clinical intervention, there is no primary indication for diagnostic imaging. In complicated cases, however, evaluation by CT or MRI is justified for treatment planning.

Laryngitis

Analogous to epiglottitis, laryngitis is associated with mucosal thickening and airway constriction. A particularly important condition is acute subglottic stenosing laryngitis in children (pseudocroup).

Laryngeal Perichondritis

Sites of predilection for perichondritis are the arytenoid cartilage and posterior commissure, where CT and MRI show enhancing areas of mucosal thickening with diffuse edema. The accurate differentiation of radiogenic perichondritis from recurrent tumor is of major clinical importance and should be accomplished by MRI.

Cricoarytenoid Arthritis

Edema of the cricoarytenoid joint area with restriction or fixation of the arytenoid cartilage is characteristic of arthritic involvement in this region.

Laryngeal Edema

Edema of the laryngeal mucosa is manifested radiologically by a thickening that may be confined to the vocal cords (Reinke edema) or may diffusely involve the entire larynx (Quincke edema).

Wegener Granulomatosis

Wegener granulomatosis is a chronic collagen disease characterized by multiple necrotizing granulomas arising from the nose and upper respiratory tract (Fig. 13.**14**). As the disease progresses, it may spread to involve the hypopharynx, larynx, and trachea, and radiographs may demonstrate foci in the lung. The diagnosis is established by otorhinolaryngoscopic examination and biopsy and by detecting autoantibodies against cytoplasmic antigens in granulocytes. MRI reveals inflammatory mucosal changes and cartilage destruction.

Degenerative Changes

The variable radiologic morphology of the thyroid cartilage depends on its degree of ossification (hyaline cartilage, fat marrow, osteosclerosis), leading to age-dependent variations in the attenuation and signal characteristics of the cartilage on CT and MRI (Figs. 13.**4** and 13.**5a**). An awareness of these physiologic changes is essential in the diagnosis of tumor invasion. Radiologic criteria of tumor involvement are asymmetric growth or enhancement, cortical plate disruption, and the visualization of extralaryngeal tumor tissue.

Traumatic Lesions

Trauma to the larynx or hypopharynx may consist of *external injuries* (gunshot, stab injury, strangulation) or *internal injuries* (caustic ingestion, foreign-body aspiration, iatrogenic trauma) (Figs. 13.**6** and 13.**17**).

In acute situations, conventional biplane radiographs can localize radiopaque foreign bodies and accompanying soft-tissue changes. But ordinary radiographs cannot exclude trauma from radiolucent objects (wood, glass, plastic, etc.), and some cases may require evaluation by CT (Fig. 14.**7**). In subacute cases, foreign bodies should be differentiated from inflammatory or neoplastic lesions of the hypopharynx and larynx.

Thyroid Cartilage Fracture

CT will generally define the fracture line through the thyroid cartilage along with associated hematoma or soft-tissue swelling. Narrowing and displacement of the trachea may also be seen (Figs. 13.**6a, b**).

Dislocation of an Arytenoid Cartilage

CT is required to diagnose dislocation of an arytenoid cartilage from its anatomic position or unphysiologic rotation of the cartilage.

Iatrogenic and Posttherapeutic Changes

Iatrogenically induced changes and posttherapeutic sequelae are an essential part of differential diagnostic considerations in the head and neck region (Fig. 14.**7**).

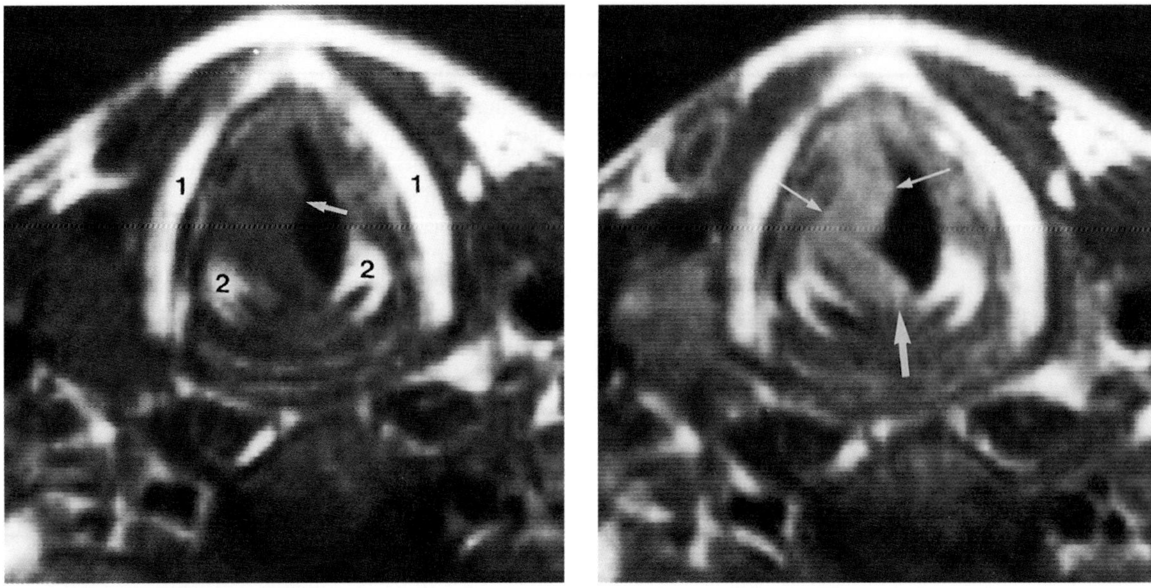

a b

Figs. 13.3 a, b **Glottic carcinoma.**
(**a**) Unenhanced T1-weighted spin-echo (SE) sequence (TR/TE = 500/17 ms) shows irregular expansion of the right vocal cord (arrow) with constriction of the laryngeal airway. Fat marrow accounts for the normal high signal intensity of the thyroid and arytenoid cartilages.
1 Thyroid cartilage
2 Arytenoid cartilage

(**b**) Contrast enhancement clearly demarcates the tumor (arrows) from the intrinsic laryngeal muscles. The tumor has already crossed the midline at the anterior and posterior commissures.

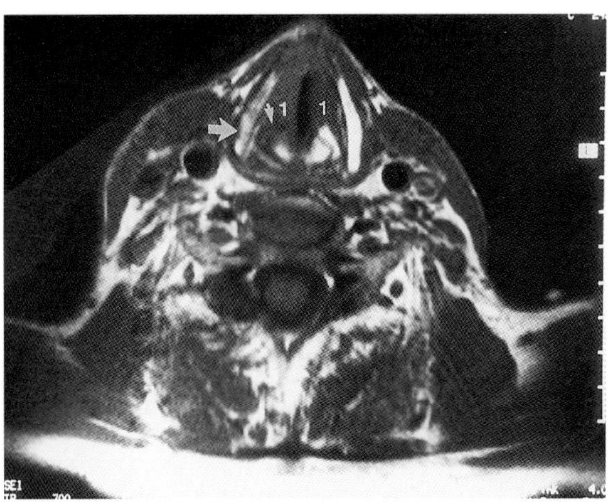

△
Fig. 13.4 **Glottic carcinoma.** T1-weighted MR image (TR/TE = 600/17 ms) shows approximate symmetry of the vocal folds, but the right thyroid cartilage has a patchy, nonhomogeneous appearance (large arrow) and there is loss of signal in the right arytenoid cartilage (small arrow) caused by malignant invasion.
1 Vocal folds

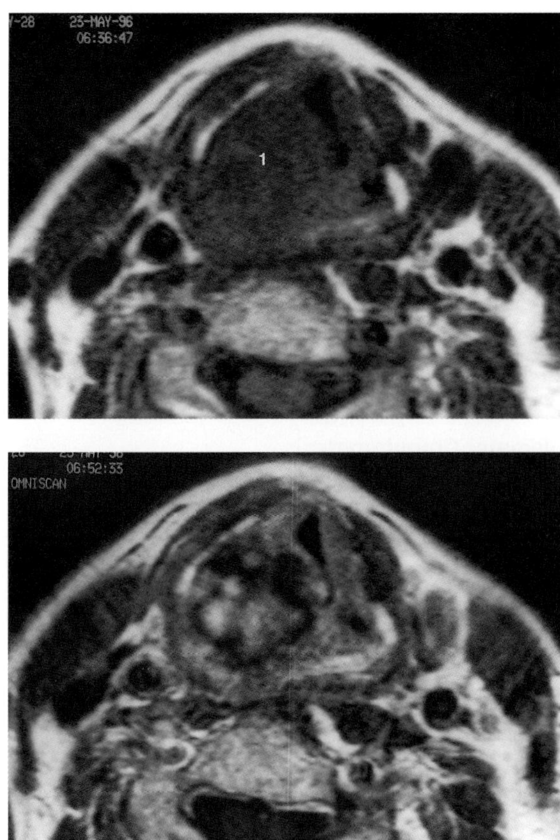

a b

Figs. 13.5 ▷

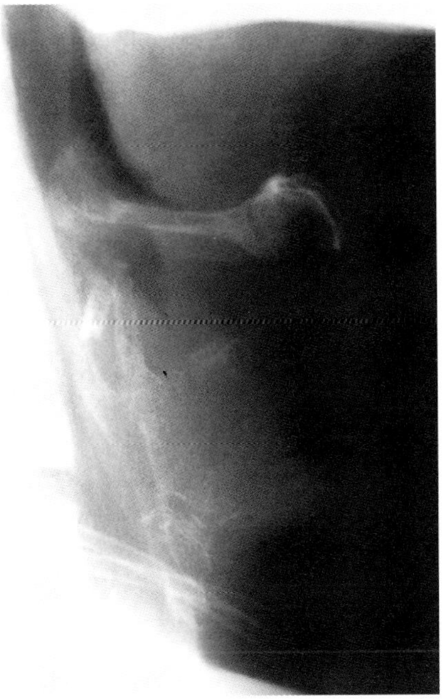

a

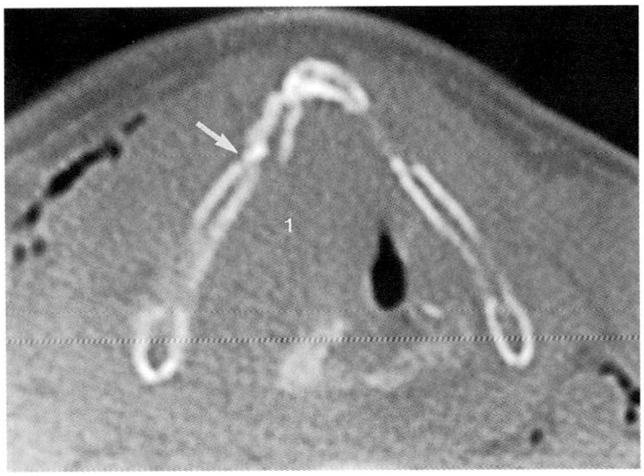

b

Figs. 13.**6 a, b** **Fracture of the thyroid cartilage.**
(**a**) Lateral radiograph following blunt trauma from a blow to the larynx shows fragmentation of the ossified thyroid cartilage with displacement of the superior pole.
(**b**) CT scan defines the fracture (arrow) in the anterior part of the thyroid cartilage along with a paralaryngeal hematoma displacing the airway to the opposite side. The scan also shows posttraumatic subcutaneous soft-tissue emphysema on the right side.
1 Paralaryngeal hematoma

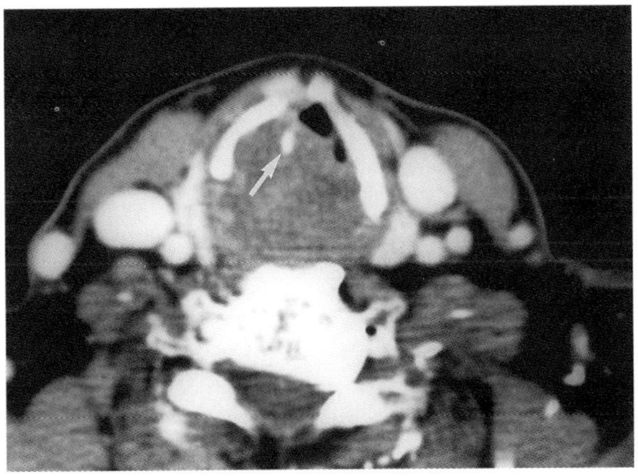

c

◁ Figs. 13.**5 a – c** **Chondroma.**
(**a**) Unenhanced T1-weighted image (TR/TE = 500/25 ms) shows a right-sided mass at the level of the glottic plane arising from the cricoid cartilage, whose fat marrow can still be partially identified on the left side following ossification. The fat marrow of the thyroid cartilage displays normal high signal intensity. The well-defined margins, typical site of occurrence, and airway constriction identify the lesion as a chondroma.
1 Mass
(**b**) After contrast administration, the mass shows a markedly nonhomogeneous internal structure with focal enhancement and areas of deficient perfusion. The tumor margins are still sharply defined.
(**c**) CT scan at a comparable level confirms anterior displacement of the right arytenoid cartilage (arrow). Lack of arytenoid cartilage invasion distinguishes the tumor from glottic carcinoma.

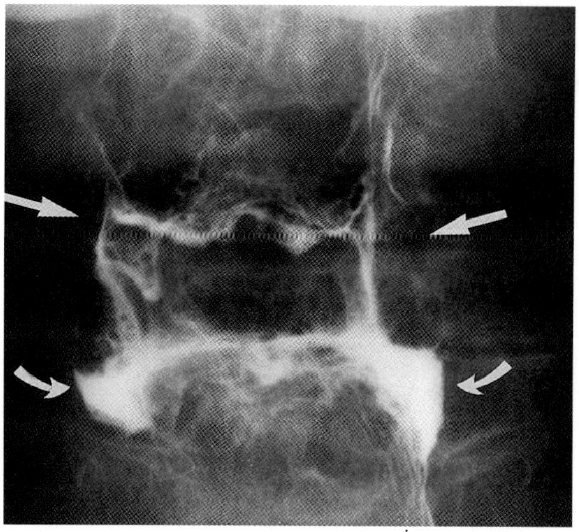

Fig. 13.**7** **Hypopharyngeal carcinoma.** Conventional barium-swallow radiograph shows asymmetry of the valleculae (arrows) and piriform sinuses (curved arrows) and limitation of pharyngeal motion during swallowing, suggestive of malignant invasion. There is an urgent indication for further evaluation by sectional imaging.

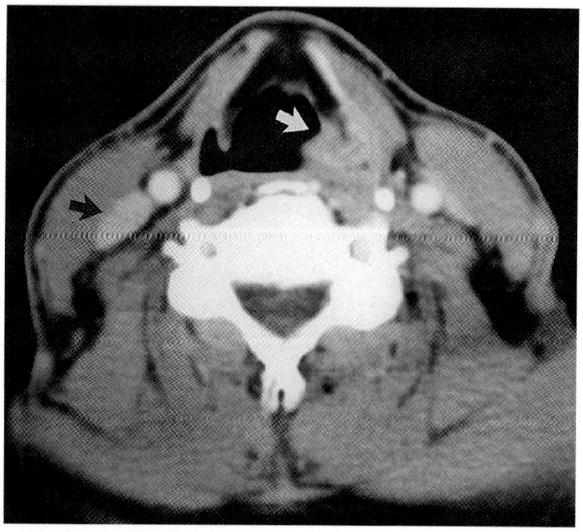

Fig. 13.**8** **Hypopharyngeal carcinoma.** CT scan shows tumor tissue (white arrow) completely filling the left piriform sinus and displacing the common carotid artery posteriorly. The enlarged parajugular lymph node on the right side (black arrow) appears reactive rather than metastatic by its morphologic features.

a

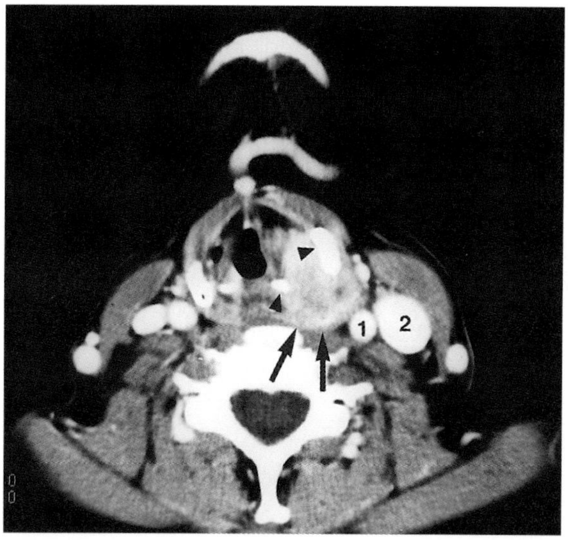

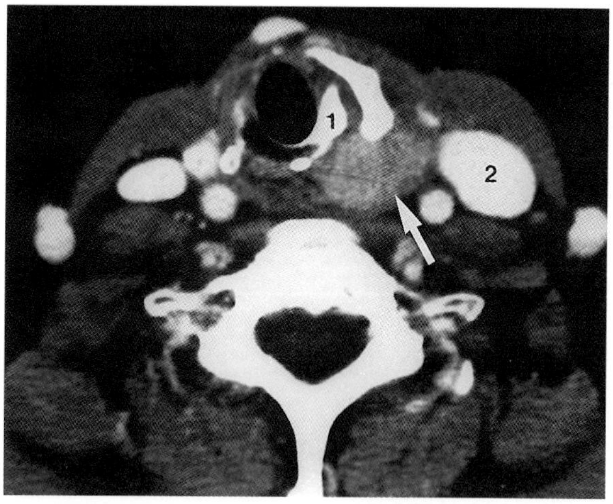

b

Figs. 13.**9 a, b** **Hypopharyngeal carcinoma.**
(**a**) Post-contrast CT shows a hypopharyngeal carcinoma (arrows) that has developed in the lower portions of the left piriform sinus in the postcricoid region near the upper esophageal sphincter. Despite its marked enhancement, the tumor is clearly distinguishable from the contrast-filled great vessels of the neck. The tumor extends anteriorly between the thyroid and arytenoid cartilages (arrowheads) toward the paralaryngeal space.
1 Common carotid artery
2 Internal jugular vein

(**b**) CT scan at a lower level shows the tumor (arrow) posterior to the cricoid cartilage and extending laterally to the internal jugular vein.
1 Cricoid cartilage
2 Internal jugular vein

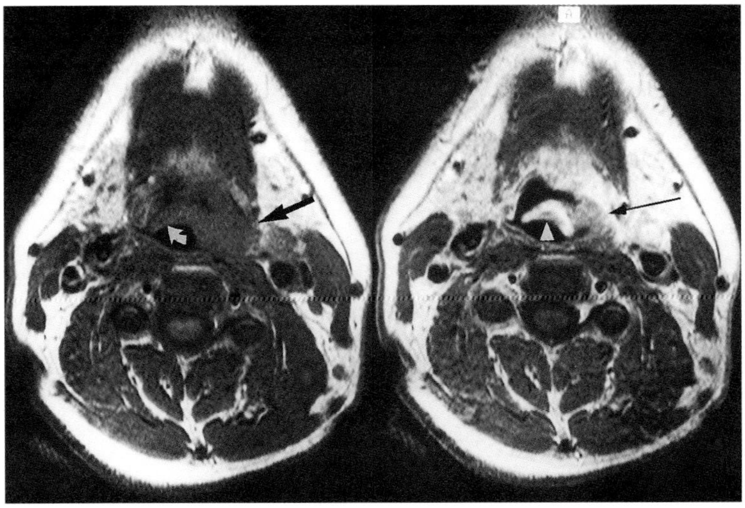

a b

Figs. 13.**10 a, b** **Hypopharyngeal carcinoma (stage T2).**
(**a**) Unenhanced T1-weighted SE sequence (TR/TE = 600/17 ms) shows a hypointense mass in the area of the left glossoepiglottic folds (black arrow) displacing the epiglottis (white arrow) to the opposite side and filling the left vallecula.
(**b**) After contrast administration the tumor (arrow) shows less enhancement than the inflamed, thickened mucosa in the epiglottic area (arrowhead).

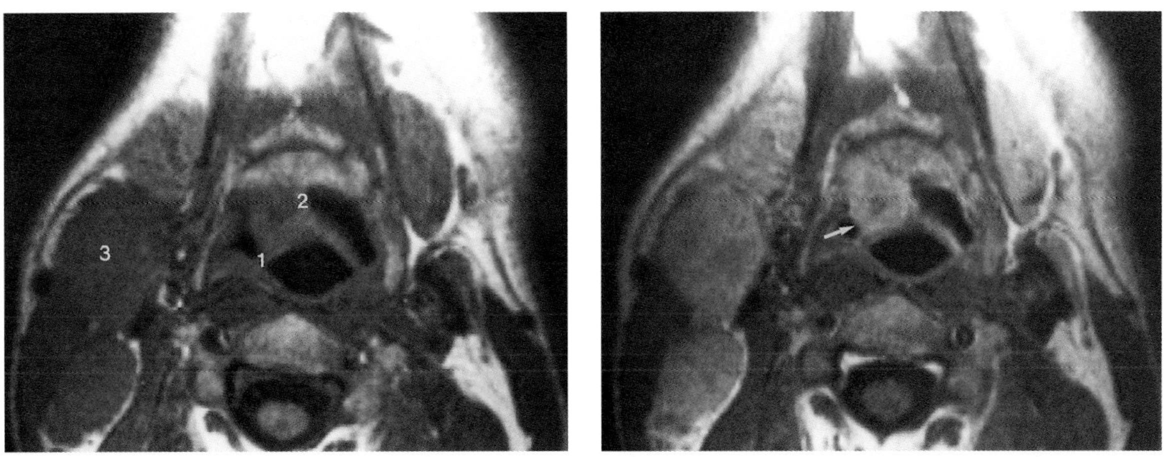

a b

Figs. 13.**11 a, b** **Hypopharyngeal carcinoma.**
(**a**) T1-weighted MR image (TR/TE = 600/17 ms) shows a hypointense mass in the area of the right vallecula abutting the lateral and median glossoepiglottic folds. A parajugular cervical lymph node on the right side is pathologically enlarged.
1 Lateral glossoepiglottic fold
2 Median glossoepiglottic fold
3 Lymph node

(**b**) Image after intravenous contrast administration accurately defines the extent of the tumor, which already shows central nonhomogeneities due to deficient vascularization.

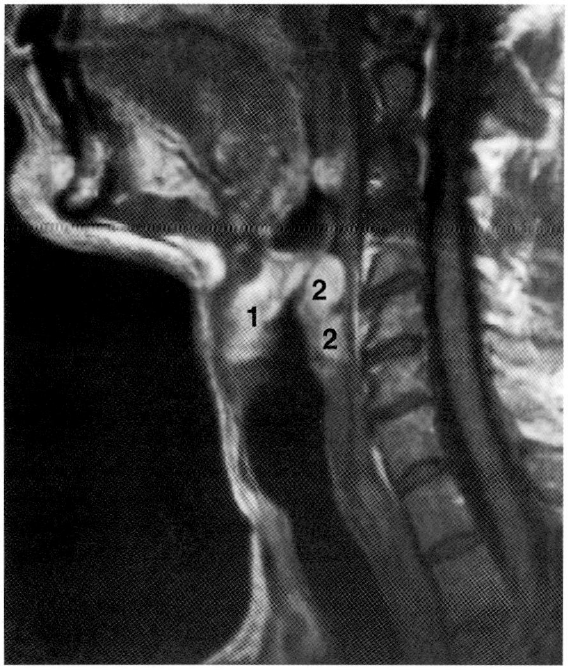

Fig. 13.**12** **Kaposi sarcoma.** Sagittal Gd-enhanced SE sequence (TR/TE = 600/17 ms) in this patient shows markedly enhancing lesions in the anterior (1) and posterior (2) portions of the supraglottic larynx. The lesions are sharply circumscribed with expansile, noninfiltrative margins. These lesions were identified as Kaposi sarcoma in a patient with HIV infection.

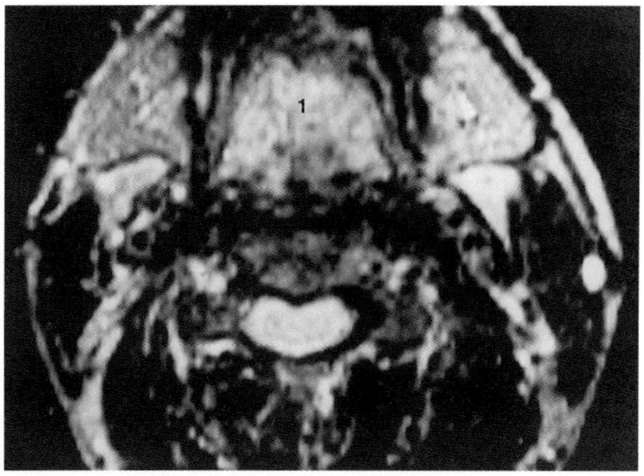

a

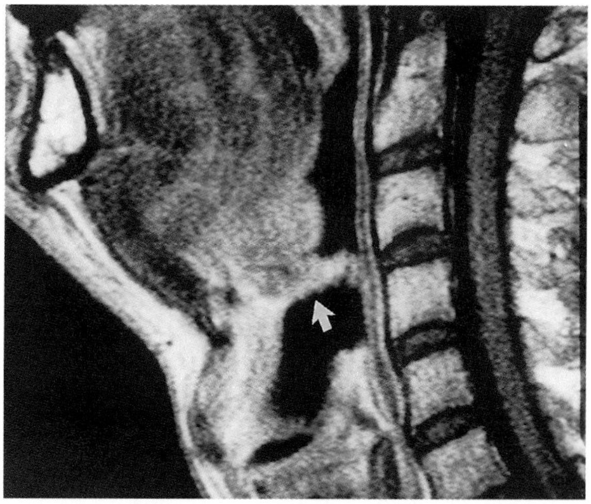

b

Figs. 13.**13 a, b** **Phlegmonous epiglottitis.**
(**a**) Axial unenhanced T2-weighted SE sequence (TR/TE = 3000/90 ms) shows a preepiglottic hyperintense area (1) with indistinct margins consistent with an inflammatory edematous fluid collection.

(**b**) Sagittal Gd-enhanced T1-weighted SE sequence (TR/TE = 600/17 ms) shows the expanded epiglottis (arrow) with increased enhancement extending into the tongue base and supraglottis. Epiglottitis was diagnosed clinically.

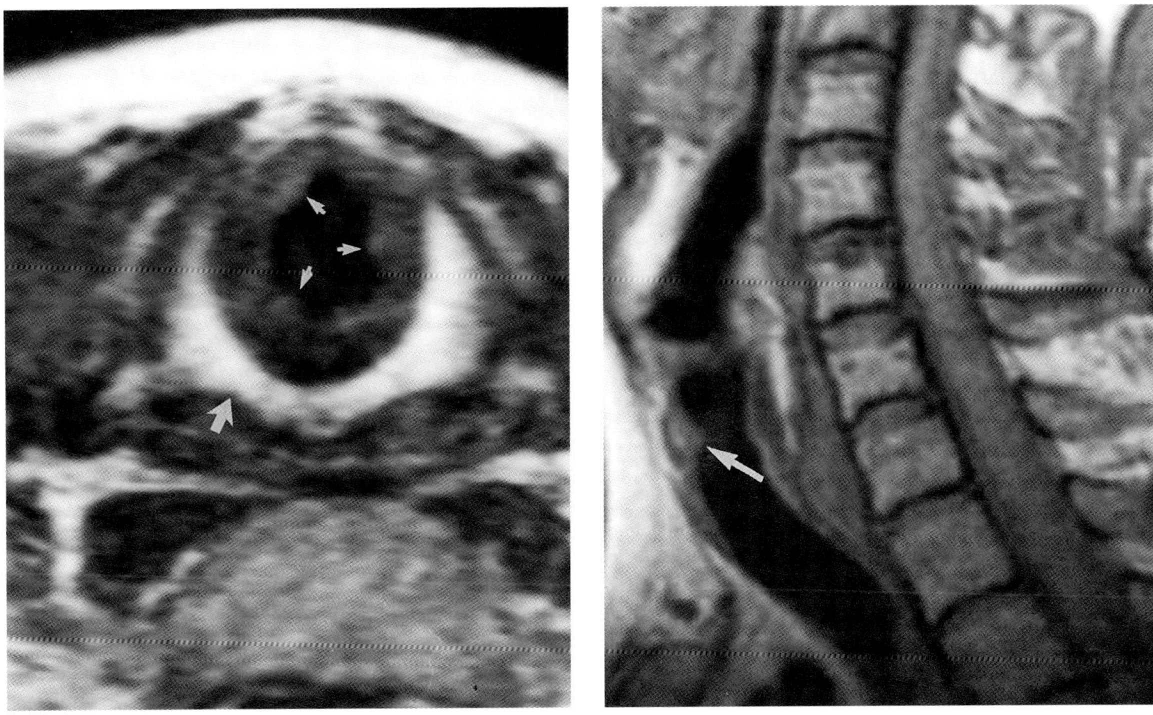

a b

Fig. 13.**14** **Wegener granulomatosis.**
(**a**) Axial T1-weighted image (TR/TE = 600/17 ms) shows the laryngeal air column irregularly bounded by hyperintense soft tissue (small arrows) at the level of the cricoid cartilage (large arrow), which displays high signal intensity and smooth margins.
(**b**) Sagittal view shows local airway constriction (arrow) caused by thickening of the mucosa. A more advanced stage would likely show granulomatous destruction of the laryngeal cartilages.

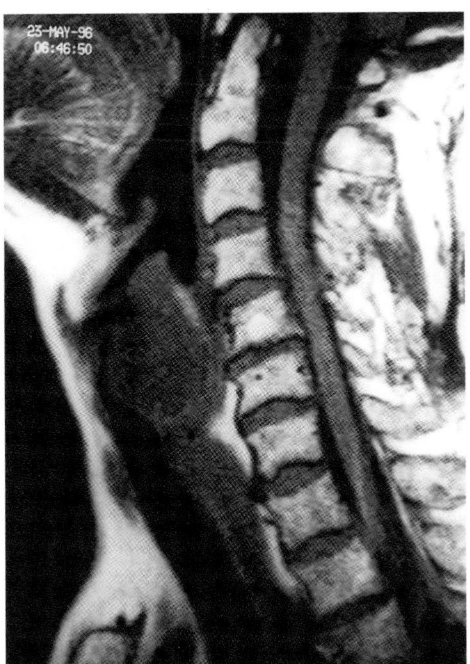

Fig. 13.**15** **Chondroma.** Sagittal MR image defines the craniocaudal extent of the chondroma and its encroachment on the laryngeal airway. The tumor appears purely expansile with no signs of infiltrative growth.

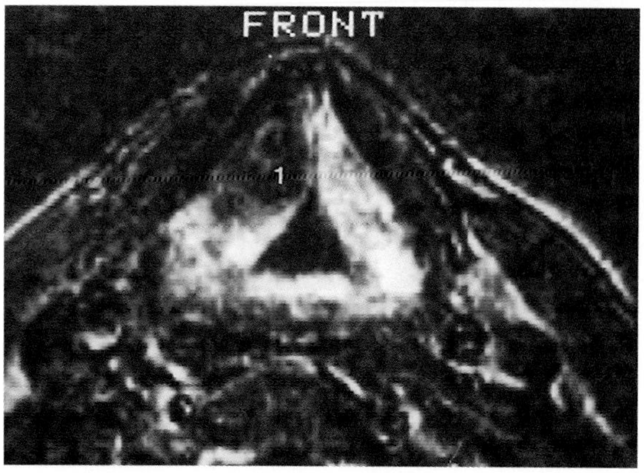

a

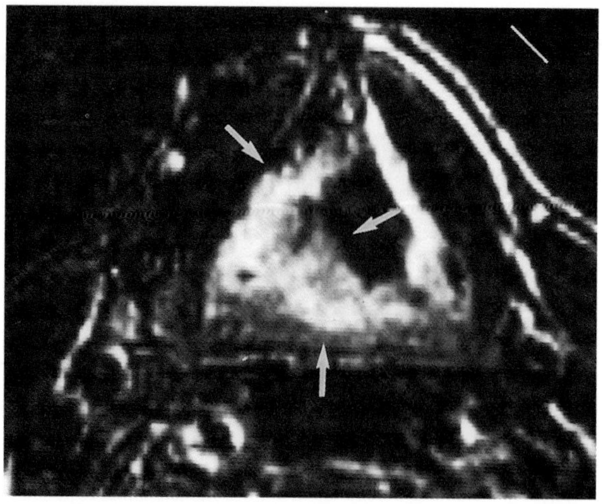

b

Figs. 13.**16** a, b **Laryngeal amyloidosis.**
(**a**) Subtraction MR images at the level of the ventricular folds before and after contrast administration document a circumscribed nonenhancing area on the right side (1) with inflammatory thickening of the mucosa. Biopsy at this site confirmed amyloidosis.

(**b**) Subtraction image at a comparable level in a patient with squamous cell carcinoma shows marked enhancement of the tumor (arrow) with constriction of the laryngeal air column.

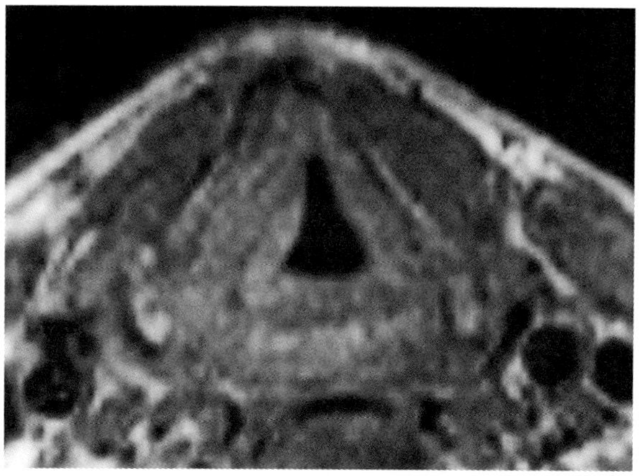

Fig. 13.**17** **Fracture of the thyroid cartilage.** MRI, like CT, can demonstrate a fracture line in the thyroid cartilage (right side). The paralaryngeal hematoma appears isointense to the laryngeal mucosa.

Postoperative Changes

Reconstructive surgical procedures using *tubed flaps*, *interpositional muscle grafts*, and *metallic implants* have considerable clinical importance and must be considered in the interpretation of findings. The accurate documentation of findings, their comparison with previous images, and interdisciplinary consultation are the most important aids to differential diagnosis. With its high soft-tissue resolution, MRI is useful for imaging these reconstructions and distinguishing them from cicatricial changes and recurrent tumor (Figs. 13.**19** and 14.**11**).

Postirradiation Changes

It is very common to find diffuse *inflammatory* and *edematous changes* in an irradiated field during or immediately after the termination of radiotherapy. Chronic changes such as *scar retraction* and osteosclerosis of cartilaginous tissue can occur months or years after a radiotherapy cycle, and CT and MRI should be used to differentiate these changes from recurrent tumor.

Intubation Injuries

Acute intubation injuries are associated with hematoma encroaching upon the airway lumen. Intubation granuloma is a chronic lesion, usually arising from the posterior part of the vocal cords, that may develop several weeks after the injury.

Figs. 13.**18 a, b** **Supraglottic carcinoma.**
(**a**) Coronal T1-weighted image (TR/TE = 600/17 ms) reveals tumor tissue in the left piriform sinus (white arrows) and asymmetry of the valleculae above (black arrows).
(**b**) Gd-enhanced image accurately delineates the tumor margins (arrows), showing extension to the arytenoid cartilage and right piriform sinus.
1 Arytenoid cartilage
2 Piriform sinus

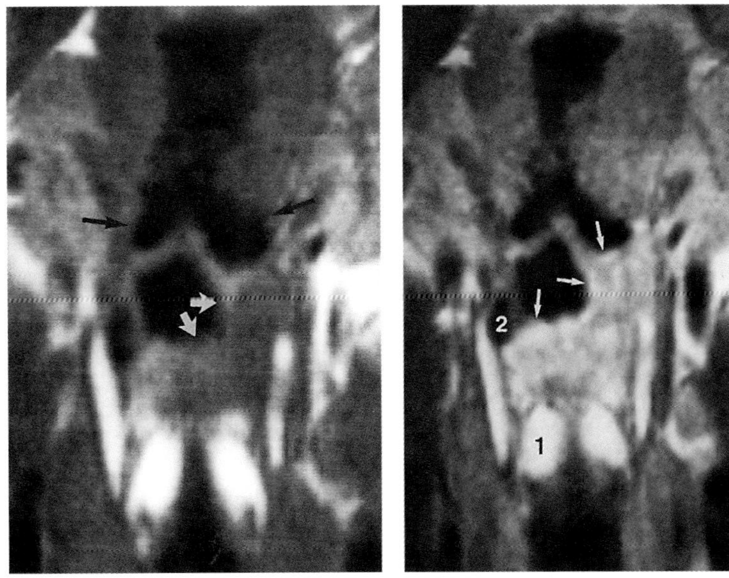

a b

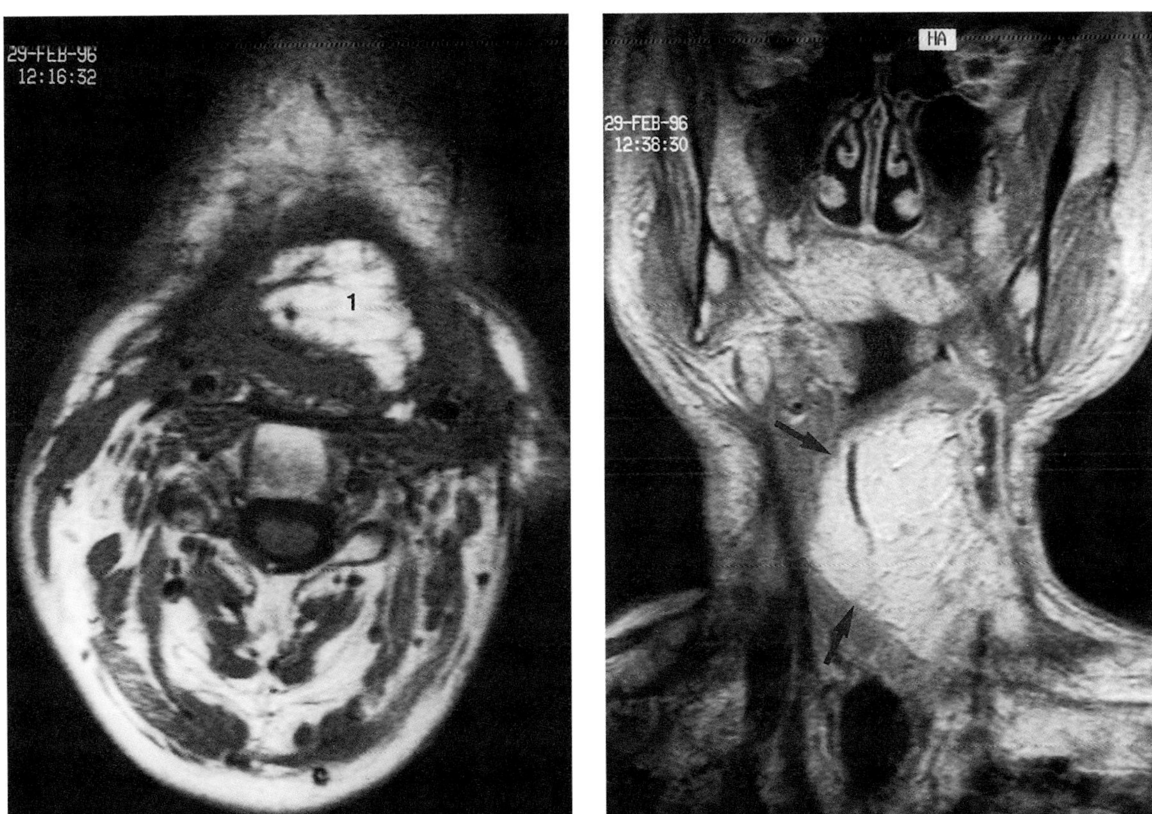

a b

Figs. 13.**19 a, b** **Postlaryngectomy fat graft.**
(**a**) Axial T1-weighted image (TR/TE = 600/17 ms) shows the interpositional fat graft as a hyperintense mass.
1 Fat graft

(**b**) Coronal view shows the smooth edges of the graft (arrows) and its attachment to the left shoulder girdle.

Imaging Criteria and Their Differential Diagnosis

Clinical incidence is a factor that should be considered in differential diagnosis. Lesions of the larynx and hypopharynx are listed in order of frequency in Table 13.**1**.

Liquid Masses

A liquid mass in the larynx or hypopharynx can be reliably detected by ultrasound, CT, and MRI. The differential diagnosis includes cysts, laryngocele, inflammatory lesions, and necrotic tumors. Topographically, laryngocele arises from the laryngeal ventricle (Figs. 13.**1** and 13.**2**) while cysts and abscesses may occur at any site (Tables 13.**2** - 13.**5**).

Table 13.**1** Differential diagnosis of laryngeal lesions

Common:
- Carcinoma (Figs. 13.**3**, 13.**4**, 13.**18**)
- Congenital lesions:
  —Atresia
  —Hypoplasia
  —Stricture
  —Stenosis
  —Laryngomalacia
- Foreign body
- Infection (Fig. 13.**13**):
  —Viral
  —Bacterial
  —Fungal
  —Retropharyngeal tuberculosis
  —Abscess
- Benign tumors:
  —Hemangioma
  —Papilloma
- Trauma (Figs. 13.**6**, 13.**17**, 14.**7**)
- Vocal cord paralysis caused by tumor (Fig. 13.**3**), trauma, or congenital defect
- Zenker diverticulum
- Laryngocele (Figs. 13.**1**, 13.**2**)

Rare:
- Amyloidosis (Fig. 13.**16**)
- Benign tumors:
  —Angiofibroma
  —Chondroma (Figs. 13.**5**, 13.**15**)
  —Rhabdomyoma
  —Fibroma
- Malignant tumors:
  —Sarcoma
- Sarcoidosis
- Wegener granulomatosis (Fig. 13.**14**)
- Endolaryngeal cyst
- Metastasis

Table 13.2 Differential diagnosis of liquid masses

Findings	Differential diagnostic criteria
Common:	
➤ Variant: —Laryngocele	Topography
➤ Mass lesion: —Cyst —Necrotic tumor	Morphology
➤ Inflammatory lesion: —Abscess	Morphology
Rare:	
➤ Variant: —Lymphocele	
➤ Vascular lesion: —Thrombosed aneurysm	

Table 13.3 Topographic and morphologic criteria for liquid masses

Topographic criteria:

- ➤ Arising from laryngeal ventricle:
  - —Laryngocele (Figs. 13.**1**, 13.**2**)
- ➤ Ubiquitous:
  - —Cyst
  - —Abscess (usually postoperative)
  - —Necrotic tumor

Morphologic criteria:

- ➤ Homogeneous margins:
  - —Cyst
  - —Laryngocele
- ➤ Narrow rim:
  - —Cyst
  - —Laryngocele
  - —Abscess
- ➤ Broad rim:
  - —Tumor with central necrosis

Table 13.4 Differential diagnostic criteria for liquid masses in CT

Attenuation between 20 and 60 HU, depending on protein content of fluid:

- ➤ Transsudate, serous fluid < 30 HU:
  - —Cyst
  - —Laryngocele
- ➤ Exudate > 30 HU:
  - —Abscess
- ➤ Nonenhancing fluid:
  - —Cyst
  - —Laryngocele
  - —Abscess
  - —Necrosis
- ➤ Narrow enhancing rim:
  - —Cyst
  - —Abscess
- ➤ Broad enhancing rim:
  - —Tumor with central necrosis

Table 13.5 Differential diagnostic criteria for liquid masses in MRI

- ➤ Low T1-weighted signal intensity, high T2-weighted signal intensity:
  - —Fluid-filled cyst
  - —Laryngocele
  - —Abscess
  - —Necrosis
- ➤ Absence of central enhancement:
  - —Cyst
  - —Laryngocele
  - —Abscess
  - —Necrosis
- ➤ Narrow enhancing rim:
  - —Cyst
  - —Abscess
- ➤ Broad enhancing rim:
  - —Tumor with central necrosis

Air-Containing Masses

The differential diagnosis of air-containing masses includes air-containing *cysts* and *laryngocele*. Air-containing cysts often result from a previous needle procedure, but air formation in cysts may occur spontaneously. Air can also form within abscesses as gas-containing vesicles undergo liquefaction.

Table 13.**6** Differential diagnosis of air-containing masses

Findings	Differential diagnostic criteria
Common:	
➤ Variant: —Laryngocele, pharyngocele —Zenker diverticulum	Morphology, density/signal characteristics Topography
➤ Mass lesion: —Air-containing cyst	Morphology
➤ Inflammatory lesion: —Abscess	Morphology, contrast enhancement
Rare:	
➤ Trauma —Air emphysema	Density/signal characteristics
➤ Iatrogenic —Postoperative, postinterventional	

Table 13.**7** Differential diagnostic criteria for air-containing masses in imaging studies

- Hypodense internal structure on CT, attenuation < 100 HU
- On MRI, internal structure hypointense or devoid of signal
- Narrow enhancing rim:
  —Cyst
  —Laryngocele
- Nonhomogeneous peripheral enhancement with solid components:
  —Abscess
  —Necrosis

Solid Tumor Masses

Squamous cell carcinoma is by far the most common solid tumor of the larynx and hypopharynx. Other malignant and benign tumors are much less frequent in this region. The primary role of diagnostic imaging is to assess topography, stage the tumor, and differentiate between primary and secondary tumor involvement.

The differential diagnosis of common and rare laryngeal masses is summarized in Tables 13.**8** - 13.**12**.

Table 13.**8** Differential diagnosis of laryngeal masses

Common:
- Malignant tumors:
  —Squamous cell carcinoma: hypopharynx (Figs. 13.**7**—13.**11**), supraglottis (Fig. 13.**18**), glottis and subglottis (Figs. 13.**3**, 13.**4**)
- Benign tumors:
  —Juvenile papilloma
  —Polyp
- Inflammatory (Fig. 13.**13**):
  —Abscess

Rare:
- Benign lesions:
  —Laryngocele (Figs. 13.**1**, 13.**2**)
  —Endolaryngeal cyst
  —Chondroma (Figs. 13.**5**, 13.**15**)
  —Lipoma
  —Fibroma
  —Rhabdomyoma
  —Hemangioma
- Malignant tumors:
  —Chondrosarcoma
  —Rhabdomyosarcoma
- Semimalignant tumors:
  —Kaposi sarcoma (Fig. 13.**12**)
- Systemic:
  —Amyloidosis (Fig. 13.**16**)

Table 13.9 Topographic and morphologic criteria for the differential diagnosis of laryngeal masses

Topographic criteria:

- Arising from laryngeal cartilages, usually cricoid cartilage
  —Chondroma (Figs. 13.**5**, 13.**15**)
  —Chondrosarcoma
- Arising from vocal cords:
  —Papilloma, polyp
- Ubiquitous, arising anywhere on the mucosa:
  —Squamous cell carcinoma
  —Kaposi sarcoma (Fig. 13.**12**)

Morphologic criteria:

- Asymmetry, nonhomogeneous internal structure, indistinct infiltrative margins, bone and cartilage destruction, airway encroachment:
  —Squamous cell carcinoma (Figs. 13.**3**, 13.**7**–13.**11**, 13.**18**)
  —Chondrosarcoma
- Homogeneous or cauliflower–like appearance, smooth margins, not calcified:
  —Polyp
  —Papilloma
- Nonhomogeneous, partially calcified, smooth margins:
  —Chondroma (Figs. 13.**5**, 13.**15**)
  —Hemangioma
- Mucous or submucous en plaque tumor with noninfiltrating margins:
  —Kaposi sarcoma (Fig. 13.**12**)
  —Hemangioma

Table 13.10 Differential diagnostic criteria for laryngeal masses in conventional oral contrast examination

- Asymmetric valleculae or piriform sinuses with mucosal irregularities, fold discontinuities, and airway constriction (Fig. 13.**7**):
  —Squamous cell carcinoma

Table 13.11 Differential diagnostic criteria for laryngeal masses in CT

- Moderately enhancing mass with precontrast attenuation of 30—50 HU, increasing to 50—70 HU after contrast administration (Figs. 13.**8**, 13.**9**):
  —Squamous cell carcinoma
- Hyperdense mass with stippled calcifications:
  —Hemangioma
  —Chondroma (Figs. 13.**5**, 13.**15**)
  —Chondrosarcoma
- Intensely enhancing, noninfiltrating tumor:
  —Kaposi sarcoma (Fig. 13.**12**)
  —Hemangioma

Table 13.12 Differential diagnostic criteria for laryngeal masses in MRI

- Low T1-weighted signal intensity, high T2-weighted signal intensity, and moderate contrast enhancement (Figs. 13.**3**, 13.**10**, 13.**11**, 13.**18**):
  —Squamous cell carcinoma
- Calcifications with central hypointense areas
  —Hemangioma
  —Chondroma (Figs. 13.**5**, 13.**15**)
  —Chondrosarcoma
- High T2-weighted signal intensity and intense contrast enhancement:
  —Kaposi sarcoma (Fig. 13.**12**)
  —Laryngitis or epiglottitis (Fig. 13.**13**)
  —Hemangioma
- High T1-weighted signal intensity and no contrast enhancement:
  —Fat graft (Fig. 13.**19**)
- Low T1- and T2-weighted signal intensity:
  —Amyloidosis (Fig. 13.**16**)

Laryngeal Cartilage Destruction

The diagnostic possibilities range from cartilage invasion by tumors including chondroma and chondrosarcoma and inflammatory processes such as Wegener granulomatosis and perichondritis to cricoarytenoid arthritis and osteosclerosis, fractures of the thyroid cartilage, and physiologic ossification (Tables 13.**13** – 13.**16**).

Table 13.**13** Topographic and morphologic criteria for the differential diagnosis of laryngeal cartilage destruction

Topographic criteria:

- Thyroid cartilage
  - Tumor invasion (T4 lesion)
  - Osteosclerosis, ossification
  - Fracture
- Cricoid cartilage:
  - Tumor invasion (T4 lesion)
  - Chondroma, chondrosarcoma
  - Osteosclerosis
  - Arthritis
  - Ossification
- Arytenoid cartilage:
  - Tumor invasion (all stages)
  - Perichondritis
  - Arthritis

Morphologic criteria:

- Symmetry:
  - Osteosclerosis
  - Perichondritis
  - Arthritis
  - Ossification
- Nonhomogeneous internal structure:
  - Chondroma, chondrosarcoma (Figs. 13.**5**, 13.**15**)
  - Tumor invasion (Fig. 13.**18**)
  - Osteosclerosis
- Cortical plate disruption:
  - Tumor invasion
  - Fracture
- Adjacent soft tissues:
  - Tumor invasion (Fig. 13.**18**)
  - Perichondritis
  - Arthritis
  - Wegener granulomatosis (Fig. 13.**14**)

Table 13.**14** Differential diagnostic criteria for laryngeal cartilage destruction in CT

- Cortical plate disruption:
  - Tumor invasion
  - Fracture (Fig. 13.**6**)
- Negative central attenuation:
  - Ossification (fat marrow)
- Intense adjacent contrast enhancement:
  - Perichondritis
  - Arthritis
- Moderate adjacent contrast enhancement:
  - Tumor invasion (Figs. 13.**8**, 13.**9**)
- No adjacent contrast enhancement:
  - Fracture (with hematoma)

Table 13.**15** Differential diagnostic criteria for laryngeal cartilage destruction in MRI

- High T1-weighted signal intensity:
  - Ossification (fat marrow)
- High T2-weighted signal intensity (adjacent):
  - Perichondritis
  - Arthritis
- Intense adjacent contrast enhancement:
  - Perichondritis
  - Arthritis
- Moderate adjacent contrast enhancement:
  - Tumor invasion (Fig. 13.**8**)
- No adjacent contrast enhancement:
  - Fracture (with hematoma)

Table 13.**16** Signal characteristics of laryngeal structures in MRI

Structure	T1-weighted sequence	T2-weighted sequence
Hyaline cartilage	Intermediate signal intensity	Intermediate signal intensity
Calcified cartilage	Low signal intensity	Low signal intensity
Ossification (fat marrow)	High signal intensity	Intermediate signal intensity
Perichondrium	Low signal intensity	Low signal intensity
Preepiglottic space	High signal intensity	Intermediate signal intensity
Tumor	Low signal intensity and contrast enhancement	High signal intensity

Unilateral Vocal Cord Paralysis

The most frequent cause of unilateral vocal cord paralysis is recurrent nerve palsy. The differential diagnoses listed in Table 13.**17** should be evaluated on the basis of CT or MR findings.

Table 13.**17** Causes of unilateral vocal cord paralysis
Aortic aneurysm
Primary neoplasms:
—Bronchial carcinoma
—Thyroid carcinoma
—Esophageal carcinoma
Secondary neoplasms, metastases
Local mass lesion or inflammation of a vocal cord (Fig. 13.**3**)
Mediastinal lesion
Postoperative sequela
Trauma

Summary and Diagnostic Strategy

The clinical examination itself should significantly advance the differential diagnosis of laryngeal and hypopharyngeal disease. Conventional radiographs and CT scans can direct treatment planning in trauma patients and can define the extent of a congenital anomaly. It is particularly important to narrow the differential diagnosis when distinguishing inflammatory from neoplastic processes. The most common neoplasm occurring in this region is squamous cell carcinoma (Figs. 13.**3**, 13.**7** – 13.**11**, 13.**18**). Using modern sectional imaging techniques and applying the above differential diagnostic criteria, the radiologist should be able to differentiate squamous cell carcinoma from less common tumors such as chondroma (Figs. 13.**5** and 13.**15**), chondrosarcoma, Kaposi sarcoma (Fig. 13.**12**), polyps, papillomas, and other rare lesions.

References

1 Castelijns, J. A., M. C. Kaiser, J. Valk, G. J. Gerritsen, A. H. van Hattum, G. B. Snow: Magnetic Resonance Imaging of the laryngeal cancer. J Comput Assist Tomogr. 11 (1987) 134–140
2 Dillon, W. P., H. R. Harnsberger: The impact of radiologic imaging on staging of cancer of the head and neck. Semin Oncol. 18 (1991) 64–79
3 Lufkin, R. B., J. D. Robinson, D. J. Castro, B. A. Jabour, G. Duckwiler, L. J. Layfield, W. N. Hanafee: Interventional Magnetic Resonance Imaging in the head and neck. Top Magn Reson Imaging 2 (1990) 76–80
4 Naumann, H. H.: Differentialdiagnostik in der Hals-Nasen-Ohren-Heilkunde. Thieme, Stuttgart 1990
5 Spiessl, B., P. Hermanek, O. Scheibe, G. Wagner: TNM-Atlas UICC. Springer, Berlin 1982
6 Steinkamp, H. J., T. Heim, J. Mäurer, M. Mathe, R. Felix: Wertigkeit von Magnetresonanztomographie und Computertomographie im Tumorstaging des Larynx-/Hypopharynxkarzinoms. Fortschr Röntgenstr. 158 (1993) 437–444
7 Vogl, Th., W. Steger, G. Grevers, M. Schreiner, S. Dresel, J. Lissner: MRI with Gd-DTPA in Tumors of Larynx and Hypopharynx. Eur J Radiol. 1 (1991) 58–64

14 Soft Tissues of the Neck

The clinical examination should always precede the radiologic evaluation of soft-tissue lesions in the neck. Clinical palpation is of key importance in classifying a lesion as soft or firm, fixed or mobile, and tender or nontender. The primary diagnostic imaging modality in the cervical region is ultrasonography (Figs. 14.**9**, 14.**17**, 14.**22**). Ultrasound is particularly useful for differentiating between cystic and solid masses. Computed tomography (CT) and magnetic resonance imaging (MRI) are available for addressing more complex differential diagnostic issues.

Normal Anatomy

The anatomic region of the neck is bounded above by the inferior border of the mandible and occipital bone and below by an imaginary plane between the suprasternal notch and the seventh cervical vertebra. Various fascial layers subdivide the neck into compartments that are important in the interpretation of transaxial images (Fig. 14.**1**).

The *visceral compartment* is the most anterior of the fascia-defined spaces in the neck and contains the aerodigestive tract including the larynx, trachea, and esophagus. The thyroid gland and parathyroid glands are also located in this compartment. The normal thyroid gland appears on MRI as a symmetric, homogeneous soft-tissue structure situated anterior and lateral to the trachea. Normal thyroid tissue has a higher signal intensity on T2-weighted images than the sternocleidomastoid and sternothyroid muscles.

The *posterior compartment* contains the cervical vertebrae and associated flexor and extensor muscles including the scaleni, longus capitis, and longus colli. These muscle groups show MRI signal intensities comparable to those of the intrinsic tongue muscles, while the fibrous fascial tissue has a low signal intensity approximating that of cortical bone. By contrast, hematopoietic marrow and bone marrow appear hyperintense on T1-weighted images. The only structures that show significant contrast enhancement are the mucosa lining the larynx and pharynx, lymphatic tissues, and richly vascularized neoplasms (Figs. 14.**13**, 14.**14**, 14.**19 b**).

The *lateral compartment* principally contains the neurovascular bundle about the common carotid artery (Figs. 14.**24** – 14.**26**). The carotid arteries and jugular veins (Fig. 14.**29**) are clearly distinguishable from surrounding fat or muscle tissue by the flow void that appears in spin-echo (SE) sequences. Even small blood vessels can be identified on axial MR images by this phenomenon and assigned to a parent vessel. Coronal images are often added to the MRI workup to give a better appreciation of topographic relationships. The lateral compartment is particularly important for determining cervical lymph-node status. Normal lymph nodes have signal characteristics comparable to those of thyroid and thymic tissue (Fig. 14.**19**).

An awareness of the anatomy and terminology of the *cervical lymph nodes* (see Ch. 12) is essential for analyzing the normal topographic anatomy of the neck. By reviewing contiguous axial MR images, the radiologist can analyze all essential nodal groups in the neck. An important part of cervical imaging is differentiating among the submental, submandibular, and deep cervical nodal groups. The deep cervical

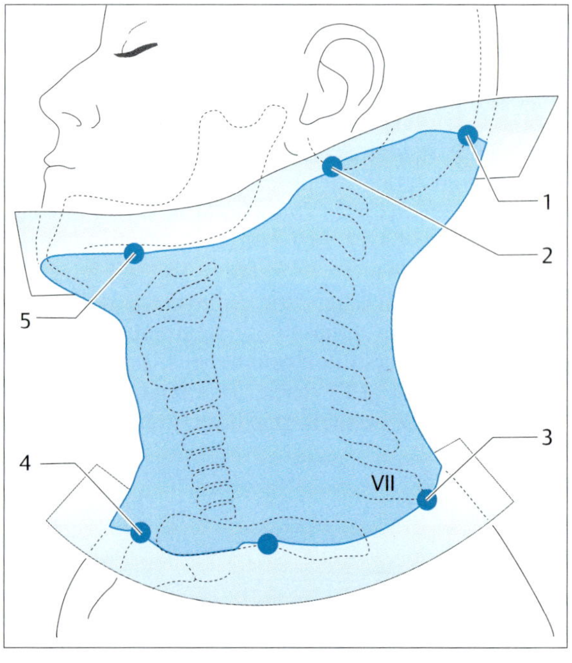

Fig. 14.**1** **Anatomic boundaries of the cervical region.**
1 External occipital protuberance
2 Mastoid bone
3 Seventh cervical vertebra
4 Suprasternal notch
5 Mandible

group is divided into three levels by the thyrohyoid, cricothyroid, and digastric muscles. The upper level, known also as the jugulodigastric group, lies between the posterior belly of the digastric muscle and the hyoid bone. The jugulo-omohyoid nodes are an important group in the lower level. Other diagnostically important nodal groups are the retropharyngeal, deep visceral, paratracheal, and paraesophageal nodes. In normal cases, the cervical nodes visualized by diagnostic imaging will be less than 5 mm in diameter. Inflammatory adenopathy is common, however, and submandibular and jugulodigastric nodes 5 to 10 mm in size may be seen even in healthy individuals (Fig. 14.**9 e**). MRI is useful for lymph node evaluation because the nodes contrast sharply with muscle and fatty tissue and because vascular signal voids clearly differentiate blood vessels from adjacent lymph nodes.

Clinical Signs and Symptoms

The most common clinical manifestations of cervical soft-tissue disease are nonspecific swelling (Fig. 14.**20**) and a solid neck mass. These findings are often associated with nonspecific inflammatory reactions or neck pain. Larger lesions may also cause dysphagia due to extrinsic compression of the hypopharynx or esophagus.

Imaging Evaluation and Differential Diagnosis

Ultrasound

Ultrasonography offers a fast and convenient method for the primary evaluation of neck masses. Most examiners use a 7.5-MHz linear probe, which is excellent for distinguishing cystic from solid lesions and detecting sonodense structures such as calculi within the salivary glands.

Ultrasound is also useful for flow investigations in the carotid arteries. First' conventional B-mode imaging is used to define vascular anatomy and atherosclerotic wall lesions (Fig. 14.**25 c**) and to determine the length and thickness of any plaques that are found. Next, color duplex sonography is performed with a 7.5-MHz linear probe to evaluate the carotid arteries for stenoses. The peak systolic flow velocity determined from spectral curves is used as a criterion for evaluating the degree of stenosis (Figs. 14.**25 d, e**). The ultrasound workup may be supplemented by MRI (Fig. 14.**25 a**), CT angiography (Figs. 14.**23** and 14.**24**), and preinterventional digital subtraction angiography (DSA) (Fig. 14.**25 b**).

Computed Tomography (CT)

If further diagnostic uncertainties exist, CT is the method of choice for further evaluation. CT scans should be obtained in all patients being evaluated for a cervical fracture or herniated disk. CT also permits the assessment of nodal involvement (Fig. 14.**8**) by malignant tumors or inflammatory lesions on axial planes from the skull base to the thoracic inlet in one examination. The slice thickness should range from 2 mm (for evaluating selected bony laminae) to 5 mm (for evaluating mass lesions or lymph nodes). Spiral CT can provide optimum contrast between vessels and lymph nodes when the proper technical parameters are used (contrast administration, slice thickness, table feed and calculated increment no greater than 5 mm). Coronal reconstructions are extremely helpful for evaluating the craniocaudal extent of lymph nodes and various other lesions.

Magnetic Resonance Imaging (MRI)

MRI is advantageous over ultrasound in that it can simultaneously image the neck and mediastinum without artifacts, and it is advantageous over CT in its ability to distinguish soft-tissue lesions from vascular structures without contrast medium (iodinated media should not be used if radioiodine therapy is anticipated). Imaging parameters such as proton density and T1/T2 relaxation times are useful for establishing the identity of various lesions. It is always important in MRI to differentiate any kind of neoplasia from postsurgical scar tissue. With its ability to image in axial and coronal planes, MRI also has a role in the evaluation and localization of lymphadenopathy. Pathologically enlarged lymph nodes that have reached a size of 5 to 10 mm are clearly distinguishable from surrounding fat and muscle tissue. Normal nodal tissue shows relatively long T1 and T2 relaxation times, thus both normal and diseased nodes have low signal intensity on T1-weighted images and are clearly demarcated from adjacent structures in the neurovascular sheath. Similar signal intensities makes it difficult to distinguish them from muscle tissue, however.

Imaging Findings

Congenital Variations and Malformations

Median (Fig. 14.3) and Lateral Neck Cysts (Figs. 14.2 and 14.4)

Median and lateral neck cysts are well-defined congenital lesions whose embryologic origin determines their site of occurrence and characteristics. The more common *median cyst* develops from remnants of the thyroglossal duct and may occur anywhere between the foramen cecum of the tongue and the pyramidal lobe of the thyroid gland. Approximately 65% of these cysts are infrahyoid and 15% are suprasternal. Most are lined by squamous epithelium and filled with lymphatic tissue. *Lateral neck cysts* are remnants of the second or occasionally the third branchial cleft. The lower sinus opening is usually sited along the mid to inferior medial border of the sternocleidomastoid muscle. The sinus tract runs upward between the internal and external carotid arteries and opens into the side of the oropharynx (Fig. 14.**2**). Large neck cysts may extend beneath the sternocleidomastoid muscle and displace nerves and vessels about the common carotid artery (Fig. 14.**4**). MRI performed after ultrasound can define the precise relationship of the cyst and its wall to surrounding structures.

Congenital Cystic Hygroma

Congenital cystic hygroma is a *cystic or cavernous lymphangioma in newborns* that presents as a subcutaneous mass and displaces surrounding tissues. It is usually sufficient to determine the extent of the mass by ultrasound imaging. MRI can be added if a more detailed evaluation is required.

Cervical Hematocele

Hematocele is analogous to cystic hygroma, arising from blood vessels rather than from the lymphatic system.

Tumors

Malignant Lymph-Node Involvement (Figs 14.9 a–e)

The criteria for malignant lymph node involvement are defined as follows:

- Nodal diameter greater than 10 mm.
- Presence of central necrosis.
- More than three clustered lymph nodes.
- Infiltrative growth.
- Fixation to surrounding structures.

Another criterion is the M/T ratio, which relates the maximum diameter of a lymph node to its transverse diameter. A value less than 2 is considered suspicious for malignancy. But all of these criteria, including the M/T ratio, are no more than relative indicators for evaluating nodal invasion. It is equally important to stage lymph nodes according to TNM criteria and describe their location based on levels to 7 (see Table 12.**8**).

Lymphadenitis

Lymph nodes affected by inflammatory changes present smooth margins and a homogeneous internal structure with a definable hilar notch. They show intense enhancement after intravenous contrast administration.

Lymphoma

In patients with multiple matted lymph nodes that individually show a homogeneous internal structure (Fig. 14.**9 f**) and are accompanied by extranodal involvement, a systemic lymphatic disease should be differentiated from Hodgkin or non-Hodgkin lymphoma. Hodgkin disease also may involve the submandibular gland, or an extranodal lymphoma may involve the parotid gland. AIDS patients commonly have lymphomatous invasion of the facial skeleton or multiple, bilateral lymph node involvement in the neck. Imaging of the anterior upper mediastinum often reveals a patchy growth but cannot differentiate Hodgkin from non-Hodgkin lymphoma.

Lipoma, Liposarcoma

Morphologic criteria for lipoma are a high signal intensity on T1-weighted MR images and low attenuation on CT scans. Lipoma has well-defined margins, whereas liposarcoma has indistinct margins and contains solid elements.

"Madelung neck" refers to a diffuse, circumferential fatty hypertrophy marked by a typical posterior notching of the neck (Fig. 14.**10**).

Neuroma, Neurofibroma, Malignant Schwannoma

These tumors typically occur along the neurovascular sheath. Common neuromas of the cervical region are vagus neuroma (Fig. 14.**12 b**) and hypoglossal neuroma. Morphologically, these tumors show a nonhomogeneous internal structure with intense peripheral contrast enhancement. Malignant schwannoma has infiltrating margins.

Fibromatosis

Fibromatosis is a *connective tissue proliferation* that shows variable biologic behavior (Fig. 14.**14**), the lesions ranging from benign fibrous masses to *semi-malignant aggressive* forms. Major sites of predilection in the cervical region are the nuchal muscles and connective-tissue spaces. The preferred imaging modality is MRI, which shows varying enhancement characteristics and degrees of invasiveness, depending on the behavior of the lesion.

Rhabdomyoma, Rhabdomyosarcoma

The mass arises from the neck muscles, but radiologic studies are seldom diagnostic. Histopathologic evaluation is generally required to make a definitive diagnosis.

Chordoma

Chordoma is usually marked radiologically by vertebral body destruction. Tumor tissue in adjacent soft-tissue spaces may show a fibrous pseudocapsule, internal septations, amorphous calcifications, and moderate contrast enhancement.

Goiter

A goiter is an *enlargement of the thyroid gland* (Fig. 14.**17**) that is unrelated to the patient's hormonal status. Diagnosis relies on serologic tests and radionuclide imaging. Diffuse goiter with homogeneous hypertrophy of the thyroid gland is distinguished from nodular goiter, which is characterized by the presence of single or multiple nodules (hot or cold). The goiter may cause tracheoesophageal displacement or compression.

Ultrasound scanning is sufficient in most patients. If the thyroid borders appear ill-defined, further evaluation by CT and MRI should be done to exclude a malignant goiter (Figs. 14.**19** and 14.**21**).

Thyroid Carcinoma

Several histologic types of thyroid malignancy are distinguished:

- Follicular or papillary thyroid carcinoma.
- Squamous cell carcinoma.
- Medullary carcinoma arising from "C cells" (Fig. 14.**21**).
- Anaplastic carcinoma (Fig. 14.**19**), which has the worst prognosis.

Finding cold nodules on radionuclide scans always warrants further investigation, which may include open biopsy, to establish a diagnosis. Imaging studies such as CT and MRI are becoming important for detecting invasion or displacement of the trachea, esophagus, and large mediastinal vessels. They are also used to evaluate local lymph node involvement and differentiate benign nodal hyperplasia from malignant invasion.

Parathyroid Hyperplasia

Imaging studies for the detection and localization of parathyroid tissue are performed only in patients with primary or tertiary hyperparathyroidism (Fig. 14.**16**) or to diagnose recurrence in patients with a history of malignant disease. With ectopic parathyroid glands occurring in up to 20% of cases, sectional imaging should cover the region from the hyoid bone to the aortic arch using contiguous slices.

MRI offers distinct advantages over ultrasound and other modalities in cases where preoperative localization is required.

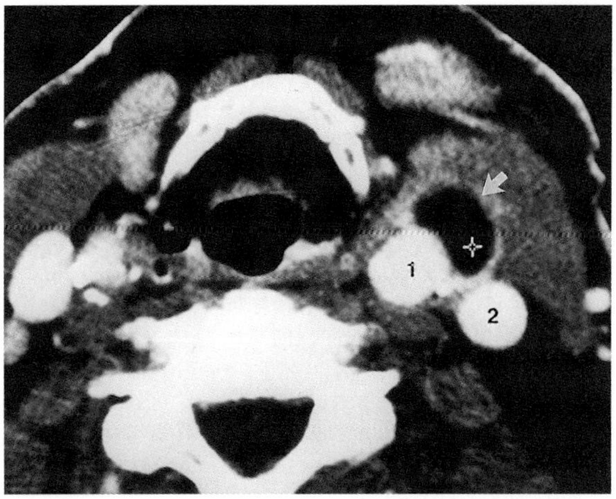

Fig. 14.**2** **Lateral neck cyst.** CT scan at the level of the hyoid bone shows marked opacification of the cervical vessels and, anterior to these, a well-circumscribed mass of fluid density consistent with a lateral neck cyst (arrow and cursor).
1 Common carotid artery
2 Internal jugular vein

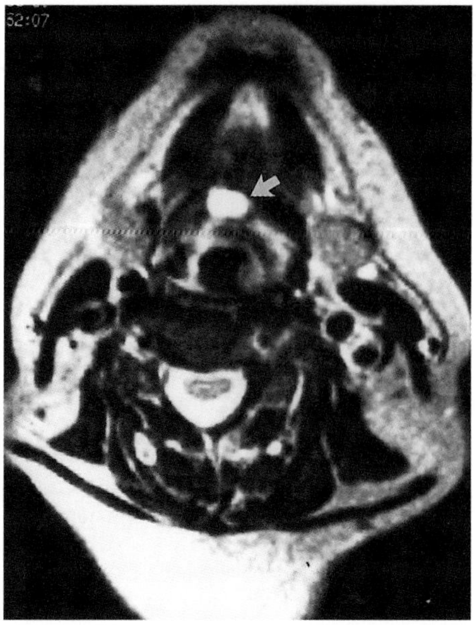

Fig. 14.**3** **Median neck cyst.** Unenhanced T2-weighted SE sequence (TR/TE = 3000/90 ms) shows a markedly hyperintense mass in the medial preepiglottic area (arrow) with well-defined margins and no signs of infiltrative growth.

a

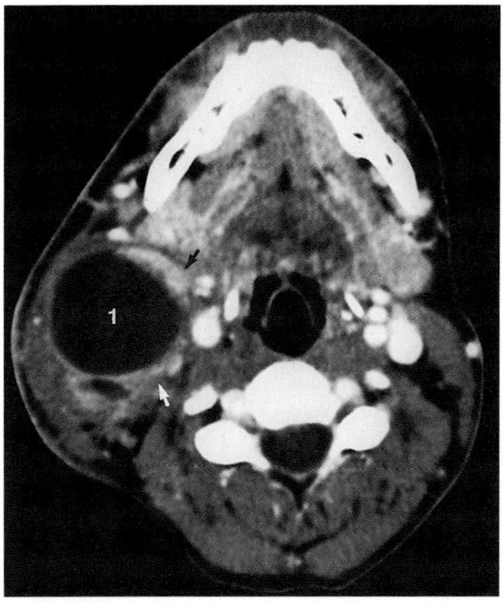

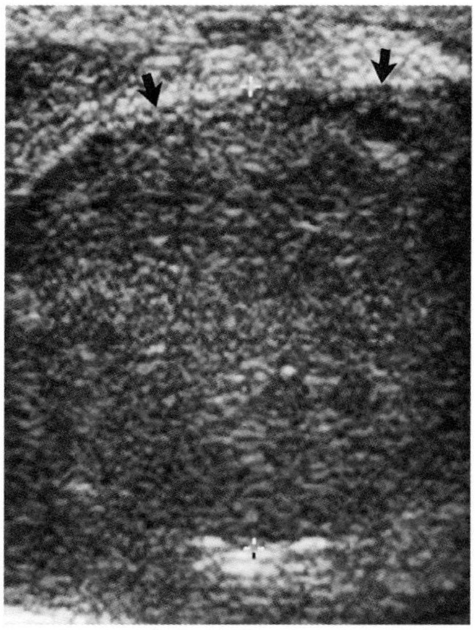

b

Figs. 14.**4** **a, b** **Infected lateral neck cyst.** CT and ultrasound.
(**a**) CT scan at the level of the epiglottis shows an extensive hypodense mass in the right cervical region corresponding to a fluid-filled lateral neck cyst. The cyst wall is thickened anteromedially and posteriorly and shows contrast enhancement (arrows), signifying infection.
1 Hypodense mass

(**b**) Ultrasound image of the cyst (arrows) shows nonhomogeneous internal echoes caused by the protein content of the intracystic fluid.

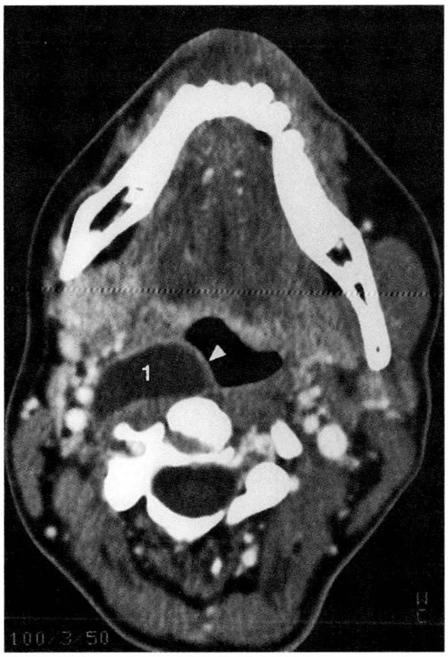

Fig. 14.5 **Parapharyngeal abscess.** Post-contrast CT scan shows a homogeneous, well-circumscribed, hypodense mass with an enhancing rim in the right parapharyngeal space. The mass is displacing and compressing the oropharynx and hypopharynx (arrowhead). The low density of the mass results from the fluid contents of the cyst.
1 Hypodense mass

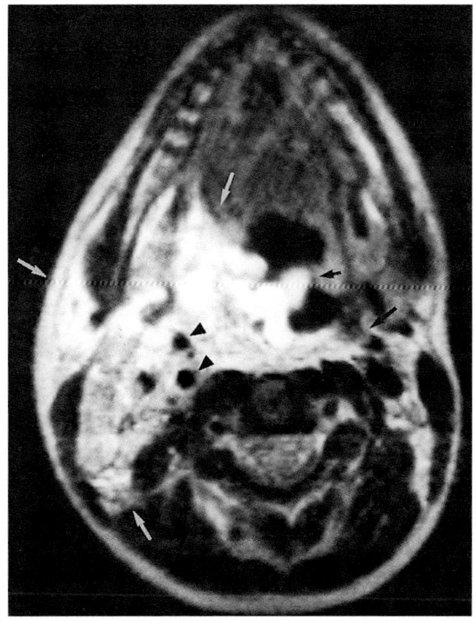

Fig. 14.6 **Cervical cellulitis.** Unenhanced T2-weighted SE sequence (TR/TE = 3000/90 ms) shows an extensive area of high signal intensity in the right parapharyngeal space (white arrows) extending into the nuchal area and enveloping the large cervical vessels (arrowheads). The lesion, which extends far across the midline to the left parapharyngeal space (black arrows), has mostly well-defined margins and has caused little mass effect in relation to its extent. Diagnosis: advanced cellulitic inflammation of the parapharyngeal space and deep cervical space.

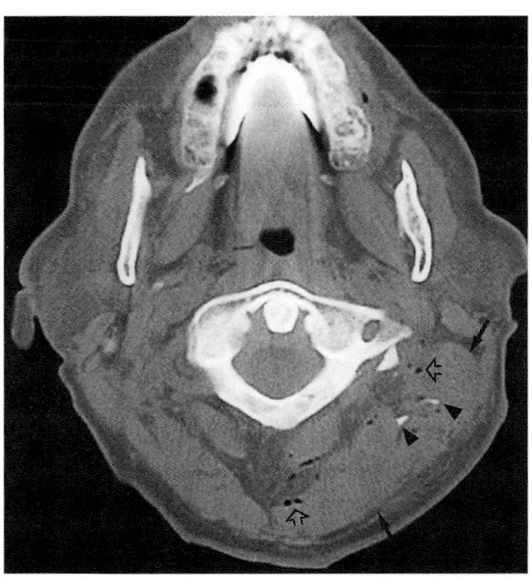

Fig. 14.7 **Trauma.** CT scan shows small densities (arrowheads) in the left nuchal area with surrounding air inclusions (open arrows) and swelling of the nuchal muscles (arrows). The lesions are caused by indriven glass slivers due to trauma. Metallic artifacts are visible in the maxillary region.

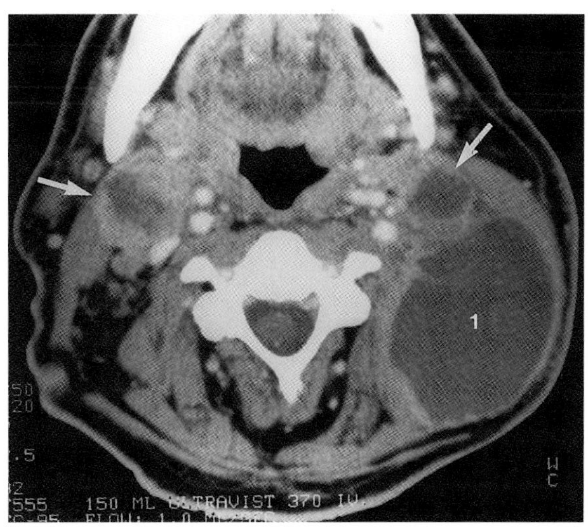

Fig. 14.8 **Lymph node metastases.** CT scan through the neck shows an extensive, well-circumscribed cervical lymph node metastasis on the left side along with other, smaller metastatic nodes anterior to the main node and in the right parapharyngeal space (arrows). All the affected nodes show peripheral contrast enhancement and central necrosis.
1 Lymph node metastases

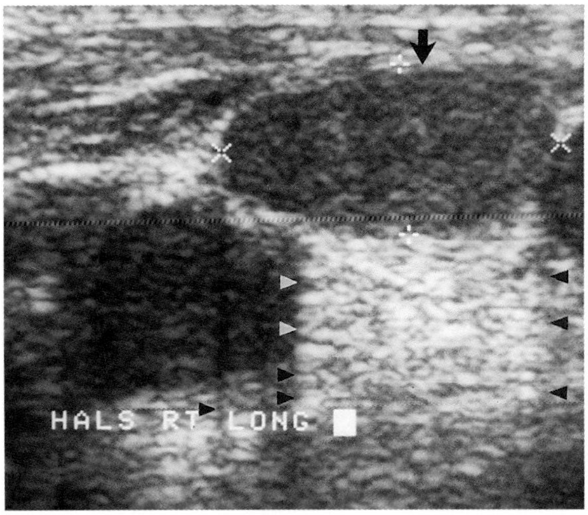

a

Figs. 14.**9 a – f** **Lymph nodes.** Ultrasound and MRI.
(**a**) Malignant lymph node (arrow) has a bulky shape and lacks a visible hilar notch. The posterior enhancement (arrowheads) is caused by central necrosis—another criterion of malignancy.

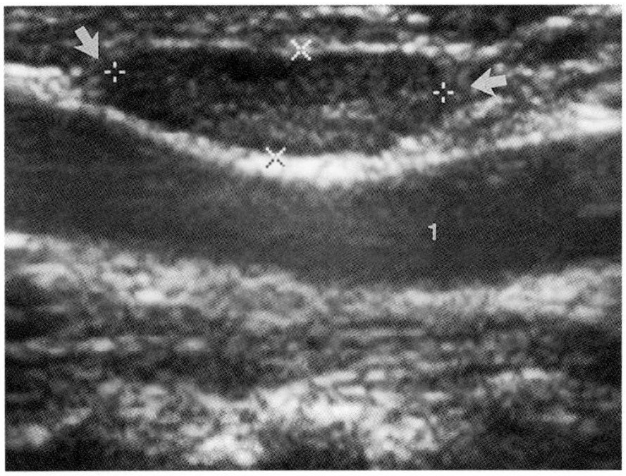

b

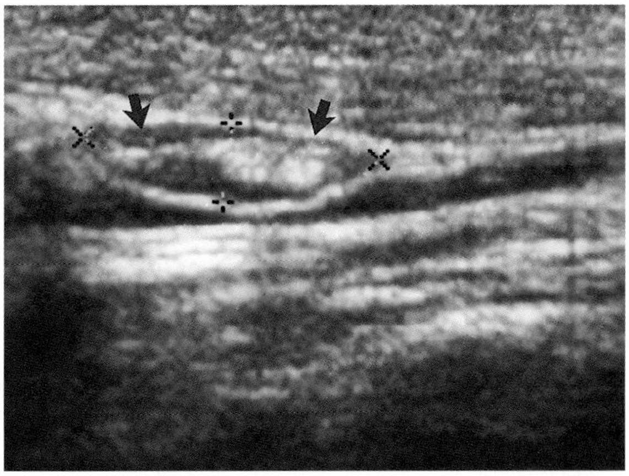

c

(**b**) This scan shows a solitary enlarged parajugular lymph node (arrows) displacing and constricting the internal jugular vein. The absence of a hilar fat sign indicates that this is a potentially malignant node.
1 Internal jugular vein

(**c**) Benign lymph node (arrows) has an elliptical shape, well-defined margins, and a hilar notch. The internal jugular vein is compressed by the node.

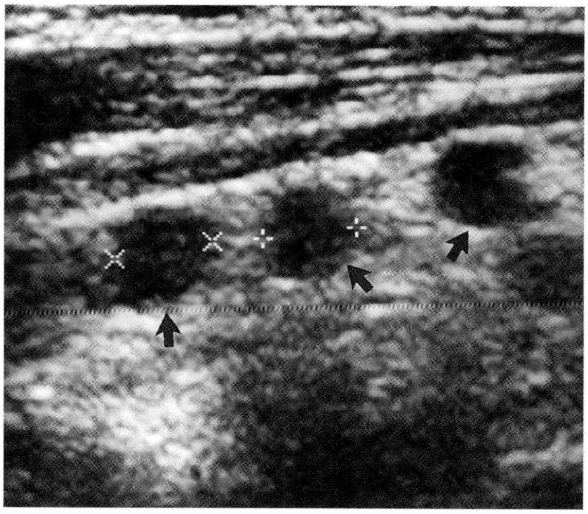

d

(**d**) Longitudinal scan through the neck shows multiple small parajugular lymph nodes (arrows). The multiplicity and rounded, bulky shape of the nodes are suspicious for malignancy.

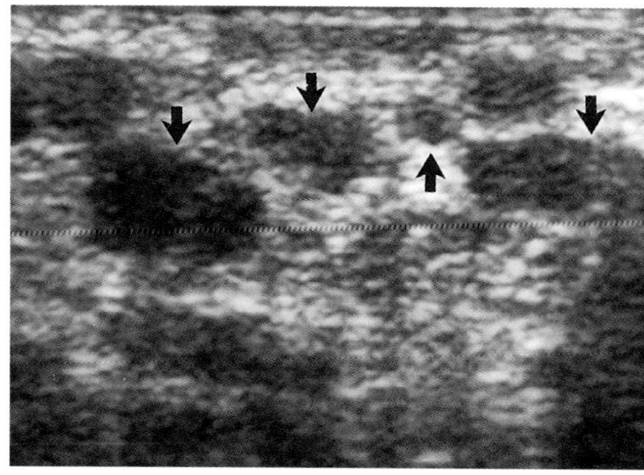

e

(**e**) Transverse scan shows multiple involved submandibular lymph nodes (arrows) in a patient with hypopharygeal carcinoma.

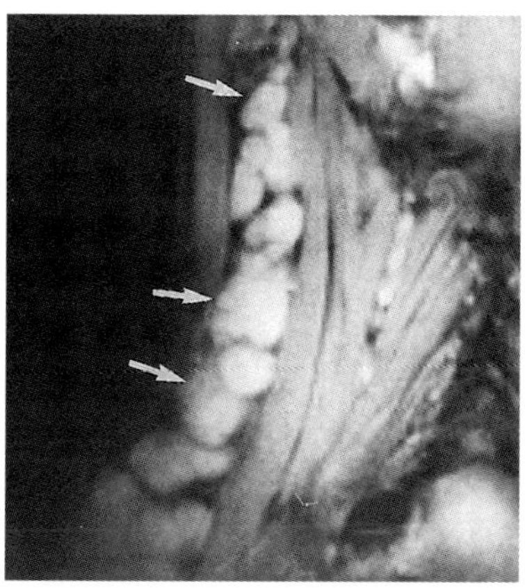

f

(**f**) Coronal MR image shows a series of matted lymph nodes (arrows) along the left side of the neck in a patient with non-Hodgkin lymphoma. Individually, the nodes appear well-circumscribed and homogeneous, contrasting with the appearance of metastatic nodal involvement.

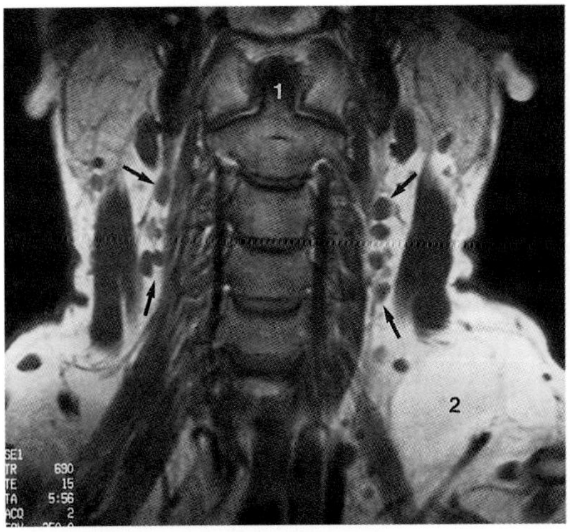

a

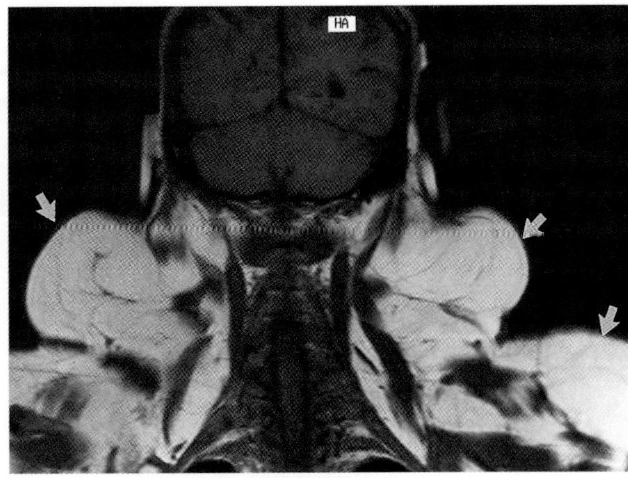

b

Figs. 14.**10 a, b** **Madelung disease.**
(**a**) Coronal unenhanced SE sequence (TR/TE = 690/15 ms) at the level of the cervical spine demonstrates a well-circumscribed hyperintense mass in the left supraclavicular space, consistent with a lipoma. Multiple small, reactive cervical lymph nodes are also visible on both sides (arrows).
1 Odontoid process of axis
2 Hyperintense mass

(**b**) "Madelung neck" consists of large, symmetric lipomas of the neck (arrows). The multiple septations within the lipomatous tissue are characteristic.

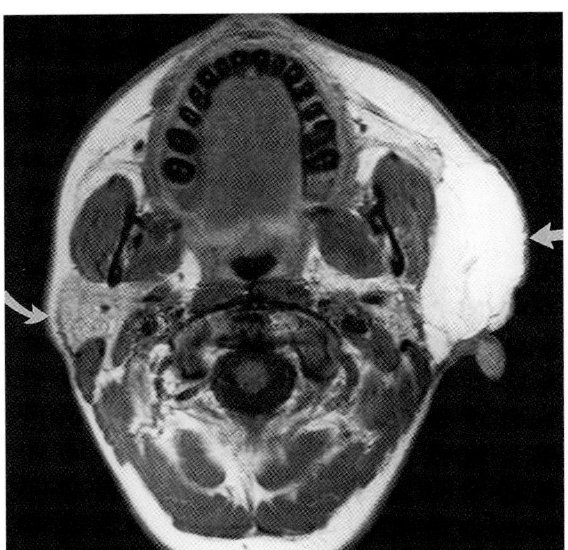

a

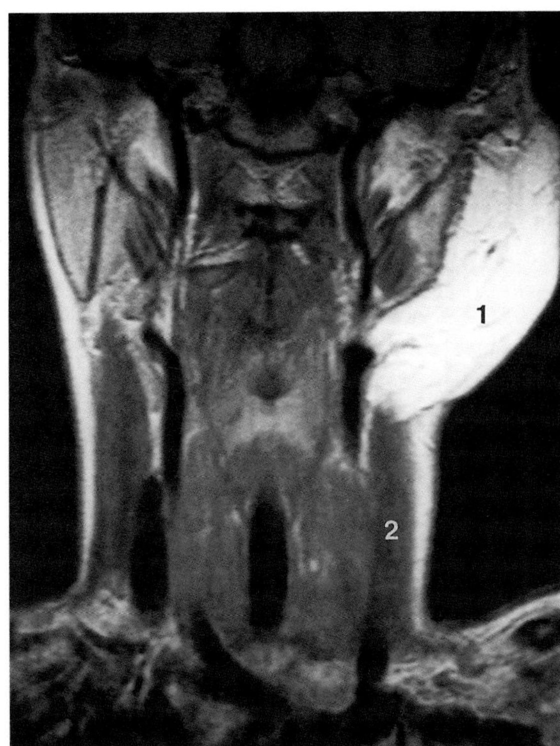

b

Figs. 14.**11 a, b** **Fat graft.**
(**a**) Unenhanced T1-weighted SE sequence (TR/TE = 600/15 ms) shows extensive hyperintense soft tissue (straight arrow) in the left buccal region of a patient who underwent parotidectomy for a malignant tumor and reconstruction with an interpositional fat graft. The right parotid gland (curved arrow) appears normal.

(**b**) Coronal image shows the full longitudinal extent of the graft, which lies above the sternocleidomastoid muscle.
1 Fat graft
2 Sternocleidomastoid muscle

Inflammatory Lesions

Abscess

Whenever an abscess is found in the soft tissues of the neck, the adjacent teeth should be examined for a possible primary focus. Other potential foci are the tonsils and oropharynx in patients with a history of sialadenitis or glossitis. The typical appearance of an abscess is that of a sharply circumscribed mass with a thin-walled capsule and serous-exudative contents (high signal intensity on T2-weighted MR images, density of about 30 HU on CT scans) (Fig. 14.**5**). Intralesional gas bubbles with a fluid level are pathognomonic for an abscess.

Cellulitis

Cellulitic lesions obscure normal anatomic boundaries due to inflammatory and edematous infiltration. They are associated with diffuse swelling and intense contrast enhancement. Advanced cases may progress to acute mediastinitis, manifested radiologically by mediastinal widening on chest radiographs and enhancing mediastinal soft tissue on CT scans (Figs. 14.**6** and 14.**20**).

Thyroiditis

The hallmark of thyroiditis is a painful, tender swelling of the thyroid gland, frequently combined with swallowing difficulties and redness of the overlying skin. The diagnosis is suggested by the clinical examination and laboratory findings, which can differentiate acute suppurative thyroiditis from the subacute forms (de Quervain and Hashimoto thyroiditis) (Fig. 14.**22**). Imaging shows edematous swelling of the thyroid gland and increased contrast enhancement.

Vascular Lesions

Hemangioma, Hemangiosarcoma, Hemangiopericytoma

Hemangiomas show an en-plaque, noninfiltrative type of growth with high signal intensity on T2-weighted MRI. Imaging also demonstrates nonhomogeneities caused by phleboliths or fibrotic elements and often reveals tortuous feeding and draining vessels.

An important imaging issue is the diagnosis of tumors that arise from vascular endothelium and undergo malignant transformation. *Hemangiosarcoma* and *hemangiopericytoma* (Figs. 14.**15** and 14.**28**) closely resemble hemangioma in their radiographic density and signal intensity but are distinguished from that lesion by their central nonhomogeneities and infiltrative growth.

Carotid Body Tumor

This tumor typically occurs in the carotid bifurcation, enhances intensely after intravenous contrast administration (see Ch. 4), and has well-defined, noninfiltrating margins (Fig. 14.**13**).

Carotid Stenoses and Aneurysms

Color duplex sonography can detect and quantify stenotic lesions of the carotid artery based on the spectral determination of flow velocities within the stenosis and at pre- and poststenotic sites (Fig. 14.**25 d**). Another criterion for stenosis at the bulbar level is the relation of the transverse luminal diameter of the common carotid artery to that of the internal and external carotid arteries. The main limitation of Doppler scanning is that it cannot cover the full length of the carotid vessels.

Doppler ultrasound can also detect carotid aneurysms, but angiographic techniques must be used to confirm higher lesions located at or near the skull base (Fig. 14.**27**).

CT (Fig. 14.**23**) and CT angiography afford the best view of calcified atherosclerotic plaques on the vessel wall, and they provide excellent sensitivity and specificity in determining the degree of stenosis (Fig. 14.**24**). Drawbacks are radiation exposure and the need for iodinated contrast medium.

By comparison, magnetic resonance angiography (MRA) is an elegant technique that can visualize the carotid arteries over their complete course without radiation exposure or contrast media. MRA may overestimate the degree of a stenosis, however, as a result of poststenotic turbulent flow (Figs. 14.**25 a** and 14.**26 a, b**).

Invasive arterial DSA is still considered the "gold standard" for preoperative investigations of the carotid system.

When all available techniques are applied, there should be no difficulty in diagnosing the complete occlusion of a carotid artery.

Thrombophlebitis or Thrombosis of the Internal Jugular Vein

These conditions most commonly result from the *spread of bacterial inflammation into the venous system*. The principal imaging techniques are CT, MRI, CT angiography, and MRA (Fig. 14.**29**). The slowing of blood flow in the internal jugular vein causes increased signal intensity on contrast-enhanced MR images. A false-positive study is ruled out by performing venous MRA, which can differentiate flow-related effects from true pathologic changes. Thrombophle-

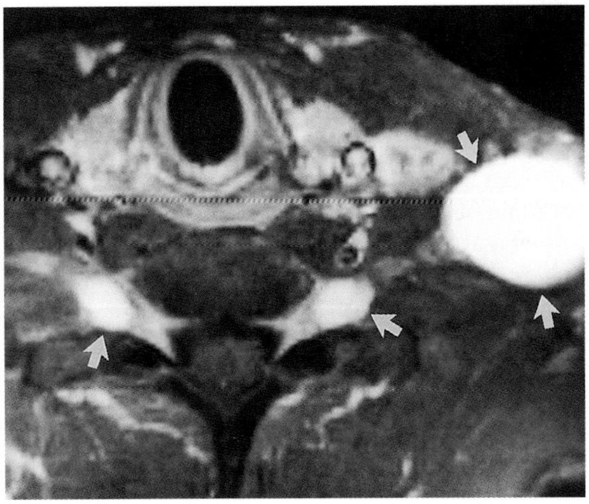
a

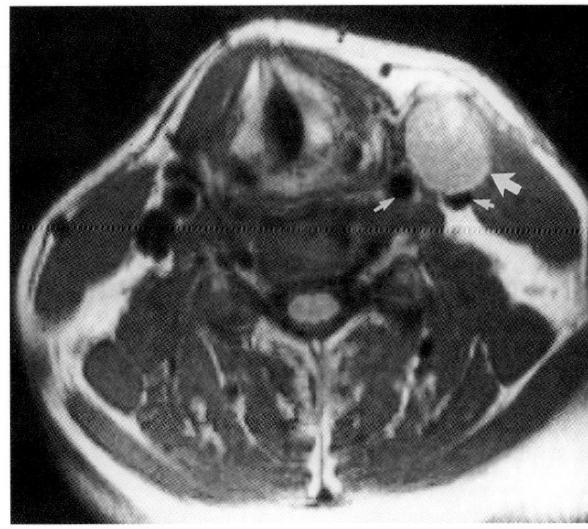
b

Figs. 14.**12 a, b** **Neuroma.**
(**a**) Axial Gd-enhanced SE sequence (TR/TE = 500/15 ms) with fat suppression shows intensely enhancing lesions in the left cervical region and both paravertebral spaces (arrows). The lesions are well-circumscribed and display a homogeneous internal structure. The conspicuous location of the lesions along nerve pathways and their multiplicity raised suspicion (subsequently confirmed) of multiple neurofibromas in a patient with Recklinghausen disease.

(**b**) Axial Gd-enhanced MRI shows a well-circumscribed, uniformly enhancing mass (large arrow) in the neurovascular sheath of the common carotid artery and internal jugular vein (small arrows). The location of the mass identifies it as a neuroma arising from the vagus nerve.

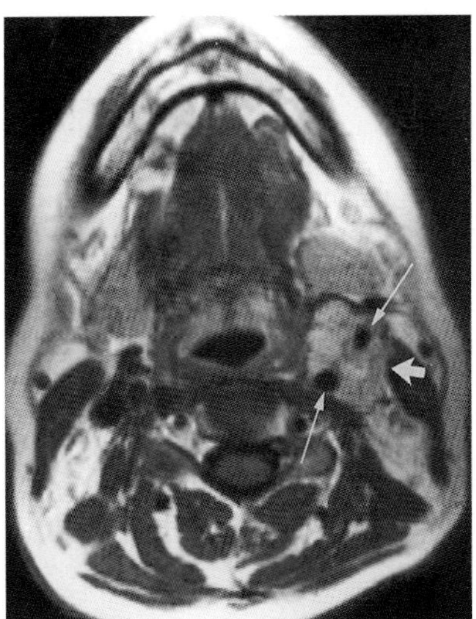
a

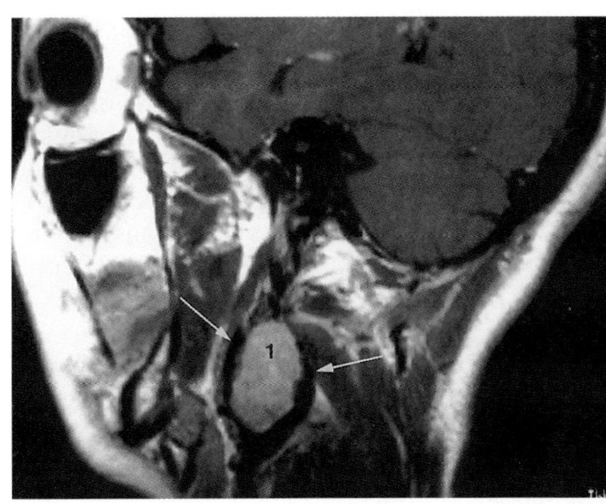

b

Figs. 14.**13 a, b** **Carotid body tumor.**
(**a**) Gd-enhanced T1-weighted SE sequence (TR/TE = 500/17 ms) shows a markedly enhancing tumor mass (thick arrow) in the bifurcation between the internal and external carotid arteries (thin arrows). The location, morphology, and enhancement characteristics of the mass are consistent with a carotid body tumor.

(**b**) Sagittal view clearly demonstrates the typical location of the tumor in the carotid bifurcation with splaying of the internal and external carotid arteries.
1 Carotid body tumor

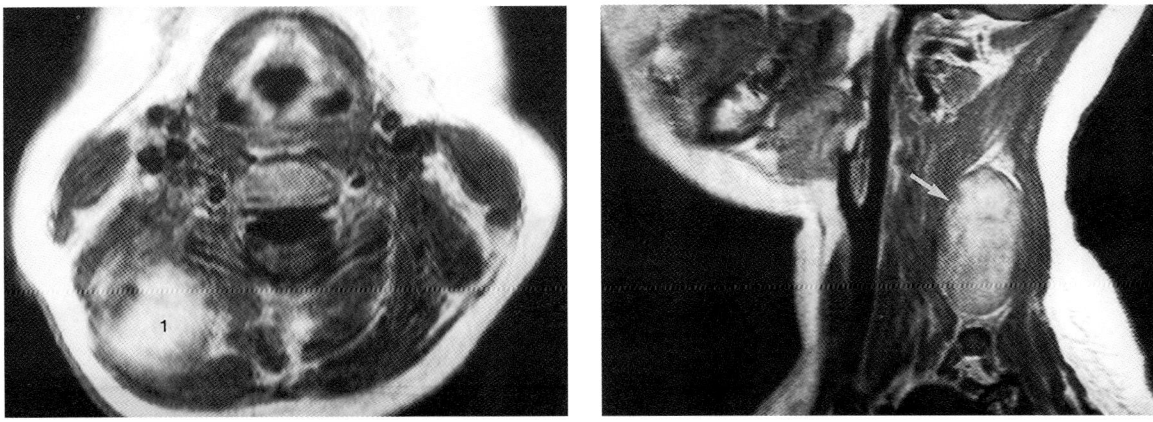

Figs. 14.**14 a, b** **Aggressive fibromatosis.**
(**a**) Axial Gd-enhanced SE sequence (TR/TE = 690/15 ms) shows a mass with ill-defined expansile and infiltrative margins in the nuchal muscles on the right side.
1 Mass with ill-defined margins

(**b**) Parasagittal image shows the nonhomogeneous internal structure of the mass (arrow) and its capsule–like superior and inferior borders. The mass was identified histologically as aggressive fibromatosis.

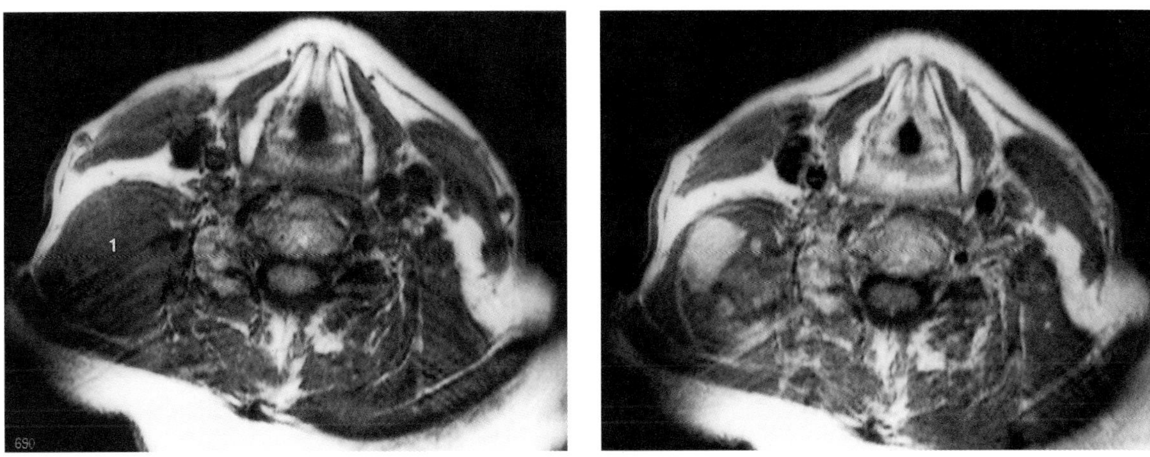

Figs. 14.**15 a, b** **Hemangiopericytoma.**
(**a**) Axial unenhanced T1-weighted image (TR/TE = 550/17 ms) shows an extensive tumor mass in the right cervical and paravertebral region. The lesion has smooth margins and uniform low signal intensity.
1 Mass

(**b**) Post-contrast image shows a nonhomogeneous enhancement pattern with greater uptake in the lateral portions of the mass and an enhancing, capsule–like boundary.

a

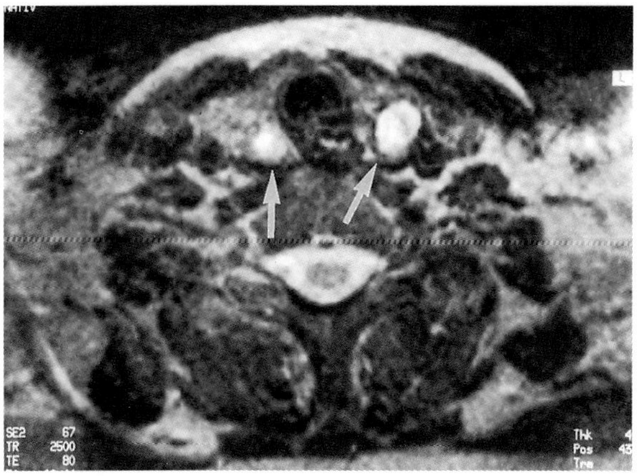

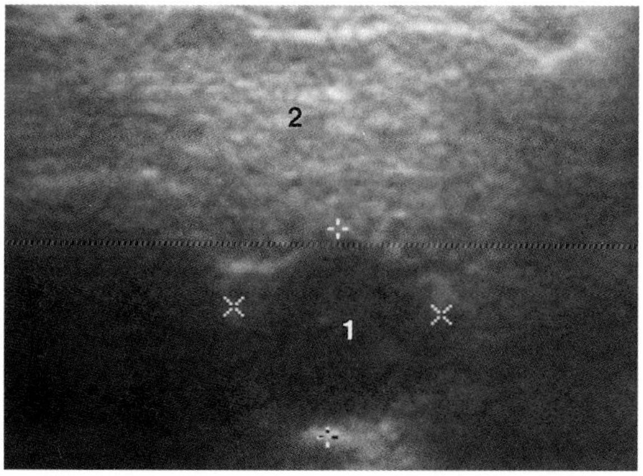

b

Figs. 14.**16 a, b** **Hyperparathyroidism.** MRI and ultrasound.
(**a**) Unenhanced T2-weighted SE sequence (TR/TE = 2500/80 ms) shows two hyperintense masses (arrows) near the inferior pole of the thyroid gland on each side in a patient with clinical signs of hyperparathyroidism. Accordingly, the masses were interpreted as hyperplastic parathyroid glands, and this was confirmed at operation.
(**b**) Ultrasound shows the hyperplastic parathyroid as a well-circumscribed hypoechoic mass posterior to the thyroid gland. By morphologic criteria alone, the mass is indistinguishable from a thyroid nodule.
1 Mass
2 Thyroid gland

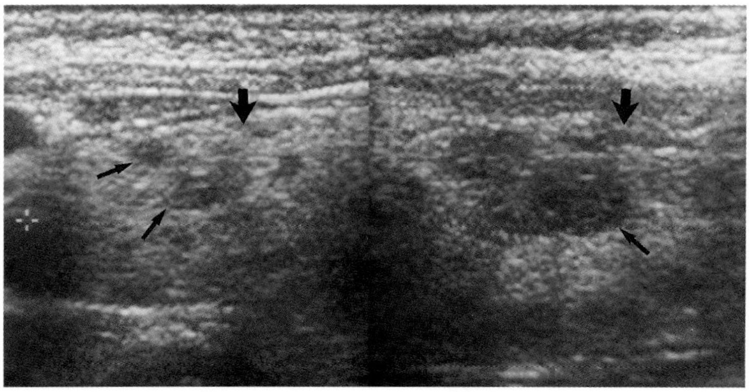

a

Figs. 14.**17 a, b** **Nodular goiter.** Ultrasound appearance.
(**a**) Longitudinal scan of a thyroid lobe (large arrows) in a patient with multi nodular goiter shows multiple hypoechoic nodular lesions (small arrows) associated with general thyroid enlargement.
(**b**) Solitary nodule (arrows) surrounded by thyroid parenchyma displays smooth margins in addition to cystic and regressive changes.

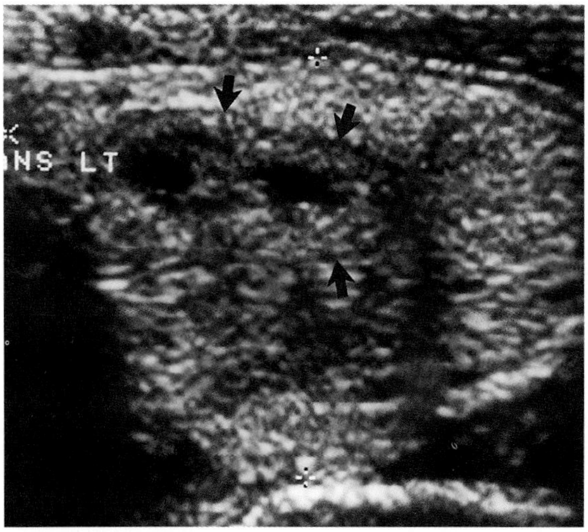

b

Fig. 14.**18**

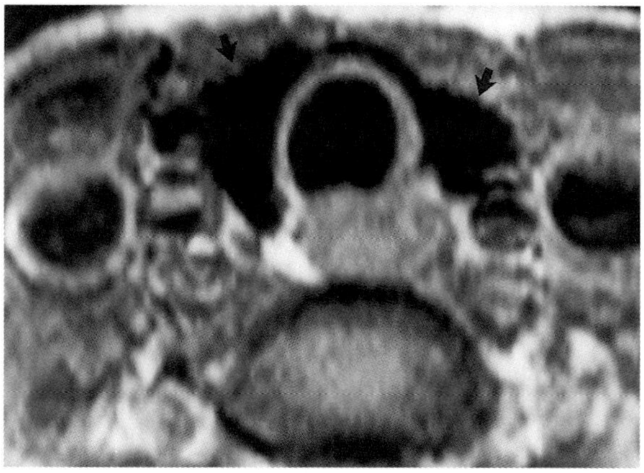

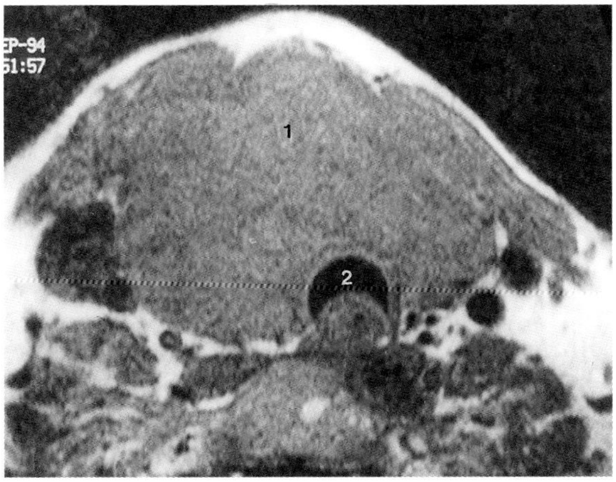

a

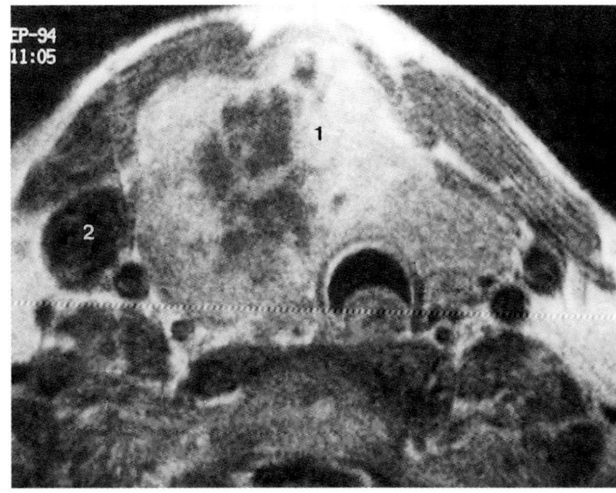

b

Figs. 14.**19 a, b** **Anaplastic thyroid carcinoma.**
(**a**) Unenhanced T1-weighted SE sequence (TR/TE = 600/17 ms) shows an extensive tumor mass displacing the trachea posteriorly and to the left.
1 Tumor mass
2 Trachea

(**b**) Image after intravenous contrast administration shows a nonhomogeneous internal structure with a moderately ill-defined anterior boundary between the tumor and infrahyoid muscles. This lesion is a thyroid carcinoma arising from the right thyroid lobe. Note the marked dilatation of the right internal jugular vein, signifying venous stasis.
1 Thyroid carcinoma
2 Internal jugular vein

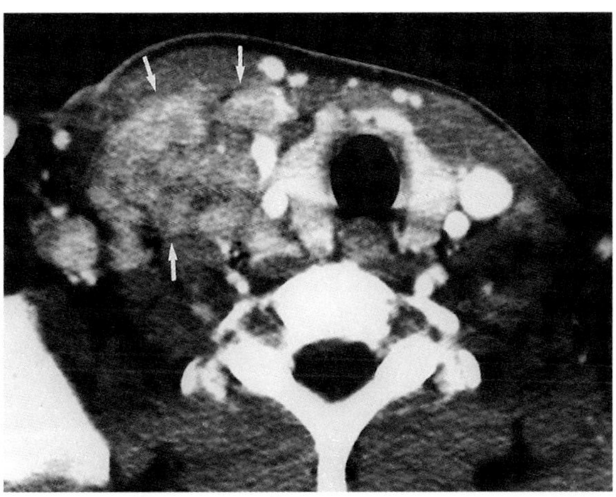

Fig. 14.**20** **Cervical cellulitis.** Post-contrast CT shows multiple enhancing foci in the right cervical region (arrows) with an associated mass effect, representing incipient areas of liquefaction in cellulitis. The patient had obvious clinical signs of inflammation.

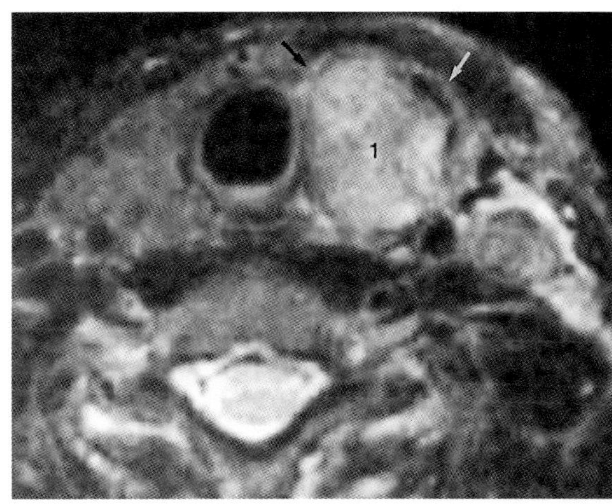

Fig. 14.**21** **C-cell carcinoma.** Post-contrast T2-weighted MR image (TR/TE = 3000/90 ms) shows a large, markedly enhancing, nonhomogeneous mass arising from the left thyroid lobe and projecting past the thyroid surface. The mass has predominantly smooth margins and an enhancing capsule (arrows). Histologic examination identified this morphologically ambiguous lesion as a C-cell carcinoma.
1 Large nonhomogeneous mass

◁ Fig. 14.**18** **Hemosiderosis.** Unenhanced SE sequence (TR/TE = 600/17 ms) shows absence of signal in a normal-sized thyroid gland with well-defined lobes (arrows). Iron deposition in the thyroid gland due to hemosiderosis created a paramagnetic effect, causing the thyroid to appear as a signal void on MRI.

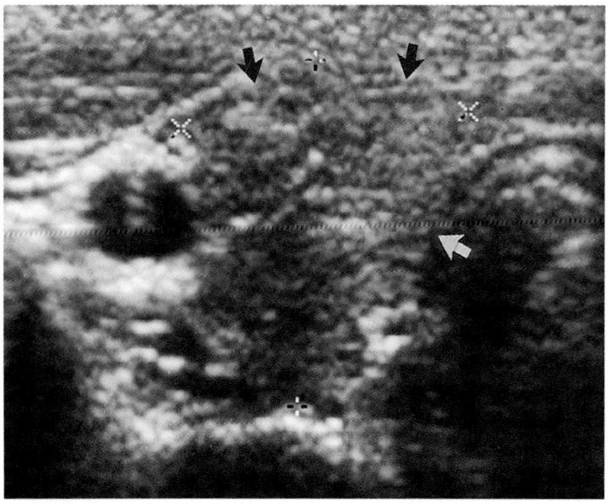

Fig. 14.**22** **Hashimoto thyroiditis.** On ultrasound examination with a 7.5-MHz linear probe, the thyroid parenchyma on the right side (arrows) appears markedly nonhomogeneous and hypoechoic with an ill-defined posterior border. The total volume of the gland is not increased. This patient had inflammatory changes in the setting of Hashimoto autoimmune thyroiditis.

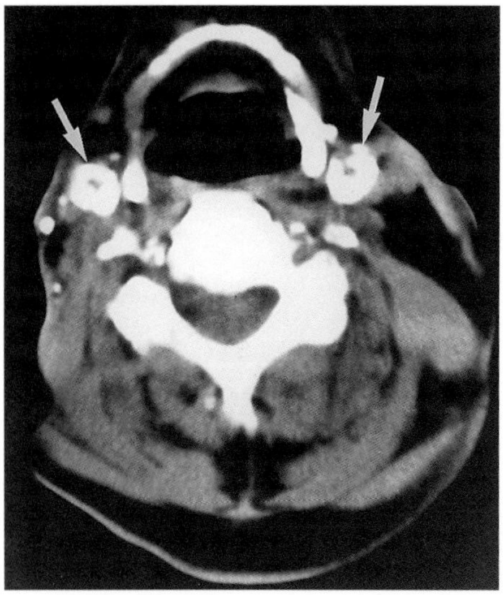

Fig. 14.**23** **Bilateral plaques in the common carotid arteries.** CT shows concentric calcifications in both common carotid arteries (arrows) causing severe luminal narrowing. The superior poles of the thyroid cartilage are visible medially.

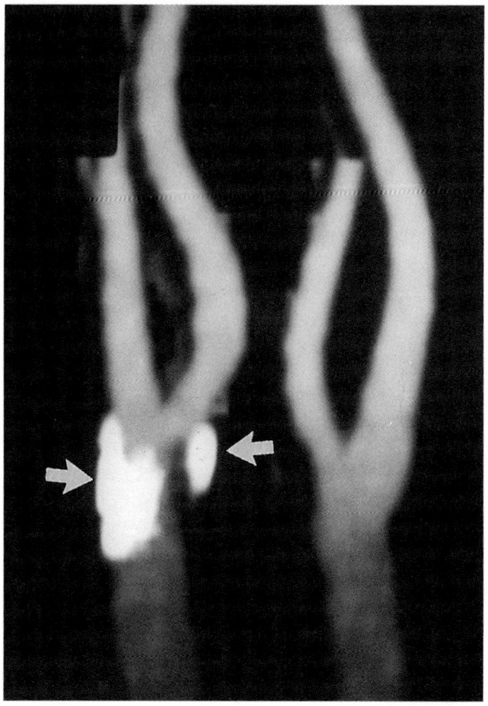

a

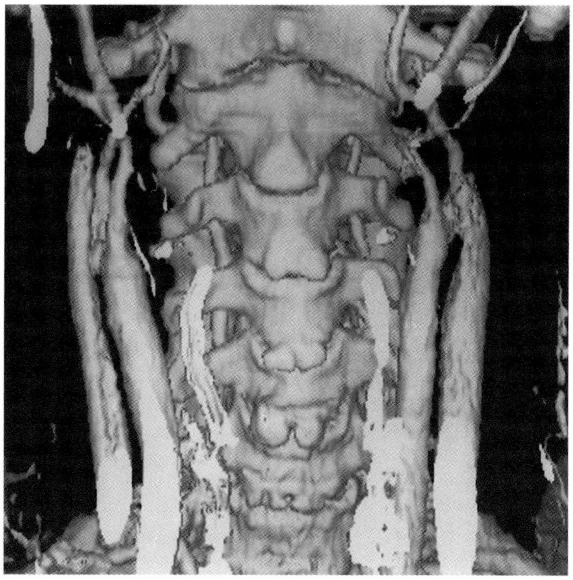

b

Figs. 14.**24 a, b** **Carotid stenosis and plaques.**
(**a**) CT angiography with maximum intensity projection (MIP) reconstruction of the data set shows calcified plaques (arrows) in the right carotid bulb accompanied by normal arterial perfusion on the left side.
(**b**) Surface-rendered view shows the relation of the major vessels to the vertebral bodies of the cervical spine and accurately defines the level of the lesions.

bitis is often associated with paravascular contrast enhancement due to an accompanying inflammatory reaction.

Traumatic Lesions

Sharp External Injury or Blunt Trauma

CT can demonstrate injury to the hyoid bone or laryngeal cartilages (Fig. 13.**6**), a foreign body with associated air inclusions, or a soft-tissue hematoma (Fig. 14.**7**). Risk of air embolism exists if the trauma has breached the internal jugular vein.

Iatrogenic and Posttherapeutic Changes

Postoperative Changes

Reconstructive procedures involving the use of tubed flaps, muscle grafts, or metallic implants can hamper diagnostic imaging and require differentiation from primary pathologic processes. MRI is the modality of first choice owing to its superior soft-tissue discrimination. A careful analysis of signal characteristics in T1-, T2- and gadolinium(Gd)-enhanced T1-weighted sequences can reliably differentiate recurrent tumor from postoperative changes (Fig. 14.**11**).

Postirradiation Changes

Diffuse inflammatory and edematous changes and scar retractions are typical postirradiation changes. MRI is best for differentiating these changes from recurrent tumor.

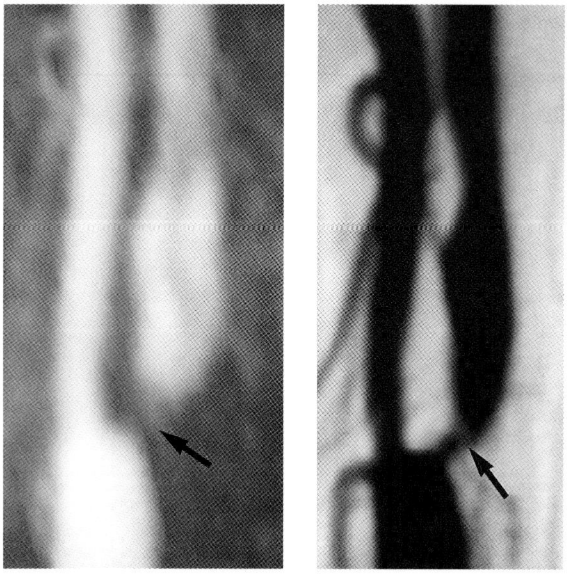

a b

Figs. 14.**25 a – e** **Carotid stenosis.** MRA, DSA, and ultrasound.

(**a**) MRA shows a signal void in the stenosed proximal segment of the internal carotid artery (arrow). The documentation of a cranial flow signal using a presaturation pulse positioned above the volume of interest excludes retrograde blood flow through the internal carotid artery. This confirms residual patency of the internal carotid artery (i.e., the degree of stenosis cannot exceed 99 %).

(**b**) Selective intra-arterial DSA documents a high-grade filiform stenosis at the origin of the left internal carotid artery (arrow) with poststenotic dilatation.

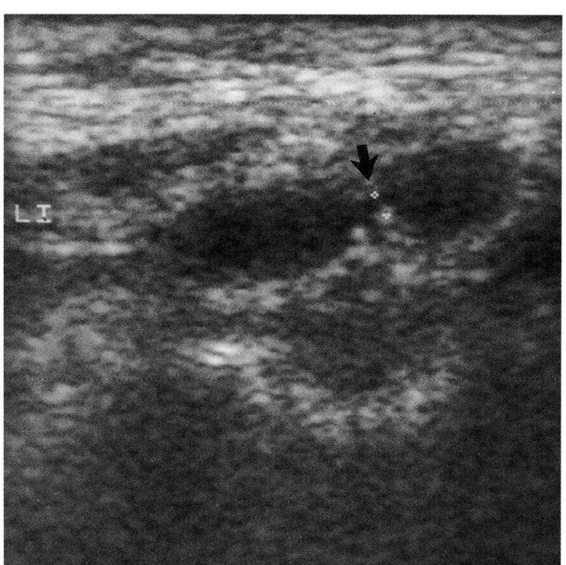

c

(**c**) B-mode ultrasound (longitudinal scan) shows plaques of mixed echogenicity (arrow and cursors) marking the location of the high-grade stenosis.

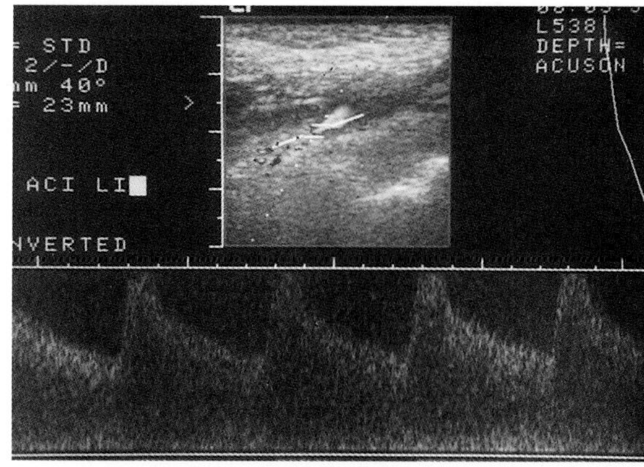

d

(**d**) Color duplex sonography shows that the flow velocity within the stenosis is increased to more than 4.0 m/s with an otherwise normal spectral waveform.

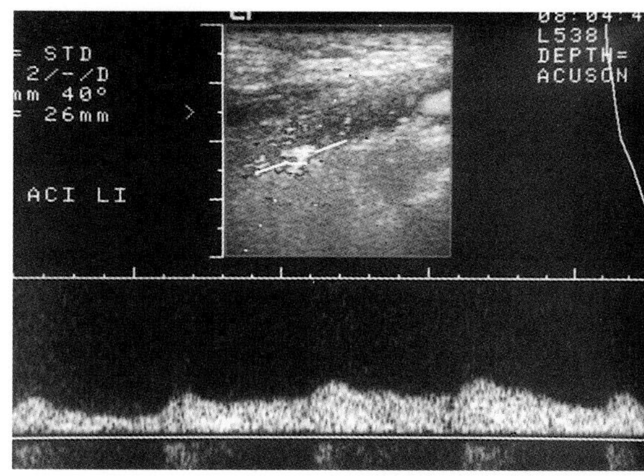

e

(**e**) The waveform shows marked poststenotic changes about 1 cm past the stenosis, where the flow velocity is slowed to less than 0.3 m/s.

Figs. 14.**26 a–c** **Occlusion of the internal carotid artery.** MRI, MRA, ultrasound.

(**a**) The right internal carotid artery is not visualized by MRI due to tumor invasion (white arrow) in a patient with recurrent tumor following neck dissection on the right side. Reduced flow velocity accounts for the high signal intensity in the right internal jugular vein (black arrow).

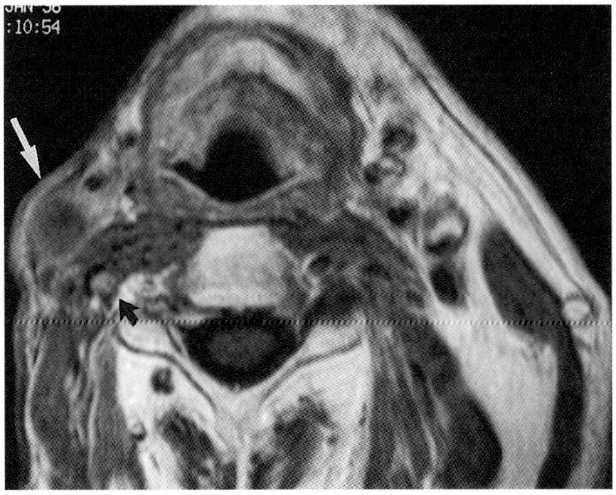

a

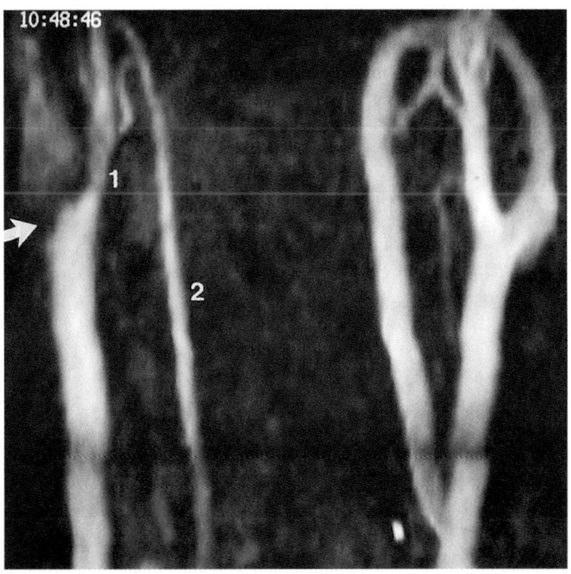

b

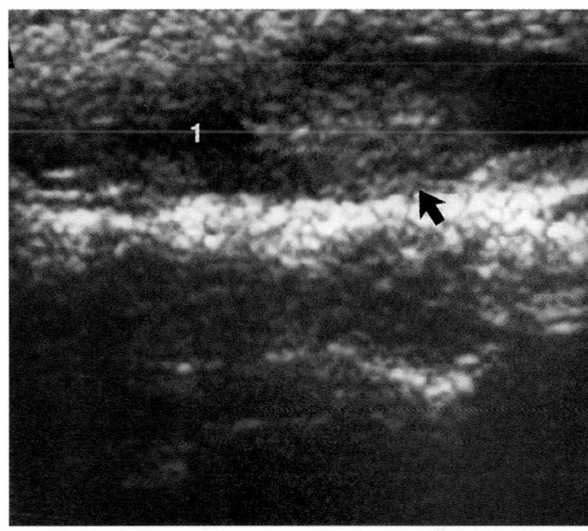

c

(**b**) MRA demonstrates the occlusion of the internal carotid artery (arrow) with normal flow in the ipsilateral external carotid and vertebral arteries and contralateral cervical vessels.

1 External carotid artery
2 Vertebral artery

(**c**) Ultrasound reveals an intraluminal mass of mixed echogenicity (arrow) at the level of the carotid bulb within the visualized segment of the internal carotid artery.

1 Internal carotid artery

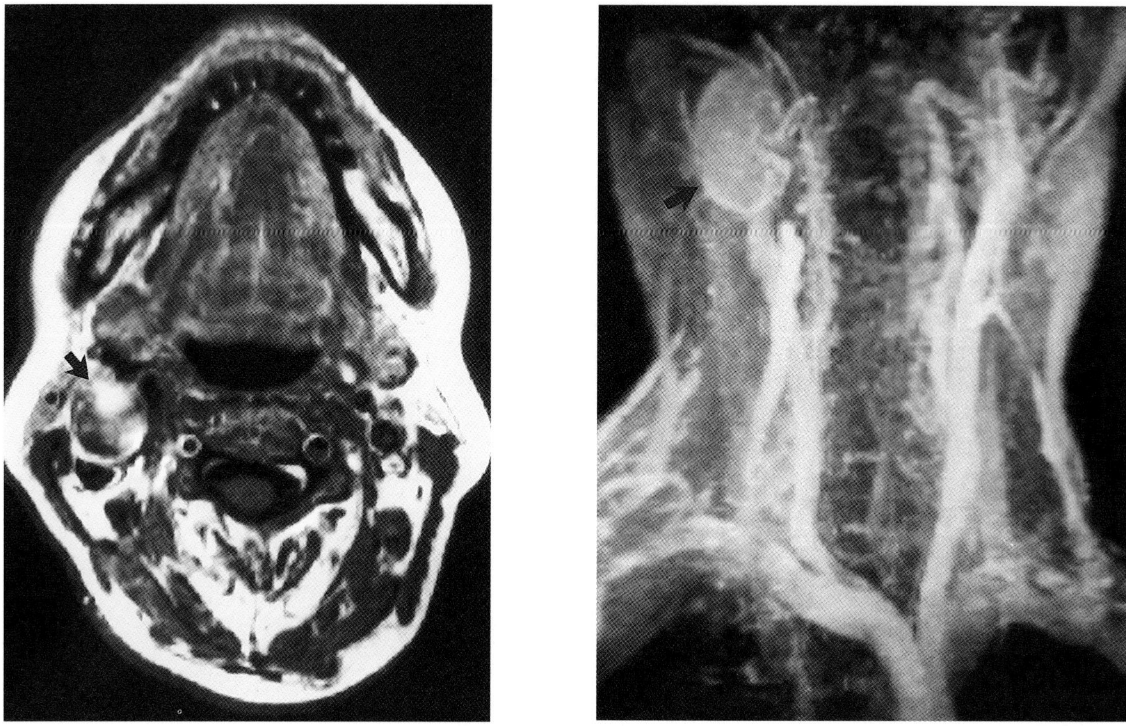

a b

Figs. 14.**27 a, b** **Aneurysm of the internal carotid artery.** MRI and MRA.
(**a**) Post-contrast MRI shows a well-circumscribed, nonuniformly enhancing mass (arrow) in the course of the internal carotid artery. The mass shows no signs of infiltrative growth.
(**b**) MRA confirms the aneurysmal dilatation of the internal carotid artery (arrow), which extends cephalad to the skull base.

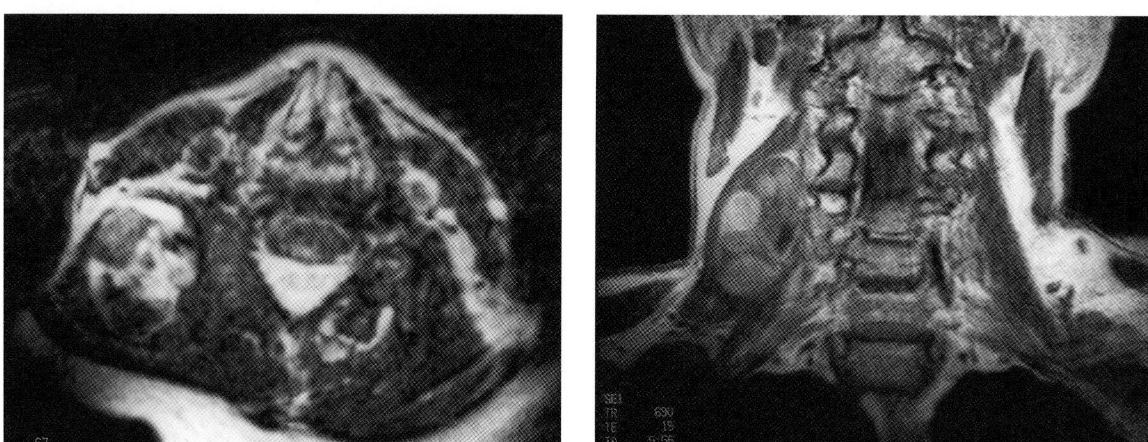

a b

Figs. 14.**28 a, b** **Hemangiopericytoma.**
(**a**) T2-weighted MR image (TR/TE = 3000/90 ms). The solid lateral component of the tumor is hypointense to the surrounding portions, which show a higher, fluid-equivalent signal intensity.
(**b**) Coronal view demonstrates the nonhomogeneous structure of the lesion, which is displacing the adjacent sternocleidomastoid muscle laterally.

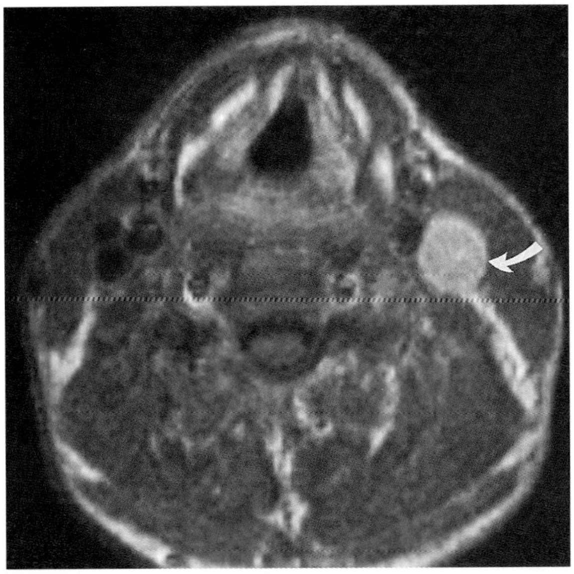
a

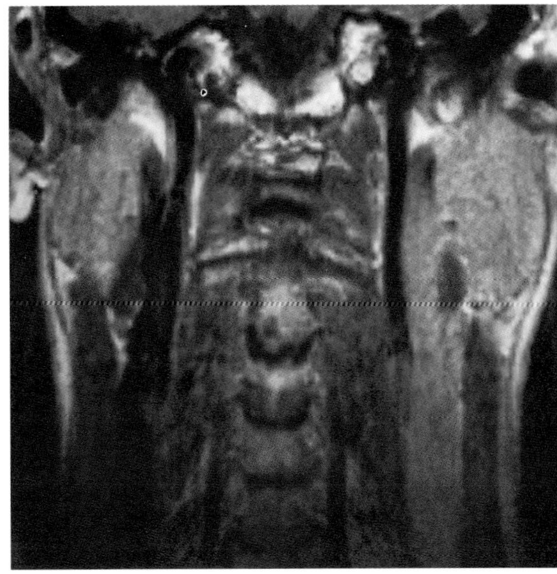
b

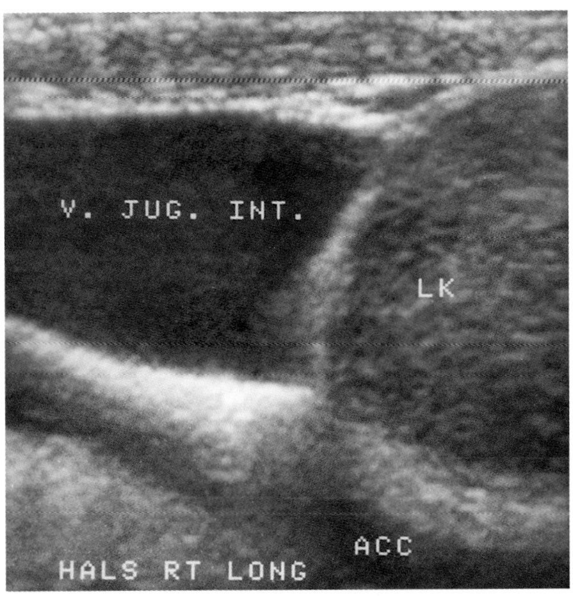

c

Figs. 14.**29 a – c** **Thrombosis vs. flow artifact in the internal jugular vein.**
(**a**) Axial MRI shows a hyperintense left jugular vein (curved arrow) with dilatation of the smooth-bordered vessel wall. There are no signs of a surrounding inflammatory reaction.
(**b**) Coronal image confirms normal bilateral venous flow with no evidence of thrombosis.
(**c**) Ultrasound scan in a different patient shows complete occlusion of the internal jugular vein by a large malignant lymph node.

LK	Lymph node
V. JUG. INT	Internal jugular vein
ACC	Common carotid artery

Imaging Criteria and Their Differential Diagnosis

Table 14.**1** lists the various cervical lesions in order of frequency.

Liquid Masses

Whenever a liquid mass is detected by ultrasound, CT, or MRI, the differential diagnosis consists mainly of inflammatory lesions such as an abscess (Fig. 14.**5**) or cellulitis, a neck cyst (Figs. 14.**2** – 14. **4**), and a necrotic tumor or lymph node (Tables 14.**2** – 14.**5**).

Table 14.**1** Frequency of various lesions of the neck

Common:
- Abscess (Fig. 14.**5**)
- Lymphadenopathy (Fig. 14.**9**):
  - Lymphadenitis
  - Metastasis
  - Systemic disease
- Salivary gland disease:
  - Mumps
  - Lithiasis (Fig. 10.**16**)
  - Neoplasia (Figs. 10.**6**, 10.**11**)
- Thyroid disease:
  - Adenoma
  - Cyst
  - Carcinoma (Figs. 14.**19**, 14.**21**)

Rare:
- Medial or lateral neck cyst (Figs. 14.**2** – 14.**4**)
- Cervical thymus
- Dilated jugular vein
- Ectopic salivary glands or thyroid tissue
- Rare tumors:
  - Glomus tumor (Fig. 14.**13**)
  - Epidermoid/dermoid cyst (Fig. 10.**4**)
  - Teratoma
  - Hygroma
  - Lipoma
  - Lymphangioma (Fig. 11.**22**)
  - Hemangioma
  - Fibroma
  - Rhabdomyoma
  - Neuroma (Fig. 14.**12**)
  - Aggressive fibromatosis (Fig. 14.**14**)

Table 14.**2** Differential diagnosis of liquid masses in the neck

Findings	Differential diagnostic criteria
Common:	
➤ Tumor:	
–Median neck cyst	Midline location in thyroglossal duct (Fig. 14.**3**)
–Lateral neck cyst	Posterior border of sternocleidomastoid muscle (Figs. 14.**2**, 14.**4**)
–Laryngocele	Arises from laryngeal ventricle (Fig. 13.**1**)
–Hygroma	Scapular region, multilocular
–Necrotic tumor	Morphology (Figs. 13.**9** – 13.**11**, 13.**18**)
➤ Inflammatory:	
–Abscess	Enhancing rim (Fig. 14.**5**)
–Cellulitis	Diffuse enhancement (Fig. 14.**6**)
Rare:	
➤ Trauma	Morphology (Fig. 14.**7**)
–Hematoma	
➤ Iatrogenic	
–Lymphocele	History

Table 14.**3** Differential diagnostic criteria for liquid neck masses in CT

Density between 20 and 60 HU, depending on protein content of liquid (Figs. 14.**2**, 14.**4**):
- Transudate, serous fluid < 30 HU:
  - Cyst (Fig. 14.**2**)
- Exudate > 30 HU:
  - Abscess (Fig. 14.**5**)
- Absence of central enhancement:
  - Cyst (Fig. 14.**2**)
  - Abscess (Fig. 14.**5**)
  - Necrosis
- Narrow enhancing rim:
  - Cyst (Fig. 14.**4**)
  - Abscess (Fig. 14.**5**)
- Broad peripheral enhancement:
  - Tumor with central necrosis
- Diffuse, intensely enhancing fluid collection with ill-defined borders:
  - Cellulitis (Fig. 14.**20**)

Table 14.4 Differential diagnostic criteria for liquid neck masses in MRI

- Hypointense on T1-weighted images, hyperintense on T2-weighted images:
  - —Cyst (Fig. 14.**3**)
  - —Abscess
  - —Necrosis
- Absence of central enhancement:
  - —Cyst (Fig. 14.**3**)
  - —Abscess
  - —Necrosis
- Narrow enhancing rim:
  - —Cyst
  - —Abscess
- Broad peripheral enhancement:
  - —Necrosis
- Lesion with ill-defined borders and high T2-weighted signal intensity:
  - —Cellulitis (Fig. 14.**6**)

Air-Containing Masses and Structures

Air-containing or gas-containing structures and masses in the cervical soft tissues most commonly have an inflammatory traumatic (Fig. 14.**7**) or iatrogenic cause (Table 14.**6**).

Solid Tumor Masses

Topographic criteria are an important consideration in the differential diagnosis of solid neck masses and especially in differentiating tumors and lymph nodes from other soft-tissue lesions (Tables 14.**7** – 14.**12**).

Thyroid Abnormalities

Pathologic changes in the thyroid gland may consist of an increase or decrease in thyroid size, increased nonhomogeneity of the thyroid parenchyma, or a change in the density, signal intensity, or echogenicity of the parenchyma (Figs. 14.**17**, 14.**18**, 14.**22**). Ultrasound is usually the primary imaging modality, and CT or MRI should be added to investigate thyroid malignancy (Fig. 14.**19**, Table 14.**13**).

Vascular Lesions

The principal vascular landmarks in the neck are the common carotid artery and the carotid bifurcation at the level of the hyoid bone and internal jugular vein. The diagnostic procedure of first choice is color duplex sonography, which can demonstrate hemodynamic changes as well as morphologic changes in the vessel walls (Fig. 14.**25**). If more detailed information is needed, ultrasound may be followed by CT angiography (for detailed evaluation of calcified plaques [Fig. 14.**24**]), MRA (to evaluate more proximal hemodynamics as far as the circle of Willis), and preoperative DSA.

MRI offers the highest sensitivity and specificity for the differentiation of tumors arising from blood vessels (Figs. 14.**25** and 14.**26**). It may be supplemented as needed by MR angiography to confirm the vascular origin of a lesion and identify feeding vessels (Table 14.**14**).

Table 14.5 Differential diagnostic criteria for liquid neck masses in ultrasonography

- Hypoechoic lesion with posterior acoustic enhancement:
  - —Cyst
  - —Abscess
  - —Necrosis (Fig. 14.**9 a**)

Table 14.6 Air-containing masses and structures in the cervical soft tissues

Findings	Differential diagnostic criteria
Common:	
➤ Variation	Arises from pharynx
—Diverticulum	
➤ Tumor	
—Cyst	Narrow rim (Fig. 14.**2**)
—Superinfection	Broad rim (Fig. 14.**4**)
➤ Inflammatory:	
—Abscess	Rim, "fluid level"
—Cellulitis	Diffuse, intense contrast enhancement (Fig. 14.**20**)
➤ Iatrogenic:	
—After puncture or perforation	Distribution
—Pneumothorax	
—Cutaneous emphysema	
➤ Trauma (Fig. 14.**7**)	
—Soft-tissue emphysema	
—Foreign body	
Rare:	
➤ Vascular:	
—Septic thrombosis of jugular vein	

Table 14.7 Topographic and morphologic criteria for soft-tissue masses

Topographic criteria

- Located along nodal pathway (jugulodigastric, submandibular, submental, deep cervical to supraclavicular):
  —Lymph nodes (Fig. 14.**9**)
- Located along neurovascular sheath in the neck, related to common or internal carotid artery and internal jugular vein, often arising from vagus or hypoglossal nerve:
  —Neuroma (Fig. 14.**12 b**)
  —Neurofibroma (Fig. 14.**12 a**)
- Arising from muscular compartments of the neck:
  —Rhabdomyoma, rhabdomyosarcoma
- Typically located at bifurcation of internal and external carotid arteries (Fig. 14.13):
  —Carotid body tumor
- Arising from notochord remnants, associated with vertebral body destruction, located in prevertebral space:
  —Chordoma
- Nuchal location (Fig. 14.**14**):
  —Aggressive fibromatosis

Morphologic criteria

- Smooth margins (benign tumors) (Fig. 14.**10**):
  —Lymphadenitis
  —Neuroma
  —Hemangioma
  —Lipoma
  —Rhabdomyoma
  —Fat graft
  —Chordoma, etc.
- Ill-defined margins (malignant tumors):
  —Liposarcoma
  —Rhabdomyosarcoma
  —Metastatic lymph node
  —Malignant schwannoma
  —Malignant goiter, etc.
- Homogeneous internal structure:
  —Lipoma (Fig. 14.**10**)
  —Rhabdomyoma
  —Lymphadenitis (Fig. 14.**9 c**)
  —Chordoma
  —Glomus tumor (Fig. 14.**13**)
- Nonhomogeneous internal structure:
  —Neuroma, neurofibroma (Figs. 14.**12 a**, **b**)
  —Nodular goiter (Fig. 14.**17**)
  —Liposarcoma
  —Rhabdomyosarcoma
  —Metastatic lymph node (Fig. 14.**9 a**)
  —Malignant schwannoma
- Presence of feeding and draining vessels:
  —Hemangioma
- Bone destruction:
  —Chordoma (vertebral body)
  —Malignant tumors, metastases
- Internal septa, amorphous calcifications:
  —Chordoma
- Diameter > 10 mm, ill-defined infiltrating margins, central necrosis, and fixation to adjacent tissue are criteria for metastatic lymph node involvement (Fig. 14.**9 a**).
- Multiple matted lymph nodes are suggestive of systemic lymphomatous disease (Fig. 14.**9 f**)

Table 14.**8** Primary tumor sites commonly associated with metastatic involvement of specific nodal groups

Upper cervical group
- Tongue base
- Paranasal sinuses
- Nasopharynx
- Tonsils

Submaxillary group
- Oral floor, tongue

Middle and lower jugular group
- Esophagus
- Larynx
- Pharynx
- Thyroid gland

Paratracheal and mediastinal group
- Larynx
- Bronchi, lung
- Thyroid gland

Supraclavicular group
- Breast
- Stomach
- Bronchi, lung
- Esophagus

Table 14.**9** Differential diagnostic criteria for soft-tissue masses in CT

- Low density (< 30 HU):
  —Lipoma, liposarcoma
- Very intense enhancement:
  —Hemangioma
  —Glomus tumor
- No enhancement:
  —Lipoma
- All other tumors show nonspecific density between 30 and 70 HU and moderate enhancement

Table 14.**10** Differential diagnostic criteria for soft-tissue masses in MRI

- High signal intensity on T1-weighted images:
  —Lipoma, liposarcoma (Fig. 14.**10**)
  —Colloid cyst
- High signal intensity on T2-weighted images:
  —Hemangioma (Fig. 14.**28 a**)
  —Parathyroid adenoma
- Very intense enhancement:
  —Hemangioma
  —Glomus tumor (Fig. 14.**13**)
- Peripheral enhancement with central necrosis:
  —Metastatic lymph node
  —Neuroma, neurofibroma (Fig. 14.**12**)
- All other tumors show intermediate signal intensity on T1- and T2-weighted images with moderate enhancement.

Table 14.**11** Differential diagnostic criteria for soft-tissue masses in ultrasonography

- Solid echogenic lesions; in most cases echogenicity is not an adequate criterion for making a specific diagnosis.

Table 14.**12** Solid tumor masses

Findings	**Differential diagnostic criteria**
Common:	
➤ Variation:	
—Asymmetry	
➤ Benign tumors:	
—Nodal hyperplasia (Fig. 14.**9 c**)	Morphology
—Lipoma (Fig. 14.**10**)	Density, signal characteristics
—Neuroma (Fig. 14.**12**)	Topography
—Glomus tumor (Fig. 14.**13**)	Contrast enhancement
—Hemangioma (Figs. 14.**15**, 14.**28**)	Vascularization
—Chordoma	Morphology
—Goiter (Fig. 14.**17**)	Thyroid tissue
➤ Malignant tumors:	
—Nodal metastasis (Fig. 14.**8**)	Morphology
—Lymphoma (Fig. 14.**9 f**)	Matted lymph nodes
Rare:	
➤ Tumors:	
—Aggressive fibromatosis (Fig. 14.**14**)	Morphology
—Soft-tissue sarcoma (Fig. 9.**6**)	Morphology

Table 14.**13** Lesions of the thyroid gland

Findings	Differential diagnostic criteria
Benign tumors:	
➤ Nodular goiter (Fig. 14.**17**)	Nonhomogeneous with cysts and calcifications
➤ Adenoma	Nodule
➤ Parathyroid hyperplasia (Fig. 14.**16**)	Topography, posterior to thyroid gland
Malignant tumors:	
➤ Malignant goiter: —Follicular carcinoma —Papillary carcinoma —Anaplastic carcinoma (Fig. 14.**19**) —C-cell carcinoma (Fig. 14.**21**)	Infiltrative growth
Inflammatory:	
➤ Thyroiditis (Fig. 14.**22**)	Swelling, edema
Systemic:	
➤ Hemosiderosis (Fig. 14.**18**)	Low signal intensity on MRI

Table 14.**14** Vascular lesions in the neck

Common:

- ➤ Stenosis of common, internal, and external carotid arteries caused by:
  - —Calcified plaques (Fig. 14.**24**)
  - —Atheromatous plaques
  - —Thrombotic deposits
- ➤ Complete occlusion of common or internal carotid artery (Fig. 14.**26**)
- ➤ Dilatation of internal jugular vein
  - —Physiologic
  - —Upper inflow stasis
- ➤ Thrombosis of internal jugular vein (Fig. 14.**29**)
- ➤ Thrombophlebitis of internal jugular vein

Rare:

- ➤ Aneurysm of common or internal carotid artery (Fig. 14.**27**)
- ➤ Septic jugular vein thrombosis

Summary and Diagnostic Strategy

Inspection and palpation of the soft tissues of the neck will often suggest an accurate working diagnosis. Ultrasound, with its ability to distinguish cystic from solid lesions, should always be the first imaging modality used. If there is continued suspicion of a soft-tissue neck tumor, MRI is preferred over CT owing to its excellent soft-tissue discrimination. There is still controversy as to which imaging modality is best for evaluating the lymph nodes. At present, none of the sectional modalities—ultrasound, CT, MRI—can distinguish nodal inflammatory change from a metastatic lymph node less than 10 mm in diameter with adequate specificity.

References

1 van den Brekel, M. W. M., H. V. Stel, J. A. Castelijns, J. J. P. Nauta, I. van der Waal, J. Valk, C. J. L. M. Meyer, G. B. Snow: Cervical lymph node metastasis: assessment of radiologic criteria. Radiology 177 (1990) 379 – 384

2 Jabour, B. A., R. B. Lufkin, L. J. Layfield, W. Hanafee: Magnetic Resonance Imaging of metastatic cervical adenopathy. Top Magn Reson Imaging 2 (1990) 69 – 75

3 Koch, T., M. Vollrath, T. Berger, P. Reimer, H. Milbradt, P. Heintz: Diagnosis of carotid body tumor by imaging procedures. HNO 38 (1990) 148 – 153

4 Lufkin, R. B., J. D. Robinson, D. J. Castro, B. A. Jabour, G. Duckwiler, L. J. Layfield, W. N. Hanafee: Interventional Magnetic Resonance Imaging in the head and neck. Top Magn Reson Imaging 2 (1990) 76 – 80

5 Naumann, H. H.: Differentialdiagnostik in der Hals-Nasen-Ohren-Heilkunde. Thieme, Stuttgart 1990

6 Som, P. M.: Lymph nodes of the neck. Radiology 165 (1987) 593 – 598

7 Sue, D. E., M. N. Brant-Zawadzki, J. Chance: Dissection of cranial arteries in the neck: correlation of MRI and arteriography. Neuroradiology 34 (1992) 273 – 278

8 Vogl, Th., S. Dresel, M. Juergens, J. Assal, J. Lissner: MR imaging with Gd-DTPA in lesions of the head and neck. J Otolaryngol. 22 (1993) 4 – 9

15 Prevertebral Space Including the Trachea and Esophagus

The prevertebral space is a connective-tissue compartment bounded by several fascial planes. It communicates with the parapharyngeal space above and the mediastinum below. The principal anatomic landmarks in this space are the trachea (Fig. 15. **11**), the esophagus (Fig. 15.**4**), and the paratracheal and paraesophageal nodal chains. Additionally, lesions such as prevertebral hematomas and abscesses commonly originate in the cervical spine (Fig. 15.**3**), and degenerative changes of the cervical spine (Figs. 15.**1** and 15.**10**) can lead to swallowing difficulties.

The radiologic diagnosis of diseases of the cervical esophagus relies on a combination of static and functional studies. Deglutition is an extremely complex process that requires the coordinated interaction of numerous neuromuscular structures. Many dysphagic complaints are caused by lesions at the level of the hypopharynx and esophageal inlet. Other sites of predilection for pathologic changes are the physiologic constrictions of the esophagus at the level of the tracheal bifurcation and aortic arch and where the esophagus pierces the diaphragm before uniting with the gastric cardia.

Based on the complex anatomic relationships of the trachea, even minor tracheal lesions are often associated with significant clinical manifestations. Tracheal lesions are rarely found incidentally at imaging, and their radiologic evaluation must include documenting the length of involvement and deep tissue extent and establishing a specific diagnosis for indeterminate lesions.

The major sites of predilection within the respiratory tract are the larynx and bronchi, but there are also a variety of primary tracheal lesions that will be discussed in this chapter.

Normal Anatomy

The trachea, esophagus, and cervical spine traverse the posterior compartment of the neck. The cervical spine consists of seven vertebral bodies and the intervening disk spaces. Lesions that involve the anterior border of the vertebral bodies can cause pain or functional disturbances in organs located in the prevertebral space (Fig. 15.**2**).

The *esophagus* is a muscular tube that begins with the union of the piriform sinuses behind the cricoid cartilage and descends through the diaphragm to the gastric cardia. Its total length is 25 to 30 cm in the prevertebral space, where it usually deviates slightly to the left. The esophagus has three clinically important physiologic constrictions that occur at the esophageal inlet in the postcricoid region, where the esophagus is crossed in its middle third by the aortic arch and tracheal bifurcation, and where the esophagus pierces the diaphragm. The combination of longitudinal and transverse muscle fibers gives the squamous epithelium-lined esophagus its elasticity and contractility. The relatively weak muscular junction in the cricopharyngeal portion of the inferior pharyngeal constrictor is a site of predilection for pressure-induced outpouching of the posterior esophageal wall (Zenker diverticulum). Behind and below the cricoid cartilage, the posterosuperior origins of the longitudinal muscular coat of the esophagus form the Laimer triangle.

The *trachea* is the portion of the respiratory tract that starts with the first tracheal cartilage just below the subglottic larynx and descends to the carina at the tracheobronchial bifurcation. It is approximately 11 cm long and generally extends from the sixth cervical vertebra to the fifth thoracic vertebra. The anterior and lateral walls of the trachea consist of a framework of 16 to 20 horseshoe-shaped cartilaginous rings. The tracheal rings are deficient posteriorly, where the wall (membranous part) is composed of transverse muscular and connective tissue fibers.

Clinical Signs and Symptoms

Diseases of the cervical esophagus present with a variety of clinical manifestations. Difficulty in swallowing, generally termed *dysphagia*, is distinguished from painful swallowing or *odynophagia*. Dysphagia is hazardous in that it predisposes to the aspiration of food or of oral contrast medium during radiographic studies. Another important clinical symptom is the "globus sensation" that is caused by the retention of food residues or foreign material within the esophagus, usually at one of the physiologic constrictions. *Hematemesis* is another symptom that requires evaluation in an emergency care setting. The bleeding may originate from esophageal varices or may signify a malignant tumor.

The most common clinical manifestations of tracheal diseases are *difficult or labored breathing* ranging to *acute dyspnea*. Patients often present with an audible inspiratory stridor as evidence of tracheal stenosis. *Dry cough* is a frequent manifestation of tracheal inflammatory disease. Pain in the trachea may result from neck trauma but more commonly originates at the bronchial level. *Recurring hemoptysis* is an alarming sign that should prompt immediate evaluation for neoplastic disease.

Today the most advanced clinical examination tools are endoscopic techniques, which permit the sampling of cytologic and histologic material and also provide access for interventional procedures.

Imaging Evaluation and Differential Diagnosis

Conventional Oral Contrast Examination

Even today, the primary radiologic procedure of choice for evaluating the hypopharynx and esophagus is the conventional oral contrast examination using barium or a water-soluble contrast medium (Fig. 15.**12**). Barium may be used unless contraindications exist (perforation, risk of aspiration, etc.). Adequate tumor diagnosis requires careful evaluation of the mucosa of the oropharynx, hypopharynx, and esophagus using single- or double-contrast technique. In cases where barium is contraindicated and in postoperative evaluations for anastomotic leak, a water-soluble contrast medium (e.g., Gastrographin) should be used. Water-soluble media can detect only sites of stenosis and contrast extravasation, however, and aspiration is still a potential hazard that may result in pulmonary edema.

Conventional Radiography

Conventional biplane radiographs with inspiratory and expiratory views still have a major role in the initial workup of tracheal disease. Plain radiography can demonstrate luminal changes during respiration as well as fixed stenotic lesions of the tracheal airway. The cervical spine may be evaluated with conventional biplane radiographs, and flexion and hyperextension views can be obtained to exclude a fracture (Figs. 15.**9** and 15.**11**).

Computed Tomography (CT)

Cases in which there is clinical or endoscopic suspicion of a tumor mass should be evaluated further by conventional or spiral CT (Figs. 15.**9** and 15.**10**). The examination follows the basic protocol explained in Chapter 14 but should cover all of the prevertebral space and, for problems involving the esophagus, should encompass the cardia.

Magnetic Resonance Imaging (MRI)

Improved imaging protocols have expanded the role of contrast-enhanced MRI in the pretreatment evaluation of tracheal and esophageal neoplasms (Figs. 15.**4** – 15.**6**). The multiplanar capabilities of MRI have proved to be a particular advantage. Initial results on pretherapeutic TNM staging by MRI confirm a high accuracy rate comparable to that of endosonography.

Ultrasound

Ultrasound scanning with a 7.5-MHz linear probe has become an established primary diagnostic modality for pediatric evaluations.

Imaging Findings

Congenital Variations and Malformations

Klippel–Feil Syndrome

Bony malformations of the cervical spine are not uncommon, but most are clinically asymptomatic. Klippel–Feil syndrome is a dysostosis characterized by the fusion of adjacent cervical vertebral bodies (Fig. 15.**2**) and a short neck of limited mobility. The differential diagnosis is usually based on conventional X-ray views of the cervical spine.

Esophageal Stenosis, Tracheoesophageal Fistula

A congenital stenosis or fistula can be visualized in newborns by instilling radiographic contrast medium into the esophagus through a feeding tube. Films often show an abrupt cutoff of the contrast column (signifying esophageal atresia), a stenotic constriction, or the passage of contrast medium into the trachea (confirming a tracheoesophageal fistula).

Congenital Brachyesophagus

Oral contrast films in this condition will usually demonstrate gastric mucosa in the distal portion of the esophagus. Often the clinical symptoms and subsequent diagnosis do not become apparent until adulthood.

Tracheal Stenosis and Tracheomalacia in Newborns

Clinical examination generally reveals labored breathing and an inspiratory stridor. The ultrasound examination is diagnostic in most cases.

Tumors

Esophageal Tumors

Endoscopic techniques and radiologic studies are mutually complementary in the detection and differential diagnosis of esophageal neoplasms. *Rare benign tumors* such as fibroma, adenoma, and leiomyoma require differentiation from the *more common malignant tumors* such as squamous cell carcinoma, adenocarcinoma, sarcoma, and lymphoma (Figs. 15.**4** – 15.**7**).

Oral contrast examination in patients with benign tumors reveals stenosis or indentation of the esophagus and the displacement of surrounding soft tissues with circumscribed filling defects. Most benign tumors present well-defined margins and a homogeneous internal structure.

The radiographic features of malignant esophageal tumors include mucosal irregularities, a rigid wall with effaced folds, and pooling of contrast medium. Sectional imaging modalities show an enhancing lesion with infiltrative margins and central nonhomogeneities (Figs. 15.**4** – 15.**7**). Lymphomatous involvement most commonly results from invasion of the distal esophagus by gastric lymphoma.

Esophageal Diverticula

Barium films can differentiate *pulsion diverticula* (Fig. 15.**12**), such as a high-sited Zenker diverticulum or epiphrenic diverticulum, from *traction diverticula*, which occur at the level of the tracheal bifurcation.

Tracheal Tumors

Intratracheal tumors are manifested initially by *stenosis of the trachea* with the displacement of surrounding soft tissues and frequent *inspiratory stridor*.

Benign tumors may consist of neoplasms such as fibroma, chondroma, and papilloma. In other cases hypertrophic scarring due to previous trauma or radiotherapy may cause a constricting mass.

Malignant tumors such as squamous cell carcinoma, adenocarcinoma, and adenoid cystic carcinoma are characterized by ill-defined margins and destruction of the tracheal cartilages. These primary tracheal tumors are distinguished from metastases (Fig. 15.**8**) and invasion by extrinsic tumor such as thyroid carcinoma.

Pseudotumors such as mucosal polyps and amyloid tumors may also occur.

Endotracheal Goiter

An endotracheal goiter consists of *ectopic thyroid tissue*, which most commonly occurs in the upper trachea. Imaging shows an intraluminal mass with well-defined, noninfiltrating margins. Once a presumptive diagnosis has been made by CT or MRI, further evaluation by thyroid scintigraphy is indicated.

Chordoma

Chordomas generally cause *vertebral body bone destruction* with radiologic evidence of adjacent soft tissue in the pre- and paravertebral spaces. The soft-tissue mass shows internal septations, a fibrous pseudocapsule, flocculent calcifications, and moderate contrast enhancement.

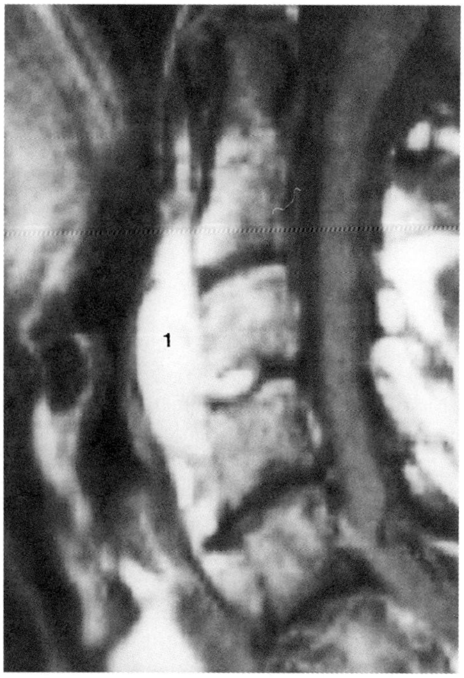

Fig. 15.1 **Degenerative spinal changes.** The fat marrow in the anterior osteophyte causes it to appear hyperintense on this sagittal T1-weighted MR image. Unlike CT, MRI cannot define the bony boundaries of the osteophyte, which causes marked indentation of the pharynx at the level of the epiglottis.

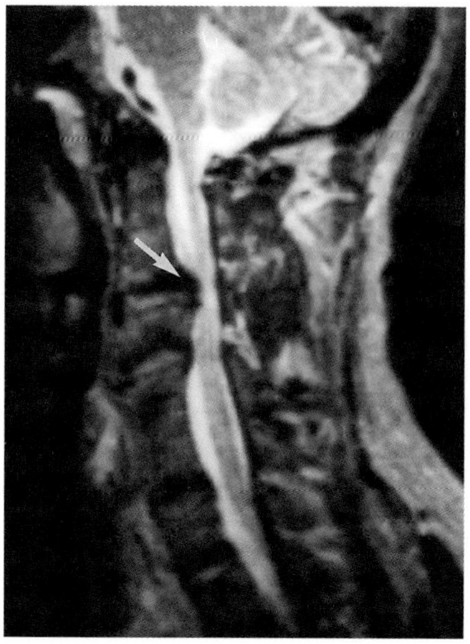

Fig. 15.2 **Klippel–Feil syndrome.** T2-weighted MR image shows a mass impinging on the spinal canal and spinal cord from the anterior side. The cause is a posterior marginal osteophyte on cervical block vertebrae in Klippel–Feil syndrome.

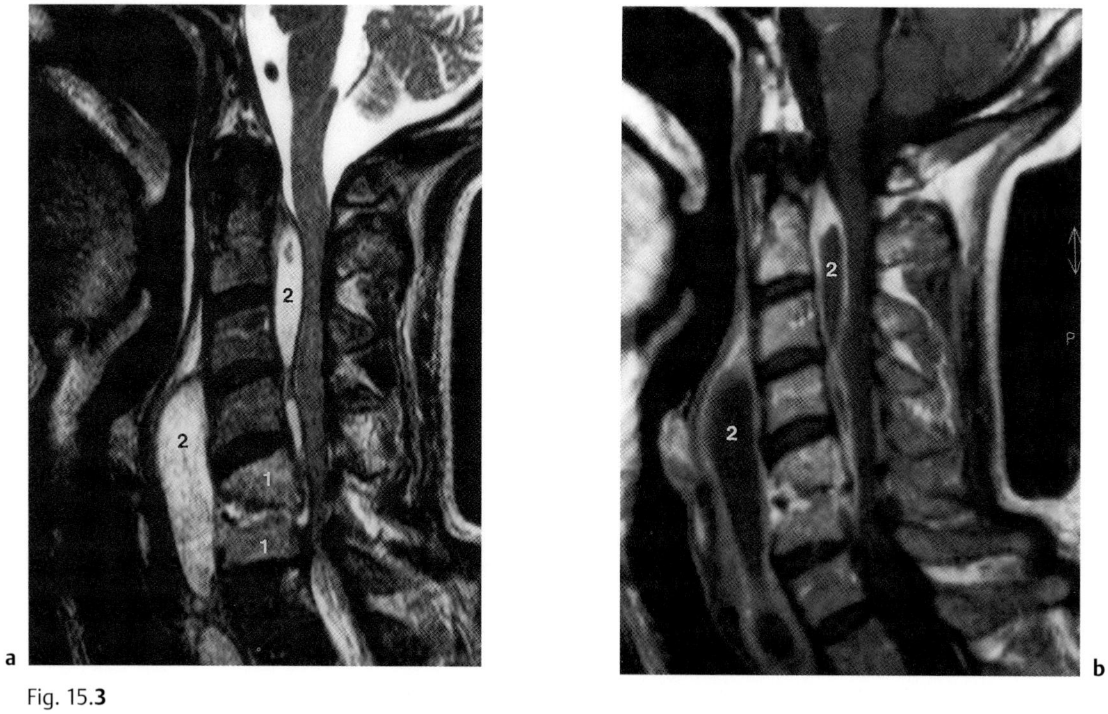

Fig. 15.3

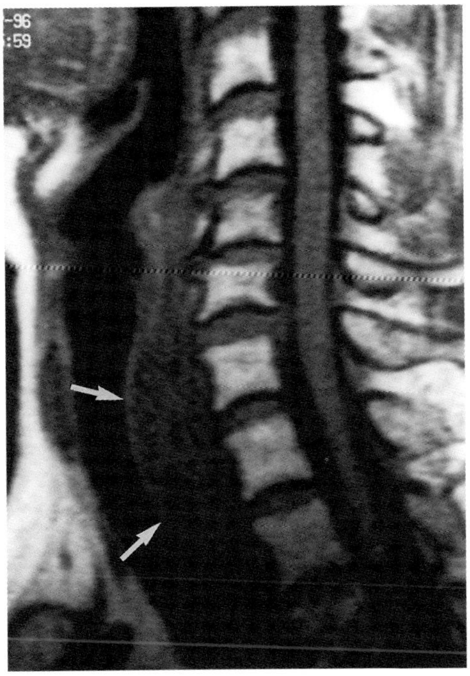

a

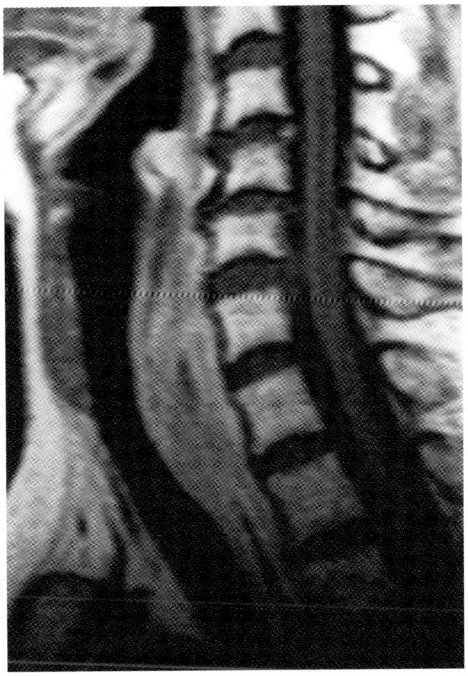

b

Figs. 15.**4 a, b** **Esophageal carcinoma.**
(**a**) Sagittal T1-weighted image (TR/TE = 600/17 ms) shows a thickening of the prevertebral space (arrows) with posterior indentation of the trachea.
(**b**) Image after intravenous contrast administration demonstrates a long, broad area of enhancing neoplastic soft tissue along the esophagus. The residual lumen appears as a central band of low signal intensity.

◁ Figs. 15.**3 a, b** **Spondylodiscitis with a pre- and paravertebral abscess.**
(**a**) Sagittal T2-weighted MR image shows increased signal intensity in the fifth and sixth cervical vertebrae and a narrowed disk space as evidence of spondylodiscitis. The image also shows prevertebral-retrolaryngeal and intraspinal masses of high signal intensity impinging on the spinal cord.
1 Spondylodiscitis
2 Spinal cord
(**b**) After intravenous contrast administration, the masses show an enhancing rim and homogeneous liquid contents, consistent with prevertebral abscesses secondary to spondylodiscitis.
2 Masses

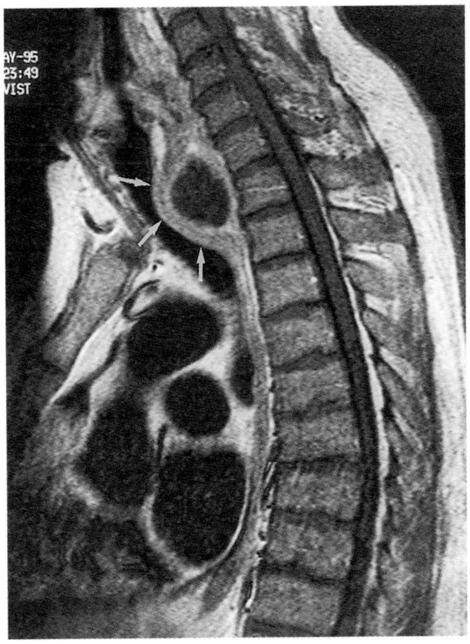

Fig. 15.**5** **Esophageal carcinoma.** Sagittal MR image demonstrates a prevertebral mass indenting the trachea and displacing it anteriorly (arrows).

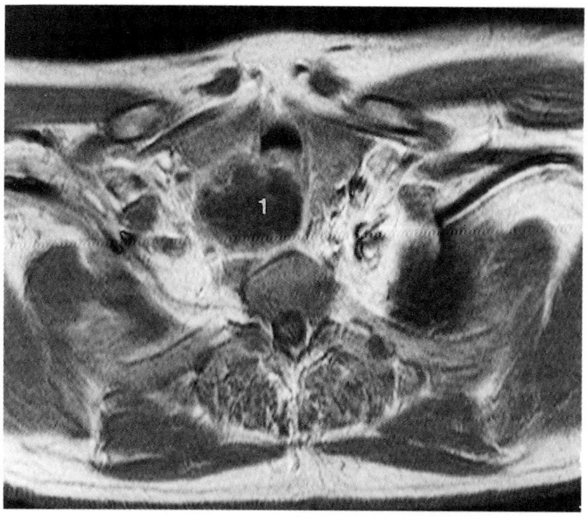

Fig. 15.**6** **Esophageal carcinoma.** Post-contrast T1-weighted SE sequence (TR/TE = 700/15 ms) shows an extensive tumor mass to the right of the midline arising from the esophagus. The signal void within the mass represents central necrosis.
1 Central necrosis

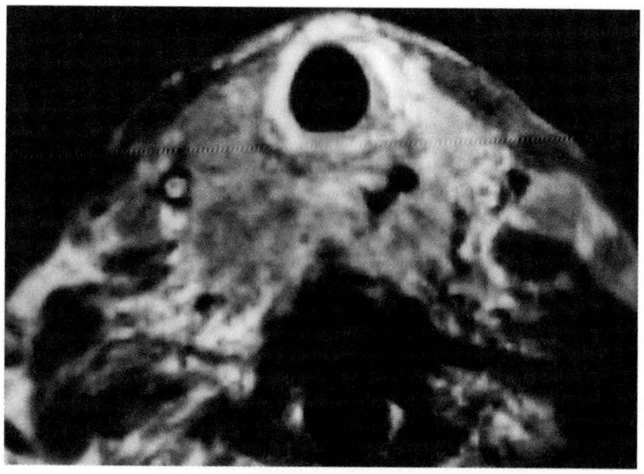

Fig. 15.**7** **Esophageal carcinoma.** Axial MR image shows an extensive tumor mass of the esophagus with bilateral invasion of the cervical soft tissues at the level of the subglottic larynx. The carcinoma shows a markedly nonhomogeneous internal structure with ill-defined margins, and invasion of the tracheal cartilage ring cannot be excluded. The distorted esophageal lumen is visible to the left of the midline.

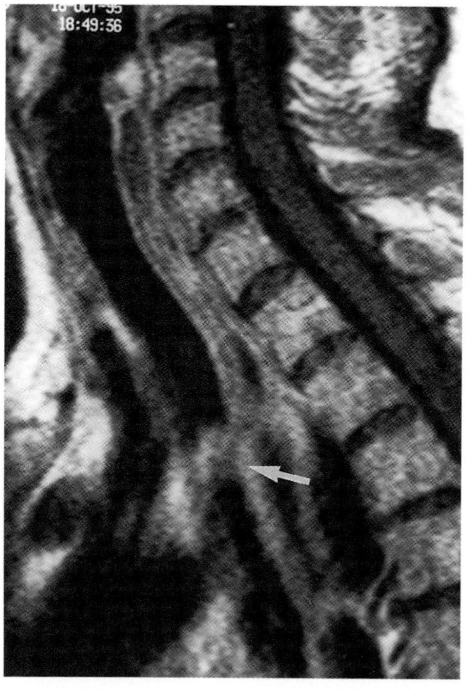

a

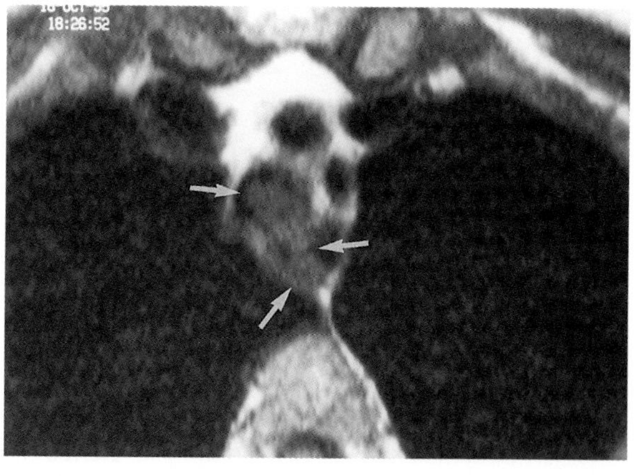

b

Figs. 15.**8 a, b** **Tracheal metastasis.**
(**a**) Sagittal MR image shows the tracheal air column filled with soft tumor tissue (arrow) at the level of the thoracic inlet. The lesion was manifested clinically by an inspiratory stridor. Endoscopic resection yielded tumor that was metastatic to a then-unknown primary.
(**b**) Axial image demonstrates subtotal stenosis of the trachea by the metastasis, which has spread to the esophagus (arrows).

Inflammatory Lesions

Spondylitis or Spondylodiscitis with a Prevertebral Abscess

Inflammations of the vertebral bodies and disk spaces tend to involve two adjacent vertebral levels due to the paired arrangement of the arterial vessels. Most cases result from the *hematogenous dissemination of a pathogenic organism* or a *postoperative complication*. A *pre-* or *paravertebral abscess* is a frequent sequela to spondylitis (Fig. 15.**3**). The preferred imaging modality is MRI owing to its sagittal imaging capability and high diagnostic accuracy.

Esophagitis

Clinically, esophagitis can have *multiple causes* including the extension of pharyngitis or gastritis to the esophagus, reflux esophagitis, and Plummer–Vinson syndrome. Candidal infection and actinomycosis are a common cause of esophagitis in immunocompromised patients (e.g., AIDS, chemotherapy). Conventional radiographs with a head-down tilt may demonstrate gastroesophageal reflux, which is often found to be accompanied by a sliding hiatal hernia. Generally, however, only a double-contrast study will permit a detailed assessment of mucosal changes. These may consist of superficial erosions that appear as dots or streaks of contrast medium, and advanced cases may show deep ulcerations and a "cobblestone" appearance chiefly affecting the lower esophagus. Abnormal contractions or segmental spasms are also commonly observed.

Barrett Esophagus

This condition is marked by a smooth, tapered stricture in the midportion of the esophagus caused by the *fibrous healing of a peptic ulcer* that has formed in ectopic gastric mucosa.

Crohn Disease

Involvement of the esophagus by *terminal ileitis* (Crohn disease) is not uncommon. The classic cobblestone appearance on radiographs is produced by ulcerations similar to those occurring in the ileum and colon.

Chagas Disease

The radiographic features of Chagas disease are very similar to those of achalasia and consist of moderate to extensive *dilatation of the esophagus* and *uncoordinated segmental contractions*. These changes are often accompanied by cardiac enlargement, megacolon, and dilatation of the ureters.

Subglottic Stenosing Laryngotracheitis

Known also as *pseudocroup*, this is predominantly a disease of small children, who present clinically with a *dry "barking" cough* and *inspiratory stridor*. Advanced cases are marked by *cyanosis* and *acute respiratory distress* with suffocation anxiety. Various causes have been postulated including viral infections, environmental toxins, and allergic factors. In most cases conventional radiographic studies will satisfactorily demonstrate the stenosis of the subglottic larynx and trachea. Otherwise MRI should be used in children, as it avoids radiation exposure.

Acute Tracheobronchitis

The most common cause is a *descending viral infection* associated with catarrhal complaints. An increasingly important cause is *bacterial diphtheria (croup)*, characterized by the formation of grayish-white deposits on palatal surfaces. CT and MRI may show thickened mucosae in the affected regions.

Tracheitis Sicca

Tracheitis sicca is a *chronic cough caused by exogenous mucosal injury*. The diagnosis is usually made clinically, and there is no primary indication for diagnostic imaging.

Degenerative and Systemic Diseases

Spondylosis, Spondylarthrosis

Anterior marginal osteophytes of the cervical vertebrae, *intervertebral disk space narrowing*, *intervertebral joint space narrowing*, and in rare cases the *"vacuum phenomenon"* are characteristic features of degenerative cervical spinal disease (Figs. 15.**1** and 15.**10**). Differentiation is required from cartilaginous exostosis (osteochondroma) (Fig. 15.**9**), a benign tumor that usually grows near metaphyses and may rarely arise from the facet joints of the cervical spine.

Achalasia

Achalasia is characterized by a *failure of relaxation of the lower esophageal sphincter* leading to esophageal dilatation and smooth conical tapering of the esophageal segment above the functional stenosis. Oral contrast radiographs and even plain chest films show an opacity with an air–fluid level in the right paracardiac or mediastinal region. Peristalsis is usually dysrhythmic and uncoordinated, delaying the propulsion of esophageal contents into the stomach.

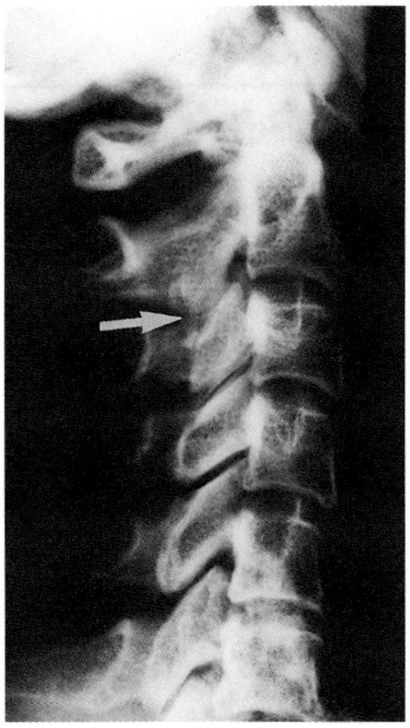
a

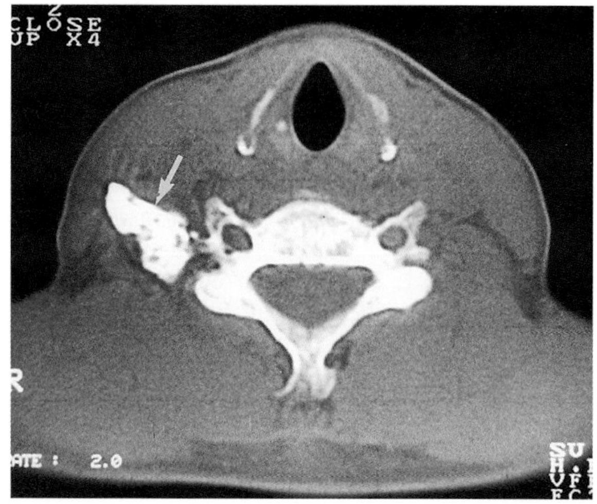

b

Figs. 15.**9 a, b** **Cartilaginous exostosis.** Conventional radiography and CT.
(**a**) Plain lateral radiograph shows a density in the intervertebral joint at C2-C3 (arrow).
(**b**) CT scan at this level shows a structure of bone density on the right side of the vertebral arch that is well demarcated from surrounding muscle (arrow). The tumor, palpable clinically as a firm, nontender mass, is identified as osteochondroma.

Scleroderma

Scleroderma may be manifested clinically by *dysphagia* and *odynophagia* with impaired esophageal motility and moderate dilatation, or there may be *gastroesophageal reflux* leading to peptic strictures. Oral contrast films demonstrate atrophy of the mucosa and a failure of peristaltic activity. Generally, there is no indication for sectional imaging procedures.

Tracheomalacia (Fig. 15.**11**)

Tracheomalacia is characterized pathologically by a softening or *chondrodystrophy* of the tracheal cartilages. Radiologically, it is characterized by a greater than 50% change in luminal diameter on radiographs taken while the patient performs a Valsalva maneuver.

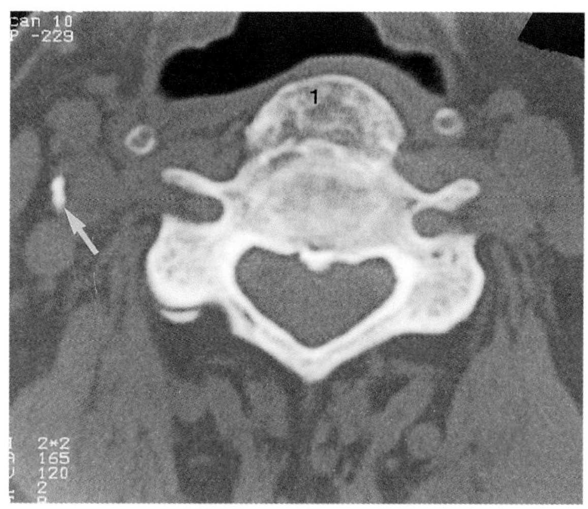

Fig. 15.**10** **Degenerative spinal changes.** Axial CT scan shows extensive anterior osteophytosis of the cervical vertebra impinging anteriorly upon the respiratory tract. The bilateral ring–like calcifications represent the upper poles of the thyroid glands. On the right side, a peripheral calcified plaque is visible on the lateral wall of the common carotid artery (arrow).
1 Osteophytic projections

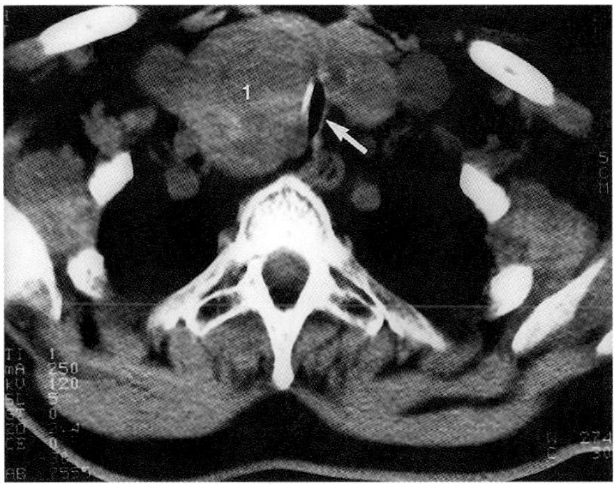

a

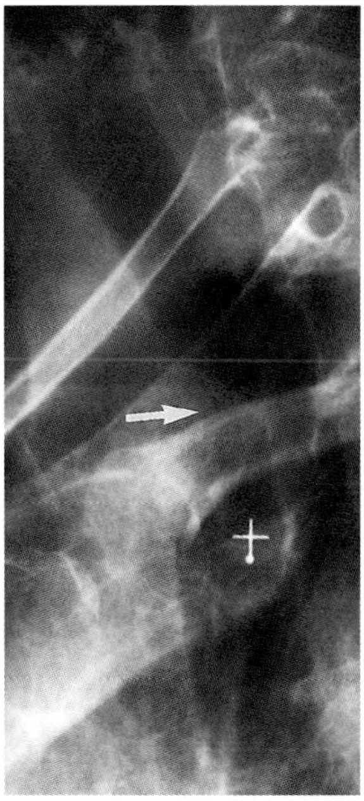

d

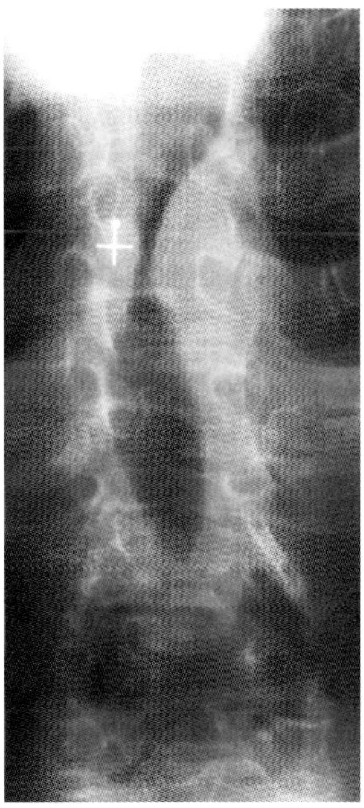

b

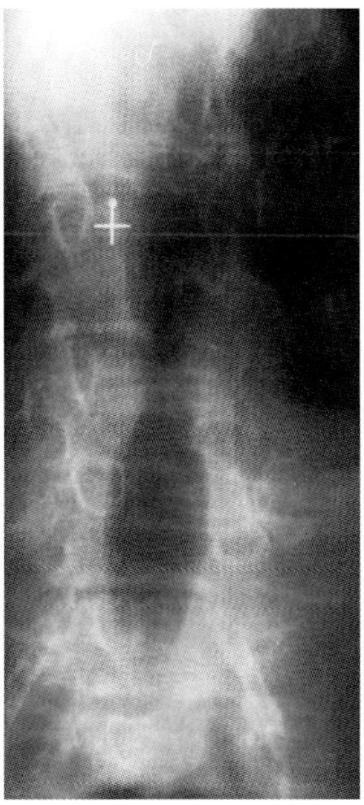

c

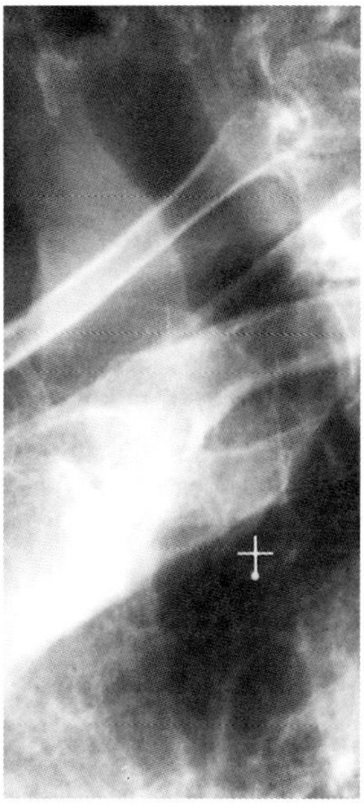

e

Figs. 15.**11 a – e** **Tracheomalacia.** CT and conventional radiography.
(**a**) CT shows a predominantly right-sided intrathoracic goiter with slit-like narrowing of the trachea (arrow).
1 Goiter
(**b, c**) Inspiratory radiograph (**b**) shows definite stenosis of the trachea above the sternoclavicular joint with more than a 50 % reduction in luminal diameter compared with the expiratory view (**c**).
(**d, e**) Lateral radiograph shows posterior indentation of the trachea (arrow) with an essentially smooth anterior border and a marked change in luminal size between inspiration (**d**) and expiration (**e**), signifying tracheomalacia.

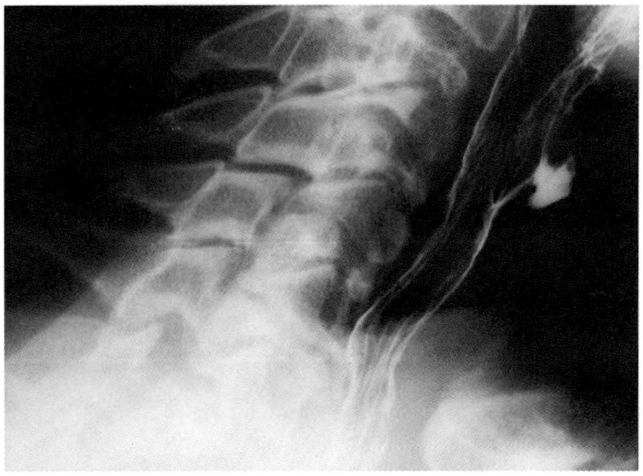

Fig. 15.**12** **Pulsion diverticulum.** Barium swallow reveals an anterior diverticulum with pooling of contrast medium. Otherwise the mucosal lining of the esophagus appears normal within the visualized segment.

a 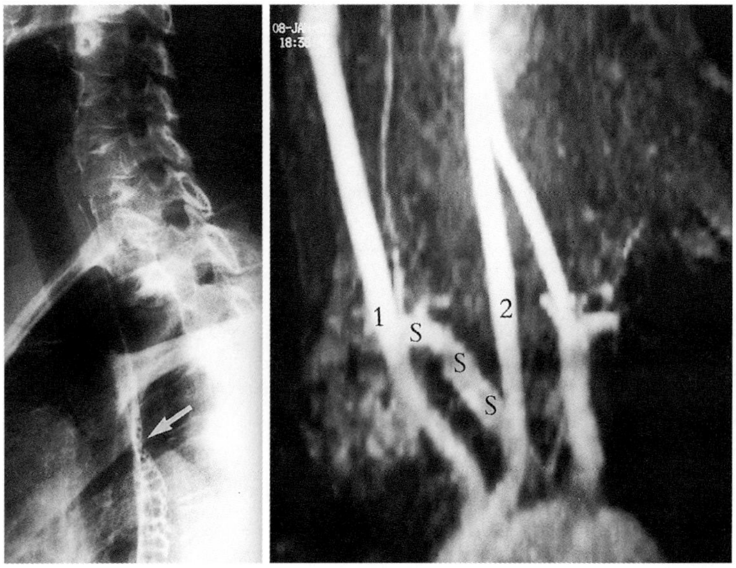 b

Figs. 15.**13 a, b** **Dysphagia lusoria.** Contrast radiograph and MRA.
(**a**) Gastrographin swallow shows localized extrinsic compression of the esophagus at the level of the thoracic inlet (arrow). Bubbles can be seen within the intraluminal contrast medium.
(**b**) MRA confirms the aberrant course of the right subclavian artery, which arises distal to the right and left common carotid arteries, then passes behind the esophagus and compresses it, producing clinical symptoms.
1 Right common carotid artery
2 Left common carotid artery
S Subclavian artery

Vascular Lesions

Dysphagia Lusoria (Fig. 15.**13**)

This type of dysphagia results from *compression of the esophagus* by an aberrant right subclavian artery. Esophagography shows the typical oblique, often pulsatile indentation of the esophageal lumen by the artery passing behind it. MRI supplemented by noninvasive magnetic resonance angiography (MRA) in the same sitting provides multiplanar views of the vascular anatomy that confirm the diagnosis and direct the planning of operative treatment.

Other congenital vascular anomalies that may cause esophageal dysfunction are a right-sided descending aorta, a duplicated aortic arch, an aberrant left pulmonary artery, and congenital or acquired dilatation of the cardiac left atrium.

Esophageal Varices

Oral contrast examination in patients with portal hypertension reveals *string-of-beads filling defects* and tortuous *ribbon-like defects* in the distal esophagus. Contrast-enhanced CT will demonstrate the opacified veins in the esophageal wall. Varices in the early stage can often be demonstrated in the right anterolateral wall of the distal esophagus.

Traumatic Lesions

Cervical Spinal Fractures with Prevertebral Hematoma

The primary diagnosis of cervical fractures can be accomplished with conventional biplane radiographs of the cervical spine. Often this is followed by CT (2-mm slice thickness) to evaluate the posterior margins and check for intraspinal hemorrhage. A hematoma in the prevertebral space can often be detected on conventional X-ray films by a thickening of the soft-tissue shadow, and CT can document its precise extent. Direct injury to the spinal cord can be diagnosed with MRI.

Direct External Injuries

When the esophagus has been perforated due to *direct injury* (e.g., a stab wound) or *blunt trauma* sustained in a motor vehicle accident, radiographs show the extravasation of orally administered water-soluble contrast medium (Gastrographin). If this type of study is not feasible, the diagnosis can be made at operation.

A stab wound or other penetrating injury that opens the trachea can cause displacement of the tracheal cartilages with soft-tissue hematoma, perifocal edema, and emphysema of the cervical soft tissues.

Whiplash Injury of the Cervical Spine

Radiographs often appear normal initially, although functional views of the cervical spine will occasionally show *segmental motion restriction*. In many cases, years may pass before *spondylotic changes* and *intervertebral disk space narrowing* can be documented.

Foreign-Body Ingestion

If a radiolucent foreign body has become lodged in the esophagus, oral contrast examination is indicated and will show a fixed, circumscribed filling defect. If there is a suspected perforating injury with risk of mediastinitis, CT should be performed to demonstrate the foreign body, hematoma, or mediastinal emphysema.

Foreign-Body Aspiration

Acute foreign-body aspiration is manifested clinically by *paroxysmal cough, stridor, pain,* and *retrosternal pressure*. Generally the foreign body is aspirated into the bronchi and frequently lodges in the right main bronchus. Roentgen evaluation consists of plain radiographs that may be supplemented by a conventional tomogram. A chest film should also be taken to exclude unilateral pulmonary hyperexpansion, and fluoroscopy may be performed to evaluate for mediastinal flutter.

Caustic Injury and Scalding

In patients with mucosal injury caused by the ingestion of *acids, bases,* or *scalding-hot liquids*, mucosal lacerations or strictures are observed on oral contrast radiographs with a water-soluble medium (Gastrographin). *Caustic ingestion* or the *inhalation of toxic or corrosive gases* causes edematous swelling of the tracheal mucosa followed by scarring and fibrosis. In severe cases, CT and MRI can document soft-tissue lacerations and complications such as perforation, abscess formation, and mediastinal cellulitis.

Iatrogenic and Posttherapeutic Changes

Postoperative Changes

In patients who have undergone *esophagectomy* with reconstruction by gastric transposition or jejunal interposition, radiographs will show corresponding changes in the mucosal relief projected over the transposed structure. An anastomotic leak is evidenced by contrast extravasation after the patient has swallowed a water-soluble iodinated medium. *Reconstructive plastic surgery* and *metallic or nonmetallic stents* implanted into the trachea hamper the detection of soft-tissue changes, especially in evaluations for residual or recurrent tumor.

Postirradiation Changes

Diffuse inflammatory and *edematous changes* and subsequent *scar retractions* secondary to radiotherapy are indistinguishable from recurrent tumor on conventional X-ray films. Contrast-enhanced MRI is generally helpful in differentiating tumor from scar tissue.

Esophageal Perforation

Iatrogenic perforation of the esophagus may occur as a result of *intubation* or *bougienage*. Oral contrast examination with a water-soluble medium can visualize the lesion, and it can diagnose a tracheoesophageal fistula by documenting the passage of contrast medium into the trachea. CT evaluation is also indicated in patients with suspected mediastinitis.

Post-intubation Pressure Injury of the Tracheal Wall

Edematous swelling of the tracheal mucosa along with *scarring and fibrotic changes* ranging to *tracheal stricture* are the principal complications of tracheal intubation and may necessitate evaluation by CT or MRI.

Table 15.1 Differential diagnosis of prevertebral masses in adults

Findings	Differential diagnostic criteria
Common:	
➤ Tumor:	
–Lymphadenopathy (Fig. 14.**9**)	Morphology
–Esophageal carcinoma (Figs. 15.**4** – 15.**7**)	Contrast enhancement
–Tracheal tumor (Fig. 15.**8**)	Topography
➤ Inflammatory:	
–Tonsillitis	Contrast enhancement
–Cellulitis (Fig. 14.**20**)	Morphology, diffuse contrast enhancement
–Spondylitis, spondylodiscitis with prevertebral abscess (Fig. 15.**3**)	Topography, contrast enhancement
➤ Degenerative:	
–Cervical osteophytosis (Figs. 15.**1**, 15.**10**)	Density, topography
➤ Traumatic:	
➤ Prevertebral hematoma	Density or signal intensity
Rare:	
➤ Tumor:	
–Chordoma	Calcification
–Retropharyngeal goiter	Density or signal intensity
–Mesenchymal tumors	

Table 15.2 Prevertebral masses in children

Common:
- Adenoids
- Lymphatic hyperplasia
- Abscess
- Tonsillitis
- Foreign body perforation
- Hematoma
- Edema (e.g., after spinal trauma)
- Lymphadenitis

Rare:
- Cystic hygroma
- Dilated jugular vein
- Cervical cyst
- Rare tumors
  - –Hemangioma
  - –Angiofibroma
  - –Neurofibroma
  - –Ganglioneuroma
  - –Neuroblastoma
  - –Teratoma
  - –Rhabdomyosarcoma
- Myxedema
- Retropharyngeal goiter
- Upper inflow stasis due to mediastinal tumor

Imaging Criteria and Their Differential Diagnosis

Expansion of the Retropharyngeal or Prevertebral Space

Expansion of the retropharyngeal or prevertebral space is an important differential diagnostic sign. Increased separation of the aerated structures of the trachea and hypopharynx from the vertebral column can be appreciated even on conventional lateral radiographs. The expansion is documented best on sagittal MR images (Fig. 15.**2**) and CT scans (Fig. 15.**9**).

The differential diagnoses for adult patients are listed in order of frequency in Table 15.**1**.

Retropharyngeal or prevertebral expansion is also an important clinical issue in children, where an even broader range of differential diagnoses must be considered (Table 15.**2**).

Tumor Masses Related to Bone

Masses that relate to bony structures generally have a vertebrogenic origin or are related to cartilaginous structures of the thyroid cartilage, cricoid, or hyoid bone. Vertebrogenic tumors may present with a destructive or expansile type of growth (Figs. 15.**1** – 15.**3**). The possible differential diagnoses are reviewed in Table 15.**3**.

Tumor Masses of the Esophagus

The differential diagnosis of a tumor mass of the esophagus includes the following:
- Benign tumors: fibroma, adenoma, leiomyoma.
- Malignant tumors (Figs. 15.**4** – 15.**7**): squamous cell carcinoma (the most common), adenocarcinoma, sarcoma, lymphoma.
- Other lesions: paraesophageal abscess, paraesophageal hematoma.

Table 15.**3** Masses that relate to bone

Findings	Differential diagnostic criteria
Variation:	
➤ Klippel–Feil syndrome (Fig. 15.**2**)	Topography
➤ Block vertebrae (Fig. 15.**2**)	
Degenerative:	
➤ Spondylosis deformans (Figs. 15.**1**, 15.**10**)	Morphology
➤ Spondylarthrosis	
➤ Cartilaginous exostosis (Fig. 15.**9**)	
➤ Herniated disk	
Tumor:	
➤ Chordoma	Calcification
➤ Vertebrogenic tumors, metastases	Destruction
Inflammatory:	
➤ Spondylitis or spondylodiscitis (Fig. 15.**3**) with prevertebral abscess	Morphology, contrast enhancement
Traumatic:	
➤ Fracture	Morphology
➤ Pre- and paravertebral hematoma	
➤ Discoligamentous instability	Limited function

Table 15.**4** Differential diagnostic criteria for tumor masses of the esophagus in oral contrast radiography

- ➤ Filling defect, smooth margins, eccentric stenosis:
  - –Fibroma
  - –Adenoma
  - –Myoma
  - –Lymphoma
  - –Paraesophageal process
- ➤ Mucosal irregularities, effaced folds, contrast pooling, rigid wall:
  - –Squamous cell carcinoma (Figs. 15.**4**–15.**7**)
  - –Adenocarcinoma
  - –Sarcoma

All of the above tumors can affect any portion of the esophagus, but lymphoma most commonly invades the distal esophagus from the gastric cardia. Morphologically, the benign tumors are homogeneous with smooth, well-defined margins and tend to cause eccentric luminal stenosis. Malignant tumors usually have ill-defined margins and a nonhomogeneous internal structure due to central necrosis. Concentric stenosis may occur (Figs. 15.**4**–15.**7**, Tables 15.**4** and 15.**5**).

Table 15.**5** Differential diagnostic criteria for tumor masses of the esophagus in CT and MRI

- ➤ Well-defined margins, homogeneous:
  - –Fibroma
  - –Adenoma
  - –Myoma
  - –Paraesophageal process
- ➤ Ill-defined margins, nonhomogeneous (central necrosis):
  - –Squamous cell carcinoma (Figs. 15.**4**–15.**7**)
  - –Adenocarcinoma
  - –Sarcoma
- ➤ Moderately enhancing, homogeneous:
  - –Fibroma
  - –Adenoma
  - –Myoma
- ➤ Irregular enhancement (central necrosis):
  - –Carcinoma
  - –Sarcoma
- ➤ Enhancing rim:
  - –Paraesophageal abscess (Fig. 15.**3**)
- ➤ Nonenhancing:
  - –Paraesophageal hematoma

All the tumors show intermediate density and nonspecific contrast enhancement. When the above morphologic criteria are combined with an assessment of regional nodal involvement, it will usually be possible to differentiate between benign and malignant tumors and between intramural and paraesophageal lesions. Further histologic classification relies on endoscopic techniques.

Tumor Masses of the Trachea

The following lesions should be considered in the differential diagnosis of tracheal tumors:

- ➤ Benign tumors: fibroma, chondroma, papilloma, scar hypertrophy, mucosal polyp, or amyloid tumor.
- ➤ Malignant tumors: squamous cell carcinoma, adenocarcinoma, adenoid cystic carcinoma.

In rare cases, a tumor may metastasize to the trachea from an extrinsic primary site (Fig. 15.**8**).

All other tumors can occur ubiquitously. With chondromas, it is usually obvious that the tumor has originated from the tracheal cartilage.

The morphologic criteria for benign–malignant differentiation are the same as described previously. In most cases a more specific diagnosis cannot be offered on the basis of radiologic findings (Tables 15.**6** and 15.**7**).

Table 15.6 Differential diagnostic criteria for tumor masses of the trachea in CT

- High density (> 50 HU):
  - Chondroma
- Cartilage destruction:
  - Chondroma
  - Carcinoma
- Intense enhancement:
  - Papilloma
  - Polyp
- Moderate enhancement:
  - Fibroma
  - Carcinoma
  - Metastasis (Fig. 15.**8**)
- Little or no enhancement:
  - Chondroma
  - Scar retraction
  - Amyloid tumor

Table 15.7 Differential diagnostic criteria for tumor masses of the trachea in MRI

- Nonspecific low T1-weighted signal intensity and intermediate T2-weighted signal intensity for all lesions indicated.
- Intense enhancement:
  - Papilloma
  - Polyp
- Moderate enhancement:
  - Fibroma
  - Carcinoma
  - Metastasis (Fig. 15.**8**)
- Little or no enhancement:
  - Chondroma
  - Scar retraction
  - Amyloid tumor

Liquid or Air-Filled Masses of the Esophagus

When a circumscribed liquid or air-filled esophageal mass is detected radiologically, the diagnostic possibilities include achalasia, diverticulum (often contains a fluid level with overlying air), and esophageal varices (Table 15.**8**).

Table 15.8 Topographic and morphologic criteria for liquid and air-filled masses of the esophagus

Topographic criteria:

- Cervical, lateral to the midline at the esophageal inlet:
  - Zenker diverticulum (Fig. 15.**12**)
- Middle third of esophagus:
  - Traction diverticulum
- Supradiaphragmatic:
  - Paramedian: epiphrenic diverticulum
  - With smoothly tapered lumen: achalasia
- Along esophageal wall:
  - Varices

Morphologic criteria:

- Smooth margins:
  - Diverticulum (Fig. 15.**12**)
  - Achalasia
- Fluid level:
  - Diverticulum
  - Achalasia
- String-of-beads configuration:
  - Varices

Primary Dilatation of the Esophagus

Besides neoplastic and inflammatory diseases of the esophagus, primary esophageal dilatation can occur as a result of Chagas disease, neuromuscular or endocrine disorders (diabetes, myxedema), or amyloidosis. No sites of predilection are known, and the entire esophagus may be affected.

Oral contrast examination shows moderate generalized dilatation of the esophagus with smooth outlining of the walls. As a general rule, imaging studies alone cannot establish a specific cause for the dilatation, and further clinical investigations are required.

Esophageal Stenosis with or without Prestenotic Dilatation

When prestenotic dilatation of the esophagus is caused by a tumor, the mucosa of the dilated segment may appear rigid and irregular due to proximal invasion. Other causes are characterized by concentric or eccentric stenosis of the esophageal wall with prestenotic dilatation and smooth margins (Figs. 15.**4** – 15.**7**).

CT and MRI can establish the location of the causative lesion as intramural, intraluminal, or mediastinal (Table 15.**9**).

Table 15.9 Topographic and morphologic criteria for esophageal stenosis

Topographic criteria:
- Entire esophagus:
  - —Prestenotic dilatation
  - —Esophageal carcinoma (Figs. 15.**4** - 15.**7**)
  - —Caustic injury, scald
  - —Paraesophageal hematoma
  - —Paraesophageal abscess (Fig. 15.**3**)
  - —Metastasis
- Upper esophagus:
  - —Thyroid goiter (Fig. 14.**17**)
  - —Spondylosis deformans (of cervical vertebrae) (Figs. 15.**1**, 15.**10**)
- Middle third:
  - —Barrett esophagus
  - —Dysphagia lusoria (Fig. 15.**13**)
- Lower esophagus:
  - —Achalasia
  - —Esophagitis
  - —Scleroderma
  - —Schatzki ring
- Physiologic constrictions of esophagus:
  - —Obstructing foreign body

Morphologic criteria:
- Smooth, eccentric luminal narrowing:
  - —Metastatic tumor
  - —Paraesophageal lesion (Fig. 15.**3**)
  - —Spondylosis deformans (Figs. 15.**1**, 15.**10**)
  - —Goiter (Fig. 14.**17**)
  - —Benign esophageal tumor
- Smooth, concentric luminal narrowing:
  - —Stricture
  - —Achalasia
  - —Scleroderma
  - —Obstructing foreign body
  - —Schatzki ring
- Irregular narrowing:
  - —Esophageal carcinoma (Figs. 15.**4** - 15.**7**)

Table 15.10 Topographic and morphologic criteria for mucosal changes

Topographic criteria:
- Entire esophagus:
  - —Esophageal carcinoma (Figs. 15.**4** - 15.**7**)
  - —Crohn disease
- Lower esophagus:
  - —Esophagitis
  - —Varices

Morphologic criteria:
- Mucosal irregularities, effaced folds, rigid wall, contrast pooling and retention:
  - —Esophageal carcinoma (Figs. 15.**4** - 15.**7**)
- Subtle filling defects, widened longitudinal folds, punctate contrast pooling, erosion, ulceration:
  - —Esophagitis
- Cobblestone appearance:
  - —Crohn disease
- String-of-beads filling defects and ribbon-like intramural defects:
  - —Varices

Table 15.11 Differential diagnostic criteria for cartilage changes in imaging studies

- Originating from tracheal cartilage, nonhomogeneous internal structure, minimal contrast enhancement, smooth margins:
  - —Chondroma
- Infiltration of tracheal cartilage or vertebral bodies, nonhomogeneous internal structure, moderate contrast enhancement, ill-defined margins:
  - —Squamous cell carcinoma
  - —Adenocarcinoma
  - —Adenoid cystic carcinoma

Changes in the Esophageal Mucosa

Evaluation of the esophageal mucosa generally has to rely on conventional barium-swallow radiographs. When a high-quality examination is performed in a cooperative patient, it should be possible to differentiate among esophagitis, esophageal carcinoma, esophageal varices, and esophageal involvement by Crohn disease (Table 15.**10**).

Cartilage Changes

Calcifications of the tracheal cartilages are consistently observed in elderly patients and usually have no bearing on the differential diagnosis. The entire trachea may be affected, including the tracheobronchial bifurcation. Accordingly, calcification of the tracheal cartilages is a frequent incidental finding on chest radiographs (Table 15.**11**).

Table 15.**12** Topographic and morphologic criteria for tracheal stenosis

Topographic criteria:
- Subglottic:
  - Tracheitis
  - (Pseudo)croup
  - Invasion or compression by thyroid tumor (Fig. 14.**17**)
  - Postintubation scar
- Supracarinal level or right main bronchus:
  - Foreign-body aspiration
- Tracheobronchial bifurcation:
  - Mediastinal or paratracheal lymph node

Morphologic criteria:
- Stenosis by extrinsic mass:
  - Tumor (thyroid gland [Fig. 14.**17**], mediastinum)
  - Paratracheal hematoma
  - Paratracheal abscess (Fig. 15.**3**)
  - Lymph node (Fig. 14.**9**)
- Eccentric thickening of tracheal wall:
  - Primary tracheal tumor
  - Post-intubation or postoperative scar tissue
  - Metastasis
- Concentric thickening of tracheal wall:
  - Tracheitis
  - (Pseudo)croup
- Instability of tracheal wall:
  - Tracheal stenosis
  - Tracheomalacia (Fig. 15.**11**)
- Intraluminal stenosis:
  - Foreign-body aspiration
  - Posttraumatic intraluminal hemorrhage

Table 15.**13** Frequency of tracheal stenoses

Common:
- Secondary stenosis:
  - Trauma
  - Intubation
  - Tracheostomy
- Primary tumors, benign or malignant:
  - Squamous cell carcinoma
- Croup or pseudocroup

Rare:
- Congenital
- Ectopic thyroid tissue
- Papillomatosis
- Amyloidosis
- Postoperative
- Postirradiation
- Rare tumors, mesenchymal tumors, metastases

Tracheal Stenosis

The differential diagnosis of tracheal stenosis includes tracheitis, (pseudo)croup, tumors, trauma, iatrogenic lesions (intubation, surgery, irradiation), tracheomalacia, an extensive goiter, congenital tracheal stenosis, foreign-body aspiration, and paratracheal disease (Table 15.**12**).

The differential diagnoses for subglottic stenosis are listed by frequency of occurrence in Table 15.**13**.

Tracheal stenosis can usually be appreciated on conventional anteroposterior (AP) and lateral radiographs. Luminal changes from inspiration to expiration (tracheomalacia) (Fig. 15.**11**) are best demonstrated by fluoroscopy.

CT and MRI are indicated for the detailed evaluation of extramural, intramural, or intraluminal stenoses, especially with an extrinsic stenosis caused by thyroid, paratracheal, or mediastinal disease.

Summary and Diagnostic Strategy

The oral contrast examination is the mainstay in the primary radiologic evaluation of esophageal diseases, and barium ingestion is generally required for the definitive diagnosis of a tumor mass. CT has assumed the greatest importance for the simultaneous evaluation of tumor extent and regional lymph-node involvement. As a rule, only esophagoscopy or gastroscopy can furnish a definitive histologic diagnosis.

Contrast-enhanced MRI is recommended for treatment planning owing to its multiplanar, 3-D capabilities. It is also used for the precise evaluation of key anatomic structures and locoregional nodal involvement.

If a tracheal lesion is immediately life-threatening, priority is given to endoscopic evaluation or, if necessary, operative intervention. For less urgent cases, the primary radiologic workup consists of conventional biplane radiographs (Figs. 15.**11 b, c**) that should include inspiratory and expiratory views in cooperative patients. Further evaluation by modern sectional imaging techniques is indicated for equivocal tumor masses and should establish whether the lesion is malignant or benign. Only endoscopy can establish a definitive histologic diagnosis and in many cases (e.g., foreign-body aspiration) may also provide the definitive therapy.

References

1 Burgener, F. A., M. Kormano: Röntgenologische Differentialdiagnostik. Thieme, Stuttgart 1993
2 Dillon, W. P., H. R. Harnsberger: The impact of radiologic imaging on staging of cancer of the head and neck. Semin Oncol. 18 (1991) 64–79
3 Naumann, H. H.: Differentialdiagnostik in der Hals-Nasen-Ohren-Heilkunde. Thieme, Stuttgart 1990
4 Vogl, Th.: Kernspintomographie der Kopf-Hals-Region. Springer, Berlin 1991
5 Vogl, Th., S. Dresel, M. Juergens, J. Assal, J. Lissner: MR Imaging with Gd-DTPA in lesions of the head and neck. J Otolaryngol. 22 (1993) 4–9
6 Wegener, O. H.: Ganzkörpercomputertomographie. Blackwell, Berlin 1992

Index

D

E

F

G

H

N

O

P

Q

R

S

T

U

V

W

Z